Y0-BDA-789

CURRICULUM AND INSTRUCTION IN NURSING

Curriculum and Instruction

in Nursing

VIRGINIA C. CONLEY, R.N., Ed.D.

Dean of the School of Nursing
The Catholic University of America
Washington

LITTLE, BROWN AND COMPANY, BOSTON

PREFACE

NURSING education is faced with challenges it has never before experienced in the development of curriculums for various educational programs. The scientific and technological advances that have been made during the twentieth century and are continuing to be made at an almost unbelievable rate have placed strenuous demands on all forms of education to reexamine the relevance of curriculums in a rapidly changing society. Nursing educators are keenly aware of the impact of the information explosion and concomitant technological developments on the lives of all persons as well as the impact of developments more specifically related to the health care of members of the society. Social and cultural events have had a considerable effect on the lives of our young people, and the youths coming to our schools are like no others in previous years. More recently, scientists, psychologists, and educators have collaborated in studying the problems of curriculum and instruction. These activities are serving as catalysts in rethinking and redefining the nature and function of curriculums.

In the past several years men have circled the earth and have landed on the moon. Terms like *Polaris submarine, radar, telstar,* and *antiballistic missiles* have become commonplace in the language of the man on the street. Likewise, *cardiac catheterizations, artificial kidneys, electronic pacemakers,* and *heart transplants* have become part of the working vocabulary of the physician, nurse, and other members of the health team. We have dared to transplant hearts, to perform delicate surgery on the brain, and to replace organs with plastic counterparts. Thirty years ago a physician who attempted these operations would have been considered a madman. At that time we were concerned with the endless series of patients whose bodies were emaciated and debilitated by racking fever and intestinal ulceration caused by the typhoid bacillus, the paralyzed bodies of polio victims being kept alive by iron lungs, and the children gasping for breath because of the ugly gray diphtheria membrane. With medical advances and public health vigilance, these diseases have been relegated to history and the annals of medicine.

Man's striving to conquer his environment has brought about phenomenal accomplishments and at the same time has revealed new and complex problems. Neither crystal balls nor fortune-tellers are needed: A variety of challenging health problems are already visible on the horizon. The relevance of our curriculums in nursing will be determined by our focus on these health needs and problems and by the identification of nursing's role in their alleviation or resolution.

Events on the national scene over the past several years have given an indication that all is not well with some of our social institutions. Schools and colleges have not remained insulated from unrest. Once havens for intellectual introspection, they have become seedbeds of discontent and disillusionment. It would be presumptuous for one to try to diagnose a single cause, for the causes are many. It serves no useful purpose to criticize an administration for not including students in budget-planning or academic appointments, or the director of student affairs for too relaxed or too restrictive policies on social living, or the director of admissions for "admitting the rebels" to the college. However, the faculty has the responsibility to examine critically its relationship to students in light of its obligations to the students, to the institution, and to society. This is suggested not as a panacea for current problems but to point out that teachers must review continually all educational offerings in view of the needs of the students of this generation and of current social institutions. Historically it has been true that when educational institutions were not in tune with society and were not responsive to the needs of students, they became ineffective as social institutions for the common good.

The ways in which students and teachers strive toward prescribed goals in their social and physical environments become the substantive materials of the curriculum of the school. The development of a curriculum not only requires a commitment to the conviction that the learning opportunities we offer are in the best interests of the student, the profession, and society, but also demands the courage to make appropriate changes when these learning opportunities are no longer useful to the goals of the curriculum. Continuous and unrelenting change has confronted man since the dawn of his experience, and it will continue as long as man exists. As John Cardinal Newman said, "To live is to change."

This text is offered as a guide for administrators, curriculum committees, teachers of curriculum, and all teachers developing courses in nursing, and as a chart of the challenges encountered in attempting to keep a curriculum abreast of social change.

V. C. C.

CONTENTS

PREFACE v

I DYNAMICS OF CURRICULUM DEVELOPMENT   1

1. THE NATURE OF CURRICULUM AND CURRICULUM DEVELOPMENT   3

CURRICULUM DEFINED—IN RETROSPECT   3
CURRICULUM CONCEPTS—CONTEMPORARY VIEWPOINTS   6
HISTORICAL PERSPECTIVE   8
APPROACHES TO CURRICULUM DEVELOPMENT   12
SUMMARY   14

2. BASIC ISSUES IN CURRICULUM DEVELOPMENT   17

ADMINISTRATION OF NURSING EDUCATION   17
FINANCING NURSING EDUCATION   19
ADEQUATE FACULTY   21
CONCEPT OF NURSING EDUCATION   22
NURSING RESEARCH   25
SUBJECT MATTER OF NURSING   27
STUDENTS   29
SUMMARY   29

3. PARTICIPANTS IN CURRICULUM DEVELOPMENT   33

INTERNAL PARTICIPANTS   33
    Students 34   Teachers 34   Administrators 35   State Boards of Nurse Examiners 36   State Departments of Education 37   State Legislatures 37

EXTERNAL PARTICIPANTS 38
    Professional Nursing Associations 38   Allied Professional
    Associations 40   Educational Associations 44   Foundations 47   Federal
    Government 50   Voluntary Associations 53   Business and Industry 55
SUMMARY   56

II SOURCES OF CURRICULUM DECISIONS   59

    4. CULTURAL VALUES AND THE CURRICULUM   61

    CULTURE—DEFINED   62
        Cultural Values 64
    CULTURAL VALUES AND SOCIAL CHANGE   66
        Cultural Change in Technological Societies 67   Cultural Stability
        Within Social Change 70   Concept of Cultural Pluralism 71
    CULTURAL VALUES AND EDUCATION   72
    CULTURAL VALUES AND THE NURSING CURRICULUM   75
    SUMMARY   77

    5. SOCIAL AND SCIENTIFIC FORCES AFFECTING
       CURRICULUM DECISIONS   81

    SOCIAL CHANGES AFFECTING HEALTH CARE   81
        Changes Affecting Individual and Group Relations 81
        Changes Within Health Care Institutions 86
    HEALTH CARE NEEDS   88
        Health Care Crisis 89   Health Care Problems 93
    PLANNING FOR HEALTH SERVICES   100
        Regional Planning for Health Care 100   Public Accountability for
        Health Care 101   Health Care in the Urban Environment 102   Role
        and Functions of Hospitals 102   Neighborhood Health Centers 103
        Consumer Participation in Health 104   Patient-Physician
        Relationships 105   Strategy for Health Planning 105
    IMPLICATIONS FOR NURSING AND NURSING CURRICULUM   107
    SUMMARY   109

    6. THE NATURE OF NURSING AND
       NURSING EDUCATION   113

    NATURE AND CHARACTERISTICS OF PROFESSIONS   113
        Purposes of Professions 115   Characteristics of Professional
        Education 116   Education for Health Manpower 121
    NATURE OF NURSING   125
        Nursing—Defined 126   Roles and Activities of the Nurse 129
        Primary Focus of Nursing 131   The Subject Matter of Nursing 133
    SYSTEM OF NURSING EDUCATION 135
        Characteristics of the System 135   Types of Educational
        Programs in Nursing 138   Career-Ladder Concepts 145
    SUMMARY   147

7. THE STUDENT AND THE CURRICULUM   153

    CHARACTERISTICS OF HIGHER EDUCATION 153
      The Student in American Higher Education 154
      The Changing Character of American Higher Education 156
    THE ASSESSMENT OF THE CHARACTERISTICS OF STUDENTS 168
      Institutional Assessment 169   Comprehensive Assessment 171
    IMPACT OF COLLEGE UPON STUDENTS 175
    THE IMPACT OF THE STUDENT UPON THE COLLEGE 180
    SUMMARY 184

8. INFLUENCE OF PSYCHOLOGICAL AND LEARNING
   THEORIES ON CURRICULUM DEVELOPMENT   189

    HISTORICAL BACKGROUND 189
    LEARNING THEORIES AND THEIR INFLUENCE ON EDUCATION 191
      Early Learning Theories 192   Gestalt and Field Theories 197
      Recent or Current Learning Theories 202
    THE NATURE OF LEARNING 211
      Generalizations from the Literature on Learning Theories 212
    INSTRUCTIONAL THEORIES 214
    SUMMARY 215

III PROCESS OF CURRICULUM DEVELOPMENT   219

9. OBJECTIVES FOR CURRICULUM AND INSTRUCTION   221

    INITIAL CONCERN FOR EDUCATIONAL OBJECTIVES 221
    EDUCATIONAL OBJECTIVES AND THE LEARNING PROCESS 224
      Reasons for Specifying Objectives 226   Process of Defining
      Objectives 229   Process of Behavioral Analysis 238
    SUMMARY 265

10. APPROACHES TO IDENTIFYING CONTENT
    IN NURSING   271

    THE NATURE OF SUBJECT MATTER 271
    THE USES OF SUBJECT MATTER 274
    SUBJECT MATTER AND THE CURRICULUM 276
    APPROACHES TO IDENTIFYING CONTENT IN NURSING 277
      Designing the Nursing Core 278   Defining and Describing Concepts 283
      Utilizing the Nursing Process 290   Analyzing Case Studies 294
      Constructing Models 297   Utilizing a Science Theory 299
    SUMMARY 300

11. DESIGN AND STRUCTURE OF THE CURRICULUM   305
    THE NATURE OF CURRICULUM DESIGN 305
    FUNCTIONS OF CURRICULUM DESIGN 308

OBJECTIVES AND CURRICULUM DESIGN   311

IDENTIFYING AND ORGANIZING CURRICULUM OPPORTUNITIES   315
  Analysis of Objectives 315   Organizing Centers 320   Examples of
  Organizing Centers 321   Continuity of Curriculum Opportunities 325
  Sequence of Curriculum Opportunities 326   Integration of
  Curriculum Opportunities 328   Balance in Curriculum Opportunity 330

STUDENT-TEACHER-COMMUNITY RELATIONSHIPS   333
  Teacher-Community Relationships 334   Student-Teacher
  Relationships 335

SUMMARY   336

12. EVALUATION OF CURRICULUM AND INSTRUCTION   341

THE EVALUATION PROCESS   342
  Evaluating the Influence of the Learning Environment 343

PURPOSES OF EVALUATION   348
  Evaluation of Instruction 349   Evaluation of Curriculum
  or Program 351   Evaluation of the System of Education 353

METHODOLOGY OF EVALUATION   355
  Goals and Roles of Evaluation 355   Roles Enacted in Evaluation 357
  Evaluation of Instruction 360   Structure of Evaluation Design 375

ISSUES AND PROBLEMS IN EVALUATION   377
  Defining Requirements for Evaluation 378   Defining Educational
  Evaluation 378   Lack of Criteria and Instruments 379

CURRICULUM EVALUATION AND RESEARCH   381
  Comparative Evaluation 383   Control-group Evaluation 384
  Research and Evaluation Methods 384

SUMMARY   385

IV THE INSTRUCTIONAL PROCESS   389

13. THE NATURE OF INSTRUCTION   391

INSTRUCTION AND TEACHING   391
  Teaching—A System of Actions 394   Teaching—As
  Decision-making 398

RELATIONSHIP BETWEEN TEACHING AND LEARNING   399

THEORIES OF TEACHING AND INSTRUCTION   402
  The Nature of Theory 403   Theories of Instruction 407   Theories
  of Teaching 412   Relationship Between Theory and Research 416

THE STUDY AND ANALYSIS OF TEACHING   417
  Dynamics of Instructional Groups 417   Classification of Teacher
  Statements 422   Interaction Analysis of Verbal and Nonverbal
  Behavior of Teachers and Students 424   Behavior of Effective
  Teachers 429

SUMMARY   431

14. VARIABLES IN THE INSTRUCTIONAL PROCESS   437

LEARNER CHARACTERISTICS   437
  Motivation 438   Previously Learned Capabilities 444

TEACHER CHARACTERISTICS 449
    Teacher Roles 449   Teacher Activities 452   Concept of
    Teacher Effectiveness 456
THE LEARNING ENVIRONMENT 461
    Physical Environment 461   Social Environment 463
    Psychological Environment 465
TEACHING STRATEGIES 469
    Setting Behavioral Goals 469   Informing the Learner of the
    Objectives 471   Presenting the Stimulus 472   Providing Cues
    for Learning 473   Controlling Attention 475   Stimulating Recall
    of Previously Learned Capabilities 476   Arranging for
    Reinforcement 477   Encouraging Generalization 478
    Measuring and Assessing Behavior 480
SUMMARY 481

15. INSTRUCTIONAL MODES AND MEDIA   487

NATURE AND IMPORTANCE OF INSTRUCTIONAL MODES AND MEDIA 487
    Rationale for Use of Instructional Modes and Media 488
    Areas of Research Needed 490
DESCRIPTION OF INSTRUCTIONAL MODES 490
    Lecture 491   Group Discussion 493   Panel Discussion 494
    Seminar 494   Demonstration 495   Laboratory Instruction 495
    Team Teaching 497   Contract Teaching 497
DESCRIPTION OF INSTRUCTIONAL MEDIA 498
    Programmed Instruction 498   Television 503   Motion
    Pictures 507   Tape and Disk Recordings 508   Computer-assisted
    Instruction 514   Simulation 516   Field Trips 520   Pictorial
    Presentation 521   Printed Language 522   Models 522
UTILIZING INSTRUCTIONAL MODES AND MEDIA 523
EDUCATIONAL TECHNOLOGY 526
SUMMARY 529

V STRATEGIES AND PROCESSES FOR
CURRICULUM CHANGE   535

16. STRATEGIES FOR CURRICULUM CHANGE   537

PROCESS OF CURRICULUM CHANGE 537
PREVIOUS APPROACHES TO CURRICULUM CHANGE 539
    Strategy of Reform 540   Efforts Toward Standard Setting 540
    Organization Efforts to Improve Curriculum 542   Activity
    Analysis 545   Establishing New Goals 547   Group Dynamics 548
    Subject Reorganization 551
RECENT STRATEGIES FOR CURRICULUM INNOVATION 553
    Implementation of Studies of Nursing 553   Strategy of Directed
    Change 558   Evaluation of an Innovation 561   Defining the Content
    of Nursing 563   Influence of the Federal Government 568
    Career-Ladder Concept 571   Systems Approach to Curriculum
    Change 576

GUIDELINES FOR DEVELOPING STRATEGIES   584
  The Student in the Learning Environment 584   The School as
  a Social System 589
SUMMARY   592

17. ROLES AND PROCESSES IN CURRICULUM CHANGE   599

  ORGANIZATIONAL PROCESSES IN CURRICULUM CHANGE   600
    Authority 600   Leadership 605   Group Dynamics 610
    Decision-making 614
  ROLES AND RELATIONSHIPS IN CURRICULUM CHANGE   618
    Environment for Curriculum Change 619   Individual
    Roles 623   Organization for Curriculum Change 636
  RESISTANCE TO CHANGE   638
    Nature of Resistance 639   Resistance in the Individual 640
    Resistance in the Organization 642   Resistance in the
    System 645   Principles Relating to Resistance to Change 649
  SUMMARY   651

INDEX   659

I

DYNAMICS OF CURRICULUM DEVELOPMENT

1 THE NATURE OF CURRICULUM AND CURRICULUM DEVELOPMENT

THE meanings that one gives to curriculum will to a large measure determine the domain and the processes of curriculum and curriculum development. There are considerable variations in the definitions of curriculum. These definitions extend from broad encompassing philosophical statements to those that are prescriptive and methodological in orientation. The general concept of curriculum has changed over the years, a fact which may be a reflection of the change in our thinking about education and the instructional process. A review of some of the definitions of curriculum as formulated by authorities in the field gives some indication of a continuous reorientation of the meaning of curriculum in relation to the nature and purpose of education.

CURRICULUM DEFINED—IN RETROSPECT

In the early history of formal education, the curriculum was often interpreted to mean the *course of study*, whether or not it was prepared in written form. For the most part, the curriculum was regarded as a written course, and revision of the curriculum consequently meant revising the course outline. Evidence reveals that frequently the preparation or revision of the course of study was done outside the school. Similar concepts refer to the curriculum as a *systematic arrangement of courses* designed for specific purposes of the student, such as the college preparatory curriculum or the vocational curriculum. On most college campuses the list of courses offered by various schools and colleges, combined into sequences for students with specific educational objectives, was identified as a curriculum. In many instances changing the curriculum involved adding or dropping certain courses and perhaps altering graduation requirements.

A curriculum guide that was prepared by the National League of Nursing Education in 1937 to assist teachers in schools of nursing in developing curriculum defined curriculum as *"any schematic and systematic arrangement of materials of instruction* extending over a considerable period of time and planned for a clearly differentiated group of students" [1]. This guide indicated that ideally a curriculum should be prepared for each student because individuals are different; they have different backgrounds, and their educational needs cannot be the same. It was further stated that since an individual curriculum is not entirely practical, a curriculum is built for a fairly homogeneous group whose members are supposed to have similar needs, and this curriculum is then adjusted to individual requirements.

A third concept of curriculum pertained to the arrangement of courses offered by the school; however, the focus was on the *subject matter content.* One of the commonly accepted definitions of curriculum was that curriculum consisted of the subject matter taught to students. The subject matter curriculum was the initial approach to curriculum in formal education, and it endured as a major focus through the 1920's. Subject matter was included in accordance with its cultural value, timeliness, and usefulness as preparation for the adult world. Changing the curriculum in this instance meant revising the content by adding new subject matter made available by scientific discoveries and social technological innovations. Some elaboration of this concept indicated that curriculum was a mammoth reservoir of ordered and accessible knowledge in banks, laboratories, and museums, ready to be drawn upon by minds capable of grasping and interpreting its content.

A change in the focus of curriculum was introduced by Caswell and Campbell's work in 1935. The definition of curriculum presented in their publication focused attention on the *experiences that students had under the guidance of the school* [2]. A general interpretation of this definition indicated that curriculum was the whole body of experiences that condition and make up the total activities of the student and for which the school assumed responsibility.

Subsequent writers interpreted this definition to include specific features and variables in the educational program. Some controversies arose over the role of teaching method in the curriculum. A summary point of view indicated that in a theoretical sense the curriculum should be those learnings independent of the method of the teacher who is to help the students attain them; however, it appears impossible to separate completely the fields of curriculum and method. Broadening this concept was the definition that indicated that curriculum is the body of experiences, stimulating environmental events, and situations, selected and arranged for instruction and learning in the schools.

Another curriculum approach described *curriculum in relation to the culture* in which the curriculum is developed. This indicated that the curriculum consists of a sequence of potential experiences that are set up in the school for the purpose of disciplining children and youth in group ways of thinking and acting. This concept states that to understand curriculum, one must understand what is meant by culture, the essential elements of culture, and how these are organized and interrelated. A similar concept introduced breadth of learning experiences, whereby curriculum was interpreted to mean all the organized courses, activities, and experiences that students have under the direction of the school, whether in the classroom or not. Finally, a somewhat different responsibility of the school was implied in the concept of curriculum that indicated that curriculum includes means employed by the school to provide students with opportunities for desirable learning experiences.

A sixth concept of curriculum indicated that curriculum is a *means to facilitate the growth of the students*. Although it is likely that this concept has not been universally applied, studies in human development have given us much useful information in relation to the appropriate types of learning activities for students in different stages of the growth processes. Human development has called our attention to the need to give consideration to the matter of individual differences among students. Within the same curriculum no two students truly ever have exactly the same experiences. When comparable opportunities are offered, there will be a range in the performance of students within a group. We have evidence that human development is greatly influenced by the sociocultural environment from which the student comes. The results of studies reported by Bloom give an indication of the impact of the environment on the stability and change in human characteristics [3]. While information about growth and development tells us what a student is able to learn at a particular stage in development, judgments must be made concerning whether certain learnings should be acquired at certain periods as opposed to others. Controversies arise in the discussions of the priorities of social versus academic learning activities in the early elementary school years.

CURRICULUM CONCEPTS—CONTEMPORARY VIEWPOINTS

The concepts of curriculum developed by contemporary authorities in the field appear to bring together many previously stated notions. Current viewpoints, with some added qualities and dimensions, utilize these notions in a more dynamic framework. The concern of the curriculum in facilitating human development implies that certain changes should be brought about in the behavior of students. Since it is not the responsibility of the school to bring about all types of behavior changes, the school selects those changes which are appropriate for the concern of teachers, leaving others for the attention of other social agencies. Curriculum becomes a means of achieving the "desired learnings" that are considered to be within the domain of the school. Problems have arisen with regard to the desired learnings for which the school is responsible. It appears that over the years schools have assumed responsibility for certain learnings that were once considered to be the prerogative of other social groups. Herein lie the fundamental issues in the discussions concerning the role of the schools in the areas of sex education, driver education, and religious training.

In describing the curriculum as the experiences that the school plans and provides so that the student may attain designated behaviors, Anderson gives attention to the *quality of experiences* as paramount [4]. The interacting factors in the learning environment that determine the quality of experiences include the teachers, the students, other adults in the school, the physical plant, the equipment, the learning materials, and the course content and procedures. Changing the curriculum in this instance involves changing the interacting focus.

A similar concept of curriculum is offered by Koopman, who extends the *educational environment to the community* [5]. This concept plays down the importance of the teacher dominating a classroom group and plays up the learner's readiness, initiative, perception, and actual experiences. It allows a more adequate role for the educational importance of the total environment, including the family, the community, and the mass media. It becomes the sum total of all of the planned and contrived learning experiences in the community, of the impact of all of the natural and man-made resources of the community. It refers to all of the creative learning experiences of the people in the community. It is a community curriculum in the sense that it grows out of the needs, interests, resources, and conditions of the community.

Two somewhat different points of view concerning the nature of curriculum are expressed by three contemporary writers. Mackenzie states that the curriculum is defined as the *planned engagement of learners* [6]. The assumption here is that engagements can be observed and to some extent controlled. The word engagement is used to mean what the learner meets face-to-face, what he attends to, or what he is involved in. There can be engagements with teachers, classmates, or others, with physical facilities, such as materials and equipment, and with subject matter, ideas, or symbols. Specific engagements may appear to be primarily intellectual, emotional, or manipulative.

A departure from this point of view is expressed by Shane and McSwain. These writers indicate that the curriculum has its being in two separate but interrelated entities: first, *in written form as a record of group consensus* as to methods, scope, and sequence; and second, *under the skin of both teachers and students* as the sum of the experiences and guides-to-action that each has interpreted for himself as the outcome of his interactive living and learning together in the school [7].

Gagné has described curriculum as a sequence of content units arranged in such a way that the learning of each unit may be accomplished as a single act, provided the capabilities described by specified prior units (in the sequence) have already been mastered by the learner. Gagné further states that a curriculum is specified when (1) the terminal objectives are stated, (2) the sequence of prerequisite capabilities is described, and (3) the initial capabilities assumed to be possessed by the student are identified. To illustrate the intent of his definition, Gagné provides several analyses of curriculums, one of which concerns mathematics [8]. The notable feature here is the hierarchy of content units that he proposes. The determination of this sequence is crucial. Each unit of content has prerequisites that must be identified and ordered so that the curriculum is a unified whole. Rather than define the term *curriculum*, Scriven prefers to speak of educational instruments [9]. These are processes, personnel, procedures, programs, and the like, that are operative when formal educational activities take place. This means that the curriculum is put to use. Necessarily, interactions exist. Content units, teachers, and the teaching environment are principal factors which interact, often in an ill-defined manner, when a curriculum is actually used.

In more recent years curriculum authorities include instructional methodology and procedures within the framework of curriculum and curriculum development. Any sharp distinction between curriculum and methods seems unfruitful. The kind and variety of learning experiences indicated by the curriculum will give direction to the methods to be employed. The appropriateness, the timing, and the design of the instructional methods will determine in a large measure the quality of the curriculum. Taba states that excluding from the definition of curriculum everything except the statement of objectives and content outlines and relegating anything that has to do with learning and learning experiences to "methods" might be too confining [10]. Curriculum is viewed in a more comprehensive reference to include all the *means employed by the school* to provide students with opportunities for desirable learning experiences. Contrasted with the more traditional concept, such a definition affects tremendously the philosophy, objectives, content, methods, and evaluation of the total curriculum.

The understanding and interpretation of the definitions and concepts pertaining to curriculum over a period of years may be facilitated by a historical review of the major purposes of education and the various sociocultural influences that contributed to the development of the twentieth-century system of education in this country. Organized nursing education made its appearance on the educational scene during the last quarter of the nineteenth century. The contributions of educational reformers have greatly influenced the system of nursing education, and now, in turn, nursing education is becoming a vital force in educational thought and action.

HISTORICAL PERSPECTIVE

Philosophers and educators have endeavored to describe the purposes of education in an American democracy since the founding of the first college in this country. The opening of Harvard College in 1636 marked the beginning of the formal educational system in the United States. The sociocultural conditions within the first colonies gave rise to the predominantly religious motives of the institutions of education. The colonists who fled Europe to seek relief from religious persecution found a fertile climate in this country to develop a way of life that was compatible with their religious views. The pattern of education considered appropriate for a gentleman, the traditional liberal arts, was transplanted from England to this country. Over one hundred years lapsed before attention was given to professional training in the institutions of higher education. Another hundred years lapsed before public education on a secondary school level was offered to the youth of this country. Because educational opportunities were initially limited in this country during the first two hundred years of the settlement in America, many young men who had the financial resources returned to Europe for their education.

The eighteenth century witnessed great political and economic rivalries conducted virtually on a worldwide scale. By 1715 the religious rivalries that marked the Reformation in Europe had largely given way to rivalries founded upon commercial interests in gaining colonies and nationalistic interests in political superiority. The Enlightenment was a reaction against the absolutistic and authoritarian regimes of the Reformation. Underlying these protests was a growing faith in common man, in science, and in human reason. This period has also been called the Age of Reason to indicate the hope and faith that man, by taking thought, could reform his institutions as a means of promoting the general welfare. Perhaps one of the most far-reaching results of the Enlightenment was the development of a new conception of education for citizenship. The political aim of education during the Reformation had been to produce a citizen who would be ready to take his place in a state that was closely allied with a ruling church. Both Catholics and Protestants believed that knowledge and truth were fixed and were revealed to man from supernatural sources; both agreed that man's primary aim in education was to arrive at a true knowledge of God's laws and commandments. Knowledge of the physical world was considered by both religious groups as far less important than knowledge of the spiritual and moral world. Both Catholics and Protestants were opposed to the implications of much of the new scientific investigations.

The Enlightenment produced a conception according to which churches were separate from the state, and the values of good citizenship were therefore entirely separate. Ideas that were to influence educational practices were voiced by Jean Jacques Rousseau, who glorified the wholesome development of all the natural powers of the individual. It seemed to many educators that Rousseau looked to the individual rather than to society to find the ultimate aims of education. Rousseau's ideas became immensely important, for he reacted violently against the conception that human nature is inherently evil, a belief which had been expressed earlier by the Moravian bishop Comenius.

Among the important thinkers during the eighteenth century was John

Locke, who formulated certain notions about the operation of human reason and the way people learn. He stressed experience and environment as the sources of knowledge and learning in that ideas, values, and knowledge have their origin in experience of the external world and of other people. It appears that some of his notions did not take root immediately in European institutions. While these institutions seemed to be unresponsive to changes in the social climate, the new currents of political, economic, and scientific thought of the European Enlightenment were entering American education and gaining considerable headway.

The ideals of science and practical utility gradually began to affect the religious outlook and the curriculums of some of the colleges. There appeared a vastly broader conception of the aim and content of liberal education, a conception which implied that college studies should contribute to the commercial and civic usefulness of the many as well as to the religious and civic leadership of the few. Because the colonists in America followed the pattern of the English universities, they established liberal arts colleges rather than universities on the medieval pattern. Therefore, the higher faculties of law, medicine, and theology were not present in the beginning of American higher education. Education for these professions during most of the eighteenth century was gained by apprenticeship to a practicing lawyer, physician, or clergyman.

Nineteenth-century United States was marked by an enormous expansion of population. There was a vast increase in building the things needed to exploit the resources of a new continent. American culture revealed the interplay of several factors: the religious tradition, humanism, democracy, nationalism, capitalism, science, industrialism, and a new psychology. The principal aims of education indicated that several conceptions were at work at the different levels of the educational system. Character and moral development, mental discipline, literacy and acquisition of information, vocational and practical aims, civic and social concerns, and individual development were considered in various forms and degrees. Throughout the century a series of specific influences from Europe were at work in American education. From Germany came the ideas of Pestalozzi, Froebel, and Herbart. To a varying degree these ideas reinforced the moral and religious aims, but they also gave stimulus to the literary, social, practical, and individual aims. Higher education during the nineteenth century experienced fundamental changes in character and purposes. Certain cultural forces that helped to expedite these changes include the gradual substitution of secular for religious authority in the spiritual, social, and intellectual activities, the growth of commerce and industry, the expansion of systematized knowledge, particularly in the physical and social sciences, and the advance of democracy and of the concept of the innate worth of the individual. One of the most important changes brought about by these factors was the decline of the prescribed curriculum. The religious-moral and disciplinary aims began to be challenged by the informational, social-civic, practical, and individual aims of education. Technical and professional education in the universities expanded to include greater attention to the professions of law, medicine, and theology. Although three independent schools of nursing were established during the latter half of the nineteenth century, they were soon absorbed by hospitals. These schools and others that were to follow for many years to come perpetuated the apprenticeship type of education.

At the close of the nineteenth century, two voices were being heard that were to help modify American education. The contributions of G. Stanley Hall to the psychological development of children and adolescents turned the attention of educators to the need for study of child development. More influential was the work of John Dewey, which proclaimed that schools should strive to elevate the aims of civic and social experience, vocational and practical usefulness, and individual development. The outline of thought contained in these works formed the groundwork of Dewey's philosophy of education, which was elaborated in form and extended into practice throughout the first half of the twentieth century. Various social and intellectual movements during the twentieth century in the United States led to a variety of approaches to education. During the first two decades of the century, the traditional religious and philosophical outlooks continued to stress moral development and mental discipline as the paramount aims of education. The rise of scientific psychology and realistic philosophy began to stress the informational and practical aspects of education. Interest in individual development was accelerated by the influence of the psychology of individual differences, and educational programs directed attention to individualized instruction. Vocational and practical aims took a paramount position closely allied to the general development of character, discipline, and knowledge. Individual development was considered an important quality of democratic education, and it was claimed that individual capacities were developed most effectively as an integral part of the social process. Curriculum began to be shaped by the needs of society as well as by the interests of students. It became evident that school experience should be planned not only with reference to good learning activities of individual students, but also with reference to the social significance of the problems that students face and must solve. The large universities, with the growth of their professional, technical, and graduate faculties, began to dominate the offerings of the undergraduate college, so that preparations for advanced specialized work became a prominent goal of college instruction.

So far, the second half of the twentieth century has experienced a multitude of technological and scientific innovations. An almost insatiable need for workers with varying degrees of skills was created in various occupational fields. The concept of the aim of education as the development of the capacities of the student for social usefulness has been generally accepted. Curriculums on all levels—secondary, junior college, and university—were ready to assume responsibility for vocational, technical, and professional education. The trend toward federal support of education that began in the nineteenth century was accelerated in the twentieth century. The efforts of the federal government in providing financial assistance to education on the various levels have been directed toward the development of programs in special occupational fields to assist the states in realizing the ideal of equality of education for all American youth. Although nursing education has found its place among other occupational education programs in the vocational schools, junior colleges, and universities, the responsibility for a large segment of nursing education has been assumed by other than educational institutions. While some divergent points of view concerning the several purposes of education are expressed by educators, one fundamental purpose appears common to all. The education for the youth of this country is concerned with the development of their capacities so that they may live personally and socially satisfying and useful lives. The characteristics of various educational programs on the different levels indicate that the citizens of this country acknowledge that there is no one pattern of education to achieve these purposes. The uniqueness of individuals to be educated in relation to their interests and abilities and the sociocultural environments in which the schools exist give direction to multiple approaches to curriculum and curriculum development.

APPROACHES TO CURRICULUM DEVELOPMENT

The review of the general purposes of education and the definitions and concepts of curriculum that have been expressed since the establishment of formal education in this country give some indication that the nature and function of curriculum have changed. More recently, curriculum appears to be concerned with assisting students to acquire certain behaviors that will be useful to them and others in the modern world. Thus, curriculum development becomes the process of selecting and offering learning opportunities that will be likely to assist the student to acquire those behaviors while he is in the school. The usual approach to establishing criteria for the learning opportunities is the analysis of the needs of society in relation to particular events in an effort to determine the types of behaviors that are expected of persons assuming specific roles in these societal events. A curriculum specialist recently stated that the behavior of the student while he is in school is of little consequence. The important behavior is that behavior the student exhibits when he is no longer under the direct influence of the school environment. Curriculum, therefore, is designed to direct and control the behavior of the students so that they may acquire the behavior required for the specific roles that they wish to assume as members of society.

What teachers do in relation to curriculum development is determined primarily on the basis of value judgments. Various learning opportunities are selected and organized in a certain way because teachers believe that the opportunities will assist the students to change their behavior in a predetermined way. The core programs in the junior high schools are planned and organized according to a certain pattern because the teachers believe that the learning opportunities included are likely to be the most useful in assisting the students in their developmental tasks as individuals and as citizens in a democratic society.

The general education components of undergraduate curriculum in colleges and universities are designed to provide the fundamental learning opportunities that are considered to be common and useful for all students regardless of their major field of study in the curriculum. A review of general education programs in undergraduate curriculums among several colleges and universities reveals some similar, but also some diverse, elements. Thomas has described the liberal arts or general education sequence of several colleges and universities, noticing the variations in the requirements as determined by the judgments of the teachers within the various schools [11]. Since institutions of higher education in this country believe and give support to the concept of diversity, the means by which the objectives of general education are obtained will vary among colleges and universities.

Nursing curriculums likewise display different patterns of organization for the preparation of the practitioner for a particular type of nursing practice. The faculties of these schools determine the pattern of curriculum events that they believe will help the students acquire the necessary behaviors in the most effective and efficient manner.

At the present time practically all curriculum planning is based upon the value judgments of teachers responsible for curriculum development in a particular school. These judgments are made with consideration given to the professional and practical experiences of the teachers and, perhaps, with some empirical investigations of curriculum activities. In this instance curriculum development is *normative* or *prescriptive* in that what is offered in the curriculum is thought to be "good" for the student in relation to the goals of the curriculum.

Another approach to curriculum development is directed by *scientific theory*. This approach indicates that curriculum decisions are made not on the basis of value judgments but on the basis of fact. Scientific theory is descriptive; it indicates what is or what exists. The research viewpoint gives attention to the observables in the learning situation. The behavior of the student becomes the dependent variable, and the conditions under which the behavior is acquired, maintained, eliminated, or shaped become the independent variables. Instruction is inseparable from curriculum, since it is the manipulation of the independent variables, and the teacher represents a cluster of independent variables. The verbal and nonverbal behaviors of the student are the only variables that can be observed and measured. Through research we learn that the manipulation of variables in a particular way yields a certain kind of behavior. The type of behavior we want students to acquire, however, is always a matter of value judgment. The ends of all curriculums must be determined by the values placed upon certain educational goals at a specific point in time. The outcomes of research will give us information upon which we can make our curriculum judgments for the purpose of attaining these goals. Sufficient research has not been forthcoming to contribute to the development of theories of curriculum and instruction upon which we can make generalizations and predictions.

SUMMARY

Curriculum development is a complex endeavor that involves many kinds of activities and decisions. Decisions must be made concerning the goals of nursing education and the specific objectives of a particular type of curriculum. The major areas or subjects of the curriculum, as well as the specific content, must be selected. Choices must be made about the type of learning activities with which to implement both content and other objectives. Decisions are needed regarding how to evaluate what students are learning and the effectiveness of the curriculum in attaining the desired ends. Finally, a choice needs to be made regarding what the overall pattern of the curriculum is to be. If curriculum development is to be adequate, all these decisions need to be made competently on a recognized and valid basis and with some degree of consistency. The complexity and multitude of decisions make it important that there be developed an adequate theory of curriculum development. Writers in the field of curriculum are presently voicing the need for a theory that will provide some basis for designing, developing, and implementing curriculum. The basis utilized in selecting curriculum opportunities are many and varied, and frequently curriculum patterns give evidence of an emphasis on one basis as opposed to another. Within a particular type of nursing curriculum, the arrangement of learning opportunities most often follows a traditional pattern of organization. Some schools have had the courage to make some modifications in the way the curriculum is organized, and a few schools have undertaken a complete breakaway from the more usual curriculum pattern. Faculties of schools of nursing in some instances ascribe to a psychological theory that is utilized in developing and implementing the curriculum; however, on occasion it is not always clear how this theory influences program planning. While many schools are making conscientious efforts to improve curriculum, there is an absence of well-defined methodology for the steady improvement of the instructional programs in nursing.

In this book curriculum is perceived as the content and processes of relationships between students, teachers, and others, and the arrangement of the physical and social environments that facilitate the attainment of specified goals that are consistent with and an integral part of the total school program. Curriculum and instruction are inseparable and involve both interaction and transaction, since all persons concerned are changed in some way during and as a result of the process. Curriculum development implies that a plan for the curriculum has been designed and a process of review and revision is ongoing for modification to achieve improvement. Curriculum improvement is more than alteration or rearrangement of student experiences according to a preconceived plan; it involves the reeducation of teachers and administrators so that they may learn to identify students' needs and desirable ways of satisfying these needs. Although attention is directed to some of the significant activities of curriculum experimentation and research in nursing, the primary focus of this book pertains to the development and implementation of curriculum by means of the thoughtful and systematic judgments of teachers working in concert in a spirit of cooperative endeavor.

REFERENCES

1. National League of Nursing Education. *A Curriculum Guide for Schools of Nursing.* New York: National League of Nursing Education, 1937. P. 13.
2. Caswell, H. L., and Campbell, D. S. *Curriculum Development.* New York: American Book, 1935.
3. Bloom, B. S. *Stability and Change in Human Characteristics.* New York: Wiley, 1964.
4. Anderson, V. E. *Principles and Procedures of Curriculum Improvement,* 2d ed. New York: Ronald, 1965. P. 6.
5. Koopman, G. R. *Curriculum Development.* New York: Center for Applied Research in Education, 1966. P. 8.
6. MacKenzie, G. N. Curricular Change: Participants, Power, and Processes. In M. B. Miles [Ed.], *Innovation in Education.* New York: Teachers College Press (Columbia University), 1964.
7. Shane, H. G., and McSwain, E. T. *Evaluation and the Elementary Curriculum.* New York: Holt, Rinehart & Winston, 1958. P. 8.
8. Gagné, R. M. Curriculum Research and the Promotion of Learning. In R. W. Tyler, R. M. Gagné, and M. Scriven [Eds.], *Perspectives of Curriculum Evaluation.* Chicago: Rand McNally, 1967. P. 23.
9. Scriven, M. The Methodology of Evaluation. In R. W. Tyler, R. M. Gagné, and M. Scriven [Eds.], *Perspectives of Curriculum Evaluation.* Chicago: Rand McNally, 1967.
10. Taba, H. *Curriculum Development: Theory and Practice.* New York: Harcourt, Brace & World, 1962. P. 9.
11. Thomas, R. *A Search for a Common Learning.* New York: McGraw-Hill, 1962.

SUPPLEMENTARY READINGS

Butts, R. F. *A Cultural History of Education.* New York: McGraw-Hill, 1947.
Krug, E. A. *Curriculum Planning.* New York: Harper & Brothers, 1950.
Smith, B. O., Stanley, W. O., and Shores, J. H. *Fundamentals of Curriculum Development.* New York: Harcourt, Brace & World, 1957.

2 BASIC ISSUES IN CURRICULUM DEVELOPMENT

THE development of nursing education in this country since the turn of the century has been determined by many forces affecting the course of events. Important among them are developments in medicine, economics, status of women, attitudes toward health and sickness, wars and conditions of living and working, and the direct impact of the hospital system, which has controlled nearly all of the education in nursing. While presenting tremendous challenges, the combination of these forces has also presented problems and obstacles to the development of nursing education. When one reads chronologically the story of this period, it appears that progress in education for nursing has been slow. Although the tremendous efforts of nurse educators is noteworthy, certain basic issues have been, and remain, evident in the development of nursing and of a system of nursing education. These issues may be classified in relation to (1) administration of nursing education, (2) financing of nursing education, (3) faculty, (4) concept of nursing and nursing education, (5) research in nursing, (6) subject matter of nursing, and (7) students.

ADMINISTRATION OF NURSING EDUCATION

The development of education for practitioners in the professions has occurred in educational institutions. While in most instances these professional schools were initially proprietary and independent, they have more recently become a part of the university family. No profession other than nursing has delegated the education of the majority of its practitioners to other than educational institutions. Repeated studies concerning the fundamental issues and the problems plaguing nursing and nursing education have pointed to the absence of an orderly system of nursing education in this country. The President's Commission in 1953 indicated that "nursing like other professional education should become a part of the general system of the nation" [1]. Although there is some indication that hospitals are beginning to relinquish their responsibilities for nursing education, there is also evidence that in hospital schools of nursing hospital administrators and trustees are not willing to delegate to the faculties of these schools responsibility for educational policies in a manner considered essential in universities offering professional preparation.

A survey of schools of nursing in 1949 revealed that of the 1,193 schools of nursing in the United States, 1,184 were controlled by hospitals and 9 were independent schools or departments of universities and colleges [2]. By 1963, the number of programs conducted by colleges and universities had increased to 196. The number of diploma programs under the auspices of hospitals had decreased to 875. During the interval of time between the survey and 1963, associate degree programs offered by community or junior colleges had been established, and eighty-four such programs were in operation. Programs leading to a certificate or diploma in practical nursing were established in public vocational education systems and hospitals. The number of these programs increased from 144 in 1950, to 737 in 1963, and most of them were administered through the public school system.

A recent reporting of the numbers and types of nursing education programs by the National League for Nursing revealed in 1971 there were:

Type	Number of Programs	Graduations
Baccalaureate degree	285	9,913
Associate degree	491	14,754
Diploma	587	22,334
Practical-Vocational	1,291	38,556

Among the various programs preparing for registered nurse licensure (baccalaureate, associate degree, diploma), the program graduating the largest number and percent of nurses was the hospital diploma program [3].

Although the American Nurses' Association has taken the position that education for nursing should be within the mainstream of American education, the fact remains that presently a substantial portion of this education is controlled and directed by hospitals.

FINANCING NURSING EDUCATION

A concomitant problem is that of adequate financing of nursing education. At the time of the first national study of nursing education, which was made by a group including representation from medicine, hospital administration, public health, education, and the lay public, concern was voiced in relation to the financial support of nursing education. The group concluded "that the development of nursing service adequate for the care of the sick and for the conduct of the modern public health campaign demands as an absolute prerequisite the securing of funds for the endowment of nursing education of all types; and that it is of primary importance, in this connection to provide reasonably generous endowments for university schools of nursing" [4]. Similar statements were made in two subsequent studies, and yet at mid-century the typical school of nursing had no budget of its own. The President's Commission on the Health Needs of the Nation reported: "Endowment money is almost non-existent in nursing education, and the amounts of public educational funds in this field are relatively small" [5].

A report of the practices of schools of nursing in 1949 was published in 1953, reporting information obtained by means of a survey of 97 percent of schools of nursing in the United States, Hawaii, and Puerto Rico. (In 1949, Hawaii was a territory of the U.S.) It was revealed that the expenditures for nursing education including the costs of instruction totaled about $25 million, or $300 per student a year. These figures do not include the cost of student maintenance or plant operation. While $300 per student a year is a low cost in comparison with other types of special preparation, this cost represents a sharp increase over the preceding decade. The major source of nursing school income, as the survey indicated, was tuition and fees, gifts and endowments, and state and local funds, representing to some degree the value of student services. Whereas most schools reported their income from tuition and fees, few reported income from gifts and endowments or from government funds. Hospital funds represented the major income in most nursing schools [6].

The report of the Surgeon General's Consultant Group on Nursing acknowledged that the cost of providing nursing education is substantially greater than the income received from the school from tuition and fees. At the time of this report, baccalaureate nursing education programs were faced with serious financial problems because of the heavy costs of providing adequate clinical teaching. The Consultant Group reported that assistance should be provided to help meet the school's educational costs and that such assistance should be tied with assistance to students. In view of the fact that nursing has not been successful in commanding adequate support for the development of its educational institutions and programs, the Consultant Group recommended that federal funds should be made available to reimburse schools of nursing for partial costs of education of students supported wholly or in part by federal scholarships or loans [7]. In addition, the Consultant Group recommended that federal funds should be provided to help pay for the construction needs for educational facilities, the development of new nursing school facilities, the expansion of nursing education facilities in colleges and universities, and the development of more efficient and effective methods of teaching. The Consultant Group also recommended the extension of the Professional Nurse Traineeship, administered by the United States Public Health Service, to cover the period prescribed for the individual trainee to complete the program of study, to provide for preparation of nursing specialists in clinical fields, and to include nurse graduates of diploma and associate degree programs for up to two years of full-time study toward a baccalaureate degree.

A response to these recommendations by outstanding nurse educators seemed to imply that the Consultant Group was somewhat shortsighted in its evaluation of the situation in nursing. Since our most critical shortage is that of the basic degree graduate, it is this group that should receive first consideration, especially since this is not only the longest and most expensive, but also the most direct, route to proper qualifications for those with the ability and interest to become leaders [8]. More recently efforts have been directed to obtain assistance from federal sources for baccalaureate nursing students; however, at present substantial progress has not been made.

Financial assistance from federal sources has expedited the improvement in the quantity of nurses and quality of nursing education and has indirectly caused us to reexamine our concept of democracy. Notable influences upon curriculum development have been visible. Whereas most of these influences have been positive in nature, faculties need to view with caution any form, financial or other, which may disturb the equilibrium of the educational program.

ADEQUATE FACULTY

Faculties of schools of nursing have shown an impressive increase in numbers, but we must remember that as late as 1911, when there were already 1,121 schools of nursing, probably not more than ten of them employed a single individual whose time was devoted wholly to teaching [9]. Even in 1929, 42 percent of the schools had not a single full-time instructor. By mid-century there were 10,477 nurse instructors, full- or part-time, but 45 percent of them had less preparation than is required for a bachelor's degree. Master's degrees were held by 1,144 instructors, and 4,581 instructors had their bachelor's degree. Approximately 30 percent of the instructors in collegiate schools held master's degrees, and in hospital schools less than 1 percent had attained this academic preparation [10].

The report of the Surgeon General's Consultant Group on Nursing, which endeavored to study the problems, needs, and goals toward providing quality nursing, indicated that teachers in all nursing education programs should have the minimum of a master's degree and that those persons holding positions of leadership in education, such as deans or directors, and faculty of graduate programs in nursing should have attained the doctoral degree [11]. This report indicated that increasing the number of well-prepared teachers in schools of professional and practical nursing is of critical importance to the future of nursing. Although a master's degree is considered a standard for teaching, almost 70 percent of the nurse educators did not have this degree at the time of this report. In diploma and in practical nurse programs, substantial numbers of faculty members did not have a bachelor's degree. One fourth of the instructors in hospital schools had little more academic background than the students they were teaching. The Consultant Group projected a need for an additional ten thousand faculty members by 1970 to make possible expansion of enrollments and to bring substandard programs up to the level required for national accreditation [12].

Some reactions to the Consultant Group's report by leaders in the profession seemed to imply that the goals set by the Group were formidable. Approaches to the problems of quantity and quality of faculty for the various educational programs in nursing were suggested. The need for quantity of faculty should not detract from their quality, and efforts should be exerted to increase the quality of graduate programs on the master's and doctoral levels. In addition, the initiation of an *active recruitment program* to interest the "students with the ablest minds" in a career in college teaching was recommended. Lastly, concern was expressed in relation to the restrictive practices that militate against students beginning graduate education early and continuing it until completion. These practices included the prerequisites of work experience, the costs to the students and to the university, the research requirement involving much time and effort, and the stifling rigidity of many graduate programs in nursing [13].

More recent projections made by the Division of Nursing of the United States Public Health Service concerning the need of nursing personnel with regard to level of educational preparation indicate that by 1975, 120,000 nurses should be prepared at the master's level, 280,000 at the baccalaureate level, 540,000 at the diploma level, and 60,000 nurses with associate degrees.

Professional teachers have been traditionally prepared in the graduate schools of our universities. It is here that the prospective teacher gains depth in his subject matter and understanding and skill in the teaching-learning process. Graduate programs in nursing have developed rapidly during the past fifteen years. The establishment of graduate programs is dependent upon the quantity and quality of our baccalaureate programs. One of the greatest bottlenecks in the preparation of teachers of nursing is that the majority of our nurses are graduating from less than college programs and must spend an inordinate amount of time equipping themselves to meet the requirements for graduate study. The problem of developing teachers of high quality is even more critical than the problem of quantity.

The lack of control of the educational program in nursing by educational institutions, the inadequate financing of schools of nursing, and the insufficient supply of qualified faculty are basic issues for review and study in ongoing curriculum development.

CONCEPT OF NURSING EDUCATION

In addition to the issues of control, finance, and faculty are those that pertain to the concept of nursing and nursing education as the content and responsibility of higher education. We are beginning to think about nursing not only as a profession but also as a learned profession. This implies that we must redirect our interests somewhat to include a concern about scholarship and, therefore, about research.

The concept of nursing as a learned profession is an exceedingly difficult one for nurses to envision as it presently exists. To achieve such a concept of nursing demands a completely new look, one that is quite different from that which we had held in the past. Nursing was initiated as a vocation and has so developed. Nursing has not bridged the gap between vocational training and learned education. The terms *professional nurse* and *registered nurse* have been used synonymously and interchangeably, a fact which may be an outward and visible manifestation of confusion concerning concepts about nursing. Recognition of nursing as a learned profession and internalization of such a concept must be followed by a clear differentiation of the occupational careers in nursing. At the present time there is a wide variety of programs preparing nurses at the vocational, technical, and professional levels. Clearer definition of the purposes and functions of these programs will be forthcoming as the phenomenon of nursing is better understood.

The concept of what nursing is continues to be the delaying force today. Judged by the literature of the nineteenth century, good nursing was generally recognized in terms of the personal qualities of the nurse. Statements about the qualities of the nurse almost invariably begin with the importance of physical strength, and they spare no detail lest some important quality be overlooked. The nurse should be neither too short nor too tall; she should not be too bulky, inclined to be slow or too heavy a sleeper. Specifications are that she should have a noiseless tread, a dextrous hand, a cheerful countenance, and substantial feet. Going beyond the physical qualities, literature states that the nurse should possess firmness, manifest prudence and discrimination, and display an unruffled temper. These nineteenth-century phrases give us practically the only terms in which good nursing was commonly recognized.

Next to personal qualities, the most frequent descriptions of nursing give details of what the nurse should wear and the etiquette or rules she should carefully observe. The most specific descriptions of what the nurse actually does are almost invariably in general phrases, such as waiting on, giving constant attention to, and comforting and cheering the sick, relieving suffering, behaving with kindness toward the patient, giving information to the doctor, and applying all the remedies prescribed. Florence Nightingale was more explicit in delineating the duties of the nurses. In addition to stressing personal qualities and appearance, she stated, "You are expected to become skillful . . . in the dressing of blisters, burns, sores, wounds, and in applying fomentations, poultices, and minor dressings . . . [in] the management of helpless patients, i.e., moving, changing, personal cleanliness of, feeding, keeping warm (or cool), preventing and dressing bedsores, managing the position

. . ." [14]. With these duties clear, education for nursing became a possibility, replacing intuition. It must be remembered that this concept of nursing came into being and existed during the time in which the provision of health care services required only patients, physicians, and nurses.

Many newcomers in the health scene have defined their specialized services for patients and families. The occupational therapist, the physical therapist, the medical social worker, the clinical psychologist, the nutritionist, and the vocational rehabilitation counselor have claimed their stake in patient care. Nursing fell heir to the responsibility of coordinating functions required to get these specialized services to patients. In addition, nursing, in a response to compelling realities within employment settings, gave attention to their medical assistant and administrative functions, giving lesser attention to the care needs of patients. We know that in hospitals more and more direct nursing care of patients was given over to practical nurses and ancillary nursing personnel, while registered nurses increasingly met the needs of physicians for help in implementing medical goals and carried the administrative elements of the hospital's operations to the point of providing direct services to patients. Nursing seems to have been left at this juncture offering three major services: caring for the needs of patients, assistance to physicians, and the administrative functions of communicating among, and coordinating the efforts of, the increasing and varied participants in health care.

The rescuing of nursing from an ill-defined state has been a continual process involving reworking and clarification as conditions in society have changed. In taking over the new concept, we have been strongly influenced by old ideas. Old ideas are difficult to shake; one of these was that personal qualities and intuition make the nurse. That this idea hung on for a long time is reflected in admission requirements, content of instruction, emphasis on manual activities, and lack of emphasis on intellectual content. It was not uncommon, even as late as the early 1950's, for high school counselors and principals to record on a student's application to schools of nursing that the "applicant is not material for college, but will make a good nurse." The fact remains that a long-outdated concept of nursing is still with us, and attention should be directed to bring it in line with what we think nursing really is or should be.

To keep up with new developments in the health field, nursing has bulged out in one new direction after another. Much of the time the nurse has had to play by ear her new roles and has been called upon for performance results before a basis for action could be laid through study. In more recent years with more and better prepared nurses available, nurses have been able to carry on research and experimentation in nursing care and in the differentiation of functions of various types of workers needed for nursing care. These studies and those to follow should serve as a basis for a clearer general understanding of the twentieth-century role of the nurse.

NURSING RESEARCH

The concept of nursing as a learned profession implies scholarship and research. No profession can fail to be concerned about the refreshment of its own knowledge, the improvement of its own standards, and the widening of its own horizons. Whitehead describes this task in a colorful manner by saying that "for successful education there must always be a certain freshness in the knowledge dealt with. It must either be new in itself or it must be invested with some novelty of application to the new world of new times. Knowledge does not keep any better than fish" [15].

Scholarship and research are those elements that create the environment within which truly higher education can exist. Research is concerned with the testing of old knowledge and the discovery of new knowledge. It is concerned with the application of knowledge from wherever it may be drawn to the present, and the ferreting out, the discovery, and the organization of new knowledge.

The field of inquiry and scholarship in nursing has to be in the area of nursing care. While the research base of nursing is not yet substantial, some relatively sophisticated studies in nursing are taking place. Studies are going on that endeavor to get at the nursing needs of the patient with specific health problems: the hospitalized child, the maternity patient, the chronically ill patient, and the orthopedic patient. Experiments have been carried out on the therapeutic role of the nurse in the care of the emotionally ill patient. Studies such as these will serve to bring up to date the concept of nursing for nurses themselves, for other related disciplines, and for the public. This research is basic to keeping our nursing services abreast of changes as well as being vital to professional education.

Studies of the preventive aspects of nursing care are helping to make clear the specific content of what the nurse can contribute in this area. This aspect of nursing is particularly in need of delineation in more concrete terms because it has been pushed out of focus by the more immediate needs of acute hospital services. Aspects of nursing other than prevention were more pressing in the hospitals that controlled the schools, and this part of nursing never really had a chance to become part of the accepted concept of nursing. A great deal of available information on prevention of illness is not being used in nursing today. Although public health nursing is recognized as including prevention, nursing in general is strongly identified with curative functions in the acute stages of the illness of the patient.

Another aspect of nursing undeveloped in the general concept of nursing, although a basic part of public health nursing, is the teaching and the guidance of patients and families. Although teachers in schools of nursing frequently indicate that health teaching is an integral part of the nursing curriculum, there is some evidence that such activities are not included in nursing practice. A recent study directed to the identification of the specific duties fulfilled by a general medical-surgical nurse in giving competent care revealed that of the total of 1,489 observations of nursing behaviors that were collected, no observations of "teaches patient care" appeared [16]. In the area of health teaching, as in prevention, studies of patients' nursing needs are helping to show concretely steps that can be taken by the hospital nurse as well as the nurse in a public health agency. Explorations are also being made that could help to extend to more nurses the role of guiding normal family life. An example of this is group leadership activities with parents in maternity and child care, centering not around disease but rather around family needs in normal family life.

Attempts are being made to reassess the various ranges of competence in nursing and to provide adequate preparation for each person in an orderly system. Studies have approached the problem from different angles. They have endeavored to differentiate the role of the aide, the practical nurse, and the professional nurse. They have examined the wide range of functions and duties now being carried by the professional nurse and have tried to find ways in which the professional nurse could become more effective and at the same time delegate certain duties. They have sought to find out exactly what distinguishes the professional from the technical or the routine aspects of nursing. There have been other efforts to delineate what should be expected of the graduate of a collegiate program as distinguished from the hospital school and junior college graduates. Particularly significant in education for nursing have been the efforts directed toward differentiation in basic and advanced preparation.

Research and experimentation in nursing care and in the functions of the different workers in nursing are essential for bringing change into the concept of nursing. The progress being made in such studies is very encouraging. Methods must change with changing conditions, and we must constantly depend upon such explorations to determine specifically what we are doing and why. We are dependent upon such research to validate a concept of nursing which then becomes the content of our educational programs.

SUBJECT MATTER OF NURSING

The contributions of the various types of nursing practitioners to nursing care is recognized; however, the more precise roles and functions of the graduates of the vocational, technical, and professional nursing programs are yet ill-defined. Our ability to state clearly what it is that the beginning professional practitioner can be expected to contribute within nursing services is essential if we hope to effect widespread understanding about distinctions between professional and technical education and practice.

In the past nursing education was not designed to encourage a search for nursing theory. Most nursing programs were then conducted outside educational institutions by instructors whose preparation in nursing went little beyond the level to which they aimed to bring their students. The format of these programs was usually a foreshortened version of the pattern followed in undergraduate medical education. Provision for preclinical sciences and future content was developed according to the clinical divisions germane to the expanding specialization within medicine. It was frequently obvious that whenever medicine defined a new specialty area and beds were set aside in hospitals, nursing curriculums added a course related to that specialty and a block of experience for reasons of staffing if not for learning nursing.

There continues to be wide differences of opinion as to what the content of various programs should be and from what the content should be derived. There is renewed attention on the need for better preparation in the natural sciences and on the interrelationships between health and disease. There is continual stress on the importance of the behavioral sciences and on the need to understand how biological, physiological, and sociocultural factors influence human behavior. There is concern in relation to understanding how individuals perceive themselves and others according to their specific roles and relationships. It is proclaimed that the nurse must learn not only to analyze the feelings and actions of patients but also to examine her own feelings and actions, and the interactions between herself and her patient.

There is considerable emphasis today on the need for nurses to learn how to diagnose nursing needs of patients and to plan, administer, and evaluate care in relation to these needs. There is attention given to the need for nurses to learn to function in group situations of varying complexity and to work with and through others in these situations. There is emphasis on the role of the nurse in working with families as well as with individual patients and in understanding the factors in the family or community that stimulate or inhibit recovery. And in all of these endeavors it is essential that the nurse relate theory to her day-to-day practice, since practice becomes the process of theory in the making.

It is said that nurses should understand the historical and present-day developments in health services and the influences of social, political, and economic trends in the United States and in a larger society. There is considerable attention given to the liberal education component of the baccalaureate curriculum, a component which contributes to the growth of the student as a person as well as a professional practitioner. While the focus and dimension of this aspect of the curriculum are usually determined by the parent organization, it has been observed that nursing curriculum may not always make available to students the breadth of learning that other students enjoy.

It is also being said that professional practitioners in nursing should have some appreciation for and competency in interpreting and applying certain research outcomes as a means of improving their professional practice. Bruner suggests that "mastery of the fundamental ideas of a field involves not only the grasping of general principles, but also the development of an attitude toward learning and inquiry, toward guessing and hunches, toward the possibility of solving problems on one's own" [17].

One of the most difficult problems facing nurse educators today is determining what the specific content of nursing is. While the basic information used by the several health professions is found within the natural and behavioral sciences, the question of what should be taught and how it should be taught poses problems for instructors in the various programs. Nursing, as in other scientific disciplines, has experienced a vast increase in the body of knowledge that it utilizes. Since all of the knowledge cannot and should not be included in any one type of program, systematic delineation must be made in relation to the type and amount of subject matter that is appropriate to attain the objectives of the specific program.

STUDENTS

A reinterpretation of the concept of democracy has enabled more students to pursue the study of nursing in the various types of nursing. Restrictive admissions policies, which were once characteristic of many nursing programs, have been relaxed. The characteristics of students of nursing display considerable heterogeneity in race, religion, sex, and socioeconomic status. In addition, many schools of nursing are endeavoring to make it possible for students who do not have the usual academic qualifications to proceed in a nursing program by means of remedial assistance in certain fundamental skills, such as reading, mathematics, and studying. The marital status of students on admission or during the years of the school program is no longer the concern of faculties and administrators of the school of nursing.

Although these changes in school policies are completely legitimate and desirable, they nevertheless necessitate appropriate planning to meet individual needs and problems while maintaining standards of education.

SUMMARY

The basic issues in nursing that have direct influence on curriculum development and implementation include administrative problems of control of education in nursing, financial support, adequate faculty, the changing concept of nursing and nursing education, research in nursing, identification of the subject matter of the discipline, and the characteristics of the student population.

While these issues may not be all-inclusive, they do appear to be ones that have persisted over the years and upon which we still focus our attention. The lack of control of educational programs is obvious, as shown by the number of nursing programs situated within the framework of the hospital. Flexibility in curriculum planning and development may be hampered by the climate of the institution whose primary responsibility is the health care of people rather than the education of the student.

The financing of nursing education is a fundamental issue that influences all aspects of the program. Support for instruction and assistance to students in the form of scholarships, grants, and loans have direct bearing on the quantity and quality of instruction and the caliber of students within the school. While marked increases in financial assistance to schools are noted, particularly in relation to federal fundings, certain phases of nursing education have been essentially deprived of resources outside the institution.

The faculty of a school of nursing probably has the most direct influence on curriculum development. At the moment the minimum preparation for teaching in any type of nursing program is considered to be the master's degree. Recent statistics reveal that many faculty members fall short of meeting this requirement. Curriculum development cannot be done in a thoughtful and systematic fashion if the teachers do not have the basic equipment for study and decision-making in this endeavor.

In addition to the issues pertaining to administration are those that are inherent in the profession. One of the most fundamental issues pertains to the development of a clear and definitive concept of the phenomenon of nursing. There is evidence that a strong vocational orientation still exists whereby practical endeavors overwhelm the intellectual pursuits. The concept of nursing as a learned profession is "catching on" slowly, and this concept implies new ways of thinking and acting. A related issue is concerned with nursing as a truly higher education. Although colleges and universities have accepted the responsibility for conducting nursing programs, frequently these programs have not required the level of scholarship that is expected of other educational programs in the university.

While some significant studies in nursing care have been published, the research base of nursing is not yet substantial. The validity of a professional curriculum is dependent upon the disciplined analysis of professional practice, and an ongoing effort to formulate, test, and validate the knowledge foundations on which the practice rests is essential. Development and identification of a substantial organized body of knowledge fundamental to nursing are imperative; however, theoretical knowledge is dependent on research. The subject matter of nursing is derived from the vast field of knowledge made available by scientific endeavors in the natural, behavioral, and medical sciences. As the knowledge base of these fields has increased both in depth and breadth, so has nursing. What information to include, how much, when, and where become questions for faculties of the various nursing programs to answer. The articulation of the subject matter within a specific program and among the various programs is a basic issue for curriculum development. Further exploration of these issues will occur in subsequent chapters of the book.

REFERENCES

1. The President's Commission on the Health Needs of the Nation. *Findings and Recommendations*. Building America's Health, vol. 1. Washington, D.C.: U.S. Government Printing Office, 1953. P. 19.
2. West, M., and Hawkins, C. *Nursing Schools at the Mid-Century*. New York: National Committee for the Improvement of Nursing Services, 1950.
3. National League for Nursing. Educational preparation for nursing—1971. *Nurs. Outlook* 20:599, 1972.
4. Goldmark, J. *Nursing and Nursing Education in the United States: Report of the Committee for the Study of Nursing Education*. New York: Macmillan, 1923. P. 20.
5. The President's Commission on the Health Needs of the Nation, op. cit., p. 19.
6. West and Hawkins, op. cit., p. 48.
7. U.S. Department of Health, Education and Welfare. *Toward Quality in Nursing: Report of the Surgeon General's Consultant Group on Nursing*. Washington, D.C.: U.S. Department of Health, Education and Welfare, 1963. P. 56.
8. National League for Nursing. *The Surgeon General's Report and Collegiate Nursing Education*. New York: National League for Nursing, 1963. P. 11.
9. Nutting, M. A. *Educational Status of Nursing* (bulletin no. 7). Washington, D.C.: U.S. Bureau of Education, 1912. P. 44.
10. West and Hawkins, op. cit., p. 45.
11. U.S. Department of Health, Education and Welfare, op. cit., p. 19.
12. U.S. Department of Health, Education and Welfare, op. cit., p. 36.
13. National League for Nursing, op. cit. [note 8], p. 17.
14. Seymer, L. R. *Selected Writings of Florence Nightingale*. New York: Macmillan, 1954. P. 305.
15. Whitehead, A. N. *The Aims of Education*. New York: Macmillan, 1929. P. 98.
16. Klaus, D. J., et al. *Controlling Experience to Improve Nursing Proficiency*. Pittsburgh: American Institutes for Research, 1966.
17. Bruner, J. S. *The Process of Education*. New York: Vintage, 1960. P. 20.

SUPPLEMENTARY READINGS

American Nurses' Association. Education for nursing. *Amer. J. Nurs.* 65:106, 1965.

Bridgman, M. *Collegiate Education in Nursing*. New York: Russell Sage Foundation, 1953.

Roberts, M. *American Nursing: History and Interpretation*. New York: Macmillan, 1954.

National League for Nursing. *The Shifting Scene—Directions for Practice.* Twenty-third Conference of the Council of Member Agencies of the Baccalaureate and Higher Degree Programs. New York: National League for Nursing, 1967.

Stewart, I. M. *The Education of Nurses.* New York: Macmillan, 1943.

3 PARTICIPANTS IN CURRICULUM DEVELOPMENT

THE participants in curriculum development are those individuals or groups of individuals who exert some influence, either direct or indirect, in determining the nature and activities of the curriculum. Participants in curriculum development may be viewed from the standpoint of their position in the social system within which the educational program exists. Mackenzie has classified participants as *external* and *internal* [1]. *Internal* participants are those who have a direct connection with the legal or social system concerned with the curriculum under consideration. Because of their direct influence, the internal participants exert a greater force in determining the nature of the curriculum. *External* participants are those individuals or groups of individuals outside the legal or social system concerned with the development of the curriculum. These participants have a greater potential for indirect action in that their efforts are usually directed toward influencing the decisions of the internal participants. This classification of participants in curriculum development is utilized in order to identify the individuals and groups that contribute to the content and process of curriculum in nursing.

INTERNAL PARTICIPANTS

Six major internal participants are identified that exert direct influence on curriculum development: students, teachers, administrators, state boards of nurse examiners, state departments of education, and state legislatures. It is likely that each of these participants influences the nursing curriculum to a different degree and that some of these participants may not have direct influence on certain curriculums.

STUDENTS

A dual role is played by students in curriculum development activities. In one role the students become the *determiners* of curriculum content and process in relation to their characteristics, such as abilities, interests, backgrounds, and goals, which influence their relationships with others in the educational environment. The role of *participants* in curriculum development is played by students when they participate actively in the planning of processes by which content, instructional methods, and materials are determined. Curriculum study groups in schools of nursing find the participation of students in cooperation with faculty and staff beneficial to all participants. Recent protests and demonstrations by students on college campuses have resulted in some positive contributions to curriculum change. Finally, the feedback from students with respect to their evaluations of particular courses in relation to content and teaching methodology has a direct influence on teachers' behavior and hence on curriculum development.

TEACHERS

A double role is also played by teachers in curriculum development. As with students, their various characteristics, such as abilities, backgrounds, personalities, become *determiners* of the curriculum event. Teachers have a direct influence in their classes and clinical activities on students, subject matter, methods and materials of instruction, and physical and social environments. That teachers serve as role models in the activities of nursing care may have a direct impact on the development of the student as a practicing nurse. In addition, the teachers individually and as a group have the major responsibility for organized curriculum development activities. They are active participants in the more formalized study of curriculum components and are directly responsible for recommending that certain changes take place in the nature and sequence of curriculum events. Hence, teachers perform three major tasks as participants in curriculum development: (1) they work and plan with students, (2) they engage in individual study, and (3) they share experiences concerning curriculum events with other teachers in group activities.

ADMINISTRATORS

The role of administrators in curriculum development may take several forms and dimensions. Because of the various types of administrative functions involved in the conduct of a school program, some different activities are required. The specifications of the administrative arrangements required for a small unit in nursing offering an undergraduate program in an independent college will probably differ from those required for a school of nursing offering graduate as well as undergraduate programs within a large, multipurpose state university. Regardless of the numbers of persons involved, there are essentially two major functions of administration that have direct bearing on curriculum. One of these functions pertains to the provision of appropriate academic resources and equipment, such as courses, laboratory activities, the library, and other instructional materials. The other function is concerned with the admission and registration of students, personnel services, and the provision of classrooms and other teaching facilities. In some instances these two functions may be carried out by the same person; more frequently, however, separate and distinct positions are established to direct and carry out these administrative responsibilities.

The administrators whose direct concern is with the numbers, types, and levels of course offering and related instructional matters include academic and clinical department heads, assistants to the chief administrative officer for academic affairs, curriculum coordinators, and supervisors. These persons have the major responsibility for establishing and maintaining the educational standards both within and among the various instructional units in the school.

The social and physical climate of the learning environment is seen as the major responsibility of those administrators concerned with the vast array of activities that have direct bearing on student life. The admissions officer selects those students who will have the opportunity for education in the school. Most frequently, however, the general admission policies are determined by the faculty. Those persons concerned with student personnel services assist the students to enjoy and profit by their school experiences. And those responsible for housing attempt to provide a pleasant and safe living environment. These administrators and those concerned with the academic affairs exert a profound influence on curriculum development.

STATE BOARDS OF NURSE EXAMINERS

The legal controlling body designated by the laws of each state is the state board of nurse examiners. The title of this group may differ among the states; however, the responsibilities and functions are essentially the same. The major purpose of this group is to protect the public by insuring safe and competent nursing care through the legal authority invested in the board. Although the composition of the board may vary among the states, the membership usually consists of registered nurses who meet the educational and professional requirements that are written into the laws of the state. The governor of the state appoints the members to the board. In most states one board handles all the legal affairs pertaining to nursing. In some states, however, one board may concern itself with matters pertaining to professional and technical nursing, and another board may handle matters concerning vocational or practical nursing. Whatever the arrangements concerning the boards and their compositions may be, there are two major functions the boards must execute to fulfill their responsibilities. One function is to license and register nurses who are qualified to practice nursing according to the specifications stated within the law. This is accomplished by examining the candidates' educational credentials and their performances in the state board examinations that are administered by this group. The second function of the board is to establish minimum curriculum requirements for the education of the practitioners. This implies that the board would prepare and distribute statements pertaining to specific curriculum events to be included in the educational programs for the professional and technical nurses and the practical or vocational nurses. The board is required to initiate supervisory activities to insure that the school meet these requirements.

Although the majority of nursing programs far surpass the curriculum requirements designated by the board, these requirements are a focus of attention in curriculum development of the faculties of schools of nursing. Also, the performance of the graduates of a school of nursing on the examination gives the faculty some indication of the strengths and weaknesses of the curriculum. Since the state boards of nurse examiners exert a direct influence on curriculum development in the schools within the state, it is of utmost importance that the most knowledgeable nurses serve on these boards.

STATE DEPARTMENTS OF EDUCATION

In the administration of state laws and regulations, the state departments of education influence directly and indirectly curriculum changes within the schools. Whether these departments operate under a state board of education or as relatively autonomous agencies, the state departments of education may require certain curricular activities to be offered in specific educational programs. In nursing education this is particularly visible in the vocational or practical nurse programs and in the technical programs in nursing that are under the auspices of the public school system. There are also instances in which the state department of education has the responsibility to execute acts of the legislature pertaining to specific curricular requirements in higher education. Most frequently these concern the teaching of the history of the state in which the college or university is located.

The state departments of education are frequently the channel through which financial support and special grants for designated educational projects and faculties are obtained. The need for training a variety of health service workers has precipitated the enactment of considerable health legislation by the United States Congress. This legislation includes funding for the education of health workers at the vocational and technical levels. Nursing has been the recipient of some of these funds through the state departments of education, enabling additional programs in nursing at this level to be established, studied, and improved.

STATE LEGISLATURES

As was previously mentioned, some state legislatures still make certain curriculum specifications. Although this practice is diminishing, the legislatures do have the responsibility to enact laws pertaining to education in general and to grant charters to institutions for the conduct of educational programs. In most instances the laws pertaining to education are directed to insure sound programs; however, they provide considerable flexibility for faculties of schools to be creative in curriculum planning. In some instances these laws have been restrictive in terms of specific requirements, thus presenting obstacles to ongoing curriculum planning. This has occurred on occasion in nursing when definitive courses and clinical requirements have been written into the laws. It then becomes the responsibility of the profession through its state association to provide the initiative for a change by the state legislature in the law.

While there may be other internal participants that are exerting a major influence in curriculum development, the six which have been described seem to represent those which have a direct relationship with the social system of which the school is an interacting constituent. More detailed consideration is given in a later chapter to these individuals and groups in relation to their specific roles and processes in curriculum activities as they pertain to the strategies for curriculum development.

EXTERNAL PARTICIPANTS

Many participants in curriculum development are found outside the social or legal system of the school situation. These persons or groups of persons are able to exert a substantial influence in determining the nature and activities of a curriculum. Although such participants are not responsible to or for the educational program, the power that they can exert cannot be underestimated. Their influence is considered to be indirect; nevertheless, it is a potent influence, particularly when it is addressed to the internal participants in curriculum development. Ten types of external participants that have some indirect influence on the curriculum are identified and include the following: professional associations, federal government, voluntary groups, academicians, educators, business and industry, prestige persons, foundations, citizens, and community action groups. A review of some of the past and present activities of these individuals and groups may indicate their contribution to and participation in curriculum development.

PROFESSIONAL NURSING ASSOCIATIONS

The professional associations in nursing having the greatest influences on curriculum development are the American Nurses' Association and its constituents on the state and local levels. Early activities of this organization were directed toward establishing legal controls on nursing education and nursing practice. The passage of state laws pertaining to nursing and the establishment of the state board of examiners of nurses by the state legislatures were the outcomes of the forces initiated by the state nurses' associations. Continuous review of these statutes is the responsibility of the group.

During the intervening years continuing efforts have focused on the standards of nursing practice for professional nurses occupying the different positions in nursing education and nursing services. Identification and description of the characteristics of the practitioners of nursing provide the programs in nursing education with essential information for the purposes of curriculum planning.

In addition, the American Nurses' Association through its committee on legislation is instrumental in obtaining public funds for nursing education. The American Nurses' Association has prepared and made available to all state nurses' associations A *Discussion Guide on Public Funds for Nursing Education,* which alerts the membership to the problems, issues, and processes of securing state and federal funds for nursing education.

The *American Journal of Nursing* provides practicing nurses and educators with pertinent information concerning nursing practice and related activities. *Nursing Research,* also published by the American Nurses' Association, reports current research in nursing practice, service, and education. The research activities of this organization have been extended to the Nursing Research Conference, which is scheduled annually. Reports of significant research activities are presented by the investigators, and critiques by fellow researchers are offered.

Whereas the National League for Nursing cannot be considered a professional organization in the same sense as the American Nurses' Association, its influence on nursing curriculum is so profound that it is included in this frame of reference for description. This organization and its predecessor, the National League of Nursing Education, was established for the purpose of improving standards of education for nurses. The organization has been persistent in its efforts to upgrade educational standards and to provide schools of nursing with information that would be useful to them in establishing, organizing, and developing curriculums in nursing. Its early efforts in providing leadership for the development of curriculum guides were monumental enterprises. Other early activities were concerned with defining the essentials of a good school of nursing and describing the duties, qualifications, and preparation of nursing-school faculty members. These were indispensable documents at the time of their preparation.

The establishment of a program for the accreditation of schools of nursing by the National League of Nursing Education prior to World War II led to the development of criteria for the evaluation of nursing education. Little progress was made in this direction because of the national war effort, and after the war ended, the accreditation activities were assumed under the auspices of the National League for Nursing. With the assistance of financial support from foundations, this organization has developed comprehensive accreditation activities for programs in nursing at the vocational, technical, professional, and graduate levels. Concomitant with the development of the criteria for the evaluation of these programs has been the identification of the characteristics of the various types of programs. These documents have been useful to faculties as guidelines for the development and improvement of curriculum. In addition to these activities, the National League for Nursing has sponsored regional curriculum conferences to enable faculties of schools of nursing to come together to discuss problems and issues in the improvement of curriculum in nursing.

The description of this organization hardly does justice to the efforts which have been exerted. When appropriate, additional attention will be directed to the work of the National League for Nursing throughout the text.

The publication of the league's *Nursing Outlook* provides the readers with useful information pertaining to nursing service and education. Curriculum activities of particular schools are reported frequently in serial form, noting the sequential developments in the specified program. This journal also offers book reviews of recent publications in the field of nursing and nursing education. The National League for Nursing maintains a communication service called *League Exchanges*, whereby materials prepared by individuals or groups that are thought to be useful to practicing nurses and/or teachers are reproduced by the league and made available for a nominal charge to interested persons. Consultation services are also available to schools of nursing. These services deal with overall administration and program planning and problems pertaining to specialized areas of the curriculum. The influence of the National League for Nursing as an organization engaged in a variety of activities has been and continues to be a forceful one in the development of curriculums in schools of nursing.

ALLIED PROFESSIONAL ASSOCIATIONS

Various allied professional groups have participated in curriculum development in nursing. At times the force that some of these associations exerted placed them into a position of direct influence whereby they performed a disservice to nursing. Perhaps the strongest and most forceful of all allied professional groups has been and still is to a great degree the American Medical Association.

Early discussions regarding the development of a system of nursing education in this country were precipitated by a committee of the American Medical Association after the Civil War. There was complete agreement that such education was needed, and the group indicated that the system for the training of nurses should be under the control of the medical profession. This notion was not and has never been acceptable to nursing. In certain instances, however, formal control was established wherein a program of nursing education was located in a school of medicine. Informally the control of nursing has been obviously under the direct influence of the medical profession, since a larger portion of nursing education has been provided by hospitals, which are essentially controlled by physicians.

The poor quality of nursing education that resulted led to the participation of the American Medical Association with the National League of Nursing Education in a study of nursing problems. In 1934 the joint committee, which became the Committee on the Grading of Nursing Schools, published the final report of the study under the title of *Nursing Schools Today and Tomorrow*. The study pointed out the shortcomings in a great number of schools of nursing and the inadequacies of the nursing curriculum.

Although subject matter was not the responsibility of the American Medical Association, individual physicians assisted greatly in the production of textbooks for nursing students. There were few outstanding authors among nurses during the early stages of nursing education, and the contributions of physicians of suitable literature was of professional character.

The dichotomy that existed in medical education between those physicians who were concerned solely with the curative aspects of medicine and those concerned with preventive medicine created problems for nurse educators. Nursing leaders were constantly under pressure to broaden the base of nursing education by those nurses who were associated with leaders in the fields of public health and preventive medicine.

The Committee on Nursing Problems of the American Medical Association, after careful study in 1948, made certain recommendations about the education of nurses. This report described the characteristics of the two groups of professional nurses as the nurse educators and the clinical nurses. The report further indicated that the nurse educator should have college training and the clinical nurse, a two-year course of training. The report also recommended a systematic form of training for the practical nurse [2].

It has been observed that the American Medical Association has been essentially opposed to forms of social legislation for health and related matters. This has had undeniable influences on nursing curriculum when federal assistance to various types of health education was included in the legislation. The American Medical Association has vigorously opposed the enactment of such legislation. However, the resources of the nursing profession have been sufficient to prevent defeat of federal support of nursing education. The American Medical Association has repeatedly demonstrated disfavor toward the extension of nursing education into higher education and concomitantly has shown a disapproving concern for the developing autonomy of nursing as a profession. Even though individuals and groups within the association have given support to the goals and activities of nursing in relation to education, the American Medical Association has been apprehensive about these developments.

The medical assistance role of the nurse expanded to such an extent that it became foremost in the minds and activities of physicians and nurses. It is understandable that the trend away from this area of responsibilities by nurses leaves the physicians uncomfortable. Considerable interpretation of the other roles that nurses must assume will be necessary to clarify to the physicians that nurses are team members in the health care services.

The official journal of the American Medical Association (*Journal of the American Medical Association*) provides valuable resource materials for teachers in schools of nursing, with reference to various aspects of medical pathology and treatment.

AMERICAN HOSPITAL ASSOCIATION

Since the majority of educational programs in nursing are controlled by hospitals, it is reasonable that the hospital association would be considered a participant in curriculum development.

The initial studies that were made of nursing and nursing education revealed outstanding weaknesses and inadequacies. Before much could be done to reconstruct the system of nursing education, it was evident that the functions of the schools of nursing and the functions of nursing service would have to be clearly differentiated. The cooperative efforts of the American Hospital Association and the National League of Nursing Education produced a publication, *Manual of the Essentials of a Good Hospital Nursing Service*, which pointed out the primary purposes of the nursing service. The publication suggested appropriate criteria for the evaluation of the service. This manual and the document prepared by the National League of Nursing Education, *Essentials of a Good School of Nursing*, offered a means for better understanding and cooperation between hospital administrators and nursing educators.

Another significant contribution of the American Hospital Association was the participation of this group with the National League of Nursing Education in a study of the costs of nursing education. The report of this activity provides a valuable economic guide for both hospitals and nursing schools [3].

The American Hospital Association has approved in principle and has been supportive of the efforts of nursing to improve its system of education, although it was not initially enthusiastic about federal assistance to schools of nursing. The concerns of the nursing profession in relation to the conduct of schools of nursing by hospitals has not met with equal concerns of the American Hospital Association. Likewise, the American Hospital Association has been vocal about the standards of nursing education as established by the various departments of the National League for Nursing. Some indication was made that the American Hospital Association should establish a means for accrediting schools of nursing under hospital control.

The publications of this association offer useful information to teachers of nursing in hospital management and services, supplies and equipment, and resources for clinical training.

AMERICAN DIETETIC ASSOCIATION

Faculties of schools of nursing have utilized the services of nutritionists and dietitians in hospitals and public health agencies for the purpose of curriculum and instruction. More recently joint activities have been initiated by the national associations, the American Dietetic Association, and the National League for Nursing. The state constituents of these organizations have also sponsored cooperative activities in the area of curriculum development in nursing. A joint endeavor of these organizations in one state resulted in the preparation of some guidelines for teaching nutrition and diet therapy in schools of nursing [4].

In addition to the cooperative activities, the publications and journals of the American Dietetic Association provide useful information for instructors in schools of nursing.

AMERICAN ORTHOPSYCHIATRY ASSOCIATION

This interdisciplinary association is concerned with a better understanding of human behavior and the more effective treatment of behavior disorders. The scientific information made available by means of meetings, workshop activities, and the official publication, The *American Journal of Orthopsy-chiatry*, has significance for nursing curriculum from the point of view of understanding students as well as patients and potential patients.

Other medical and health groups attend to various specific areas or problems. The influence of these associations on nursing curriculum is primarily through the information revealed through organizational activities and publications.

EDUCATIONAL ASSOCIATIONS

Several professional educational associations participate indirectly in curriculum development in nursing, and their contributions throughout the years are notable.

The American Council of Education, a council of educational associations and institutions of higher education, assisted nursing in the development of collegiate programs. A report of these activities was published under the title of *Nursing Education and National Service* in 1942 [5].

The Association of Collegiate Schools of Nursing, which was organized for the purpose of promoting, studying, and improving collegiate education in nursing, became a member of the American Council of Education. This association was dissolved with the restructuring of nursing organization in 1950. The relationship of these organizations provided opportunities for the interpretation of nursing education to educators in the fields of general education and sought assistance from them.

Regional Accrediting Associations

The six regional accrediting associations have provided the faculties of college and university nursing programs with educational standards and criteria for the purpose of self-evaluation. These associations cooperate with the accrediting service of the National League for Nursing for joint review and evaluation of nursing programs. The accrediting associations will be considered more fully in the chapter dealing with evaluation of the curriculum.

Regional Education Association

Regional planning for higher education was initiated after World War II. At that time heavy demands were created in the South for professional, technical, and graduate education. An expanding industrial economy called for more highly trained manpower, and the industrial expansion in the South appeared to be greater than in the nation as a whole. The increasing number of students desiring to attend college required more and better schools. The governors of fourteen southern states called on college and university leaders in the South to help devise ways of supplying the education that the region needed. The Southern Regional Compact was signed by the governors, which permits the states to share the educational resources of the region, relying on the facilities of the neighboring states instead of attempting to provide every type of education within their own borders. The compact created a central agency to coordinate their efforts—the Southern Regional Education Board, with headquarters in Atlanta, Georgia.

At the time of the organization of the Southern Regional Education Board, there were no programs for the preparation of nursing teachers, administrators, or clinical supervisors. The faculties and administrative personnel for the undergraduate programs in nursing had to be recruited from the northern and western states, or the southern nurses had to go to institutions in other areas for their advanced education and training. A subcommittee on nursing education of the Southern Regional Education Board recommended the establishment of several regional programs for graduate study in nursing. This recommendation was accepted, and six universities in the South were selected to establish graduate programs in nursing.

The committee and the schools together decided on the curriculum offerings in the six universities. Funds were provided by the W. K. Kellogg Foundation for a five-year project, and a project director was appointed. Deans and faculty members of the 126 colleges and universities in the region worked cooperatively, creatively, and experimentally toward common goals. Six months before this project terminated, the W. K. Kellogg Foundation approved a grant for a second five-year project, which began in 1967 [6].

A very recent activity of the nursing group of the Southern Regional Education Board was the sponsorship of a series of seminars for psychiatric nursing instructors for the purpose of developing behavioral concepts in nursing that would be useful in teaching. Other ongoing activities pertain to the exploration and use of multimedia technology in instruction.

As in the South, the western governors came together to seek solutions to common problems. One of the most urgent appeared to be a gap in the development of educational facilities to prepare highly specialized technical and professional personnel.

These governors reviewed the activities and progress of the Southern Regional Education Board, and in November, 1949, they endorsed the principle of closer cooperation for higher education. The Western Regional Education Compact, which created the Western Interstate Commission for Higher Education (WICHE), became operative in 1951 [7]. Nurse educators in the West were in agreement with the WICHE premise that there is a definite relationship between the quality of the educational system for the preparation of professional workers and the quality of services they render.

Although collegiate nursing education had "taken root" relatively early in the West, nurse educators were concerned that the pattern of this education reflected the characteristics of the "training school." They also recognized that a successfully designed and executed curriculum demands a faculty of outstanding stature. In an effort to have such faculty available to schools of nursing, graduate programs in nursing would need review and upgrading. It was recognized that a new type of graduate program in nursing could not come into being without cooperative planning, and a device was needed that would facilitate the working together for the achievement of a common goal.

The Western Council on Higher Education for Nursing was organized in 1957 and provided a means whereby nurse educators could exchange ideas and share experiences, could undertake cooperative planning for educational programs, and could stimulate research in nursing. One of the most significant projects in the area of graduate education was the curriculum project concerned with defining clinical content of graduate programs in nursing [8]. The baccalaureate program has also been a focus of attention, and this group has endeavored to identify essential content in these programs [9]. Other activities were concerned with the formulation of guidelines for the development of baccalaureate programs in the West.

In an endeavor to identify the major needs for education in the West, the Western Council on Higher Education for Nursing made a survey of the needs of, the present supply of, and the training facilities for nurses. On the basis of data obtained, certain recommendations were made to strengthen existing programs, expand specific programs, and develop new programs in nursing education [10]. Particularly significant for curriculum development was a study that endeavored to validate the baccalaureate nursing curriculum by means of the critical incident technique [11]. Other projects of this group that have implications for curriculum were concerned with teaching and leadership effectiveness.

A third regional association is the New England Council on Higher Education for Nursing, which is a constituent of the New England Board of Higher Education. Although the New England group does not have the same governmental organization as the other two regional groups, some of its purposes are similar. The New England Council on Higher Education for Nursing has been concerned with the various aspects of curriculum development in colleges and universities. Five interuniversity faculty work conferences have been held which have given attention to the various components of the undergraduate curriculum, the utilization of resources for teaching, and the use of newer instructional methods and teaching aids. This cooperative endeavor of the faculties of baccalaureate programs in nursing in the Northeast has provided an opportunity for the sharing of ideas and experiences and the generation of new ideas, an opportunity which has brought considerable refreshment and stimulation to the faculty members involved.

NATIONAL EDUCATION ASSOCIATION

Although not directly concerned with nursing education, the National Education Association and its various constituents have aided nursing primarily through conference groups and publications. Particularly useful are the reports, yearbooks, and other published literature of the Association for Supervision and Curriculum Development. Although the association gives attention to both broad, general areas and specific topics, much of the information is pertinent to curriculum development in nursing.

AMERICAN JUNIOR COLLEGE ASSOCIATION

The rapid development of community junior-college programs in nursing has been facilitated by the close association of the American Junior College Association with the National League for Nursing. Before organizational arrangements were provided for communication with this association, the National League for Nursing employed a member of the American Junior College Association as a consultant. The consultant served to interpret the purposes and roles of the junior colleges and provided assistance to those schools that were interested in developing nursing programs. More recently the state constituents of the American Junior College Association and the National League for Nursing have continued this service on the state and local levels.

FOUNDATIONS

Nursing and nursing education has been the recipient of foundation support for several types of projects and activities. When substantial private philanthropy was no longer available for educational endeavors, contributions from foundations were forthcoming. The assistance from the various foundations has been used for financing studies, programs, and students and has been made available to schools of nursing and to nursing organizations.

Efforts to improve nursing education were initiated by the Rockefeller Foundation in 1918 in cooperation with the National League of Nursing Education. This foundation agreed to finance a comprehensive study of the nursing situations at that time, especially as it related to the education of nurses. This study was published in 1923 under the title of *Nursing and Nursing Education in the United States*, and because of the objectivity and impartial presentation of the findings, it became an important event in nursing. The Rockefeller Foundation also prepared a summary of the work of schools of nursing in several countries for the development of collegiate nursing programs abroad. During its formation and development, the National Organization for Public Health Nursing received financial assistance from the Rockefeller Foundation. This foundation financed a five-year experiment in methods of educating nurses at Yale University, and at the termination of the experiment an endowment of one million dollars was provided to insure the continuation of the school. This foundation has contributed substantially to the movement for collegiate schools of nursing through its financial help to several pioneer schools, its staunch support of the collegiate type of organization, and its fellowships. Because of the success of the endeavor at Yale University, a second experiment was initiated at Vanderbilt University, and another million-dollar endowment was forthcoming [12]. In an effort to prepare nurses who can undertake research in nursing, the Rockefeller Foundation contributed a grant of $100,000 to the Division of Nursing Education of Teachers College at Columbia University. This center administers a program of research, experimentation, and field service in nursing directed toward the improvement of nursing services [13].

The contributions of the W. K. Kellogg Foundation to nursing and nursing education through financial assistance were initiated during World War II. The National Nursing Council, which was established in 1942, assumed responsibility for the plans for nursing service and programs so that military needs could be met without undue disruption of civilian service. For a period the principle source of income for the work of this council came from the W. K. Kellogg Foundation, which contributed over $300,000 to the program [14]. During the postwar period the W. K. Kellogg Foundation gave grants to a number of universities to develop advanced programs in clinical nursing. These courses were directed to nurses interested in becoming teachers, supervisors, head nurses, consultants, or expert practitioners in specific clinical areas [15].

The increased demands for nursing services following World War II made it necessary to examine the system in existence and the educational programs preparing the practitioners. The National Committee for the Improvement of Nursing Services assumed this responsibility and the W. K. Kellogg Foundation granted $200,000 for a three-year program [16]. The continuing influence of this foundation on nursing and nursing education is described by Roberts, who said that "the most specific action taken by any national body to improve the administration of nursing services was that of the W. K. Kellogg Foundation, which, in 1950 invited 14 universities to participate in a two-to-five-year program for the improvement of the preparation of administration of nursing service" [17].

Significant also were the contributions of the W. K. Kellogg Foundation to individual schools and to various states for the establishment of practical nurse education within the public school systems. Also contributory to nursing education was the systematic evaluation of the experiment in community junior-college education for nursing, which was conducted by Bernice Anderson and financed by the W. K. Kellogg Foundation. As with the Rockefeller Foundation, the W. K. Kellogg Foundation has provided grants to individual schools for specific projects and scholarship assistance for students.

One of the most significant studies of nursing and nursing education was made by Esther Lucille Brown, and the report of the study was published under the title of *Nursing for the Future*. This study was made possible by the combined efforts of the Carnegie Corporation and the Russell Sage Foundation. The findings of this study indicated that the educational needs of nursing were not well understood by colleges and universities. In an effort to interpret and advise institutions of higher education in relation to matters pertaining to nursing education, Margaret Bridgman, Dean of Skidmore College, was engaged by the Russell Sage Foundation. Her publication, *Collegiate Education for Nursing*, which was addressed primarily to educators, was published by this foundation in 1953.

The generous efforts of the various foundations in nursing and nursing education has been outstandingly noteworthy. The impact of the activities financed by these groups is immeasurable; however, it can be safe to assume that these groups were vital catalysts in the improvement of nursing services through the upgrading of nursing curriculum at all levels of education.

FEDERAL GOVERNMENT

Early in the development of the system of education in this country, the federal government became involved primarily through financial support to higher education. The land-grant movement in 1862 was a response to the rapid industrial and agricultural development in the United States, and the university assisted in this development through training and research. Universities became involved with the daily life of society as students came to the university from all walks of life.

During World War II universities were asked to assist in national defense and scientific development. Major support for nursing education began at this time in response to a national demand for more nurses. The participation of the federal government in curriculum development has and continues to be in the nature of giving funds for the support of nursing education. In June, 1943, the Seventy-eighth Congress enacted the Nurse Training Act, which provided for the organization and development of the United States Cadet Nurse Corps. This act also provided for postgraduate preparation for graduate nurses. The five-year program cost the federal government approximately $160 million. In addition, the Lanham Act of 1940 authorized expenditures of over $25.5 million for new facilities, such as classrooms, demonstration rooms, and library space.

In 1956 additional federal funds were provided through the enactment of the Health Amendments Act. This legislation provided funds for (1) the preparation of public health nurses, (2) advanced preparation for graduate nurses in teaching, supervision, and administration, and (3) the expansion of vocational education for the training of practical nurses. In 1959 this program was extended for a period of five years.

The Manpower Development and Training Act of 1962 provided funds for the development of a vast array of educational programs for careers in health occupations. This not only includes practical nurse programs but also provides funds for refresher courses for nurses who desire to return to professional activities after their home responsibilities are less demanding.

Some of our nursing programs have developed more rapidly than others, and some areas of clinical specialization have expanded tremendously as a result of federal support. The critical need for qualified psychiatric nurses to service both the civilian and military population during World War II led to the establishment of advanced programs in psychiatric nursing for graduate nurses, with emphasis on teaching, supervision, and administration. Mental health training in the United States has improved both in quantity and quality during the period of federal support. This support provides opportunities for training, curriculum development, and instruction at the master's and doctoral level.

The Children's Bureau has provided financial support to programs of graduate study in maternal and child health. That other areas of clinical specialization have not expanded to the extent that psychiatric nursing and maternal and child health have is due in good measure to the fact that traineeship support is available for other specialties, and funds are not available for training grants to develop new programs. Federal support has helped to raise the standards of preparation for nurses in hospitals as well as in schools of nursing and in general has heightened interest in graduate education in nursing. This support has produced most of the faculty engaged in nursing education today.

The involvement of the federal government in nursing education has served to improve our programs. It has supported faculty, encouraged curriculum study and innovation, aided in recruiting and retraining students, and promoted research. Since 1955 the nursing research grants and fellowship programs of the Public Health Service have allocated approximately $11 million for nursing research project grants, $2 million for nursing research fellowships, and $700,000 for the nurse-scientist training grants.

Although we need federal grants to support our programs, these grants do not always enhance the financial health of our schools. Tuition payments do not pay the cost of education. In general, universities absorb approximately two thirds of the cost of a student's education. Although the administration of the traineeship program increases the need for bookkeeping, there is no support for such essential services.

Faculties of schools of nursing must be careful to avoid academic imbalance as a result of funds being available to some programs and not to others. Federal support for one program and not for others can create some distortion in the educational program. Program expansion should be in accordance with the goals of the school irrespective of financial support. More funds are urgently needed for curriculum study. Federal funds should support the efforts of the faculty to change the curriculum, which forms the basis of the nurses' professional knowledge and skill, rather than force the faculty to meet built-in requirements for the purpose of funding.

UNITED STATES OFFICE OF EDUCATION

From the time of the enactment of legislation for federal funding for vocational education, the United States Office of Education encouraged the state boards for vocational education to promote the organization of programs in practical nursing. In 1949 the United States Public Health Service detailed a professional nurse to the Office of Education to assist states to organize and improve curriculum for practical nurse training.

Through the combined efforts of vocational education organizations and national nursing and health organizations, useful information was made available in a document, *Practical Nursing, An Analysis of the Practical Nurse Occupation with Suggestions for the Organization of Training Programs*. A second publication, *Practical Nursing Curriculum*, outlined a curriculum pattern that might be used by schools. Both of these documents were published by the United States Office of Education and became valuable tools for educators.

The Health Amendments Act was passed in 1956 and made it possible for interested states to develop, expand, or improve practical nurse curriculums. Funds appropriated each fiscal year were distributed by the United States Office of Education to state boards for vocational education. In the same year the United States Office of Education established a Practical Nurse Education Section, with a staff of three professional nurses to work with the states in extending and improving their programs. A publication *Guides for Developing Curricula for the Education of Practical Nurses*, was prepared and made available to interested educators [18]. It can be assumed that the principles, policies, and standards set forth in the publications of the United States Office of Education and the funds allocated through federal legislation opened the way for the widespread development of practical nurse programs.

AMERICAN RED CROSS

The American Red Cross may be considered a quasi-governmental agency, although its initial responsibilities and services were to the federal government. The organization developed as a response to the need for an official agency to select and assign nurses to military hospitals for wartime services. These responsibilities necessitated the agency in cooperation with American Nurses' Association to establish standards and criteria for the selection of graduate nurses for military services. The professional standards for enrollment and other policies had a powerful influence on the development of nursing and nursing education. The requirements for enrollment in the American Red Cross in regard to professional preparation were well above the minimum requirements of many state boards of nurse examiners. This fact served as a stimulus to the state nurses' associations to activate improvement in state legislation.

The civilian activities are primarily concerned with providing nursing services to supplement those offered through other agencies. The programs, demonstrations, and materials prepared by the local chapter of the American Red Cross provide vital curriculum experience for students in all types of nursing programs.

VOLUNTARY ASSOCIATIONS

A voluntary association develops when a small group of people, finding that they have a certain interest or purpose in common, agree to meet and to act together in order to satisfy that interest or achieve that purpose. Frequently their action requires that they urge other like-minded persons to join them, so that some associations may become very large and extend throughout the country. Contemporary Western society is noted for the tendency for voluntary groups to form that contribute to the well-being of the community. Readily visible are the voluntary associations that dedicate themselves to the alleviation of specific health and social problems. Some of the older, well-established, and productive associations have served indirectly as participants in curriculum development in nursing.

The National Tuberculosis Association (NTA) was the first of many voluntary associations whose programs influenced the evaluation of public health nursing. The employment of special tuberculosis nurses demonstrated the need for specialized training in this area and the contribution to health care of families and communities of these nursing services. The activities of the NTA alerted schools of nursing to the need for curriculum experiences in the area of tuberculosis nursing as a means of alleviating a growing social and health problem in this country. The ongoing activities of the NTA have continually directed the focus of nursing toward a wider community service than that of the hospital environment. The various studies and publications of the NTA stress the need for improvement in the preparation of the public health nurse.

The Joint Tuberculosis Nursing Advisory Service of the National Organization for Public Health Nursing (NOPHN), the National League of Nursing Education (NLNE), and the National Tuberculosis Association (NTA), which was organized shortly after World War II, provided nursing services and schools of nursing with handbooks, annotated lists of publications, and visual aids, all of which were useful in educational programs. With the restructuring of the national nursing organizations in 1953, the activities of this joint enterprise became the responsibility of the cooperative efforts of the National League for Nursing and National Association for Tuberculosis and Respiratory Diseases and is financed by the latter organization. The nursing advisory services of the National League for Nursing is diligent in its efforts to provide schools of nursing and citizen groups with consultant services, materials and resources for instruction, and funds for local projects.

Similarly, the establishment of the Joint Orthopedic Nursing Advisory Service by the NOPHN, the National Foundation for Infantile Paralysis, and NLNE in 1941 focused attention on the preventive and therapeutic nursing care of patients as opposed to home, hospital, or public health nursing. It became apparent that greater attention should be given in the development of curriculums to clinical nursing care of patients and families. As with the Joint Tuberculosis Advisory Service, this group provided schools of nursing and nursing services with abundant instructional resources in the area of preventing crippling deformities and of restoring patients to maximum usefulness.

With the reorganization of the national nursing associations, the activities of this group were allocated to the Nursing Advisory Service for Orthopedics and Poliomyelitis of the National League for Nursing, which was financed by the National Foundation for Orthopedics and Poliomyelitis.

The American Cancer Society and its local constituents are making significant contributions to curriculum development through a variety of ways. Many local groups cooperate actively with nursing organizations and schools of nursing in conducting workshops and short courses.

The American Heart Association is concerned with promoting a better understanding of heart disease and the treatment and rehabilitation of persons with a specific disease of the heart. Since 1959 the association has conducted nursing education programs on nursing problems in heart disease. More recently it has established a Council on Cardiovascular Nursing to disseminate reliable information in the field and to help achieve the association's objectives for improved patient care. The association publishes a journal, *Circulation*, which includes technical papers on various aspects of heart disease. It also publishes a quarterly, *Cardio-Vascular Nursing*, which offers a variety of educational materials in nursing.

The National Association for Mental Health is a coordinated citizens' organization working for the improved care and treatment of the mentally ill and handicapped. It also is concerned with improved methods and services in research, prevention, detection, diagnosis, and treatment of mental illnesses as well as the promotion of mental health.

The influence that this association may have on nursing curriculum is primarily through its communication media, presentation of papers at meetings, and the official publication *Mental Hygiene*. This information is addressed to professionals as well as to the general public concerned with the care of the mentally disturbed patient. In addition, this society is also generous in furnishing educational, community, and professional groups with instructional materials about mental health and the nursing implications of caring for patients with mental and emotional problems.

The preventive aspects of health and the responsibilities of health workers in this area have been the concern of the American Public Health Association. This association participated in a study that was concerned with the grading of schools of nursing and made substantial contributions to it. The influence of the association in expanding the role of the nurse was visible in the instruction in public health nursing in curriculums of schools of nursing.

The American Public Health Association may be considered to be a voluntary organization rather than professional. This group has always been concerned with public involvement in the health affairs of the community, and membership into the association is open to lay citizens. The nursing section of the American Public Health Association has provided opportunities for nurse educators and practitioners to discuss problems relating to the quantity and quality of professional nurses who are engaged in the various activities of public health nursing.

BUSINESS AND INDUSTRY

The major activities of business and industry in curriculum development have been initiated by the dairy and food industries and the drug companies. The efforts of these enterprises have been primarily directed toward the preparation and distribution of teaching materials and aids that have some relationship to the products that the companies produce. These teaching resources are usually of high quality, and the advertising motive is not paramount.

These firms frequently prepare films and film strips pertaining to subjects that have no direct bearing on the companies' products and are made available as a service for educational purposes. In addition, there have been occasions when particular industries have financed experimental programs for the training of personnel.

SUMMARY

The individuals and groups that exert influence on curriculum development in nursing are identified as internal or external participants. The *internal* participants have direct connection with the social or legal system and are responsible to and for the curriculum under consideration. The *external* participants are the individuals and groups of individuals who are outside the social or legal system, and their influence is considered to be indirect.

The major internal participants in the development of nursing curriculums include students, teachers, administrators, state boards of nurse examiners, state departments of education, and state legislatures. Each of these individuals or groups has a vital but different role to play in the formulation and implementation of the curriculum.

The external participants in curriculum development exert a substantial power in determining the nature and activities of curriculum development primarily through their influences on the internal participants. External participants are usually considered as groups of individuals with special interests and may be classified as professional associations, allied professional associations, and business and industry.

The activities of the external participants over the years seem to indicate that these groups have made valuable contributions to the development of curriculums in nursing. The forms of these contributions include research studies, financial support, workshops, publications, and collaborative endeavors in nursing projects. A variety of particular groups are identified; however, not all groups that have made some contribution have necessarily been included. There is an indication that nursing education has been accepted as a responsibility of society and is closely knit within the activities of the social system.

REFERENCES

1. Mackenzie, G. N. Curricular Change: Participants, Power and Processes. In M. B. Miles [Ed.], *Innovation in Education.* New York: Teachers College Press (Columbia University), 1964. P. 409.
2. Committee on Nursing Problems. The report of the committee on nursing problems. *J.A.M.A.* 137:877, 1948.
3. American Hospital Association, and National League of Nursing Education. *Administrative Cost Analysis for Nursing Service and Nursing Education.* New York: National League of Nursing Education, 1940.

4. Joint Committee of the Maryland Dietetic Association, and the Maryland League for Nursing. *Guidelines for Teaching Nutrition and Diet Therapy in Schools of Nursing.* New York: National League for Nursing, 1962.
5. American Council of Education. *Nursing Education and National Service.* American Council on Education Studies, vol. 6. Washington, D.C.: American Council of Education, 1942.
6. Carnegie, M. E. Interstate cooperative in nursing. *Nurs. Outlook* 16:49, 1968.
7. Coulter, P. P. *The Winds of Change.* Boulder: Western Interstate Commission for Higher Education, 1963. P. 3.
8. Western Council on Higher Education for Nursing. *Defining Clinical Content—Graduate Programs.* Boulder: Western Interstate Commission for Higher Education, 1967.
9. Western Council on Higher Education for Nursing. *Essential Content in Baccalaureate Programs in Nursing.* Boulder: Western Interstate Commission for Higher Education, 1967.
10. Western Council on Higher Education for Nursing. *Nurses for the West.* Boulder: Western Interstate Commission for Higher Education, 1959.
11. Coulter, P. P., and Leino, A. *Validation of the Collegiate Nursing Curriculum Through Use of the Critical Incident.* Boulder: Western Council on Higher Education for Nursing, 1965.
12. Roberts, M. M. *American Nursing, History and Interpretation.* New York: Macmillan, 1955. P. 180.
13. Ibid., p. 531.
14. Ibid., p. 355.
15. Ibid., p. 424.
16. Ibid., p. 504.
17. Ibid., p. 506.
18. Orem, D. E. *Guides for Developing Curricula for the Education of Practical Nurses.* Washington, D.C.: U.S. Office of Education, 1959.

SUPPLEMENTARY READINGS

Anderson, L. G., and Ertell, M. W. Extra-institutional Forces Affecting Professional Education. In *Education for the Professions.* Sixty-First Yearbook of the National Society for the Study of Education. Chicago: University of Chicago Press, 1962.
Ayers, A. L. Role of interested groups in curriculum planning. *Educ. Leadership* 19:35, 1961.
Bartholf, M. Regional planning for nursing education in the South. *Nurs. Outlook* 3:538, 1955.
Belcher, H. C. *Nursing Education and Research; A Report of the Regional Project, 1962–1966.* Atlanta: Southern Regional Education Board, 1968.
Bixler, G. K., and Simmons, L. W. *The Regional Project in Graduate Education and Research in Nursing.* Atlanta: Southern Regional Education Board, 1960.
Brandt, J. A. Licensing Legislation. In *Social Legislation and Nursing Practice.* New York: American Nurses' Association, 1960.
Committee on Education. *The Nursing School Faculty—Duties, Qualifications*

and Preparation of Its Members. New York: National League of Nursing Education, 1933.

Committee on Education. *Curriculum for Schools of Nursing.* New York: National League of Nursing Education, 1927.

Committee on Education. *Standard Curriculum for Nursing Schools.* New York: National League of Nursing Education, 1917.

Committee on the Grading of Nursing Schools. *Nursing Schools Today and Tomorrow.* New York: National League of Nursing Education, 1934.

Committee on Standards. *Essentials of a Good School of Nursing.* New York: National League of Nursing Education, 1936.

Curriculum Committee. *A Curriculum Guide for Schools of Nursing.* New York: National League of Nursing Education, 1937.

Doll, R. *Curriculum Improvement: Decision-Making and Process.* Boston: Allyn and Bacon, 1964.

Griffin, W. This I believe. About regional nursing education programs. *Nurs. Outlook* 17:24, 1969.

Ingmere, A. E. *Effectiveness of a Leadership Program in Nursing.* Boulder: Western Interstate Commission for Higher Education, 1968.

National Society for the Study of Education. *Social Forces Influencing American Education.* Sixtieth Yearbook, Part II. Chicago: University of Chicago Press, 1961.

New England Council on Higher Education for Nursing. *The First Inter-University Faculty Work Conference.* Stowe: New England Board of Higher Education, 1964.

New England Council on Higher Education for Nursing. *The Second Inter-University Faculty Work Conference.* Cape Cod: New England Board of Higher Education, 1965.

New England Council on Higher Education for Nursing. *The Third Inter-University Faculty Work Conference.* Cape Cod: New England Board of Higher Education, 1966.

New England Council on Higher Education for Nursing. *The Fourth Inter-University Faculty Work Conference.* Cape Cod: New England Board of Higher Education, 1967.

Robinson, G. Legislation influences curriculum development. *Educ. Leadership* 19:26, 1961.

Smith, C. E. Nursing education—a public responsibility. *Nurs. Outlook* 1:96, 1953.

Spalding, E. K. *Nursing Legislation and Education.* Washington, D.C.: Catholic University of America Press, 1963.

Stewart, I. M. *The Education of Nurses.* New York: Macmillan, 1949.

Sugg, R. S., Jr., and Jones, G. H. *The Southern Regional Education Board; Ten Years of Regional Cooperation in Higher Education.* Baton Rouge: Louisiana State University Press, 1960.

U.S. Department of Labor. *Training Health Service Workers: The Critical Challenge.* Washington, D.C.: U.S. Department of Health, Education and Welfare, 1966.

Western Council on Higher Education for Nursing. *Toward More Effective Teaching.* Boulder: Western Interstate Commission for Higher Education, 1964.

II | SOURCES OF CURRICULUM DECISIONS

4 CULTURAL VALUES AND THE CURRICULUM

MAN is inventive by nature. However, his greatest invention is noninvention, that is, his skill in transmitting, intact and unchanged, from one generation to the next, the fundamental ways of doing things that he learned from the generation which preceded him. Within any society there must be ways of getting food, clothing, and shelter. Ways of dividing the work must be developed. There must be some patterning of the relationships of men, women, and children, of old and young members of the group, and of kin and nonkin. There must be some means of aesthetic expression and some kind of value system with ways of maintaining it. Means by which children are brought into the world, cared for, and taught social customs in order to maintain conformity in the life of the society must be adopted. In all societies there is some degree of interrelationship in cultural patterns, so that change in any one pattern may well affect changes in others.

From the perspective of those in each generation, and for the society as an enduring, historical entity, this process of cultural transmission yields enormous economy. Each new generation need not discover, at great cost in time and subject to great risk of failure, what those coming before have already learned. Since all those in each generation receive more or less the same cultural heritage from the preceding generation, they can more easily relate to one another and more effectively coordinate their actions. The grand total of all the objects, ideas, knowledges, ways of doing things, habits, values, and attitudes that each generation in a society passes on to the next is what is often referred to as the culture of a group.

CULTURE—DEFINED

The concept of culture relates to a stable system of standardized ways of thinking and acting. It also refers to the simultaneous occupation of the minds of many individuals with certain beliefs, precepts, maxims, and facts. It is the sum total of all the patterned ways by which a people live.

Culture was described by Edward B. Tylor, who was considered to be the father of cultural anthropology, as that complex whole which includes knowledge, beliefs, art, morals, law, custom, and any other capabilities and habits acquired by man as a member of society. More recently Simpson described culture as (1) the ways of life or designs for living common at any one time to all mankind, (2) the ways of living peculiar to a group of societies between which there is a greater or lesser degree of interaction, (3) the patterns of behavior peculiar to a given society, and (4) the special ways of behaving that are characteristic of the segments of a large and complex society [1]. Thus, culture may be defined broadly as a shared design for living that guides the actions of men in groups and that is passed on through the family, education, and other avenues of communication.

The concept of culture is made necessary by the observed fact of the plasticity of human beings. Newborn members of different groups are taught to carry out the same acts in an almost infinite variety of different ways. It is virtually impossible to discover a single act that is carried out in precisely the same manner by the members of all societies. If whole groups or societies learn to do certain things in a more or less uniform fashion, we can make some sort of general statement concerning the group. This kind of learned behavior that is common to a group of people, transmitted by the older generation to its offspring or transmitted in some portion by any members of one group to a member or members of another group, is called culture.

Cultural patterns of social groups have been studied and described by a number of cultural anthropologists. These studies indicate how knowledge is conserved and how the basis for communal life, which rests upon common information and understanding, is established. Among those individuals who share a particular culture, certain specialized and standardized ways of doing things are established. These social acts are referred to as *customs* and are routinely carried out according to a generally accepted pattern in a given group. Definite sets or complexes of customary ways of doing things, organized about a particular problem or designed to attain a given objective, are readily identified in any human community. Such a cluster of customary ways of doing things is designated as a *role*. Roles are generally recognized and defined by the participants in a social system. A role has certain normative rights and duties which we may call role expectations.

Certain roles are open and can be assigned to anyone; however, certain broadly defined sequences of acts are followed. Other roles are more highly specialized and become specific to particular individuals. When this degree of formalization exists, in particular when we use a specific name, title, or similar designation for certain individuals, then a social position has been created. The social position, more frequently referred to as a *status position*, is a socially recognized role, a position in social as opposed to geographical space, to which individuals may be assigned and which confers on the individual a set of rights and obligations, defined and assigned by a particular cultural group.

Just as social acts may be aggregated into customs, and sets of such actions aggregated into roles, so a more complex structure of roles organized around some central activity or social need may be aggregated into an institution [2]. Institutions constitute the main building blocks of society. The number of institutions and the degree of their specialization vary from society to society. Highly developed civilizations and large-scale industrial societies are characterized by the intensive specializations of institutions organized around defined problems of social life. At least four major sets or complexes of important institutions are recognized by most sociologists. These include the political institutions, which are concerned with the exercise of power and which have a monopoly on the legitimate use of force. Second, there are the economic institutions, concerned with the production and distribution of goods and services. A third category includes the expressive-integrative institutions, which deal with the arts, drama, and recreation. Also included in this group are those institutions that deal with ideas and with the transmission of values, such as scientific, religious, philosophical, and educational organizations. The last group includes the kinship institutions, which are focused on the problems of procreation and provide for caring and rearing of the young [3]. Each major institutional complex participates in and contributes to a number of ways to the life of the community. Just as roles are defined and assigned to individuals who are sharing a particular culture, the roles that are assigned to these major institutions and the various component institutions within each category are determined and defined by the cultural group. Institutions are the means by which a particular culture group transmits the system of values that is important to them for the purposes of human relations, interaction, and survival. Various religious groups organize to perpetuate and transmit theological doctrines, and to provide for interaction among members who support the group as a viable social institution.

In societies that are undergoing change made possible through scientific endeavors, some patterns of culture are changed more rapidly than others. The concept of "culture lag" developed by William Ogburn dealt with the acceleration in the rate of growth of material culture and indicated that changes in our nonmaterial culture—our ideas and social arrangements—always lag behind changes in our material culture—our technology and invention [4]. From a functional frame of reference, the various institutions within any society operate as they do because they fulfill some strong drive in those who make up the society. Some cultural anthropologists believe that the major institutions are repressive to individuals, curbing their energies, stifling their creativeness, and splitting their purposes. They indicate that cultures become bundles of conflicting and even contradictory tendencies. A living culture, however, may strive to resolve its contradictions and deal with the clashes of purpose, the overlapping, and the sense of paradox [5].

CULTURAL VALUES

Individuals, groups, organizations, societies, and cultures are spoken of as having, expressing, and pursuing values. In the many definitions of values proposed by sociologists and anthropologists, a common element lies in the recognition of values as an expression of the ultimate ends, goals, or purposes of social action. Values deal not so much with what is but with what ought to be. Almost any conceivable aspect of any relationship can be, and somewhere probably has been made, an object of value. Honesty and duplicity, silence and loquaciousness, stoicism and emotionality, and restless activity and passive acceptance have all been valued in different societies.

Values do not consist of desires but consist rather of the desirable, that is, what we not only want but feel is right and proper to want for ourselves and for others. Values precisely are abstract standards that transcend the ephemeral situations and the impulses of the moment. The matter of values is certainly the prime intellectual issue of the present day. The practical implications of this problem also are of the most intense importance. Our cohesiveness and strength as a people depend upon the achievement of greater clarity and force in making explicit among ourselves and to the outside world what we conceive to be good, what we hold to be right or wrong in private acts, what our official duties are, and what are those responsibilities of our nation in its dealings with other nations.

Much the same range of human qualities and aspects of relationships are recognized in most societies, the main difference between cultures being in the value they put on these qualities as important or minor, or good or bad. One culture values aggressiveness and deplores passivity; another emphasizes the virtue of sobriety over emotionality. In an effort to measure the nature and distribution of values, Florence Kluckholm discovered through a complex undertaking that all societies adopt some value position with regard to man's relation to other men, to nature, to time, and to activity [6]. She indicated that all cultures have discovered pretty much the same range of positions or alternatives with regard to the solution of certain basic common human problems, but she found that different cultures placed different values on the various alternatives. Kluckholm found that groups were indeed different, and no two of the cultures chose exactly the same pattern of preferences on any of the value orientations.

The basic similarities in human biology the world over are vastly more numerous than the variations. Equally, there are certain necessities in social life for man, regardless of where or in what culture he lives. Cooperation in order to live and for other ends requires a certain minimum of reciprocal behavior, of a standard system of communication, and, indeed, of mutually accepted values. The broad outline of the ground plan of all cultures is and has to be approximately the same because men always and everywhere are faced with certain unavoidable problems that arise out of the natural living situation. Since most of the patterns of all cultures crystallize around the same forces, there are significant respects in which each culture is not wholly isolated and self-contained but is related to and comparable to all other cultures.

There are at least some broad resemblances in content, specifically in the value content. Considering the exuberant variation of cultures in most respects, the circumstances in which in some particulars almost identical values prevail among mankind is arresting. No culture tolerates indiscriminate lying, stealing, or violence within the group. No culture places a value upon suffering as an end in itself. There is no known culture in which the fact of death is not ceremonialized [7].

The fact that a value is universal does not make it necessarily absolute. It is possible that changed circumstances in the human situation may lead to the gradual disappearance of some of the present universal values. The mere existence of universal values after so many millennia of cultural history and in such diverse environments suggests that they correspond to something deep in man's nature or are necessary conditions to social life.

In all cultures men are constantly talking and arguing about what is true and good, what is better and worse, what is right and wrong. Although no individuals and no tribes or nations unqualifiedly live up to their own abstract standards that transcend all times and situations and human impulses, there is abundant evidence to support the assertion that values not only count as ultimate goals in human life but also directly influence human conduct and everyday existence.

CULTURAL VALUES AND SOCIAL CHANGE

In the study of attitudes and values, sociologists seek to discover the forces that produce changes in the important and generally stable personal orientations and dispositions. The changes in people's values brought about by the changes in social relations, technology, urbanization, and economic systems are well documented.

When one speaks of political or social changes in a society, one must bear in mind that men instituted these changes in the expectation of certain benefits and that these changes did in fact have an effect on man, although perhaps not the same as those anticipated. Change can be forced upon men as a result of changes in the natural environment, or it can be forced on him by other men. In any case, man will react to change in a definite way. He is conditioned to respond by at least two identifiable factors: (1) his inherent nature, and (2) the immediate basis of his present expectations. It is one of the features of so-called primitive societies that when the environment is stable and contacts with other cultures are limited, they tend not to change, at least not with any appreciable speed. But from its very inception Western culture has been given to continuous and rapid change, at times with explosive speed. It is therefore very difficult to take one period and insulate it from its past, particularly when some of the factors active at this period can be identified as having continuity from the twelfth century. We cannot therefore talk of things in the nineteenth century apart from the time that preceded it and that followed it. Concepts such as democracy and freedom have no absolute definition, except in terms of existing values, choices, opportunities, and available forms of security. The values that were devised when power was in the hands of the aristocracy had the effect of creating what seemed to be an atmosphere of stability and serenity. The use of force as a social agent to insure the dominance of one group over another has insidious consequences on the whole fabric of life. Human relations are governed by rules and not by feelings. Correctness takes the place of truth, and maxims of expediency and prudence take the place of wisdom. Spontaneity of feeling is lost and is replaced by affection. Human relatedness is controlled entirely by an institutionalized formalism. Men being what they are, however, feelings cannot be controlled forever. Given the opportunity, men will eventually break the bonds of emotional constriction.

CULTURAL CHANGE IN TECHNOLOGICAL SOCIETIES

From the Reformation onward the institutional framework of Western culture changed in such a way as to give more opportunity for individual expression. In the changing institutional framework, man had more opportunities for responsibility for himself. He had new opportunities for enterprise, more risk and more choice. With more opportunity for activity and enjoyment, the general level of aspiration became tied to goals that were concrete and attainable with effort. New social opportunities loosened one of the most powerful influences for social stability. The Romanticists emphasized risk and venture. They did not want to endorse the evils of a fixed and implacable social hierarchy, and in the light of the newly created opportunities, they proclaimed the rights of the individual to aspire, risk, and fail. They denied that society was a fixed order and a law of nature. They advocated a change. The Romantic Movement was the manifestation of an emotional breakthrough occasioned by the effective alteration of a certain social patterning.

Although this was a Western phenomenon, its effects varied in different places. The people of this period saw the fall of dynasties and the rise of a new social order. They were therefore not inclined to place unlimited confidence in the stability of an old social order. Moreover, the idea had been planted in the minds of people that they had something to say about the kind of order they wanted. At the very least, they knew that it changed. The greatest of all changes took place in the domain of man's relation to himself. The new order, based on liberalism as a political creed and a way of life, altered the feeling of responsibility for oneself. One's status in life was determined only in part by one's status at birth. It could be altered by will and enterprise. One's fate depended one one's character and ability, and the latter was influenced by the former. Character became recognized as the implementation of social interaction; institutions were not divinely decreed, but were created by man.

Some observations of the changing characteristics of the culture of the American society have been made by J. Robert Oppenheimer, who identifies the unresolved problems as those of survival, liberty, and fraternity [8]. This scientist states that the world is being held together by a system of mutual threats that have been made possible by the science and technology of the twentieth century. In the place of the brotherhood of man, Oppenheimer indicates that the world is experiencing the compulsory brotherhood of the bomb. The attitudes of America toward itself have moved away from that time when seventy-five years ago the United States was isolated from world policies and seemed to care little that European governments set about to destroy each other in small wars and petty disputes, as long as they did so without America's involvement. The anxiety about security has distracted the American people from the true concerns that should engage them—the problems of social change and education. Right now this country is concerned with those problems that involve the effort to become invulnerable—invulnerable to attack, invulnerable to contrary political ideas, invulnerable to all experiences that are exciting or dangerous. In an effort to achieve invulnerability, America has become conservative in politics, in culture, and in social enterprise. Oppenheimer indicates that conservatism in this sense is anti-democratic and reactionary in nature as opposed to the theory that defines conservatism as a belief in preserving the traditional values and retaining the existing system. The present brand of conservatism seems to imply that those persons who appear to have answers to pressing problems should control the many persons who do not have these answers.

The basic need of individuals for freedom of movement is related to Oppenheimer's second unresolved problem, that of liberty. The political, economic, social, and personal dimensions of liberty require a liberation of spirit, which can occur when a person has sufficient self-confidence that enables him to be himself. The concept that one has of his own liberty reflects the social setting in which the individual finds himself. In a class system large sectors of the society, having been taught to adapt to existing conditions, may hold no conception of a personal liberty. The activities of different governments do not negate the desire for personal liberty and freedom. In societies that subscribe to rigidity of class structure and in those whose governments practice autocratic procedures, there appear to be universal desires for personal liberty.

In the great succession of discoveries it appears that man has become re-moved from one another. The high degree of specialization of activity has created a situation whereby man neither has the time nor the skill to tell one another what he has learned, nor can he listen or hear or welcome the enrich-ment of the common culture and common understanding. Thus it seems that the public sector of men's lives, what he has and holds in common, has suf-fered, as have the illumination of the arts, the deepening of justice and virtue, and the ennobling of power and of common discourse. While specialized traditions flourish, all men have essentially lost the ability to talk with one another.

The discoveries and actions of great men in a technological society contrib-ute directly to the evolution of social and value systems. Each new form arises from that which preceded it in a gradual unfolding and reflects the interaction of inevitable change and the human desire for stability. This evolution is brought about when the impulse to create change through the uses of tech-nology and science impinges directly upon the relatively inelastic framework of the institutions and values that shape society. The impact of a technology is readily seen in the changing characteristics of the society and its system of values. In urban areas the masses of people, in terms of numbers and density, place a premium upon privacy. The existential problems of aloneness and alienation are intensified in men who must lead their lives in the new urban environments.

The changing nature of work brought about by science and technology has increased the material well-being and provided a higher standard of living for a larger segment of the population. Not only has the energy of machines become available in personal and everyday life, but machines and technology have a profound effect in changing the productivity of the total economic system. As machines do more work and are integrated into complex produc-tion systems, the quality of individual work is changing; man-work relationships are increasingly abstract and symbolic. Men and women must now learn to work in an environment of machines and systems. The values traditionally inculcated concerning work, the expectations and rewards, and a host of other attitudes that can be grouped in the work ethos must be reappraised. The scientific and technological community deals with things and processes and moves faster than human affairs can normally or easily accommodate. It is much easier to plan a program for landing on the moon than it is to change the attitudes and institutional practices of people involved in human rights issues.

Technology has been referred to as the art of organizing the world so it need not be experienced. Not only can man travel faster, but he sees magnificent extension of muscular systems in huge engines capable of the work of a thousand men or in delicate machines capable of performing tactile operations with far greater ease and speed than that of the human hand. Information-processing computers perform marvels of computation and analysis in fractions of minutes. It has been noted that with the extension of man's senses made possible by technology, his self-conscious has become dulled and his life has become depersonalized.

The characteristics of the technological society as it now exists give indication of the characteristics of the society that will be most determinate in shaping the quality of life in the future. These characteristics give directions to the goals and control of education and to the responsibilities of the education for effecting change.

CULTURAL STABILITY WITHIN SOCIAL CHANGE

Within advanced technological societies, one finds instances where subcultures endure and perpetuate the way of life of their ancestors that appears to reject the world of today. That the Amish have endured so long, adhering to the past, carving out their separate world, is awesome indeed. The Amish themselves give one the feeling that for the most part they have no desire for change, for their behavior patterns are deeply rooted in their religious values and beliefs. Life among this group is pastoral but not without problems. They struggle to find good farm land, to compete commercially using archaic farm methods, and to keep people from moving out of the religion. The Amish families cling to each other in a secure, close-knit way of life. More frequently theirs is a security paid for by total conformity in dress, style of living, and family and social behavior. The Amish realize the danger of educating their young into dissatisfaction with their way of life, and they conduct their own schools to perpetuate their philosophy and ideals. In spite of this the youth bring anachronisms to the scene: a boy harvesting tobacco by hand, wearing sunglasses; an Amish teenager clattering through a covered bridge in his courting buggy, his arm around his date, listening to modern music from his hidden transistor radio. There is wonderment by outsiders about the Amish way of life. Their answer is their religion and their respect for the way their ancestors did things.

While the Amish have remained relatively stable in their geographic setting, another and similar cultural group finds that urbanization and concomitant technology are forcing them from their original area of establishment. A Mennonite community in Virginia finds that the communication media of the twentieth century, superhighways, movies, television, and airports are threatening their spiritual values. This community is leaving Virginia to seek a rural setting more compatible with their agrarian way of life. Like the Amish, the Mennonites feel that they cannot change their way of life and remain loyal to their beliefs. Many shun the material things of life, are conscientious objectors, and will not participate in politics even to the extent of casting a vote. While the Mennonites may obtain employment in semiskilled and clerical occupations outside the group, they must marry within their group if they are to remain true to their faith. The Mennonite group conduct their own schools to transmit their beliefs so that their children will not be "corrupted by the devil."

CONCEPT OF CULTURAL PLURALISM

The belief in individual expression of man and the right of men to determine their social order has given rise to the concept of cultural pluralism. The struggle for self-identity or ethnic pride is not solely the property of our black brothers, though we need to be grateful to them for their leadership. We read accounts of the poor treatment of Italian-Americans in the history of this nation. Our Jewish neighbors have been denied certain rights and privileges, and the voices of the American Indians have been loud and strong. Each of these cultural groups are striving for self-identity and the opportunity to live in a cultural environment that they know and understand. We are faced with the reality of cultural pluralism and the recognition that a multiculture nation demands a change in some basic values and new learnings for all of America.

Cultural diversity has always existed in the United States. We have boasted of our ability to live side by side with those of varying ethnic backgrounds. But all too frequently in this process of living side by side, we have tended to eliminate differences. Cultural pluralism appears to be regarded as a threat. This has been particularly evident when individuals decide to leave the basic ethnic identity and to Americanize completely. For those persons who are part of a subculture in order to better oneself and to assume different roles, they must cast off their separate culture and become assimilated in the dominant culture.

This phenomenon raises the question, Can a pluralistic cultural society exist? At the moment it appears that we have no experience to give us direction. While societies have always displayed cultural diversity, it appears that a dominant cultural group and several subservient subcultures are in continuous interaction. To recognize that there are many cultures existing in the United States is not enough. It is too easy to say that we have many cultures, but mine is the best one, the superior one. Man must face cultural pluralism without placing the various people in a rank order and distributing emoluments in accordance with that order.

CULTURAL VALUES AND EDUCATION

Formal education is often thought to be a characteristic of "civilized" or advanced societies and to take place only in organized institutions known as schools. Yet education, both formal and informal, is as old and as universal a phenomenon as man. The interpretation of education solely in terms of intellectual written traditions has limited the perspective of education by ignoring the variety of educational practice associated with the "primitive" societies brought to our attention by research of anthropologists. In many primitive cultures, formal education is carried out in the form of initiation ceremonies by special classes of people, priests, wizards, or shamans. Every individual in the specific tribe is required to pass through such ceremonies before he becomes a member of that tribe. In its social functions, initiation ceremonies in primitive cultures are as formal and as important as educational institutions in advanced cultures.

Through the initiation ceremonies, which are frequently critical tests of endurance, the youth are inducted into the culture of the society. They are also trained in the appropriate skills to reproduce the mode of life in that society. In primitive societies that are relatively homogeneous, where there is little division of labor and a simple system of social stratification, education is largely a process by which the individual is inducted into his cultural inheritance. Leadership status is achieved rather than ascribed. There are no special classes from which leaders are recruited, and no assumed innate distinctive traits among people from different households or classes. Although those who become leaders have to go through certain educational experiences, such experiences are not the sole prerogatives of a special group. There seems to be a respect for the uniqueness of the individual that leaves no room for measuring the worth of one against the other. There is no educational concept that places a higher premium on the gifted, rewards and differentiates him from the dullard, and goads the latter to perform faster than he is able.

In such societies concepts of equality and equal opportunity have no substantial meaning. The principle of equality in the Western tradition dates back to the origins of democratic institutions in ancient Greece, and in the modern times it has emerged as a basic principle of democracy. In both ancient and modern times equality has signified the possession of certain rights, mostly legal and political, by every member of the body politic. It was introduced as a means to eliminate or lessen existing inequalities whereby certain individuals or groups were treated differently, possessed more advantages, or exercised undue authority over others. Equality has also been justified on the grounds that it is necessary to attain the goal of the worth of the individual. Equality of opportunity, educational or otherwise, has been applied similarly to situations in which certain people, by virtue of their wealth, have more chances to acquire certain things than their fellowman and are treated specially.

In primitive societies there are no classes or groups that receive preferential treatment by virtue of birth or wealth, there are no special strata from which people are recruited to high positions, and rights are not distributed according to ascriptive criteria. What actually differentiates these primitive cultures from Western culture is that in the former the worth of the individual supersedes his specific social status. The rapidly developing technological societies of Western civilization are creating conditions and processes that operate in opposition to the attainment of the ideals of democracy. The full participation in American society is being denied to a large segment of the population as a result of the tidal wave of cultural change that follows swiftly the explosive advances of science and technology. The advance of technology has all but destroyed the tasks at which the poorly educated could be profitably employed. The most shocking incongruity in this nation today is the presence of serious cultural deprivation in great urban centers, with cultural resources unmatched by any previous age in quantity, variety, and richness. The contrast of poverty with riches, cultural and spiritual as well as material, is not new in the history of mankind. The contrast, however, is even more disconcerting and dangerous today than in any past period because in this society the city is not merely the brightest facet of the culture and the major generation of cultural change, it is the heart of the culture.

The decay at the core of the cities of Western civilization is so extensive that the remedy is to be found, not in piecemeal attempts at rehabilitation, but in a magnificently imaginative reconceptualization of the place of the city in an evolving technological society and in an equally imaginative planning to enable all the inhabitants of the city to share fully in the benefits such a society can offer. The great metropolitan center will not cure its ills or attain its promise unless the urban schools and universities play their proper role in creating understanding of the conditions of modern man and the kinds of action through which those conditions may be modified so that every man has the opportunity and the motivation to live as fully as the state of culture and the resources of the planet permit.

Studies have suggested that the incapacity for education may be as much a function of environment as of genetic inheritance. Schools are expected to find means to overcome cultural deprivation and other handicaps to learning, to rise above the prejudices and follies of the society that supports them, and to break up the ghettos created by avarice, discrimination, and other forms of social exclusiveness. Education is not only charged with responsibility for overcoming cultural and other environmental barriers to learning, it is also expected to find means of developing the creative potential for contribution to the arts, sciences, and public service. Some universities are beginning to contribute significantly to the necessary redefinition of the culture to be transmitted and are starting to grapple with the problem of how the capacity to learn can be rescued from cultural blight.

Public disputes over the aims of education are not likely to be resolved because they are disputes of total outlooks in opposition to one another. They are the cultural disputes that prevail among well-organized social units when each is trying to extend the scope of its influence by urging assent to its own vision of the world. Schools have social, political, and moral responsibilities of perpetuating what others have invented and given to ensuing generations. The challenge to the educator, specifically to the American educator, scarcely requires elaboration. From primitive tribes to Egypt, China, Greece, and the Christian world, the task of education has been first and foremost that of transmitting, expounding, and in some cases refining the great values of each culture.

Until recently the need for literacy was considered to be the most pressing in underdeveloped countries. But the concept has now been broadened, and literacy is regarded as the tool of education in all areas of life. As long as the function of education was to maintain and pass on to the new generation the traditions of a culture, its skills, knowledge, and principles of interpersonal conduct—its religious tenets and values—there was no need for literacy or for education provided and stimulated by outsiders. Parents and other relatives educated the child in his cultural heritage by giving him increasing participation in the work of making a living, in community work, and ceremonies, as well as giving him specific instruction [9].

In either case, the function of education was the innoculation of the established tradition. With the impact of civilization, the function of education has necessarily changed. The need now is to move away to new knowledge and skills, to a new place in a new social order; education is now not with maintenance of the old, but for change.

CULTURAL VALUES AND THE NURSING CURRICULUM

Students today are becoming increasingly aware of social needs. They are demanding that their education be relevant. Colleges and universities are exploring ways to fulfill their traditional role as well as to keep abreast of rapid changes in society today. The same problems exist in the health fields. Our systems of education and delivery of health services are being questioned as never before. The challenge for relevancy was never greater for nursing—to meet "nurse-power" demands, to educate for the future, and to revise our methods of the delivery of nursing services to the public.

Institutions of higher education have three major functions: advancing organized knowledge, transmitting it from one generation to the next, and extending these central functions beyond the campus into the community. The issue today is not so much the relevance of the functions of teaching, research, and public service as it is their application in a rapidly changing society. In relation to the role of the schools midst social change, Cohen has said:

> The key word of the younger generation is relevance. The questions they are concerned with are oriented toward goals, purposes, and values. They are no longer satisfied with fragmented knowledge leading to improved skills and techniques as ends in themselves. They want greater articulation of what they are learning to the attainment of this goal. They are turned outward to the problems of contemporary society, to a collective concern, rather than inward toward a series of skills and disciplines which insure upward mobility [10].

The health professions have not been exempt from criticism and student dissent. In 1966 the development of the Student Health Organization formed the nucleus of an organization now represented in most medical schools and in many schools of nursing. At the 1968 convention of the American Medical Association, a medical student accused the American Medical Association of racial and economic discrimination, antiquated medical education, maldistribution of patient care, and poor delivery of services. He presented a series of demands for change. His wife, a navy nurse, was courtmartialed for dropping antiwar leaflets onto the decks of navy ships in San Francisco Bay.

Part of the blame for lack of relevance can be placed on professional educators, including nurses, who many times believe that there is a discrete body of technical knowledge that once learned by an individual, enables him to perform as a professional under any circumstances. He can work anywhere as long as he is equipped with the techniques of his trade. Hand in hand with this goes the factor of time; for the more technical the knowledge that must be imparted, the less time there is for exploring the social issues of the profession.

All relevant curriculum planning must begin with the recognition that students are greatly differentiated from each other, not only in their abilities and interests, but also in their purposes, learning styles, backgrounds, and personalities. Problems of consequence include how to treat a student as an individual, as a unique human being in the midst of the student body. Another fundamental issue is voiced by Clark Kerr, who indicated that "we, as educators, are being asked to prepare the generalist as well as the specialist in an age of specialization looking for better generalization" [11].

Are the schools graduating nurses who are informed about the distribution of health services in the United States, who are appraised of rural and ghetto needs, who understand relationships between social and psychological deprivation and physical illness, who are aware of the institutional needs that exist or are needed to provide adequate sociomedical care to the aged and infirm, or who know the political and administrative systems which surround research and practice? Are we offering opportunities so that our graduates can provide leadership to their fellow health workers? Students (or new graduates) often complain about the gap between the reality of practicing their profession and the ideal experiences they had as nursing students. Many times they are criticized for not being a change agent, for not instituting or effecting changes in patient care. Yet they are expected to assume responsibilities for which they are not always prepared.

The unfortunate outcome of the graduate's lack of awareness is a feeling of frustration and inadequacy. These feelings all too often are basic to the nurse's decision to leave certain areas of practice in search of the somewhat unrealistic world of her student experience. Encounters with neophyte graduates of baccalaureate programs in nursing reveal their frustration with hospital nursing. Many of these nurses have this type of nursing practice and give the following reasons:

"I am not able to practice the type of nursing I was taught."

"I am so busy with the nonessential requirements set up by the bureaucratic structure that I have no time to get to the bedside of the patient."

"In training we were told to use initiative, be creative, use good judgment, and our concerns should always be first for the patient. Here I am not able to do any of these things. I don't know what is expected of me."

"I wish that while we were in training we would have been helped to handle some of the problems which would confront us as a graduate nurse."

The dilemma of preparing practitioners for undefined roles is indeed great; however, educators have the responsibility of assisting the student to bridge the gap between the idealistic form of practice and that which is realistic in relation to the social climate and environment.

Another relevant aspect may be of a geographical nature and is best described by a young nurse who worked as a VISTA volunteer in a small rural town when she revealed:

> My student nursing program taught me the human side of nursing—not just irrigating catheters and changing dressings. It taught me, too, about underdeveloped countries and their sick, starving inhabitants, but I saw my first starving child in Illinois. Please, educators, bring the teaching, the information, closer to home [12].

SUMMARY

The curriculum is always in every society a reflection of what the people think, feel, believe, and do. To understand the structure and function of the curriculum, it is necessary to understand what is meant by culture, what the essential elements of a culture are, and how these are organized and interrelated.

What happens to the curriculum when the culture is changing is important. Since the curriculum is interwoven with the whole cultural fabric, it follows that as the culture undergoes serious modification, the curriculum will become an object of concern. The rapidly changing cultural characteristics of a technological society have been observed, and their impact on every facet of human life has been noted. The role of education in such a society has acquired a new dimension, that of educating the members of the society for change. This applies no less to the curriculum of the schools of nursing, which endeavors to prepare nurses for the broad fields of health care and health services. The basic concerns that man has for his fellowman has brought into sharp focus the health problem inherent in a rapidly changing society and the means by which these problems can be studied and alleviated. The young people of this generation are reacting and responding to these issues. Although they do not deny the desirability of attaining certain elements of the material culture, it appears that for many these elements are seen as means to build a richer cultural environment whereby all members of the group have essentially the same rights, obligations, privileges, and responsibilities. The curriculum of the school of nursing must be sensitive to the cultural changes in a society that is markedly affected by scientific and technological advances, and it must provide the student with learning opportunities that will enable him to be an effective participant in the change process. The appropriateness of the curriculum will be determined in a large measure by the value judgments of teachers and all others who contribute to the development and implementation of the curriculum.

REFERENCES

1. Simpson, G. *Man in Society.* New York: Random House, 1954. P. 30.
2. Reuter, E. B. *Handbook of Sociology.* New York: Dryden, 1941. P. 113.
3. Inkeles, A. *What Is Sociology?* Englewood Cliffs, N.J.: Prentice Hall, 1964. P. 67.
4. Ogburn, W. F. *Social Change with Respect to Culture and Original Nature.* New York: Viking, 1950. P. 3.
5. Lerner, M. *America As a Civilization.* New York: Simon and Schuster, 1947. P. 42.
6. Kluckholm, F., and Strodtbeck, F. L. *Variations in Value Orientation.* New York: Harper & Row, 1961. P. 10.
7. Kluckholm, R. (Ed.). *Culture and Behavior; Collected Essays of Clyde Kluckholm.* New York: Free Press of Glencoe, 1964.

8. Fields, M. R. *Encounters with Reality*. New York: Center for Applied Research in Education, 1967. P. 2.
9. Mead, M. (Ed.). *Cultural Patterns and Technical Change*. New York: Mentor, 1955. P. 252.
10. Cohen, N. E. The university and social change. *School and Society* 97:479, 1969.
11. Kerr, C. The Frantic Race to Remain Contemporary. In R. S. Morison (Ed.), *The Contemporary University: U.S.A.* Boston: Houghton Mifflin, 1966. P. 36. Originally appeared in *Daedalus*, Fall 1964, © 1964 by the American Academy of Arts and Sciences.
12. Musalino, M. They are dying. *Amer. J. Nurs.* 69:2429, 1969.

SUPPLEMENTARY READINGS

Conant, J. B. *Slums and Suburbs*. New York: New American Library of World Literature, 1964.
Gardner, J. W. *No Easy Victories*. New York: Harper & Row, 1968.
Gardner, J. W. *Self-Renewal*. New York: Harper & Row, 1963.
Gordon, M. *Assimilation in American Life*. New York: Oxford University Press, 1964.
Grambs, J. D. *Schools, Scholars and Society*. Englewood Cliffs, N.J.: Prentice-Hall, 1965.
Hickerson, N. *Education for Alienation*. Englewood Cliffs, N.J.: Prentice-Hall, 1966.
Honey, J. C. Education for public service: Challenge to the universities. *J. Higher Educ.* 40:297, 1969.
Kardiner, A., and Preble, E. *They Studied Man*. New York: Mentor, 1963.
Kilzer, E., and Ross, E. J. *Western Social Thought*. Milwaukee: Bruce, 1954.
Kiser, C. Cultural pluralism. *Ann. Amer. Acad. Polit. Soc. Sci.* 262:117, 1949.
Kluckholm, C., and Kelly, W. H. The Concept of Culture. In R. Lenton (Ed.), *The Science of Man in the World Crisis*. New York: Columbia University Press, 1945.
Kramer, M. Collegiate graduate nurses in medical center hospitals. *Nurs. Res.* 18:207, 1969.
Paul, B. D. (Ed.). *Health, Culture and Community*. New York: Russell Sage Foundation, 1955.
Russman, F. *The Culturally Deprived Child*. New York: Harper & Row, 1962.
Whitehead, A. N. *The Aims of Education*. New York: Mentor, 1929.

5 SOCIAL AND SCIENTIFIC FORCES AFFECTING CURRICULUM DECISIONS

THE institutions of health and education occur in a social context, and they affect and are affected by the elements and the processes within this social context. Changes that may occur in one or more of the social institutions or in the processes through which these institutions achieve their goals affect other institutions and their processes. It has been previously noted that changes do occur, and in some societies they occur radically and rapidly. These changes are seen most frequently in situations in which the inventions and ingenuity of man devise new ways of living, working, and playing. During the past several decades in the United States, technological advances have created the need and opportunity for multiple changes in our relationship with our fellowman and various social groups, and in our arrangements for living, including work and leisure-time activities. While in many instances the social changes provide the means for improved conditions, they also precipitate or aggravate conditions in society that become detrimental to the health and well-being of segments of society. The problems that develop become the focus and attention of a variety of social institutions, health and education in particular, for study, analysis, and resolution.

SOCIAL CHANGES AFFECTING HEALTH CARE
CHANGES AFFECTING INDIVIDUAL AND GROUP RELATIONS

Six broad changes in the social order that have either direct or indirect bearing on health care are identified. In each of these changes the fundamental issues pertain to the alterations that occur in staff (health personnel)–patient relationships. These changes include (1) population mobility, (2) general sophistication of the population, (3) commercialization of the professions, (4) shifts in age composition and disease prevalence in the population, (5) changes from a religio-philosophical orientation toward a scientific outlook, and (6) growth and spread of organized interest groups.

Population Mobility

The people of this country are traveling over the earth at a rate and pace that man has not known before, shifting their home sites repeatedly in the course of a lifetime. Such constant movement complicates the issue of continuity in health care and in the interpersonal relationships involved in health care. When one tries to analyze what it is people are criticizing in the health and hospital care system, one finds that we have today a medically disengaged population. The population is no longer latched onto the medical system, and it does not know how to get "plugged back" into the system.

Specialization eliminated the family doctor. And the geographical mobility (it is estimated that we change residences five times and change jobs nine times in a lifetime) means that we are always breaking our connections with the health care system. Studies have been made in the last few years on what happens because of this social mobility, for contrary to what we hear, people actually do get off welfare and on the employed lists. For the people in this category, the big city hospital used to serve a real function as the central port of entry into the health care system. If the welfare or "free" patient could make it to the big city hospital doorway, he was in the system of care. He also had the help of a social worker, who could guide him and keep him latched onto the system. But once he moved above a certain income level, then he became lost on this medical landscape because the guidance he had is also lost. One strong indication of how large our medically disengaged population really is, is the rate at which emergency-room visits at our hospitals are increasing. It is estimated that if things go on as they are at the present time, by 1975 there will be more medical care delivered in the emergency rooms than in all the doctors' offices in the country. Moreover, studies repeatedly indicate that only about one in ten patients coming to the emergency room is there for purposes for which the emergency room was set up. They are people who are medically lost and who are trying to find their way into the system. They know that if they make it to the emergency-room door, they will get to see a doctor. There is, in my opinion, no other excuse or reason or cause for this phenomenon than the fact that the mobile American public does not know how to assimilate itself into the rapidly changing health care system that we have in this country.

GENERAL SOPHISTICATION OF THE POPULATION

The second broad social change affecting the health care system is the increasing sophistication of the potential patients. There was a time when the physician, nurse, and other health professionals knew more about almost anything than did anybody else. Medical personnel have enjoyed a kind of intellectual aristocracy. This is no longer true. Now almost any physician, even in the semicivilized spots of America, face people who know or think they know more about many things than their doctors can possibly know.

The quantity and quality of health care is now a concern of the general population, whose voice will be loud and strong in the future. The educational level of the population is rising very rapidly in the country. The education average has moved in just a decade from nine years of public schooling to eleven years. The number of college graduates grows almost geometrically. Moreover, we are educating the public in public health through television, popular journals, and science sections in our newspapers. With a more highly educated patient population, one that is going to know more than a nurse knew thirty years ago about health matters, it seems reasonable to expect greater demands for services of professionals and to expect the participation of the consumers of health services at various levels of planning and action. Greater understanding and satisfaction will probably be forthcoming when the patient participates in his own care; moreover, the changes in relationships between health personnel and patients will also be forthcoming.

COMMERCIALIZATION OF THE PROFESSIONS

Another change affecting health service is what has been called the commercialization of the professions. At one time there were people known as professionals, whose services seemed beyond a price in any sense. There were physicians, clergy, professors, and nurses who pursued careers almost irrespective of the incomes and who refused to move when offered several times their earnings to go elsewhere.

These dedicated professionals have become substantially commercialized. We now think of a professor less as an academic longhair and more as a sharp businessman.

The health service system was at one time pervaded by an atmosphere of altruism, however carried out to meet peoples' needs, and money was a dirty word. The health services system is now an extremely large and very expensive enterprise and a very technical one; hence, it is now forced to compete in the labor market on equal terms with industry and government. The health field now offers a variety of opportunities for men and women, especially for women in nursing and supporting personnel. Employers in the health field now face this fact, and it influences their labor force recruitment orientation to the work world and also has direct bearing on the relationships that are established and maintained with patients.

SHIFTS IN AGE COMPOSITION AND DISEASE PREVALENCE
IN THE POPULATION

Population statistics reveal now that polarization of the population occurs at very young and very old ages. Both of these groups have dependency needs that must be met by others. The 2.1 million persons receiving old-age assistance have a median age of seventy-six years. Although much can be done for this group to promote self-care and to make their remaining years comfortable and secure, these aged people—two thirds of them elderly women—cannot realistically be expected to achieve full independence.

The communicable diseases are on their way out, and the chronic, long-term illnesses are gaining attention in medical and hospital practice. In coping with communicable diseases, the health professions did things mostly to or for patients. With the chronic diseases the professionals have to depend much more upon the patient cooperating in the therapeutic programs. This calls for many modifications in the old norms of staff-patient relations.

CHANGE FROM A RELIGIO-PHILOSOPHICAL ORIENTATION

There is a transition on our part from a religio-philosophical orientation to a materialistic and scientific attitude toward life and its problems. We seem to have unlimited faith in the notion that science can do almost anything for us. Notwithstanding the abundance of information that science has provided to assist us in solving our problems, science does not make the judgments. The users of scientific information must make the value judgments as to how the information will be used. These decisions depend upon our religio-philosophical orientation, that is, man's relations with himself, his relationships with his fellowman, and his relationships with his God. Without this orientation we may find ourselves distraught by the limitations of science.

It is not uncommon to hear persons in all walks of life quoting the findings of research to justify or give support to their activities. Whether this is sales talk or whether such information contributes substantially to the common good must be determined. Overattentiveness to the scientific orientation reduces or dilutes staff-patient relations, since it overlooks to a great extent the person as an individual, with certain undeniable rights and privileges.

THE GROWTH AND SPREAD OF ORGANIZED INTEREST GROUPS

American people have become a highly organized people—organized labor, organized professionals, organized producers, and organized consumers as well as organized salesmen. This development has entered the health field and is altering old norms and patterns in health care. Governments, unions, and other organized interests are engaged in bargaining for health services and are interested in building their own hospitals, hiring their own personnel, and shaping up their own system of health care. The interest and activities of organized labor have been and will continue to be influential in the relationships of health personnel and patients. The primary objective of the labor movement in hospital affairs is to wipe out dead-end jobs. The unions have begun negotiations, with the assistance of governmental agencies, to set up training programs whereby nursing aides can become licensed practical nurses. Attention is focused on the career-ladder concept that we all hear so much about, and the union has been foremost in breaking through in this area. Because society discriminates and exploits, one discovers that in all the aide categories there is a large group of blacks and Puerto Ricans who have been forced into lower economic jobs. Citizens who have been deprived of opportunity, but who have potential, have been denied access to higher education and access to higher hospital and health services.

Social progress and social change are fraught with difficulties and problems, and social scientists have reflected that it is easier to engineer a complicated piece of technical equipment than to engineer a new concept in social security or in education or in health care. Walter Reuther observed this struggle during the election campaign of 1936, when the question of initiating a social security system was before the American people. A week before the election, tens of thousands of automobile workers had propaganda against social security stuffed into their pay envelopes. The workers were warned that if social security was enacted by the Congress, every worker would wear a dog tag around his neck with his number on it and that he would cease to be a human being; he would lose his personal freedom. The voice of organized medicine, like the voice of backward sections of organized labor, has not been characterized by social enlightenment or by the spirit of social pioneering that is so essential for social change [1].

CHANGES WITHIN HEALTH CARE INSTITUTIONS

In addition to the broad social changes that are affecting to a considerable degree the health care of the citizens of this country, there are changes occurring within health care institutions that have direct impact on the relationships between health personnel and patients. Six major changes are noted.

EXPANSION OF MEDICAL EQUIPMENT

The vast expansion of medical equipment is visible to the patients, the professional, and to the public, who pays the bills for these new devices. The skills, functions, and relationships of the health professionals have had to keep pace with the expanding equipment and techniques. Personnel attend to gadgets and documents as much as or more than to patients directly, and in the eyes of the patient, doctors and nurses resort more and more to forms of remote control in their ministrations. There are literally one-hundred diagnostic and therapeutic procedures being performed in the modern hospital today that did not exist twenty years ago. An obvious and outward indication of the expansion in the need for and utilization of medical equipment is the fact that the estimated requirements in relation to floor space within the hospitals per patient has increased about fivefold in the past several decades.

ELABORATION OF INSTITUTIONALIZED MEDICAL CARE

The doctors, nurses, and others, along with the patient, have become something like cogs in the wheel of an evermore tightly structured system. Today hospitalization requires 2.6 employees per occupied bed, whereas twenty years ago the figure was about one half of this. The number of people working in hospitals has increased because of new scientific developments. Our developments keep creating new processes, creating more jobs, for many of these processes are not automatic. The behaviors of these persons become patterned and interlinked, chainlike, into procedure processes somewhat similar to production-line developments in industry. The freedom of the physician is restricted, the ingenuity and the spontaneity of the nurse is limited, and the patients feel that their uniquely personal characteristics are slurred over, neglected, or squelched.

INCREASE IN USE OF MEDICAL AND PARAMEDICAL SPECIALISTS

A third change in medical institutions has been the rapid increase in the use of medical and paramedical specialists in varied types of patient services. We are still in the throes of readapting medical care in terms of the increasing host of specialists who gather together around the patient, and to whom the patient is expected, as a model patient, to adapt each in turn. At one hospital last year it was reported that more open-heart surgery was performed than appendectomies. Each open-heart case required ten to fifteen times more highly specialized man hours than any appendectomy requires.

If the patient can gain sufficient composure to observe carefully what is going on around him, he will recognize two kinds of specialists. First there are the scientific specialists, who have learned more and more about less and less in the field of disease and patient problems. They are the experts and are of course indispensable and expensive. And then there are the factory-shaped specialists, who have been quickly taught just a little about a small task in order to do it passably well and cheaply. These specialists are now moving up to more dignified titles and labels with more prerogatives and pay.

INTERDEPENDENCY OF PERSONNEL

A natural component of specialization is the interdependency of personnel that results in a sharp splitting up of individual responsibility. Any breakdowns or failures in the linked segments of responsibility bring into play the phenomenon of placing blame. The practice of placing blame on hospital personnel has been identified by Leo Simmons as a built-in part of the system, with checks and counterchecks, maintained largely by the system. The pinning down of blame may help to insure discipline, but the pattern does not help in enlightening the understanding of individual behavior or group relationships.

BROADENING PERSPECTIVES IN MEDICAL CARE

A fifth important change within medical service has been the broadening perspectives in medical care or what is considered to constitute good patient care. The old perspective was focused on the treatment of acute illness, and, as a matter of fact, the modern hospital arose to provide treatment for such emergency ailments and for the mentally ill and indigent persons. The new horizon in patient care has extended itself greatly. What we have done is to expand the concept of patient care to preventive measures on the one hand and rehabilitative provisions on the other. More than that, we are making room in the new concept of comprehensive patient care to include all the services that the varied specialists can contribute for the well-being of the patient. This expansion in our ideas of improved patient care overrides the more traditional views.

GROWTH OF PREPAYMENT HEALTH PLANS

A sixth change has been the rapid growth of prepayment plans, the rise of group medical practice, and the greater involvement of the government in health services. Heretofore, most of us, when we went into the hospital as patients under the old system of payments, were subjected to the full authority of the staff. Where an issue arose and became sharply drawn between the patient and the hospital authorities of various ranks, it not infrequently was resolved in the following manner: Hospital, or medical authorities said to the patient, "If you don't like it here, you can go elsewhere." If the patient left, "discharged against medical advice" could then be written into the record. This may have been in order if the patient was a charity case or if he was a private patient paying his way. It carries an intolerable connotation when the patient under consideration has been paying for this service for ten, fifteen or twenty years and has now come to get his prepaid medical care. He has a stake in the firm. Also through the federal government, increasing amounts of medical care for growing segments of the population are being covered and measurably controlled on a national or state basis. These controls and regulations have a definite influence on patient-staff relationships.

Social changes in relation to health care services have been instituted in the expectation that these changes would facilitate better health care to more persons. The public is somewhat cognizant of a great gap between what is actually done for patients and what could be done by use of the full health potential of this country; the public is dissatisfied with present medicine and health service practices, and there are mounting pressures for improvements.

HEALTH CARE NEEDS

There is growing awareness of the gap between our performance and our potential in health. The contrasts are startling and are made even sharper by the promises of science and technology. John Gardner has so aptly portrayed the dilemma whereby the revolutions, social, economic, and scientific, have greatly enhanced and have also complicated our ability to provide health services [2]. He indicates that the results of this revolution have provided a vastly more sophisticated society, one taught to seek the benefits that progress has made possible, a society that lives longer and is more vulnerable to disease and dependency in later life, a society in which the gap between what is possible for some and inaccessible to others has widened and deepened, a society in which our performance lags far behind our potential.

It is known that the United States health record is inferior to a number of European nations. This unfavorable position does not arise because the research programs of our National Institutes of Health are inferior, nor is the medical ability of the individual physician worse in the United States than elsewhere. In recent decades we enjoyed hearing that ours was the healthiest nation in the world and that our health program was the greatest. The data now consistently reveal that we have fallen substantially behind other countries in health progress. Information based on such hard criteria as infant mortality, the mortality of middle-aged men, and the health records of long-neglected segments of our population, shows that America is a health laggard among nations of the world. It has long been known by the public health worker and it was evident to the Eighty-ninth Congress that problems of the American health care system are now most clearly seen in the urban ghetto. Health is inextricably linked with life as a whole.

In describing the American health care system, Walter Reuther indicated that what we have is a disorganized, disjointed, antiquated, obsolete non-system of health care. The American people—the consumers of health care—are being required to subsidize a nonsystem that fails to deal with their basic health care needs, and the cost of that system is continuing to skyrocket at a rate that is two and one-half times faster than the increases in the general price level. Reuther further indicated that health care in America is in deep crisis, not because we lack the resources, not because the medical profession lacks the competence; we are in crisis because we lack a sound, modern, universal system for financing and providing comprehensive, high-quality health care [3]. Fundamental progress in health depends on solving the major issues challenging our entire national life.

HEALTH CARE CRISIS

A whole new set of health problems has emerged largely as a result of the industrial revolution. While the pattern of health conditions changed slowly during the nineteenth century, the rate of change has speeded up during the twentieth century, corresponding to advances in industrial technology. Persons responsible for vigilance of the health of this country have indicated that a crisis in health care is eminent. This health crisis manifests itself in the following ways:

1. *A breakdown of the health care delivery system.* Gardner indicates that most health services have developed in a chaotic fashion, unrelated to each other or to the reality of the need [4]. Some areas are rich in hospital or clinics, but essential laboratory and supporting services may be nonexistent. Little thought has been given to the homebound patient or to the patient who needs to move freely or frequently from the hospital to the convalescent home to his own home. Community programs are focused on disease categories instead of on people. The result is a fragmentation of services, an inefficient use of resources, and worst of all, inferior care for the individual. Everyone seems to agree that the existing system or lack of system for the delivery of health care has serious shortcomings. But there is not yet any agreement as to what the perfect system should be. It seems likely that we will go through a period of experimentation, and in true American fashion end up with several variations in different parts of the country, suiting local preference and conditions.

2. *Severe discrepancy in health between the poor and affluent living in the same cities.* Those who are least able to cope with the system, the disadvantaged, are the very ones most in need of medical care. The results show up sharply in our mortality statistics, particularly for blacks in urban ghettos. Maternal and infant deaths have gone down rapidly in the United States in the early past twenty years. But the differences between white and nonwhite groups have increased. Maternal mortality among nonwhite mothers is now almost four times that for white mothers, and infant mortality is two or three times higher for nonwhite than for white infants. That is not because we do not know how to reduce infant mortality, but because we have not been able to make adequate information and care available. Often the only care available to the poor is fragmented, impersonal, and of inferior quality. But the medical situation can be almost as frustrating for those who are better off economically. Too often they are bounced from one specialist to another, with their identity getting lost in the shuffle. Rich and poor alike are inconvenienced by crowded waiting rooms. Rich and poor alike are threatened by shortages of people and equipment. And no one is happy about the steep rise in medical prices.

3. *Man-made environmental hazards.* We are living during a period unique

in human history in a generation when man has achieved the capacity to control his environment. Man can tap and use vast quantities of energy and conduct great chemical operations, producing millions of new compounds. He has achieved great personal mobility with the automobile and the airplane. He has created some difficult environmental problems, which seem to be growing more serious and affecting mankind to an increasing degree. A hundred years ago infectious diseases were the major source of concern. Today infectious diseases play a minor role in the United States, and a new group of environmental health hazards is appearing. We are an increasingly affluent society whose activities give rise to massive pollution of a limited living space.

One of the major sources of pollution is the symbol of affluence to many citizens—the automobile. The products of imperfect combustion of motor vehicle fuel are a cause of air pollution in every urban area. Other major air pollution contributors are the sulfur oxides. The source of these is the combustion of sulfur-containing fuels, such as coal and residual oil. Particulate matter, an important factor in air pollution, is a product of the operation of motor vehicles. Airborne particulate matter may affect health directly when it is inhaled in the lungs and when it contains toxic substances. The combination of the chemicals, together with particulate matter, sunlight, and adverse meteorological conditions can produce an annoying situation in the form of smog.

Pollution that is due to sewage is still with us. Many cities still dump untreated wastes into streams or provide only the rudimentary primary treatment. And human waste is overshadowed by the contribution of animal wastes in some streams. Industrial activity is another great source of waste. Excessive organic matter overburdens the capacity of streams to purify themselves by oxygenation. It is speculated that many sources of potable water are now becoming increasingly contaminated with a variety of chemicals that probably exert delayed toxic effects [5].

Another source of possible physiologic insult for man is radiation. This may come from several sources, but all are a product of our highly technological society. When one speaks of radiation, attention is usually directed to radioactive isotopes accompanying nuclear weapon fallout. This source of radiation for the moment is not an important contribution to radiation damage. The largest source of radiation damage is Xrays: The major problem derives from the X-ray units used in connection with the healing arts. It has been estimated that about 90 percent of the excessive radiation is being administered out of carelessness or ignorance [6].

As a result of exploiting science and technology, man has created new patterns of affluent living. At the same time, however, he has carelessly, even foolishly, degraded his environment. In an effort to control or monitor the environment so that the body will not be continuously subjected to insults, attention should be directed to the origins of the problems that have precipitated the health crisis.

Failure to comprehend long-term adverse health effects can result from the application of certain technological innovations. The machine production of a novel, attractive form of tobacco early in the century led to expansion of an industry that had been highly profitable but that had taken its toll in the lives of millions of consumers. In the case of heavy smokers the life span is being shortened, so that the effects of beneficial medical advances has been cancelled. Hopefully by the end of the century we will have succeeded in controlling the colossal impact of this single technological development on the health of our nation and of other nations. Another contributing factor that has bearing on the origin of health problems is the continuing reliance on industry to find simple, technological solutions to problems that are identified. But frequently searching for the technological solutions means not interfering with industry—production and profits must continue whatever the cost in health. This blind faith in industrial technology as the only path to solution is increasingly unjustified, especially when damage to health and life as a whole lies in the balance. Finally, we have not developed adequate social mechanisms for the control of current health problems. This becomes obvious when we note the differences in the ratio of physicians to population in various communities. The unique distribution of physicians in certain areas is a contributing factor in the origin of health problems. The alarming conditions under which many persons reside, in rodent, and insect-ridden housing, with broken plumbing, stairs, and windows, is seen in the ghettos of all of our major cities. Away from the urban areas the farm workers frequently report that the exposure to pesticides which are sprayed from airplanes on the fields leads to illness. Lastly, the dead fish floating in the dirty water of the Potomac as it flows through our nation's capital imperils the health of those in the surrounding area. So polluted is the Potomac by untreated and inadequately treated sewage that fish cannot live there, people cannot swim or enjoy boating; and the distribution by the fish of human disease-causing bacteria is appearing to be a serious hazard. This situation most likely can be seen in many of our rivers and streams across the country.

HEALTH CARE PROBLEMS

The health problems to be faced must be viewed in the frame of reference of comprehensive community health. Total community health includes mental and physical ailments, environmental hazards of health, and the social components of both problem areas. Demographic variables, such as age and sex distribution, concentration of population, geographic and cultural differences, and varying socioeconomic states, influence each of the health problem areas. Projections can be made for many of these variables on both a national and a local basis. Population estimates in the United States project 225 to 250 million people by 1980. Women will predominate over men by a ratio of 100: 70. About one half of the population will comprise those under eighteen and over sixty-five years of age, largely unproductive members of society requiring costly education for the young and extensive care for the old. Life expectancy at birth will probably hover around seventy years for men, with a five-year bonus for women. Life expectancy after fifty-five years of age will be relatively unchanged unless a breakthrough occurs in the causes and cure of heart diseases, cancer, and other degenerative diseases.

In viewing the changes that are likely to occur in health problems during the next decade, Hilleboe identifies seven major problem areas. These problem areas are (1) physical and mental disorders, (2) environmental dimensions of health, (3) poverty and health, (4) resources to meet health needs, (5) finances, (6) health manpower, and (7) facilities, supplies, and equipment [7].

A brief review of each area will indicate some of the inherent problems.

PHYSICAL AND MENTAL DISORDERS

It is anticipated that through the development of new antibiotics, many of our current surgical problems will become medical problems. The treatment of respiratory diseases will include the use of more effective vaccines. After immunological difficulties have been overcome, transplants of vital organs will become commonplace. Institutional facilities will continue to be overtaxed because of the prolongation of life of disabled persons. Hopefully the now sharp distinction between public preventive medicine and private clinical medicine will become blurred.

The chronic illness, especially among older people, will require the continued concentration of research. The etiological causes of coronary artery disease, cancer, high blood pressure, and arthritis are yet to be revealed. Rehabilitation will continue to be the preventing of the progression of diseases and the minimizing of their ill effects. New protheses developed by means of biomedical engineering will enable many severely disabled people to get out of bed, to take care of their personal needs, and to be more productive. The number and percentage of older people in our population increase regularly, and more money, manpower, and facilities are needed to keep people reasonably happy and healthy. Resources expended on research in geriatrics and rehabilitation are good investments for the future, that is if society is now ready for an extension of people's productivity.

Mental disorders will command more attention in the future in diagnosis and treatment. Community programs to care for the mentally ill and retarded persons are beginning to break down some of the personal fears and prejudices against those affected. The shift away from providing care in the institution to providing care in community facilities and private homes will continue. With the development of the community mental health programs and ambulatory care centers, services of high quality are being extended to people regardless of social and economic status. Prevention of occurrence of mental illness presents many difficulties. Social scientists are making available some useful information concerning the social characteristics of those who have mental breakdowns. In addition, excessive violence should be the concern of social scientists, criminologists, and health workers, since this is indeed an extreme form of social and personal behavior.

Infant mortality, accidents, handicaps, and dental diseases can be reduced. More attention needs to be given to the problems of growth and development of adolescents, for we must try harder to see youth as they see themselves. Environmental determinants play a role in shaping individuality probably as great as or greater than genetic determinants. It appears that through experimental work with animals, the conditioning of the organism by the environment begins during intrauterine life, and such factors as temperature, type of housing, infection, nutrition, variety and extent of stimuli, degree of crowding may have profound and lasting effects. If these experiments are confirmed through observations of growing children, it may be necessary to redirect our health resources to the prenatal period and the first few years of life.

In all parts of the world signs and symptoms of malnutrition appear in many patterns. Although the impact of the problems of malnutrition appear greatest in the large cities, many impoverished families in the rural areas reflect the diverse effects of inadequate diet. All health workers will need to take forceful initiative in stimulating community awareness and action and in mobilizing community resources.

In many parts of the world acute infections and parasitic diseases present problems, particularly in the economically depressed rural areas. Tuberculosis, hepatitis, and the common cold continue to drain people and their communities of their resources. A major factor in the recurrence of these diseases is the low standard of living of deprived families.

Accidents have both medical and environmental aspects that deserve attention. The problem areas of accidents include transportation, the home, the place of work, and recreational sites. Health education is one means of prevention and control; however, this must be complemented by a whole array of health services. Occupational diseases and hazards need greater attention.

The health agencies should join forces with labor unions to insist on the application of modern methods of protecting workers against physical, chemical, and biological hazards. Space flight and submarine explorations will add new environmental and health dimensions to occupational health.

Environmental Dimensions of Health

The environmental dimensions of health were mentioned previously as they related to man-made hazards. The problems are mammoth in scope, since the environment of the community contributes to the social, medical, and economic welfare of the people. Industrialization and urbanization have changed the environment so drastically that reorientation will be necessary for professional personnel concerned with health and welfare and for community leaders. Health leaders and their colleagues who are concerned with human resources will need to involve themselves in every aspect of the relationship between environment and health. The specific environmental problem areas in health are grouped in six main areas, with some overlap. *Water resources* are concerned with water pollution and the problems of water uses for human consumption, for industry, and for recreation. Efforts need to be concentrated on preventing new pollution as well as on the reduction of existing pollution. The problems of *air resources* have broad social and economic implications as well as those of personal health. The physical and chemical pollutants pour into the lungs and permeate the bodies of city dwellers every day. In addition, it causes the destruction of property. *Food and pharmaceutical resources* are concerned with the purity and quality of food and drugs. Advances in the packaging and storing of foods should enable us to reduce food wastes and at the same time provide us the means of getting the right foods to the right people at the right time. The control of pharmaceuticals pertains to the safe and appropriate use of drugs, biologic products, hormones, and therapeutic devices, all of which continue to be troublesome problems. Resolution of these problems will require the cooperation of the professionals, industry, and government. *Ionized radiation* will probably be under strict federal and state control as we gain more information about its genetic effects on future generations. Efforts will be directed toward the principal sources of human exposure, diagnostic X-ray machines, by enforcing higher standards for equipment and X-ray technicians. Training of medical personnel will urge physicians to limit X-ray examinations to a minimum. The medical aspects of civil defense that are concerned with atomic weapons testing will continue to be an important responsibility of health agencies.

Public health workers have been interested in the *hygiene of housing* for many decades. Improved housing is not going to change the lives of the poor until more is done about unemployment, lack of education, and medical care. Low-cost housing developments in the future will require medical care within housing complexes, especially for the convenience of older citizens. *Solid wastes* rank with water and air pollution as major environmental contaminants. The problems of disposing of the enormous quantities of refuse is perplexing and will continue as a major health problem as the population increases. Rat and vermin population multiply in proportion to the accumulation of wastes. In addition, the excessive use of pesticides and insecticides affects the safety of living things and of food sources. Environmentalists and the government will need to develop new approaches to dealing with the problems of solid wastes and general sanitation.

POVERTY AND HEALTH

Poverty affects and is affected by every one of the health problems that have been reviewed. It was estimated in 1966 that thirty million people in this country lived in poverty and an additional fifteen million were near poverty level. Studies have shown how much more severely diseases, defects, and injuries affect the poor than their more affluent neighbors. Negro and other nonwhite families suffer more than three times higher prevalence rates of poverty than white families. The mental, physical, environmental, and social aspects of human well-being are interdependent. A comprehensive approach to health problems, therefore, requires equal consideration to mental and physical ailments, to the environmental dimensions, and to the social components.

RESOURCES TO MEET HEALTH NEEDS

The principal resource that makes manpower, facilities, equipment, and supplies available is money. In addition, large amounts of money will continue to be needed for research and for the education of health professionals, technicians, and auxiliaries. Some determination of goals and patterns of services and some utilization of personnel is essential before an estimation of essential resources can be made.

FINANCES

Inflation, population growth, greater use of services, and advances in medical science contribute to the rising costs of the American health care system. Because of the pluralistic society in which we live, few controls are exercised in the expenditure of funds. In this country health services are owned, operated, and financed under a multitude of institutions. The federal government has been raising its contributions to health programs in service, research, and education, and this trend is likely to continue. James has indicated that federal legislation has enabled the poor people to obtain the same poor quality of medical care as those who can afford to pay for it [8]. A major priority in all health planning must be to consider reducing the cost of health services to the American people. Hospital and medical costs have skyrocketed alarmingly. It has been projected that in the near future a hospital room will cost $100 a day. Health services have risen from 7 to 8 percent per year in the past two decades and jumped from 14 to 16 percent each year in the last two years. Concentrated effort in planning must be undertaken to solve this problem.

To bring some degree of order out of chaos and to eliminate waste and duplication, a national system of comprehensive health services seems inevitable. The financial barriers to good health must be removed, and a more equitable system of distributing funds for education and research is essential for ongoing developments of health services.

HEALTH MANPOWER

Health manpower studies have been revealing figures that give indications of the numbers of various professional and nonprofessional workers which will be needed to provide services to 200 million Americans. The total number of health workers is estimated at over three million. The President's National Advisory Commission on Health Manpower, in referring to our system of health, stated that our health care is characterized by multiple, inadequately coordinated subsystems, some of which are totally independent of each other [9]. The concept of a national system of comprehensive health services will probably imply new roles for the various health workers. Professional staff will need to be trained for these new roles, and schools will have to reorganize their curriculums to meet the diverse needs as the system changes. The teaching of the environmental dimensions of health services should have equal time with that of personal health services. Continuing education for existing health workers is a necessity in a period of rapid social, political, and technological change. The recruiting, training, and retraining of health personnel should give attention to the minority groups. This is a relatively untapped pool of labor forces.

Traditionally there has been underutilization of qualified manpower by capital-poor institutions, such as universities and hospitals, in the service section of our economy. Hospitals, the major employers of health manpower, generally are unable to afford supportive clerical and administrative personnel in the numbers needed to free their professional and technical staffs from routine and repetitious tasks. Innovations and imagination are needed in the utilization of health manpower if we are not to waste this resource and are to realize the fullest margin of our manpower potential. New means must be devised and tested, new avenues must be followed, and old methods must be applied in new areas in our efforts to improve utilization.

FACILITIES, SUPPLIES, AND EQUIPMENT

Since 1946 a network of hospitals has sprung up over the country, an event that has been made possible through federal funding. In addition, federal funds have assisted in the construction of nursing homes and in rehabilitation, diagnostic, and treatment centers. Community mental health centers have been established for the care of the mentally ill.

If a definitive label could be given to the major thrust in health care now and as it is entering into the future, the label might read "outreach health services." From the point of view of many health professionals, it appears that our most pressing national health needs can be best met by this type of endeavor. It is predicted that substitute health services outside of the inpatient institutions, which will relieve a good deal of the pressure on the acute inpatient services, are going to assume a much greater importance in the near future.

Meeting the challenge of the preventive health problems will require much greater emphasis upon health services, such as satellite services at varying distances from the base hospital, coordinated institution-based or community-based home-care assistance, expanded diagnostic activities, self-care units, and expanded emergency and outpatient services at the base hospital.

The development and operation of these various outreach health services will change the institution we have grown to know as the hospital. Basic elements of the traditional United States hospital have made it the center of quality health care in the community. Frequently this came by chance and often in spite of the hospital, simply because there was no other quality health organization to fill this role. As the hospital developed, it became the center of expensive equipment, the workshop for specialized health professionals, and the training and research center for health personnel. The hospital became the one quality health resource in the community.

Because of this success, the hospital is going to be thrust into a position of community health leadership. It is going to become more involved in ambulatory health care, home health services, neighborhood health centers, and preventive and restorative health services. In the next twenty years nursing services are going to be much more involved in these affairs and the new challenges they bring. Professional workers in hospitals and related institutions will be participating in the shift of the health focus from treating diseases to disease prevention, with proportionately greater emphasis on health maintenance and restoration.

Many individuals are saying that the hospital is the only institution or community agency that possesses the resources, has the necessary organizational arrangements and know-how, and has the enthusiasm and drive to serve as a port of entry into the health care system. It may be that in the future most health care will be hospital based, and that people will join a hospital as they join a church today. This would be a way of getting everyone in the community latched onto a medical care and hospital system, and it would be a way for the system to know just whom it was responsible for within that system. The hospital is fast giving up many activities around the hospital not directly or intimately related to the patient's care. There will come a time in the early future when no hospital will do for itself anything that does not require contact with the patient. Service industries are being created to provide for food service, for housekeeping, and for laundry. More and more, hospital care will get down to the essential services in which there must be contact among the patient and professional and paramedical personnel, and industry will take responsibility for those services that, given industry's profit drive and great accent on efficiency, it can do far better than the hospital can.

PLANNING FOR HEALTH SERVICES

Health care needs will continue to change at an even more rapid rate. Scientific discoveries of the space age will lead to new health practices. The era of transplanting organs of the human body will call for moral, ethical, and legal reevaluations. The public will be more involved and more aware of medical advances than ever before. Increased expenditures for medical research in university medical centers will siphon more and more doctors-in-training away from community medical centers. By 1975 the federal government will be paying well over one half of the total costs of medical care and health-science research.

REGIONAL PLANNING FOR HEALTH CARE

Regional planning is not unique to the health field or to the United States. Many nations have emphasized this approach to the delivery of health services, and the implementation of the theory usually reflects the unique cultural characteristics of the groups involved. The underlying philosophy of regional planning is the acknowledgment of the fundamental rights of all men to health and health services. Governmental action is making possible funding to develop and make available to the people in designated regions of the country the necessary resources, facilities, services, and equipment to enable them to obtain health care. A basic premise of regional planning is that it encounters problems which are characteristic of that region. Regional planning focuses on these problems, which may be different among the several regions.

The democratic environment provides for free enterprise and equality of opportunity and is characterized by a plethora of voluntary agencies concerned with all sorts of activities reflecting the special interests of segments of the community. It is assumed that regional planning will utilize the energies and efforts of all existing agencies in the community toward resolving the problems in that region. It appears that some obstacles have been encountered in the efforts of voluntary agencies trying to maintain their own independence in terms of deciding how they will spend volunteered time and money [10]. In spite of the inherent difficulties, it seems that the regional approach has substantial merits and justifications. The more specific objectives of the regional program are developed by those most directly concerned; and these objections reflect the value orientation of the people within a region. Legislative enactments require consumer participation in decision-making and approval of plans for health activities. In this instance the society directly decides (1) how much of its total resources will be spent for its health, and (2) what priorities will be established with reference to how these resources will be spent. These decisions are too broad to be made by any one profession. If plans and objections are based upon the values of those who plan, then the values of planners should be made clear and acknowledged by those who plan and those who make decisions [11].

PUBLIC ACCOUNTABILITY FOR HEALTH CARE

Already an overwhelming percentage of today's medical and hospital care is being purchased by buyers who are growing increasingly sophisticated. As the direct financing of institutional health services shifts from the patient to another party, this third party assumes a great interest in what is provided to patient beneficiaries. The large institutions that provide financial insurance for these services have developed great sensitivity about the matter of dollars they spend for health care on behalf of their beneficiaries. We move, therefore, into a new era of public accountability. Providers of care now report to sophisticated buyers. Not only the administrative staffs but also the medical and nursing staffs will be involved in this reporting.

The public is demanding that the medical care system reverse its outlook, that its perspective be turned outward rather than inward, and that the medical care and hospital system serve the patient where the patient is, economically and geographically, moving the system within reach of the individual. The medical care and hospital system will be expected to become more consumer oriented. The seller's market that has prevailed for several generations in the field of medical and hospital care has enabled medical and hospital services to suit physicians and hospitals rather than patients and the public. Services that have been organized and provided are in terms of what physicians and hospitals decided patients should have, what physicians and hospitals wanted, and what best suited the aspirations of physicians and hospitals.

The hospital has keyed its policies and practices to increase its own internal efficiency rather than to make the changes needed in the market it is supposed to serve. It has set the specifications for its product and asked the consumer to fit those specifications. The hospital has set the conditions under which its services were available and to a large extent ignored the conditions that were unattended. The participation of the consumer in the financing of health programs, through private and public agencies, will stimulate the interest in and demand for health services that they consider to be adequate in quantity and quality.

HEALTH CARE IN THE URBAN ENVIRONMENT

We will need to develop a better understanding of the urban environment and its effect on the urban resident as an individual, in his neighborhood, at his place of work, or in any of the special situations composing the urban environment. We will also need to learn much more about the symptoms and the true extent of urban problems. In the rural setting a distressed family is visible and as such, is more likely to receive some attention from the community. In the urban ghetto, a disadvantaged family is not usually visible, except as a member of a community in which their problems are the same as those of the tens of thousands of disadvantaged neighborhoods. Better techniques must be developed to measure health effects of urbanization, which reflects a worldwide population redistribution no less clearly than the worldwide population explosion. Heart disease is the major cause of death, and thus deserves the priority of interest and effort. But for the patient with acute coronary occlusion, that national priority is valueless except as he is provided with a complex set of facilities, devices, drugs, and specially trained personnel. Analogous to heart disease, urban health requires priority. However, we lack the equivalent of the National Heart Institute, and we have only the bare beginnings of the refined technologies that are needed to deal with the health problems of man in an urban environment. Hospitals must assume a responsibility in the community for more than just health care services. They must assume responsibility for trying to improve the total environment, especially the immediate environment in which they serve. They need to be concerned about housing and education and health and transportation; they must think about more than just delivering health care services. Hospitals should regard themselves as health agencies and not simply as medical care agencies.

ROLE AND FUNCTIONS OF HOSPITALS

Hospitals will become more and more the center of the delivery of health services in the future. This includes not only the general hospitals of today but also the extension of these hospitals into other kinds of care, such as ambulatory care, extended care, and nursing home and convalescent care. The hospital will become the center for the delivery of these health services. More and more hospitals are building nursing homes. Another aspect of health care services is the trend toward hospital mergers and shared services. If four hospitals in the same area all have emergency rooms, they can agree that instead of four there will be only one emergency room open twenty-four hours a day, seven days a week. Costs are reduced through the operation of one large, efficient emergency room instead of four small ones. This technique is evident in obstetrical units. Some hospitals are closing their maternity units in order to centralize operations. Another possibility is to merge children's hospitals, which are very expensive to operate, so that one facility provides all pediatric care in a community.

The hospital will tend more and more to be the geographic center and the service center for health care. The hospital will be doing more outside its walls and is going to be drawing to itself more of the things related to hospital care that are now being taken care of elsewhere in the community. The hospital may come to dominate a conglomerate campus, containing many activities, with control centered within the hospital. It may be that many small rural hospitals will close or merge with others. With modern highways the patient can travel large distances rapidly so that two hospitals may find themselves unable to support a full range of medical and surgical care. The United States has over eight thousand hospitals, but less than three thousand hospitals could more than serve the whole nation if they were well planned, expanded, and well located so that no one would have to endanger life by traveling far. Hospitals are now a set of very small-scale enterprises, poorly located in part because of bad planning, in part because of a rapidly moving population. In many instances the urban sprawl has caught hospitals in the central city rather than out where the people are.

NEIGHBORHOOD HEALTH CENTERS

The neighborhood health center is a useful concept. Services can be performed most effectively in a medical center type of campus in which all resources are of the highest quality. This health center attempts to avoid the need for transportation in order to serve those for whom transportation is difficult and who have health needs related to housing, sanitation, and nutrition. The neighborhood health center represents a radical reorganization of health services, which are extended to deliver better care and are directed to primary care. An assumption underlying the organization of these units is the notion that primary health care must be optimally rendered in a primary location.

The neighborhood health center stands in the middle of its community and is affected by the same forces that affect all aspects of community living. A coordinated home-care program is woven into the fabric of the health center program, and the technical advances that have been made available in hospitals can be applied in health centers. The health programs are family-centered, and although the various specialists are available, all health workers work as a coordinated team. It is the belief of many health professionals and community residents that the concept of the family health care group, with an array of professionals working together in a collegial manner, is a far more fundamental approach than a single physician versus an internist-pediatrician model for family care [12].

CONSUMER PARTICIPATION IN HEALTH

The medical profession, like all professions, has steadfastly denied the nonprofessional person any access or any right to say anything about the professional person's business. The physician now is being challenged from all sides, and he is being challenged by people who know what they are talking about—in the areas of costs, quality, and equality. The pressure for consumer participation in policy determination in many fields is a very important, new development, and a very troublesome one in the sense that it does necessarily inject into the process people who are inexperienced, that is, they have no background in what frequently are highly technical matters. We have always had compromises between the technicians and the general public in organizations such as school boards, but the current pressure is for more active participation, not only in policy formulation, but also in the particulars of operation. Consumer representation is not going to disappear. The hope is that over a period of time we will develop some sort of consumer representation that is more sophisticated than it is at present. As this process goes on, the consumer groups should become better organized and more willing to utilize the spokesmen who have become experts. The public is going to become increasingly enlightened about what it wants and needs in terms of health services. Health is going to be perceived by people as a need and a right and as something that they can logically demand. The major problems in health care as perceived by the public at the moment include (1) costs, (2) discontinuity of care and lack of comprehensiveness, (3) increasingly impersonal nature of the medical encounter, and (4) the fact that very few people seem to be trying to prevent disease and keep people out of hospitals.

PATIENT-PHYSICIAN RELATIONSHIPS

Already visible is the development of a new type of patient-physician relationship, falling somewhere between the one that existed with the old-time personal physician who made house calls and the prevailing mechanical, impersonal relationship that is the target of so many complaints today. The new relationship is being made possible by group medical practice and multidiscipline group practice.

The nature of the physician's practice inevitably reflects the manpower shortages. More and more of the recent graduates of medical schools are going into specialty practice, group practice, and institutional practice. Fewer of them are going into general practice. There is some indication that there is increasing interest among medical students in public health as a focus for their work, that is, working in areas, such as the urban inner city that are presently bereft of medical service. The practice of medicine in the urban health centers will probably bring about the development of patient-physician relationships that have never before existed. The dimension of this relationship will be different, for the physician in this setting will be concerned with the health of the community, which is a collective activity involved in health education, school health programs, and detection and prevention of disease.

The concept of the physician's assistant is vague and confusing to many. According to some authorities in the medical profession, the purpose of introducing this worker into medical practice is not yet clear. Does it mean that this assistant will enable the physician to see more patients, and therefore the quality of care will increase? Will the costs of health care go up or down as a result of this new worker? What will the introduction of the physician's assistant on the health team do to the patient-physician and nurse-physician relationships? And finally, what may be the legal implications? At the moment the concept of the physician's assistant is new, and there appear to be as many different concepts as there are persons concerned about this health worker.

STRATEGY FOR HEALTH PLANNING

A strategy for health planning must be based on improvement in the quality of life for all people. This necessitates a critical examination of whether an individual and corporate freedom in use of property or a devotion to the common good shall be the guiding force of social life. Such a strategy requires divorcing ourselves from exclusive reliance on technological progress, since this seems to generate health problems at a rate that is accelerating faster than the hoped-for solutions to these problems. This does not mean abandoning the search for technological progress. It does mean, however, controlling its application in the interest of human values. This value system places human needs above protection of present economic interests.

A commitment to comprehensive health planning in no way implies a monolithic form. While the federal government authorizes the state to establish or designate a single agency for comprehensive health planning, to appoint an advisory council, and to complete a state plan that will form the basis for federal support to state and local health activities, the state assumes the responsibility to stimulate, support, and coordinate planning activities within its regions. Without denying the substantial contribution of a variety of governmental and nongovernmental agencies to the health of the American people, a better molding of these and related efforts is required if we hope to make progress toward attainable goals of quality, efficiency, and equality of health services. While no one has fashioned a blueprint that will be acceptable to all regions (and this is probably not desirable) some new patterns of responsibilities and relationships are needed to close up the great gaps in our present system. Priorities in tackling these problems will undoubtedly hinge upon feasibility, since relationships among agencies of a single state or local government will usually be more susceptible to organizational change than broader intergovernmental relationships or those involving the public and nonpublic sectors.

Planning for health care, which requires some reorganization of services, will be greatly facilitated by attitudes and beliefs that are supportive of comprehensive planning. Genuine beliefs in the need for and feasibility of comprehensive planning on a national, state, and community basis are essential. Positive attitudes can be engendered if visible manifestations of success can be demonstrated. Health leaders need to exchange convictions, to talk to others who may not be of the same persuasion. Health leaders need to be articulate in making known the concepts, values, and goals of health planning among political leaders and the public, who are the sources of their ultimate sanction and support. Planning advice emanating from the federal government should be unified and clarified, and alternative models of organization and conduct of the planning process should be developed and presented in terms understandable to those who will make decisions.

The concept of regionalization provides for the expertise and unique contributions of federal and private sectors, providers, and consumers organized by communities to come together through cooperative interaction. It does not call for discarding of investments in present programs and facilities but a coordination and utilization based on reassessment. Three levels of health services are envisaged: primary, secondary, and tertiary. Although each level can be identified more or less distinctly, there will be some overlap; but more importantly, there must be a high degree of coordination among the various levels.

In the trilevel approach primary care is received at a neighborhood health center, where simpler diagnostic procedures and treatment can be performed. Other sources of primary care within the same center might be independently practicing physicians, a medical group, and a hospital outpatient department. Primary level of care is the point at which the patient enters the health care system. The more complex diagnostic and therapeutic medical and surgical services would be available in secondary care centers, that is, the community hospital, including pediatric and maternity care. Tertiary care is provided at major medical centers for people requiring diagnostic, therapeutic, and rehabilitative services beyond the capabilities of the average community hospital. All levels are equally necessary for a comprehensive system of health care, and a large number of decentralized primary sources of care must be available so that all people have easy entry to the system.

A strategy for health planning will require attention to the upgrading of existing professional personnel for the accomplishment of comprehensive health planning and to the recruitment and training of new personnel with specialized capabilities. Technology has invaded all domains of living, including community health agencies. While various forms of technology can enable more persons to profit by new knowledge, highly specialized manpower is necessary to make this possible. The achievement of the community goals for improved socioeconomic well-being, to which health contributes, is most likely to occur when all health workers seize their new opportunities to shape the kind of world in which we would all like to live.

IMPLICATIONS FOR NURSING AND
NURSING CURRICULUM

The history of civilization reveals the concerted endeavors of men to alleviate the ills of society. The efforts of groups of persons with similar interests and skills and with altruistic motives have been directed toward improving the well-being of fellow citizens. As specialized groups have increased their knowledge and became more competent in the use of their skills, they became identified as professionals. The members of the various professions established codes of behavior that were acceptable to the group and consistent with the social values of a larger group.

Professions, such as medicine, law, and nursing, have addressed themselves to the current social ills and problems, and since these change from one period of time to another, the focus and emphasis today is not the same as yesterday. The major health problems have been identified and reviewed as they affect and are affected by the social and technological innovations of the past several decades. The impact of these problems becomes increasingly penetrating as the innovations gain momentum in quantity and breadth of influence. It is inevitable that all professions, especially those concerned with health, must be sensitive to and knowledgeable about those ills that are most disruptive to man's mode of living. Once the professional does not display the appropriate knowledge and skills, he ceases to be an effective, or even a safe, practitioner.

In order that the beginning professional practitioners can be competent, the curriculums of the schools must be relevant and must make it possible for students to gain the necessary professional equipment to practice. Students of the health professions are demanding to know more about man and society and the impact of one on the other. They want to know and understand individuals and personal problems and the ways society has attempted to help people, to understand cultural differences and the degree of society's acceptance of these differences. Students know that they must be prepared to practice in a dynamic, changing, and often frightening world of people who have feelings, ideas, and differences, which are finally reaching expression and are being heard. Students want to know how to work with and through these searching, powerful pressures and sincerely hope to contribute to an effective solution to today's social and health problems. The curriculum can prepare the practitioner to begin his practice, but the professional must accept the responsibility for lifelong learning. The school must instill in the student that professional practice requires a continuous study that is for the most part self-directed. For those practitioners who desire depth of knowledge in specialized areas of practice and some additional skills, formal study on the graduate level is appropriate.

All professions have acknowledged and accepted the concept that the practitioner must utilize others in an effort to benefit a larger client group. This implies team work among the various professions working toward the goal of optimal health care. Physicians have a colorful record in the allocation of specific responsibilities to others as medical practice became more complex. The X-ray and laboratory technicians and others have relieved the physician of some highly specialized and routine activities. Other professions have found that various types of assistants have enabled them to extend their professional practice to a larger group. Likewise, nursing has accepted the role of the technician and nursing assistant in designing and implementing nursing care. Thus, the nursing profession has the responsibility of determining what these roles will be and developing appropriate curriculums for the different areas of nursing. In this endeavor, the prime concern of the educator is the development of the student as a competent practitioner at a specific level of practice and as a person who may live a richer, fuller, and more satisfying life because of her educational experiences.

SUMMARY

The social and scientific innovations of the twentieth century have had their positive and negative influences upon the health of the American people. The changes in the social order that have had direct or indirect bearing on health have been described and include population mobility, general sophistication of the population, commercialization of the professions, shifts in age composition and disease prevalence, change from a religio-philosophical orientation toward a scientific outlook, and the growth and spread of organized pressure groups. In addition to these social changes, there are changes occurring within health care institutions that have an impact on the relationships between health personnel and patients. These changes are identified as the expansion of medical equipment, elaboration of institutionalized medical care, increased use of medical and paramedical specialists, interdependency of personnel, broadening perspectives on medical care, and growth of prepayment health plans. These changes appear to have direct bearing on the quantity and quality of health care available to the public.

While science and technology have provided us with abundant know-how, there is evidence of a widening gap between our performance and our potential in health. Health leaders have expressed alarm that this country is approaching a health crisis. The essential lack of a health care system, the discrepancy in the health of the poor and of the affluent in the same city, and the environmental health hazards that have been created by man are seen as manifestations of a health crisis, which has deep and insidious social, economic, and political origins.

An approach to resolving the issues precipitated by the health care crisis involves comprehensive health planning. In order for all persons to have the care that they need when they need it, attention must be directed to the major health problems plaguing the country. Seven problems which will likely persist over the next decade include physical and mental disorders, environmental dimensions of health, poverty and health, resources to meet health needs, finances, health manpower, and facilities, supplies, and equipment. It is apparent that planning for health in the future will require continuous vigilance of these problems and others that may arise. In developing a strategy for health planning, consideration must also be given to certain social processes that are developing in the area of health care. Regional planning is envisioned as a means to make available to the people of a geographical area better resources for health care. The participation of consumers with and purchasers of health care will cause these consumers to have voice in the kind and amount of care they desire and need. The arrangements for the delivery of health services will probably change the role and function of the hospital and the neighborhood health centers. Finally the relationships between the patient and physician will no doubt have somewhat different dimensions as medical care becomes intertwined with the vast array of social and health problems.

It is indeed obvious that the total health care system is in a state of rapid change. For the beginning nursing practitioner in all health fields to cope with change and to be effective in directing change, the curriculum of the professional nursing schools must provide the necessary equipment. Nursing curriculums must be relevant in terms of the needs of society to provide for optimal health care and the needs of the student to provide appropriate educational experiences. The responsibilities of nurse educators in developing a system of nursing education must take into consideration the contributions which nursing can make in comprehensive health care. As changes occur in the arrangements for health care, so will changes occur in the roles and functions of the various health workers. So that gaps do not continue to occur in services to people, planning for care and the educational preparation of those giving the care must be seen as a cooperative enterprise of all health professions.

REFERENCES

1. Reuther, W. P. The health care crisis: Where do we go from here? *Amer. J. Public Health* 59:12, 1969.
2. Gardner, J. W. *No Easy Victories*. New York: Harper & Row, 1968. P. 53.
3. Reuther, op. cit., p. 14.
4. Gardner, op. cit., p. 54.
5. Abelson, P. H. Man-made environmental hazards. *Amer. J. Public Health* 58:2047, 1968.
6. Ibid., p. 2048.
7. Hilleboe, H. E. Public health in the United States in the 1970's. *Amer. J. Public Health* 58:1588, 1968.
8. James, G. Critique of the System of Health Care in the United States in Terms of Delivery of Services by the Professions. Paper read at the Council of Baccalaureate and Higher Degree Programs, National League for Nursing, March 11, 1970, at Kansas City, Missouri.
9. *Report of the National Advisory Commission on Health Manpower*, vol. 1. Washington, D.C.: U.S. Government Printing Office, 1967.
10. Lewis, C. E. The thermodynamics of regional planning. *Amer. J. Public Health* 59:773, 1969.
11. Ibid.
12. Gibson, Count D. The neighborhood health center: The primary unit of health care. *Amer. J. Public Health* 58:1188, 1968.

SUPPLEMENTARY READINGS

Anderson, O. W. *Toward an Unambiguous Profession. A Review of Nursing.* Chicago: Center for Health Administrative Studies, Graduate School of Business, 1968.
Berke, M., and Hahn, J. A. L. What are the issues? *Hospitals* 44:46, 1970.
Breslow, L. The urgency of social action of health. *Amer. J. Public Health* 60:10, 1970.
Bryant, J. *Health and the Developing World*. Ithaca: Cornell University Press, 1969.
Crosby, E. L. Hospitals as the center of the health care universe. *Hospitals* 44:52, 1970.
Domke, H. R. The city and the changing American health system. *Amer. J. Public Health* 60:38, 1970.
Hochbaum, G. M. Consumer participation in health planning: Toward conceptual clarification. *Amer. J. Public Health* 59:1699, 1968.
Katz, A. H., and Felton, J. S. *Health and the Community*. New York: Free Press, 1965.
Kissick, W. L. Effective utilization: The critical factor in health manpower. *Amer. J. Public Health* 58:23, 1968.
Knowles, J. The physician in the decade ahead. *Hospitals* 44:57, 1970.

Health Care Needs—Bases for Change. Report of the 1968 Regional Conferences, Council of Hospitals and Related Institutional Nursing Services, National League for Nursing. New York: National League for Nursing, 1968.

Lenzer, A.   New health careers for the poor. *Amer. J. Public Health* 60:45, 1970.

Odoroff, M. E.   Measuring progress of regional medical programs. *Amer. J. Public Health* 58:1051, 1968.

Willard, W. R.   Diverse factors in regional medical planning. *Amer. J. Public Health* 58:1026, 1968.

6 THE NATURE OF NURSING AND NURSING EDUCATION

THE nature of nursing practice and of the education of the practitioners of nursing is directly related to the general development of a society and its institutional arrangements for the health and well-being of its members. The history of the growth of nursing as a profession portrays the fervent efforts of groups of individuals to provide a service to mankind that was not offered by other groups in society. The need for such services was recognized early, for the origins of nursing are deeply rooted in the history of man. The development of nursing as a profession and its status at the present time can be viewed in relation to and as a part of the existing social milieu. The nature and design of education for nursing reflect the growth of nursing as a profession and the characteristics of the social relationships of a particular society. The curriculum worker in nursing will need to give attention to certain fundamental issues and questions that have bearing upon the form and content of nursing programs in relation to the social climate at a particular time. General information is provided that pertains to the nature and characteristics of professions, the nature of nursing, and the educational system in nursing.

NATURE AND CHARACTERISTICS OF PROFESSIONS

Professions are the outgrowths of society's needs or desires to provide special services to prevent, resolve, and alleviate the problems of a given society. Society in its early, simplified form required few special services for its people;

therefore, few special groups were necessary. As society's complexity increased, the number of professions grew, and the activities of a given profession became more highly specialized. The growth and proliferation of the various professions are manifestations of society's recognition of its problems and of its desire to overcome these problems.

The term *profession* has been used to designate the activities of many groups of people. Frequently the way in which the word is used by one group will bear little relationship to the way in which the word is used by another. It is likely that professional plumbers and professional physicians have few characteristics in common. There is not complete agreement about those characteristics that designate a profession; however, considerable attention has been given to the identification of the characteristics of professional activities. One of the earliest and best known definitions setting forth criteria for distinguishing professions from other kinds of work was that of Abraham Flexner. Professional activity, as viewed by Flexner, was basically intellectual and carried with it great personal responsibility; it was learned in that it was based upon fundamental knowledge and not merely routine; it was practical in nature rather than essentially academic or theoretic; the technique of the activity could be taught; it was strongly organized internally; and it was motivated by altruism [1].

Flexner used these criteria to classify various occupations and at that time found that medicine, law, engineering, writing, painting, and composing music were professions. In an effort to place the appropriate emphasis on the characteristics of professional activities, Flexner said that "the unselfish devotion of those who have chosen to give themselves to making the world a fitter place to live in can fill social work with the professional spirit and thus to some extent lift it above all the distinctions which I have been at such pains to make" [2].

In more recent years others have attempted some refinements of the distinguishing characteristics of a profession. Tyler describes the two essential characteristics of a true profession to be the existence of a generally recognized code of ethics supported by group discipline and the basing of technical operations on general principles rather than rule-of-thumb or routine skills [3]. Blauch includes a quality dimension in designating the earmarks of a profession as specialized skills requiring long study and training, success measured by quality of service rendered rather than by any financial standard, and the organization of a professional association to maintain and improve service and also enforce a code of ethics [4].

PURPOSES OF PROFESSIONS

Although the various descriptions of professions emphasize one characteristic as opposed to others, all definitions and criteria seem to imply a fundamental purpose of all professions. The underlying purpose for a profession is to supply the society with services, skills, and facilities that satisfy important needs or desires of the members of that society. Although the services of the various professions arose to satisfy needs of individuals, professions have found it necessary to extend their attention from individuals to groups. Through the use of other people in the helping process, the professions can reach and attend to larger numbers of people. In addition, professions have expended considerable effort to reduce problems by modifying the causes rather than by limiting themselves to treating effects. Medicine has instituted and supported prevention of disease through public health programs, dentistry has actively encouraged cities to fluoridate their water supplies to prevent dental decay and disease, and pharmacists have engaged in a variety of activities to prevent the misuse and abuse of drugs and pharmaceuticals. Thus the social usefulness of a profession is extended beyond the immediate concerns of an individual or a group to the concerns of the environment, modifying it in such ways that problems are reduced or prevented. Professions remain vital by extending their social usefulness beyond the more immediate problems to those activities that benefit the larger society [5].

Professions are generally considered to be occupations that possess a monopoly of some esoteric body of knowledge. This knowledge is considered to be necessary for the ongoing functioning of the society. What the members of the profession know and can do is important, but no one else knows or can do these things. Medicine is supposed to have an absolute monopoly of the knowledge necessary to heal the sick. Healing the sick and maintaining the health of the society is seen as one of the important functions that must be performed if the society is to maintain its equilibrium. Professional practice is based upon a body of knowledge. No profession, however, is ever completely satisfied with that body of knowledge, and each professional group strives to advance the knowledge of its field through systematic observation and experimentation. The search for new knowledge enables the profession to develop more effective methods of practice. To a greater or lesser degree, all professions have accepted the responsibility of advancing knowledge in their fields. A professional who does not utilize new knowledge revealed by research in his practice may be judged to be incompetent by his peers.

One purpose of a profession is to protect its members against individuals and groups that endeavor to practice without the competence to do so. The professional has special competencies that the ordinary man does not have to contribute to the well-being of society. Thus the profession protects society from dishonest persons who may do damage to the trust that society has in the profession. Through the efforts of professional associations, legal sanctions are awarded whereby a profession is given exclusive rights to practice in the field of its competence. Legal controls are used to limit those who will enter the profession in an endeavor to exclude those who are considered to be incompetent. Through the enforcement of a code of ethics, the profession exerts internal control over its members to insure ethical and competent practice.

CHARACTERISTICS OF PROFESSIONAL EDUCATION

The characteristics of education for professional activities reveal the stage of development of a profession in accepting and attaining the purposes previously described. It cannot be assumed that the precise objectives of professional service and concomitantly that the objectives of education for that service are always clear or immutable. The objectives of the older and more stable professions change with time and as conditions change. For the newer professions a major task in achieving status and stability is that of formulating objectives that are acceptable to members of the profession and to the society the profession serves.

The objectives of a professional school are determined to a great degree by the type of service the graduates are supposed to offer. This service implies the attainment of a body of knowledge and technical skills. In addition, the profession is expected to have altruistic motivations, as the professional activities are governed by a code of ethics that heavily emphasizes devotion to service for the good of the client. The stage of development of the profession and the demand for its specific services by society help to define the activities of practice. Definitions of practice of almost all professions are formulated by the professional organizations of its members and are incorporated into the laws of the state, and these give direction to the formulation and content of the educational program.

AIM OF PROFESSIONAL EDUCATION

The primary objective of professional education is to assist students to obtain the knowledge and competence that are peculiar to the field. Education must help a prospective dentist to learn how to prevent and treat dental problems, a prospective social worker to learn now to intervene to preserve the integrity, well-being, and resources of a family, and a prospective engineer to learn how to build a bridge. Each of these professions requires complex actions; however, they are based on the competencies that are peculiar to the profession.

Educators and practitioners agree that graduates of the professional schools should be able to demonstrate that they are competent practitioners when they enter the profession. The word *competence* is broad and vague and provides little guidance to the professional school. Although practitioners and educators do not always agree on the definition of competence, they do agree that it means the ability to execute tasks with a minimum of energy. They also probably agree that competence means the ability to solve problems peculiar to the profession with some degree of creativity and ingenuity. Educators and practitioners do not always agree on what the specific tasks are and what the special required competencies are. Educators in the professional schools focus their attention on preparing the student to be able to solve the problems that he will confront after the initial stages of his career have been completed. Practitioners frequently claim that the school should prepare the student to be able to begin practice immediately after graduation so that little time is needed for insuring competence and self-confidence. This position is usually justifiable when the professional education is lengthy and a period of supervised practice follows the educational program, such as the internship in medicine. Educators and practitioners frequently disagree on the amount of practical experience the school should provide. The educator is more likely to be concerned that the student acquire principles and concepts rather than specific facts and skills. While the educator places a high value on knowledge, the practitioner values early competence in his field of practice.

Competence in professional practice is essential; however, the usefulness of this competence is directly related to contemporary conditions in society. The practitioner must be able to anticipate the directions in which these conditions may change and make the appropriate adaptations in his practice to cope with these changing conditions. The professional school has the responsibility to assist the student to acquire sensitivity to social climate so that his work may contribute to the social changes for human welfare. This implies that the student should acquire necessary information about society, the conditions and problems within society, and the efforts of social institutions to remedy or alleviate the undesirable conditions. The practitioner will need to relate his practice to the issues and problems that face society.

A third objective of professional education relates to the concern of the school to stimulate and encourage students and beginning practitioners to continue study in their fields after graduation from the professional school. Graduation is not the end of study; a professional practitioner is a lifelong learner. Although his basic formal education prepares him to enter the profession, his continuing education, formal or self-directed, permits him to rise in his profession. The body of knowledge of a profession changes so rapidly that what the practitioner learned while a student may be out of date in a few years. To remain competent and safe in his practice, he must continue to study throughout his professional career.

These objectives of education are common to all professions. Each profession, however, must describe them more specifically as they relate to individual professional requirements. The activities of each professional group are different, and these give direction to the appropriate focus and emphasis of the curriculum. The knowledge orientation, as well as the skills, will differ among professional groups as will the status and types of research activities. Educators within each profession must relate their objectives to the more specific needs of the professional service to be rendered.

COMPONENTS OF PROFESSIONAL EDUCATION

The nature and purposes of professional education give direction to the formulation of various components of the curriculum. The professional curriculum rests upon three bases: (1) involvement of the student in the liberal studies as basic preparation for any profession and for the life of citizenship and personnel fulfillment, (2) the pursuit of professional studies to the point of developing the knowledge and skills necessary for competent practice at a minimum level, and (3) the art of application, or the process of combining knowledge and skills in activities that are directed to alleviating the problems of society [6].

General education or liberal studies have received considerable attention in undergraduate curriculums in recent years. The fundamental objective of this phase of the curriculum is to provide the student with learning opportunities that will assist him to develop personally, socially and intellectually. Introducing the undergraduate to basic information in the broad fields of knowledge may assist him to gain some resources to live a richer and fuller life. The specific fields of knowledge to be included and the amount of each varies widely among institutions of higher learning. Since all students regardless of their occupational interests are required to select a sequence of courses within the basic disciplines, the concept of some common learnings for all students seems to hold forth. Historically the notion of general education became prevalent after the free-elective system in higher education was determined ineffective. In response to the inadequacies of this system, undergraduate curriculums have been structured to provide breadth of learning through the study of several disciplines and depth of learning through the study of a specific area of knowledge. The depth of learning can occur in one of the liberal arts or sciences or in an occupational or professional field. The sum total of the general studies offering breadth of learning and the specialized study offering depth of learning may be considered to be liberal education.

The areas of study included in the general education component vary widely among institutions and seem to relate to the mission of the school as a social institution. Public institutions, that is, state or municipal colleges or universities, frequently demonstrate their responsibility to prepare enlightened citizens by including requirements in the areas of history, government, and politics. Church-related schools prescribe some learning opportunities in religion and philosophy appropriate to a specific religious group. Private institutions, those without governmental or religious affiliations, display a range of interests and requirements that reflect the particular orientation of the college or university (that is, humanities and natural or social sciences). It is obvious this component of the curriculum will display some diverse elements among the various educational institutions.

The general education base of the undergraduate curriculum may offer fundamental information in the basic sciences. These learning opportunities are usually related to the revelation of knowledge of the various sciences, and they also deal with the modes of inquiry that made the knowledge possible. In this frame of reference, the scientific information has no value orientation other than that of stimulating ongoing efforts to add to the body of knowledge or to refine that which has been made apparent. The scientific information may be used by individuals in ways in which they deem it to be useful to them in the broad activities of living. Professionals have the responsibility of drawing from the basic sciences appropriate concepts and principles and utilizing them in their professional activities.

Professional studies is the second component of the undergraduate curriculum. This includes (1) the professional or applied science, (2) the body of knowledge of the profession, and (3) learning opportunities directed toward the professionalization of the student. The professional sciences become that body of knowledge drawn from the basic sciences that have direct applicability to professional practice. This implies a value dimension, since the science information that is selected and organized will assist the practitioner in his efforts to prevent or alleviate the problems of man and society. The various health professions will probably describe the professional sciences in ways that reflect their major purposes and activities. The practitioners of social work may see a greater need for a behavioral science orientation, whereas pharmacists may require a focus and emphasis upon the biological sciences. Nursing has experienced thrusts in two specific directions: toward the biological sciences, and more recently toward the behavioral sciences. A reasonable balance may be appropriate to provide the necessary scientific base for nursing actions. Although the basic and professional sciences support some common purposes, each has a unique contribution to the goals of the curriculum.

The professional studies component of the curriculum also relates to the specialized body of knowledge of the particular professional group. This pertains to the accumulation of the facts, concepts, and principles revealed through scientific endeavors which gives direction to the practice of the discipline. This body of knowledge is the theoretical base of the curriculum, which provides the practitioner with the necessary information that may enable him to practice safely and competently. The professional knowledge base is different for all professions, since goals and responsibilities of the various professions are different. The content of this knowledge is developed through research, which yields necessary data pertaining to the effectiveness of various therapeutic approaches on the health and well-being of individuals and families. From this frame of reference it might be said that present professional knowledge in nursing may be considered a priori rather than scientific in nature. Questions are being raised as to whether there is a body of knowledge unique to nursing, separate and distinct from that of other health professions.

All professions have developed skills specific to their practice activities. Highly professionalized occupations such as medicine and law have seen to it that through legal constraints many of their skills have been rendered unduplicable. True unduplicability may be more a function of legal safeguards than of actual skills. This process, however, insures exclusive rights of performance to a particular profession. Skill is the precision in analyzing a situation and in intervening in such a way as to bring about the desired result. Skill is not routine, repetitive performance. It is based upon diagnosis and analysis, which requires a full understanding of all critical factors in a situation. The understanding must come from knowledge underlying the practice. The skills unique to a profession can be taught, and these become an essential basis of professional education.

The professional study sequence provides opportunities for the student to become identified with a professional group. During the process of professionalization, insights may be gained into the role expectations of practitioners of the profession. The socialization process does not imply the neglect of personal identification. Philosophical and historical perspectives of practice become the frame of reference for the code of ethical behavior of the professional practitioners. The legal sanctions and constraints provide the mechanisms for protecting the profession from those incompetent to practice. The professional studies provide the appropriate knowledge and skills necessary for safe and competent practice.

The professional school shares with the profession the concern of application of knowledge and skills. In some fields the student learns most of the art of application after he leaves the professional school. In general, those professions in which the practitioners begin their practice in relatively independent circumstances expend much time on application during the educational process. Medicine, dentistry, nursing, and social work usually devote as much time on application as they do to professional studies. Other professional fields, such as teaching, engineering, and architecture spend considerably less time on the art of application. These practitioners usually begin their work under the close supervision of others. The art of application becomes the process of combining knowledge and skills in activities and procedures that will solve or reduce the problems of the professional. The development of the art of application requires continuous application of the knowledge of the particular field, tempered by philosophy, the arts, and humanities. The internalization of these elements, along with the ideology and the values inherent in the profession, gives the practitioner the necessary professional expertise appropriate to his field.

These components, liberal studies, professional studies, and the art of application, are the bases upon which professional education and practice rests. The way in which these are woven into the curriculum is a matter for the faculty of the school to determine. The type or degree of competency that the student attains while in the professional school is related to the overall development of the profession and the way in which the professional school articulates with the practice field and other social institutions.

EDUCATION FOR HEALTH MANPOWER

All professionals have accepted the responsibility of extending their services to a large group by means of using other workers in a team relationship. In one instance this includes the specialist and the research scientist, who contribute highly specialized knowledge and skills developed through the efforts of scientific investigations for the resolution of problems encountered by the profession. In addition, practitioners use other than professional workers to carry out activities of a technical or vocational nature. The professional, however, is always responsible for the plan and delivery of health care to individuals or groups. By delegating certain activities and tasks to others who have the competence to perform these activities, the professional worker concentrates his time and efforts on the functions of the profession that require precision in judgment and decision-making.

The complexity of health problems confronting this country and in fact the world require the development of new knowledge and skills. The activities of the researcher are imperative in order to provide new information that is useful in preventing and combating illness and in restoring those afflicted to a state of optimal health. The knowledge created by the researcher and scientist can be utilized by the professional practitioner to improve and extend his practice. The educational preparation for the research worker and for those holding positions of leadership is offered at the graduate level of study. The basic function of the graduate schools of our universities is to preserve, transmit, and advance knowledge. The orientation of graduate study is the development of research skills in highly specialized fields. Frequently, but not in all instances, graduate education focuses on the acquisition of administrative and teaching competencies. Initial preparation for these activities takes place in programs leading to the master's degree, which can be supplemented by self-development in specific professional positions. The research scientist and those persons assuming major administrative and teaching responsibilities are prepared in doctoral programs. Although the earlier doctoral programs gave primary consideration to the arts and sciences, more recently various professions have gained entry into the graduate schools and have established programs of study in specialized areas leading to the master's and doctoral degrees.

The rapid industrialization of this country has created a need for the development of technology in practically all social endeavors. This is no less true in the area of health, which is experiencing an explosion of knowledge and related technological innovations. To incorporate new knowledge and technologies into health care activities, new types of workers are necessary. Technicians have been trained and used by professionals to work with them in a team relationship in order to make more and better health services available to greater numbers of people. American education has responded to the social and technological forces and has modified its educational patterns to meet the needs created by these forces. Technical education is an example of the changing focus of education and has evolved as our society has attempted to keep abreast of changing needs. At the turn of the century a new institution emerged that was destined to play an important part in education at the technical or semiprofessional level. This institution is the community junior-college. In the beginning this new two-year college tended to limit its offerings to those courses of study usually included in the first two years of a four-year liberal arts college. Preparation for transfer was its primary function, although many of its students terminated their formal education at the end of the two-year period. But the insistent demand for men and women trained to enter the expanding semiprofessional occupations caused community junior-colleges to develop curriculums of the technical institute type. A variety of technical workers in health-related occupations are prepared in programs offered by these colleges and include X-ray technicians, inhalation therapy technicians, dental hygienists and assistants, occupational therapy assistants, medical records technicians, operating room technicians, biomedical engineering technicians, public health technicians, medical emergency technicians, and nurse technicians. These technical assistants work side by side with their professional colleagues to complement and supplement their activities in health care services.

Major social events have created the need for workers with vocational competencies. World War I established the need for specific job training because of the retraining requirements for veterans that existed when the "dough boys" returned to a world of work which had changed rapidly from the one that they had left. It was during the years immediately following World War I that tremendous headway was made in the area of vocational training. The second emergency that intensified our understanding of the effectiveness of vocational education was the depression of the 1930's. During this period vocational training became a part of the emphasis of the National Youth Administration and the Civilian Conservation Corps, wherein our youth were provided with work experience opportunities in which they were able to develop skills that later were to help them when they sought employment. The period of conflict during World War II cemented our understanding of the contribution of vocational education to our nation's welfare. It was during this period that over seven and one-half million men and women were taught skills that were needed to maintain the effort in preparing for an all-out world war. Once again, at the close of this war, there was established a great vocational effort for the retraining of veterans. More recently, with rapid technological changes occurring, training and retraining were necessary to provide workers with the skills that are demanded for holding jobs. Vocational education programs have been organized at the high school and adult education levels in various occupations including nursing.

The development of educational programs to prepare various workers within an occupation reflects the nature and complexity of the activities and services offered by the particular occupations. The urgent demands for health manpower require all professions to give attention to an analysis of their services and to develop educational programs to prepare the appropriate workers to

TABLE 1.   Theory-Skill Spectrum in the Health Fields

THEORY	Research scientist
	Physician and Dentist practitioners
	Paramedical—Paradental Registered nurse (B.S.) Dietitian Pharmacist Medical record librarian Occupational therapist Physiotherapist
	Technical assistant X-ray technician Registered nurse (A.D.N.) Medical record technician Dispensing optician Occupational therapy assistant Inhalation therapy technician
SKILL	Practical assistant Licensed practical nurse Psychiatric aide
	Aide Orderly-nurse's aide Dietary aide Housekeeping aide

From R. E. Kinsinger. *Education for Health Technicians—An Overview.* Washington, D.C.: American Association of Junior Colleges, 1965. P. 9.

contribute to these services. The focus and structure of the different types of programs are dependent upon the goals and objectives of these programs. The professional, who has the responsibility for discriminating judgments and decision-making, needs a substantial theoretical educational base, whereas the vocational worker greatly needs the development of manipulatory skills.

The theory-skill spectrum (Table 1) by Kinsinger gives the curriculum worker some general ideas pertaining to the relationship of the theoretical base and skill component of the various programs in relation to the objectives and nature of the activities of the different workers in the health occupations. This can serve as a guide for curriculum development.

NATURE OF NURSING

Nursing has been described as an occupation in which the professionals are assisted by several types of workers, each trained for differentiated tasks. The functions of nursing require activities, which can be thought of as spread along a continuum, extending from the simple or elementary type of nursing tasks to the highly complex activities associated with the full professional role. Simple tasks can be learned through on-the-job training; those tasks of a complex nature require extensive technical and broad general and professional education. McManus has identified factors that determine the placement of these activities on the continuum.

These factors include (1) the degree of responsibility the worker has for deciding about what nursing action to take, (2) the kind and amount of skill required in nursing activities, (3) the demands these activities make upon intellectual capacity, (4) the scope of responsibility for directing the work of others, and (5) the type and amount of training and education, technical and professional knowledge, and the quality of judgment required [7].

Nursing provides a service to society. In providing this service, it becomes a social system within the larger system of health care. It affects and is affected by other subsystems, such as medicine and social work, as well as the total system. It has been observed that nursing has been oriented to medical care and to agency administration to a greater degree than to its own goals and objectives. As the medical, social, and nursing participants in health care have developed, and other participants, such as physical and occupational therapists, nutritionists, and rehabilitation workers, have been instituted, it has become important that the various practitioners identify their special roles and activities in the delivery of health services. Further delination of the practice is necessary when more than one type of practitioner works within a particular practice area. Thus, not only is it appropriate to describe the goals and domain of nursing in relation to other helping professions, but it is also necessary to identify the activities of various workers—professional, technician, assistant— within the practice of nursing.

NURSING—DEFINED

Definitions of nursing that were acceptable to the profession were formulated during the time when the delivery of health was the primary responsibility of the physician and the nurse. With the proliferation of specialized health workers, which began to take place following World War II, these definitions seemed to place nursing in an ambiguous position. The definitions which described the nurse's function were so general that any health worker might claim that it was also his function. Most of the definitions of nursing practice incorporated into the nurse practice acts by the state legislatures failed to identify the independent or self-directed activities of nurses.

The American Nurses' Association, responding to the discontent over the ambiguous position of nursing, engaged in an investigation of the nurse's functions during a five-year period beginning in 1950. Studies were conducted in seventeen states, which were summarized by Everett and Helen MacGill Hughes and Irwin Deutcher under the title of *Twenty Thousand Nurses Tell Their Story* [8]. As a result of this study, the definition of the practice of nursing formulated by the American Nurses' Association provided an empirical approach to the identification of the nursing function. The official statement, which was first published in 1955 and was reaffirmed in 1962, reads as follows:

The practice of professional nursing means the performance for compensation of any act in the observation, care and counsel of the ill, injured, or infirm, or in the maintenance of health or prevention of illness of others, or in the supervision and teaching of other personnel, or the administration of medications and treatments as prescribed by a licensed physician or dentist; requiring substantial specialized judgment and skill and based on knowledge and application of the principles of biological, physical and social science. The foregoing shall not be deemed to include acts of diagnosis or prescription of therapeutic or corrective measures [9].

The practice of practical nursing means the performance for compensation of selected acts in the care of the ill, injured, or infirm under the direction of a registered professional nurse or a licensed physician or a licensed dentist; and not requiring the substantial skill, judgment, and knowledge required in professional nursing [10].

Noteworthy attempts have been made to clarify the legal functions and prerogatives of the professional nurse. Lesnik describes seven categories of professional nursing functions that are supported by the case decisions of judicial review. He divides these into "independent functions which require no prior medical order for their validity" and "dependent functions which do require such order" [11]. Observation of symptoms and reactions, including the limited responsibility or diagnosis without the right to prescribe treatment or medication, is considered to be an independent legal function of nursing. The analysis of the legal functions through court decisions gives attention to the independent practice of nursing based upon training and experience. Lesnik and other legal authorities indicate the weaknesses of the nurse practice acts in that they describe the practice of nursing in a very general way.

Professional nurse educators have endeavored to define more explicitly the practice of nursing. McManus states that the function of the professional nurse is parallel somewhat to that of the professional physician. The unique responsibility of the physician recognized by law is to identify the medical problem and to diagnose, plan, and prescribe treatment. Similarly, the unique function of the professional nurse may be conceived to be (1) the identification or diagnosis of the nursing problem and the recognition of its interrelated aspects, and (2) the deciding upon a course of nursing action to be followed for the solution of the problem in light of immediate and long-term objectives of nursing, with regard to prevention of illness, direct care, rehabilitation, and promotion of the highest standard of health possible for the individual [12].

This interpretation of the practice of nursing implies that the patient may present nursing problems which are distinct from but related to his medical problems. While nursing practice is concerned with observation of the patients' symptoms and reactions that are directly related to the medical problem and participation in the medical regimen, this practice is essentially concerned with the diagnosis of nursing problems and with the determining of appropriate nursing action in the instance of the individual and his family.

Another interpretation of nursing practice is offered by Kreuter, who attributes the unique contribution of nursing to its ministrations to the basic human needs of patients. This author defines nursing care as acting and interacting with the patient through physical and personal contact for his welfare, and intervening on his behalf between him and those stresses in the physical environment and the social climate that impinge on him [13]. Kreuter's definition of nursing directs the focus of nursing to assisting the patient in meeting the fundamental needs that all persons have for survival and living. A definition of nursing that is compatible with Kreuter's definition but more definitive and explicit is that by Virginia Henderson. This well-known nurse describes the unique function of the nurse as assisting the individual, sick or well, in the performance of those activities contributing to health or recovery (or to peaceful death) that the patient would perform unaided if he had the necessary strength, will, or knowledge, and to do this in such a way as to help him gain independence as rapidly as possible [14]. According to Henderson the nurse is and should be legally an independent practitioner, able to make independent judgments as long as he or she is not diagnosing or prescribing treatment for disease. Basic nursing care is concerned with helping the patient with activities pertaining to respiration, elimination, nutrition, maintaining normal body temperature, mobility, safety, and communication through both social and psychological modes of expression. Even though these are seen as the major focus of nursing, the nurse also has a therapeutic role in carrying out the physician's prescriptions.

Henderson says that "In certain situations the nurse may find it necessary to assume the role of a physician—in hospitals with no medical resident or intern, for instance, or in emergencies. First aid, which has elements of diagnosis and therapy, is expected of all informed citizens under certain conditions."

A similar approach is taken by Abdellah, who defines nursing as a service to individuals and families—therefore to society. This service involves (1) recognizing the nursing problems of the patient; (2) deciding the appropriate courses of action to take in terms of relevant nursing principles; (3) providing continuous care of the individual's total health needs; (4) providing continuous care to relieve pain and discomfort and provide immediate security for the individual; (5) adjusting the total nursing-care plan to meet the patient's individual needs; (6) helping the individual to become more self-directing in attaining or maintaining a healthy state of mind and body; (7) instructing nursing personnel and family to help the individual to do for himself that which he can within his limitations; (8) helping the individual to adjust to his limitations and emotional problems; (9) working with allied health professions in planning for optimum health on local, state, national, and international levels; and (10) carrying out continuous evaluation and research to improve nursing techniques and to develop new techniques to meet the health needs of people [15]. Abdellah and her colleagues further delineate the nature and focus of nursing problems as those basic concerns of all persons regardless of the specific health problems, the problems that are related to normal and disturbed physiological processes, the concerns of persons that involve mainly emotional and interpersonal difficulties, and those problems of a sociological or community orientation [16]. This careful and detailed analysis of nursing also indicates that the nursing problems of the patient may be overt or covert and that the action taken by the nurse requires a direct or an indirect approach. These additional dimensions of nursing problems and nursing approaches have been the focus of attention of scholars in nursing and other related disciplines.

ROLES AND ACTIVITIES OF THE NURSE

The phenomenon of nursing is described in a general way in the several definitions that have appeared in literature. It is obvious that nursing needs to be defined more precisely before identification can be made of the basic elements that the nurse needs to master so that she can practice competently and effectively.

Sociologists have had an enduring interest in the role of the nurse in patient care. They suggest that the action taken by nurses in the care of patients can be classified under two roles. One, the therapeutic role, includes all those actions directed toward the prevention and treatment of disease. The other is called the expressive role by some and the mother-substitute role by others. It includes all those activities directed toward creating an environment in which the patient feels comforted, accepted, protected, cared for, and supported. The emphasis in the performance of the expressive role is not on cure but on the manner in which care is provided. The physical care of the patient is important because these acts performed by the nurse communicate to the patient her concern for his welfare.

Johnson and Martin state that the objective of the expressive role is the relief of tension in the group. The group referred to here is composed of the doctor, nurse, and patient. Though they do not so state, the group actually consists of all those who have some relationship to the patient, including the members of his family and his friends. The authors further state that in any social system certain problems must be solved if the system is to maintain itself. It must move forward toward the accomplishment of a common goal, and it must maintain internal equilibrium. Relationships among the social system members must be harmonious and integrated, and each member must feel good both within himself and toward other group members. They emphasize the importance of the nurse in this role by suggesting that here she is the expert and as such should give leadership. She stands as an intermediary between the patient and the doctor and what he does for and to the patient. If this view is accepted, the nurse also stands between the patient and other persons who participate in his care. To fulfill this role, she must know what the common goal or objective is and give leadership to those working toward its achievement. Johnson and Martin emphasize that the physical care of the patient is important because it gives the nurse an opportunity to reduce the tensions of the patient and to promote good feeling. But the expressive role of the nurse can be carried too far. The patient can be so gratified that he prefers sickness to health. The nurse has the responsibility for recognizing the signs indicating that the patient is finding the secondary gains of illness preferable to returning to the healthy state and for supporting the physician and the patient when the physician decides the time has come to help the patient move toward recovery [17].

Schulman compares the feeling that the nurse should have for her patient as being similar to the feeling that a mother has for her child [18]. The early phase of the mother-child relationship is largely physical and marked by tenderness and compassion. The mother tends her child and stands between him and harm. She comforts and soothes his hurts. As the child grows and develops in his ability to care for himself, she encourages him to become independent of her.

Johnson indicates that "the achievement and maintenance of a stable state is nursing's distinctive contribution to patient welfare, and the specific purpose of nursing care. . . . Change of any magnitude toward recovery from illness or toward more desirable health practices depends upon the periodic achievement and maintenance . . . of this stable state [19]. Nursing care presents at least two major avenues for assisting the patient to maintain or reestablish equilibrium. First, stimuli which are stressors can be reduced in many instances. It is for this reason the management of the environment—both the physical and psychological environment—is of major importance. Secondly, nursing can support through promotion and sustaining measures the patient's natural defenses and adaptive processes. The primary focus and objectives of nursing care have to do with the immediate situation; activities center on those human needs for food and fluids, for rest and exercise, for warmth and shelter, for approval and esteem, for love and affection and the like [20]."

The interpretations of the roles and activities of the nurse in the practice of nursing seem to indicate a strong tendency to place primary focus on patient care. Nursing practice has developed in bureaucratic institutions and has been distracted from its essential purposes by the forceful demands of medical practice and hospital administration. By abandoning the patient to become a medical assistant and a high-level administrator, the nurse has created confusion in her role orientation. Also, her flight from the bedside has created a vacuum in patient care that has been filled to some degree by nonprofessionals. Only recently has attention been directed to the return of nursing to its primary function and mission. The emergence of the nurse-clinician is an identification of the shift in the direction of nursing practice. The activities of these practitioners should provide information that can assist in defining more precisely the practice of nursing.

PRIMARY FOCUS OF NURSING

The endeavors of scholars in various disciplines to study the roles and activities of the nurse in the practice of nursing has facilitated the efforts of the organized profession to formulate concepts pertaining to the primary focus of nursing that are agreeable to the profession. In 1967 at a meeting of the Council of Agency Members of the Department of Baccalaureate and Higher Degree Programs of the National League for Nursing, Mary Tschudin stated:

If we are to work together effectively as a team—as colleagues—we must understand each other's unique contributions to the joint goals and efforts of the team. We must understand each other's particular competencies and the frame of reference from which each approaches his professional responsibilities. We must also understand how our individual roles and functions interrelate and support one another in the achievement of a common goal [21].

This noted nurse educator indicated that it was of immediate importance to delineate a central nursing role that would be flexible enough to accommodate both the present and the future in nursing. A redefinition and reformation of purpose should give us a renewed sense of direction as we move to the future for nursing practice and nursing education [22].

Continuous thoughtful deliberations and discussions among members of this organization have resulted in a statement of position on the primary focus of nursing [23]. Fundamental premises underlying this statement indicate that a profession has an obligation to delineate the unique contribution it makes to the society it serves. It is the establishment of the unique contribution of the profession that guides the development of the body of knowledge and the design of the systematic programs of professional education. The organized profession has the responsibility to define the boundaries of practice of its members and to assure the society of the competence of its members. Based upon these premises, and utilizing the components of nursing as proposed in the American Nurses' Association position paper on nursing education [24], the Council of Member Agencies of the Department of Baccalaureate and Higher Degree Programs of the National League for Nursing accepts care, cure, and coordination as the major components of nursing practice. This group accepts that nursing has the responsibility to participate in the curative and coordinative functions, even though it agrees that the primary focus of nursing is care.

It is likely indeed that professional practitioners and educators in nursing will view these components differently. These components—care, cure, and coordination—are general concepts, and more definitive roles and activities encompassed by the components need continuous exploration and refinement.

The lack of a clear consensus as to a definition of nursing practice has presented difficulties in attempts to differentiate the practice of the professional nurse and that of the nurse technician. Matheney has identified some essential elements of technical nursing practice that are in agreement with the American Nurses' Association position paper, which indicates that technical nursing practice is unlimited in depth but limited in scope. Technical nursing practice is concerned primarily with the direct nursing of patients with health problems, patients who present common, recurring nursing problems. This nursing care includes both the immediate care of patients with acute illnesses or acute phases of chronic health problems and long-range planning for nursing and health care for patients with long-term illnesses. Matheney describes the major focuses of the technical nurse as the concerns of physical comfort and safety, physiological malfunction, psychological and social difficulties, and rehabilitative needs of patients. This nurse is also responsible for the provision of nursing care and for the performance of medically delegated techniques that are required to meet patients' needs. The technical nurse is able to use appropriately a wide range of physical and psychological measures of nursing intervention. In addition to providing a high quality of direct nursing care, the technical nurse coordinates nursing care with other health services. She functions as a member of a nursing team under the leadership of a professional nurse [25].

Although at the present time the differences in the practice of professional and technical nursing are not decisive nor clear, some general substantive and methodological issues emerge. Johnson suggests two desired attributes of the professional practitioner: sensitivity to a broad range of cues in the problematic situation, and intellectual command of a large selection of alternative explanatory and predictive interpretations to bring to bear on the situation [26]. A third attribute of importance in the practice of the professional is the consistent evaluation of the wisdom of the decisions made and of the use of practice as a means of gathering data for the refinement and the extension of the scientific rationale for practice. In this instance practice is a means for validating nursing knowledge and obtaining additional knowledge for further validation. The professional practitioner has obtained knowledge in wide areas, alerting her to the cues and variables in the nursing situation. Her nursing actions are those of a continuous nature, concerned with prevention of illness, as well as those of an immediate nature, involved in complex health problems. The focus of professional practice goes beyond the immediate care situation to a variety of community agencies and the patient's or client's home. The professional nurse is responsible for the nursing care given by other members of the nursing team; therefore, she must plan and make appropriate decisions concerning the delegation of nursing care to other team members. The professional nurse plans with other professionals in developing long-range planning for health care.

The analysis of the roles and activities of the technical and professional nurse provides only a general orientation. Continuous exploration needs to be done to determine how these practitioners can utilize their individual knowledges and skills in a team relationship to make the best possible contribution to the health care of individuals and families. The reader is urged to remain alert to forthcoming studies and surveys that may give additional information concerning the components of professional and technical practice.

THE SUBJECT MATTER OF NURSING

Nursing, in its drive toward professionalization, is confronted with the need to develop a scientific body upon which nursing practice can be based. The rule-of-thumb procedures, the empirical approach, and the use of stereotyped patterns of response to situations are no longer adequate in practically any phase of modern living. They are particularly inadequate in nursing, where expanding scientific knowledge and the overwhelming need for change in practice require the use of judgment and the ability to make rational decisions. All occupational fields today require an increasing degree of competence, and nursing is no exception. Competency in nursing, as in other fields, must be based on a sound theoretical background of appropriate knowledge. One of the major stumbling blocks in developing a body of knowledge uniquely applicable to nursing has been the failure to define clearly the practice of nursing itself. At the present time nursing has no well-delineated theoretical framework nor does it have conceptual basis to give it meaning or direction.

The practice of nursing as it ought to be necessarily dictates the source of the theoretical background it requires. Nurse practitioners and educators are attempting to formulate some notions about nursing that can be utilized in the development of nursing theories. Nursing theory may be said to represent that aspect of theoretical knowledge which differentiates nursing from other professional disciplines. It develops through synthesis and patterning of knowledge for new theses, which lead to resynthesis and further patterning. The process is ongoing as additional knowledge is revealed, for this knowledge then is incorporated into the patterning and synthesis. Theories of nursing emerge from the same base as do the theories of other disciplines, but the configuration of knowledge that contributes to nursing theory is unique in kind and amount. The social ends for which nursing theory is to be used are in themselves different from those of other disciplines.

Theoretical knowledge is dependent on research. Although some useful nursing research is being reported, nursing has been late in responding to this professional mandate. The slow development of academically situated schools of nursing has been responsible for the lack of a climate and environment for scientific investigations of the practice of nursing. In some instances nursing has recapitulated the experiences of medical education. Medicine, however, associated itself with universities in 1910; nursing did not. Medicine knew that a body of knowledge had to be developed through research and that the university provided the resources for these activities. It is indeed incumbent upon nursing to demonstrate the existence of a body of knowledge that is exclusive to it, founded on science, communicated through a precise, universally accepted language, constantly extended through rigorous research, and shared with an appropriate peer group.

The development of a body of knowledge of nursing will give direction to the organization of learning content in accordance with the same stratification as other academic pursuits: the undergraduate, the master's and the doctoral levels. And this will be done according to the objectives of each program of instruction. Until this scientific approach can be used, nursing faculties on the various levels must arrive at some a priori consensus about the nature and focus of nursing practice, the delineation of appropriate content compatible with their views about the unique contributions of nursing to health care, and the role of the various types of nurse practitioners in health services. The curriculum is dependent upon a careful analysis of the substance and methods of nursing practice.

SYSTEM OF NURSING EDUCATION
CHARACTERISTICS OF THE SYSTEM

The system of nursing education in the United States displays some unique characteristics that are not seen in education for other professions. Nursing is the only profession that allocates to other than educational institutions a portion of its education. The hospital diploma programs are presently graduating the largest number of registered nurses. While educational programs have been developed at the vocational, technical, and professional levels, there is presently no clear differentiation as to the levels of responsibility for which the graduates of each type of program are prepared. There is a strong belief that the baccalaureate program should be the minimal requirement for nurses who will assume leadership roles. Although the length and nature of training differ markedly in the diploma and the associate degree programs, graduates of both are presently expected to carry the same responsibilities. The situation is aggravated further by the fact that almost all kinds of nurses must carry responsibilities for which they are not adequately prepared.

A careful examination of the system of nursing education is necessary in an effort to create order out of the present confusion. We also need to determine how these systems can be merged or related in a pattern that will adequately prepare the nurses of the nation to render better patient care and at the same time allow them to advance professionally in an orderly manner. Nursing and allied professional groups have periodically made studies of the problems of nursing and nursing education, beginning fifty years ago with the publication of the study, *Nursing and Nursing Education in the United States*, by Josephine Goldmark [Reference 4, Chapter 2]. The various concerns pertaining to nursing education at that time focused on (1) the control of nursing education by service agencies, (2) the lack of adequate financing of nursing education, (3) the narrow scope of the nursing curriculum, and (4) the need for prepared nonprofessional nursing personnel in the care of patients.

These same problems have continued to plague nurses, and more recent reviews of the educational system have suggested specific directions for present and future considerations. Following World War II, when the war emergency had ended, hospitals and health agencies found that they were unable to operate their services with sufficient personnel either in quantity or quality. The nursing profession concluded that there was something drastically wrong with a system of education that could not meet the demands for service. The National Nursing Council undertook a study of the educational system in nursing in 1948. This study was directed by Esther Lucille Brown, a sociologist, and the report of the study was published in *Nursing for the Future* [27].

One of the major recommendations of the study indicated that the term *professional*, when applied to nursing education, be restricted to schools (whether operated by universities, colleges, hospitals affiliated with institutions of higher learning, medical colleges, or independent institutions) that are able to furnish professional education as that term has come to be understood by educators [28]. Two types of nurse practitioners were identified by Dr. Brown: the graduate bedside nurse and the professional nurse. The graduate bedside nurse would receive her education in the diploma program. The study recommended that the good hospital schools be strengthened through curriculum experimentation, which might lead to shortening the program. The report recommended that the education of the professional nurse be in an institution of higher learning and that these schools be established as autonomous units within the university. Finally, Brown recommended that all sources, private and public, be tapped for making available the largest possible sums for creating and strengthening college or university programs in nursing [29].

Although the study initially evoked considerable discussions and controversy within the profession and among physicians and hospital administrators, it also provided guidelines for the continuous review and reordering of the system of nursing education.

The Consultant Group on Nursing was appointed in the spring of 1961 by the surgeon general of the Public Health Service, to advise him on nursing needs and to identify the appropriate role of the federal government in assuring adequate nursing services for our nation. This group recognized that nursing is an essential element of health care and that there are major problems confronting the nursing profession which can best be solved with the help of constructive public understanding and support. After a substantial review of the needs and goals for providing quality nursing care, the group recommended that a study be made of the present system of nursing education in relation to the responsibilities and skill levels required for high-quality patient care. In addition to this recommendation, the group indicated that the federal government should endeavor to expand its present program of support and assistance to nursing and nursing education [30]. During the time the consultant group was at work, the American Nurses' Association Committee on Education was engaged in formulating statements that would present the position of the association toward the educational preparation for those who render nursing care. The statements were prepared and adopted by the organization in 1964 and became known as the American Nurses' Association's first position on education for nursing. The position taken by this association indicated that education for those who work in nursing should take place in institutions of learning within the general system of education. More specifically, the association stated that the education for all those who are licensed to practice nursing should take place in institutions of higher education. The committee recognized the complexity of nursing and identified those practitioners who would engage in professional nursing practice and those who would engage in technical practice. The position of the American Nurses' Association in regard to educational preparation of these practitioners revealed that the minimum preparation for those beginning professional practice at the present time should be a baccalaureate degree in nursing. Also, the minimum preparation for those beginning technical nursing practice should be an associate degree in nursing. Lastly, the committee reported that education for assistants in the health services should be short, intensive preservice programs in vocational institutions rather than an on-the-job training program [31].

The recommendations of the Surgeon General's Consultant Group on Nursing that pertained to the conduct of a national investigation of nursing education was endorsed by the two major organizations in nursing—the American Nurses' Association and the National League for Nursing. These two groups appropriated funds and established a joint committee to study the ways to conduct and finance such a national inquiry. Funds were made available by the American Nurses' Foundation, the Avalon Foundation, and the W. K. Kellogg Foundation to support this investigation. Although the commission was a direct outgrowth of the interest of the American Nurses' Association and the National League for Nursing, it was set up as an independent agency and functioned as a self-directing group. The study yielded much useful information, and fifteen recommendations were forthcoming. The recommendations directed to the issues of nursing practice and nursing education include the following:

Each state have, or create, a master planning committee that will take nursing education under its purview, such committee to include representatives of nursing education, other health professions, and the public, to recommend specific guidelines, means for implementation, and deadlines to ensure that nursing education is positioned in the mainstream of American educational patterns.

Federal, regional, state and local governments adopt measures for the increased support of nursing research and education. Priority should be given to construction grants, institutional grants, advanced traineeships and research grants and contracts. Private funds and foundations support nursing research and educational innovations where such activities are not publicly aided.

A National Joint Practice Commission, with state counterpart committees, be established between medicine and nursing to discuss and make recommendations concerning the congruent roles of the physician and the nurse in providing quality health care with particular attention to: the rise of the nurse clinician; the introduction of the physician's assistant; the increased activity of other professions and para-professions in areas long assumed to be the concern solely of the physician and/or the nurse.

Two essentially related, but differing, career patterns be developed for nursing practice: A. One career pattern (episodic) would emphasize nursing practice that is essentially curative and restorative, generally acute or chronic in nature, and most frequently provided in the setting of the hospital and inpatient facility. B. The second career pattern (distributive) would emphasize the nursing practice that is designed essentially for health maintenance and disease prevention, generally continuous in nature, seldom acute, and most frequently operative in the community or in newly developing institutional settings.

No less than three regional or inter-institutional committees be funded for the study and development of the nursing curriculum in order to develop objectives, universals, alternatives, and sequences for nursing instruction. These committees should specify appropriate levels of general and specialized learning for the different types of educational institutions, and should be particularly concerned with the articulation of programs between two collegiate levels [32].

A closing statement of the report of the commission indicates that "nursing may well be the key to whether our entire system for health care will remain viable and responsible to the demands placed upon it" [33].

TYPES OF EDUCATIONAL PROGRAMS IN NURSING

The various studies and activities of the profession have provided direction and guidelines for future developments in nursing education. Although the system is somewhat fluid at the moment, three types of educational programs are preparing nurse practitioners: the diploma, the associate degree, and the baccalaureate nursing programs. In addition to these are the programs preparing nurse assistants, those who perform certain nonprofessional tasks in nature delegated by the registered nurse. At the other end of the continuum are the programs preparing the teachers, administrators, and researchers in nursing. A brief description of these programs is provided.

PROGRAMS PREPARING THE NURSE TECHNICIAN

The nurse technician is presently being prepared in two types of programs: the hospital diploma program and the community junior-college program. The hospital diploma program has been the typical nursing program preparing for licensure. These programs grew rapidly in number and in enrollment to meet the nursing needs of hospitals. The first schools of nursing to be established in the country followed the pattern of the school of nursing developed by Florence Nightingale, in that they were supported and controlled by lay societies. Because of the lack of adequate financing, these schools soon came under the control of hospitals. During the period from 1873 to 1893, approximately one hundred schools of nursing were opened in this country. This new system of education proved useful and profitable to hospitals; it was evident that patients received better care by better educated women. In the next twenty-year period, over one thousand new schools were established. Standards of education varied as did the products these schools provided. Although in many instances the curriculum increased from two to three years, there was no increase in the hours of instruction, only an increase in the amount of nursing service given to the hospital. The professional organizations, which came into existence in the early 1900's, were deeply conscious of the danger to society and to the profession of inadequately prepared nurses. It was through the efforts of the state nurses' associations that legislation was enacted which established standards for the profession. The laws set the minimum standards for the practice of nursing and for educational programs and became the first means of standard setting.

In more recent years, the hospital diploma programs have made substantial strides to improve their curriculums. Attempts have been made to separate the educational programs from the nursing service activities of the hospital. Attention has been directed toward providing learning opportunities to meet the needs of students rather than those of nursing service, with greater faculty control of the learning environment. In many instances this allowed a reduction in the length of the program. Quality of instruction in the natural and behavioral sciences has been made possible by means of affiliations with junior or senior colleges. Although these schools have made desperate efforts to improve the programs of instruction, the graduates of these programs experience some disadvantages. The present lack of relationship among the types of nursing education programs carries penalties for the student who begins as a nurse trained in a hospital school and who then wishes to advance. Such a student usually cannot seek a baccalaureate degree without sacrificing two or more years because credit for training and experience in a hospital school is severely discounted by colleges and universities. There were approximately 1,100 hospital diploma programs, and presently there are about 587 such programs. The admission of new students to these programs has been steadily declining. This trend might indicate that as educational institutions become willing and able to offer programs in nursing, there will be less need for the hospital to assume this responsibility. Although the National Commission for the Study of Nursing and Nursing Education recommends that nursing education be channeled into the mainstream of American education, the commission suggests that no hospital school should close or collegiate program open until the state master-planning committee is assured that an orderly transfer of functions and facilities has been developed [34].

The second type of program preparing the nurse technician is the community junior-college program. The participation of junior colleges in nursing education prior to 1950 was primarily concerned with the provision of general education courses to students enrolled in hospital nursing programs. In 1952 there were in all probability no more than four or five nursing programs leading to an associate degree that were conducted by institutions authorized to grant such a degree. Today there are 491 such programs, and the numbers of the new programs and the admission of students to these programs are increasing at a rapid rate. The curriculum is offered within a two-year period, and it provides the student with a general and nursing education, including clinical experience, developed in accordance with college policy and the regulations of the state licensing authority. Graduates are prepared to give care to patients who have health problems, and they are concerned to a major extent with restorative or care-and-cure aspects of nursing. Performances on state board examinations and evaluations of work records give indication that the graduates of the community junior-college programs are making a valuable contribution to nursing. Community junior-colleges serve two major purposes: (1) They provide those educational experiences that are comparable to the freshman and sophomore years in a four-year college and enable the student to transfer into the junior year of a senior college for specialized study. (2) They provide technical or semiprofessional education within a two-year period, enabling the student to obtain employment immediately upon graduation.

The programs in nursing education fall within the framework of the latter objective. The associate degree programs, unlike all other programs in nursing education, have been planned and administered by utilizing the results of an extensive research project [35]. The basic assumptions guiding the direction of these programs indicate (1) that the functions of nursing can be differentiated and that most nursing be in the intermediate area, the semiprofessional or technical; (2) that education for nursing belongs in educational institutions; (3) that the community junior-college is the logical institution within organized education for this nursing program; and (4) that if a program for nursing were education centered, less time would be required to reach the objectives. Community junior-colleges are expanding at a phenomenal rate, and it is likely they will continue to assume an increasingly greater responsibility for the education of nurses.

PROGRAMS PREPARING THE PROFESSIONAL NURSE

The professional nurse practitioner is prepared in baccalaureate programs in senior colleges and universities. Graduate programs at the master's and doctoral levels offer educational opportunities for professional nurses preparing for positions of leadership in teaching, administration, clinical specialization, and research.

Baccalaureate degree programs are presently conducted by approximately 285 colleges and universities. These programs are not new in nursing, as the first collegiate program was established at the University of Minnesota in 1909. During the past ten years, however, the growth of these schools in relation to numbers of schools and total enrollment has been significant. The objectives of baccalaureate education may be stated generally as (1) to prepare the individual to live a richer and fuller life by gaining some knowledge of the cultural, social, and physical environment in which he lives; and (2) to prepare the individual to contribute to socially desirable activities and services of that society by gaining some specialized knowledge and skills.

The curriculum in nursing comprises liberal arts and sciences as well as the professional sequence. Appropriate knowledge is drawn from the basic disciplines and certain applied fields of study for a foundation for nursing education. The nursing content offered provides a reasonably sound and broad basis in knowledge that is sufficient to enable the future practitioner to cope adequately with the common nursing problems in patient care wherever she may practice. Graduates of baccalaureate degree programs are broadly prepared to give nursing care, to interpret and demonstrate such care to others, and to plan, direct, and evaluate nursing care provided by members of the nursing team.

Many baccalaureate nursing programs grew out of diploma programs and frequently carried with them the characteristics of the apprenticeship type of education. In a number of instances faculty members of baccalaureate programs had many years of experience teaching in diploma programs and were lacking in the approaches to and methods of higher education. Consequently, for some time baccalaureate programs in nursing reflected a change in name and location rather than a substantial change in character. More recently, however, the new curriculums being developed and the revisions being made in existing programs are demonstrating creative and courageous innovation on the part of the faculties. It appears evident that the faculty members are truly addressing themselves to the nature and function of higher education and the requirements of professional education at the baccalaureate level.

Modifications in the structure of these programs reflect the impact of a technological society on patterns and content of education. Attention to the science component indicates the concern of the faculty for the natural and behavioral sciences as essential foundations for professional study. The identification and resolution of nursing problems, as opposed to medical or administrative problems, as the focus of nursing and nursing education is apparent. The acknowledgment that the professional practitioner improves his practice by utilizing the findings of research has motivated faculty to delineate certain research competencies appropriate for the beginning practitioner. Appropriate training for these competencies is included in many baccalaureate curriculums. The more traditional subject matter that indicated a medical orientation is giving away to clinical courses and content that suggest a nursing focus. Flexibility is a key factor in curriculum implementation and is demonstrated by the variety of means by which students' attainments are assessed. Individualized planning takes into consideration students' needs, abilities, and interests in an effort to facilitate completing the program requirements as expeditiously as possible. Baccalaureate curriculums reveal the sensitivity of the faculty to the social and scientific forces of this century. The mobility of the student population reflects that of a larger society, and a great number of students graduate from colleges different from those they entered as freshmen. Greater attention is being given to planning curriculums that will not greatly penalize the student who transfers to another program because of a change in geographical location or change in career goals. It appears that nursing is well within an era of radical review, reform, and revision of baccalaureate nursing education.

Graduate programs in nursing developed as a response to the need for faculty to teach in the increasing number of baccalaureate programs. The initial purpose of the graduate programs was the preparation of teachers and administrators. Although this initial purpose has not changed, the emphasis has shifted to include a substantial foundation in clinical nursing and a concern for research. The development of highly complex nursing services called for administrators with considerable know-how in designing and implementing nursing services in health agencies, which were undergoing changes in purposes and programs. Advances in medical, biological, and social sciences have precipitated concern for the preparation of the clinical specialist in nursing who can apply these kinds of knowledge in nursing intervention in the care of individuals and families having complex health problems. Programs at the master's level provide opportunities for the student to design and conduct individual research activity.

Professional nurses seeking positions of leadership in the profession, such as deans of schools of nursing, directors of large and complex nursing services, faculty for graduate programs in nursing, and independent researchers, obtain preparation in doctoral programs. Only recently have these programs been made available in schools of nursing. At the present time the majority of nurses holding doctoral degrees have obtained these degrees through the study of disciplines other than nursing (natural and behavioral sciences, education, philosophy). For many nurses this is a circuitous route that must meet the rigorous demands of another field of study. As more doctoral programs in nursing develop, the pathway will be shorter and more appropriate to the concerns of nursing practice and research. The major focus of doctoral programs in nursing is the development and testing of knowledge through research in an effort to build nursing theories.

PROGRAMS PREPARING THE NURSING ASSISTANT

The simple, elementary nursing tasks that are delegated by the professional nurse are the responsibility of the practical nurse and other nursing assistants. The preparation of these workers takes place in organized education programs or, in the case of nursing assistants, in on-the-job training programs. Before 1900 only one school for the training of practical nurses was reported in existence in the United States. The early schools of practical nursing were organized and financed by interested individuals and organizations, not primarily by the nursing profession. These were an outgrowth of community efforts to supply some training to women who wished to work as practical nurses in homes. Eventually the courses were developed into more formal training programs that included clinical instruction and supervised clinical practice in hospitals.

During the period between 1920 and 1940, the public showed less interest in practical nursing than it had shown in the preceding twenty years. The preoccupation of graduate nurses with their own progress toward professional status, the mass unemployment during the depression years, and the trend toward hospital care as opposed to home care were sufficient reasons to account for the lack of progress in practical nurse education. Although the Goldmark Report in 1923 called attention to the urgent need for training a group of nonprofessional workers to assist the professional nurse in rendering bedside care to the sick, no nationally organized effort was made to carry forward this recommendation for about twenty years.

The years from 1940 to 1960 were quite different. They revealed a story of unparalleled and unprecedented progress in the establishment of educational programs for practical nurses. Federal legislation for vocational education made it possible to establish and conduct practical nursing programs in the public schools. The combined efforts of federal agencies, vocational education, and the national nursing organization sought to improve the quality of practical nurse education. These programs have developed at a phenomenal rate since 1950, and approximately two thirds of them are under the supervision of public education in vocational schools. By 1960 all jurisdictions that license professional nurses also provided for practical nurse licensure. Where at one time the focus of practical nursing was home care, the major portion of the curriculums today are directed toward the tasks involved in the care of acutely ill, hospitalized patients.

In a little more than a decade, employment in health occupations jumped 40 percent while total employment increased 14 percent. More than two million persons work in health services. Most of these are professionals; however, nearly three quarters of a million persons serve as practical nurses, orderlies, nurses aides, hospital attendants, and other subprofessional occupations. The preparation for nurses' aides, hospital attendants, and nursing unit clerks is provided by service institutions by means of on-the-job training. Federal assistance by means of the Manpower Development and Training Act is facilitating the preparation of these workers for participation in nursing activities, thus relieving the professional nurse of many time-consuming tasks.

CAREER-LADDER CONCEPTS

Students select and engage in programs of study in nursing for a variety of reasons. With full knowledge of all of the types of curriculums, many students select a particular one because it seems most useful to them for their career interest and goals. For some students their selections may depend heavily upon available resources of time and money. Students enroll in certain programs of study because their capabilities seem to indicate that they will be successful in one program as opposed to another. Selection may also be made on the basis of recommendation or suggestion by family, physician, and friends. Finally, the student may also select a particular program because she is lacking information about other available career opportunities. For a number of students their choice will be a suitable one for both short-term and long-range goals. A significant number of students will, however, desire to make some change in their career orientation within the field of nursing or within the complex of the health professions. In an endeavor to facilitate the attainment of career goals by students, and at the same time approach the problems of health manpower, the concept of career ladders has been developed.

The development of the concept of career ladders has taken three general approaches: (1) a single career ladder encompassing all health professions; (2) multiple career ladders, identifying the mode of progression within each profession; and (3) career ladder within a profession, identifying progression in relation to level of practice, professional and technical. The interpretations of the career-ladder concept require the statement of assumptions underlying them before decisions can be made and appropriate action taken [36]. The single career-ladder concept seems to require acceptance of the assumption that all health occupations can be ordered on a single continuum of mission, purpose, content, importance, significance, difficulty, and reward. This interpretation suggests that the career ladder should permit nurses to move easily into medicine. The concept also assumes that one of the health professions represents the epitome of aspirations for those who seek careers in the broad fields of health and that at least some knowledge and skills are shared by all health workers. The single career-ladder concept seems to deny the several determinants of career choice and the motivations that lead some persons to seek careers in medicine, while others chose nursing, social work, dentistry, and the like. There are questions in the minds of the various professionals as to whether medicine should be considered to be the summit of the ladder, with other professions assuming the roles of rungs or steps toward the top position.

A second concept or interpretation of the career ladder is that there are, and always will be, several different occupations within the broad field of health. Each of these has unique and distinguishing characteristics, and within each, careers can be ordered on a continuum of mission, purpose, content, importance, significance, difficulty, and reward. This interpretation suggests that career ladders be devised to permit the practical nurse to move into professional nursing and the dental hygienist, into dentistry. The concept projects a single career ladder within each health occupation, with the most highly specialized professional representing the epitome of aspiration to those within each. This concept assumes basic differences among the several health occupations, even though it recognizes that some knowledge and skills may be shared by practitioners in all fields. It does, however, deny differences in motivation and abilities of the persons seeking preparation for different careers within any one field of work.

A third possible interpretation of the concept of career ladder is that there are now and will probably always be opportunities for many different careers that are intrinsically rewarding in each of the health occupations. These careers are of equal importance and significance, although they differ from each other in relation to the native ability needed, the nature and content of education required, and their intrinsic reward. This interpretation projects several career ladders within each of the health occupations. It also assumes basic differences among the health occupations and among professionals, technicians, and assistants in each, although it recognizes that some knowledge and skills may be shared by practitioners in all.

Basic to the concept of career ladders is the effort of nurse educators to facilitate the attainment of career goals of students in the quickest and most economical way. Inherent in this effort is the realization that some students will change their goals; therefore, programs should be flexible enough to provide for change without undue hardship to the student. No educational program is considered to be terminal to the degree that other opportunities will not be made available to a graduate of a specific program who is qualified to continue her educational endeavors. Faculties of schools of nursing offering various types of curriculum are exercising much imagination and creativity in developing means to expedite students' attainment of necessary knowledge and skills for a specific type of nursing practice. Reexamination is being made of the more traditional prerequisites, such as numbers of credits for courses and amount of time for clinical practice. More realistic approaches are being developed for the assessment and evaluation of the student's knowledge and skills for the purpose of continuous guidance and educational planning. More recently the National League for Nursing has agreed to undertake a nation-wide study to evaluate the ways nursing schools, colleges, and universities are experimenting with curriculum plans to allow students who change career goals to move rapidly from one type of program to another. The statement of this organization concerning an open curriculum indicates that this curriculum is a system that takes into account the different purposes of the various types of programs but that recognizes common areas of achievement. This system permits student mobility in the light of ability, changing career goals, and changing aspirations. This system requires clear delineation of the achievement expectations of all nursing programs, from practical nursing through graduate education. It also recognizes the possibility of mobility from other health-related fields. The open curriculum reflects an interrelated system of achievement in nursing education with open doors rather than quantitative serial steps [37].

SUMMARY

Nursing is evolving as a profession and is reflecting those characteristics that have been considered essential for full professional status. Efforts of the profession to contribute to and be a part of the total health care system are evidenced by the endeavors to define more precisely the unique role of nursing in the care of individuals and groups. The focus of nursing on direct care of patients, as opposed to medical assistance and agency administration, are salutary efforts to return nursing to its original purpose and mission. If this were not the case, nursing might eventually find it difficult to justify its existence as a health profession.

The attention to the independent functions of nursing, those that are performed without direct medical authority or sanction, is providing opportunities for nurses to study more intently the impact of nursing care on the health and well-being of people. It is extremely difficult at the moment to obtain evidence that the quality of care rendered by professionally prepared nurses makes a positive difference in the welfare of patients in the extent or rate of recovery, in constructive response to illness experience, in adapting to continuing disability, or in learned behavior that will forward optimal health. This is indeed a major concern of a profession that offers a service to society. The acceptance of care as the primary focus of nursing opens the avenues for the study of the phenomenon of care as it relates to nursing. Through informal and formal investigations, notions can be subjected to test, a priori knowledge can be validated, and more specific hypotheses can be formulated. The practice of nursing becomes theory in the making, which eventually will lead to the development of a body of knowledge called nursing. As this becomes evident, a more rational approach can be identified that will assist us in the stratification of this knowledge for the various types of nurse practitioners.

Nursing is an occupation requiring activities that can be arranged on a continuum, ranging from the elementary type of nursing tasks to the highly complex activities associated with the professional role. It is incumbent upon the profession to delineate the roles and activities of the various types of practitioners—the professional and the nurse technician—and to determine the best possible means of utilizing these practitioners in nursing care. Not only will this facilitate more efficient care and effective nursing service to patients and families, but it will also contribute to greater job satisfaction, which becomes a powerful intrinsic reward.

The educational system in nursing for preparing the different practitioners is in a state of transition. The baccalaureate program in nursing at the moment is the basic preparation for the beginning professional practitioner. Beyond that, at the graduate level are the programs of specialized study for clinical specialization, teaching, and administration. In the last decade we have experienced rapid development of curriculums in community junior-colleges for the preparation of the nurse technicians. Although the hospital diploma programs offer educational opportunities for this type of practitioner, these programs are declining in number and in the admissions of students to the programs. This transition is a manifestation of the need and desire of the profession to channel its educational programs into the mainstream of education. The nursing assistant, who performs the elementary nursing tasks, is prepared in vocational programs within the secondary schools or adult education programs.

Each of the nursing programs has specific goals and objectives and is committed to prepare a certain type of worker in nursing. Although the student makes her own career choice in relation to a particular program of study, there are instances when career goals are changed. If the student appears to possess the necessary equipment to continue her education in another type of program, opportunities should be made available. No educational program should be thought of as terminal in that the doors are closed for continued study. In the past the journey on the educational ladder in nursing has been beset with many problems and obstacles. More recently, however, nurse educators are giving serious attention to developing ways and means to expedite the movement from one level of education to another. As we view the characteristics of students as they relate to and reflect a society in rapid change, we become aware that our curriculums must be flexible and in tune with the capabilities, motivations, and aspirations of those who select a career in nursing.

REFERENCES

1. Flexner, A. Is Social Work a Profession? In *Proceedings of the National Conference of Charities and Correction*. Chicago: Hillmann, 1915. P. 576.
2. Ibid., p. 583.
3. Tyler, R. W. Distinctive attributes for the professions. *Soc. Work J.* 23:52, 1952.
4. Blauch, L. E. [Ed.]. *Education for the Professions*. Washington, D.C.: U.S. Government Printing Office, 1955. P. 1.
5. McGlothlin, W. J. *The Professional Schools*. New York: Center for Applied Research in Education, 1964. P. 6.
6. Ibid., p. 32.
7. McManus, R. L. Nurses want a chance to be professional. *Mod. Hosp.* 58:2, 1958.
8. Hughes, E. C., et al. *Twenty Thousand Nurses Tell Their Story*. Philadelphia: Lippincott, 1958.
9. American Nurses' Association. ANA board approves a definition of nursing practice. *Amer. J. Nurs.* 55:1474, 1955.
10. American Nurses' Association. ANA statement on auxiliary personnel in nursing service. *Amer. J. Nurs.* 62:72, 1962.
11. Lesnik, M. J. The board of nurse examiners and the Nurse Practice Act. *Amer. J. Nurs.* 54:1484, 1954.
12. McManus, R. L. Assumptions of functions of nursing. *Regional Planning for Nursing and Nursing Education*. New York: Teachers College Press (Columbia University), 1954. P. 54.
13. Kreuter, F. R. What is good nursing care? *Nurs. Outlook* 5:302, 1957.
14. Henderson, V. *The Nature of Nursing*. New York: Macmillan, 1966. P. 15.
15. Abdellah, F. G., et al. *Patient-Centered Approaches to Nursing*. New York: Macmillan, 1960. P. 24.
16. Ibid., p. 163.

17. Johnson, M. M., and Martin, H. W.   A sociological analysis of the nurses' role. *Amer. J. Nurs.* 53:373, 1952.
18. Schulman, S.   Basic Functional Roles in Nursing: Mother Surrogate and Healer. In E. G. Jaco [Ed.], *Patients, Physicians and Illness*. Glencoe, Ill.: Free Press, 1958. P. 530.
19. Johnson, D. E.   The significance of nursing care. *Amer. J. Nurs.* 61:64, 1961.
20. Ibid., p. 66.
21. Tschudin, M. S.   The Redefinition of Nursing: A Critical Need. In *The Shifting Scene—Foundations for Strength*. New York: National League for Nursing, 1967. P. 3.
22. Ibid., p. 4.
23. Department of Baccalaureate and Higher Degree Programs.   Statement of Position on the Primary Focus of Nursing. In *The Shifting Scene—Directions for Practice*. New York: National League for Nursing, 1967. P. 4.
24. Committee on Education.   *Position Paper: Educational Preparation for Nurse Practitioners and Assistants to Nurses*. New York: American Nurses' Association, 1965. P. 5.
25. Matheney, R. V.   Technical Nursing Practice. In *The Shifting Scene—Directions for Practice*. New York: National League for Nursing, 1967. P. 19.
26. Johnson, D. E.   Professional Practice in Nursing. In *The Shifting Scene—Directions for Practice*. New York: National League for Nursing, 1967. P. 26.
27. Brown, E. L.   *Nursing for the Future*. New York: Russell Sage Foundation, 1948.
28. Ibid., p. 77.
29. Ibid., p. 173.
30. Consultant Group on Nursing.   *Toward Quality in Nursing: Needs and Goals. Report of the Surgeon General's Consultant Group on Nursing*. Washington, D.C.: U.S. Department of Health, Education and Welfare, 1963.
31. American Nurses' Association.   American Nurses' Association's first position on education for nursing. *Amer. J. Nurs.* 65:106, 1965.
32. American Nurses' Association.   National Commission for the Study of Nursing and Nursing Education. *Amer. J. Nurs.* 70:279, 1970.
33. Ibid., p. 294.
34. Ibid., p. 287.
35. Montag, M.   *Community College Education for Nursing*. New York: McGraw-Hill, 1959.
36. Editorial.   The surgeon general looks at nursing. *Amer. J. Nurs.* 67:64, 1967.
37. Editorial.   Board approves statement on open curriculum. *N.L.N. News* 18:1, 1970.

SUPPLEMENTARY READINGS

American Nurses' Association.   Principles governing professional nursing education. *Amer. J. Nurs.* 62:56, 1962.
Boyle, R. E.   Critical issues in collegiate education. *Nurs. Outlook* 10:165, 1962.
Bridgman, M.   *Collegiate Education for Nursing*. New York: Russell Sage Foundation, 1953.

Bueschel, J. F. M. Why junior college education for nursing? *Nurs. Outlook* 4:450, 1952.

Dressel, P. L. *The Undergraduate Curriculum in Higher Education.* New York: Center for Applied Research in Education, 1963.

Ethical Standards Committee of the American Nurses' Association. Code for professional nursing. *Amer. J. Nurs.* 52:1247, 1952.

Frank, Sr., C. M., and Heidgerken, L. E. [Eds.]. *Perspectives in Nursing Education.* Washington, D.C.: Catholic University Press, 1963.

Hassenplug, L. Nursing education in universities. *Nurs. Outlook* 8:92, 1960.

Henry, N. B. *Education for the Professions.* Chicago: University of Chicago Press, 1962.

Hershey, N. The law and the nurse: Nurses medical practice problems, part I. *Amer. J. Nurs.* 62:82, 1962.

Hillway, T. *The American Two-Year College.* New York: Harper & Bros., 1958.

Landis, B. Y. *Ethical Standards and Professional Conduct.* Annals of the American Academy of Political and Social Sciences, vol. 297, 1955.

Lesnik, M. J. Nursing functions and legal control. *Amer. J. Nurs.* 53:1210, 1950.

Levine, E. Nurse manpower—yesterday, today and tomorrow. *Amer. J. Nurs.* 69: 290, 1969.

McClure, W. The challenge of vocational and technical education. *Phi Delta Kappan* 43:212, 1962.

McGrath, E. *Liberal Education and the Professions.* New York: Teachers College Bureau of Publications (Columbia University), 1959.

Mussallem, H. K. The changing role of the nurse. *Amer. J. Nurs.* 69:514, 1969.

Pfnister, A. O. The professions and education. *Nurs. Outlook* 12:28, 1964.

Roberts, M. M. *American Nursing, History and Interpretation.* New York: Macmillan, 1958.

Russell, C. *Liberal Education and Nursing.* New York: Teachers College Bureau of Publications (Columbia University), 1959.

Schwier, M. E. Junior college education and nursing education. *Junior Coll. J.* 2:88, 1955.

Stevenson, N. M. Perspectives on developments in practical nursing. *Nurs. Outlook* 8:34, 1960.

Tschudin, M. Educational preparation needed by the nurse in the future. *Nurs. Outlook* 12:32, 1964.

7 THE STUDENT AND THE CURRICULUM

THE greatly increased attention to the assessment of the students in schools and colleges can be attributed to the generally accepted purpose of the curriculum as facilitating the growth of the students. Growth of the student refers not only to academic and professional attainments but also to personal and social development. If curriculum opportunities and materials are to be developed to enhance the growth of the student, it appears obvious that we must know what the student is like before curriculum plans can be developed. Periodic assessment of selected student characteristics may provide pertinent information indicating the effectiveness of curriculum events and processes. Thus, viable sources of information that can assist the faculty in making curriculum decisions are the characteristics of the students who select and who are admitted to particular schools. The diverse characteristics of students reflect those of the general population of this country and of its social institutions.

CHARACTERISTICS OF HIGHER EDUCATION

A basic feature of American higher education has been its decentralization; groups of people have always been free to start schools and colleges in accordance with their needs and their ideas about the road to a better life. It seems that virtually every objective that could reasonably be conceived of is somewhere represented, although diversity seems to be yielding somewhat in the face of the increasing organization of our society. The objectives of higher education have their roots in the American ethos and they show a tendency to change as the American situation changes. It is characteristically American that our institutions should be as diversified as they are. They differ in respect to all the features and dimensions that describe a particular college: in size, in the quality of faculty, in standards, in curriculum offerings, in the climate of culture in the school, and in the characteristics of the student population. Although this diversity is still evident, it appears that some changes are occurring. Even though the characteristics of students within a particular school have been somewhat homogeneous among various types of schools, these characteristics have displayed considerable heterogeneity. There are indications that greater homogeneity of characteristics is occurring among the various schools and an increased heterogeneity is developing within individual schools. Some exploration of this notion seems appropriate. Schools are becoming more alike in respect to some student characteristics. However, within a particular school students are more diverse.

THE STUDENT IN AMERICAN HIGHER EDUCATION

The American formal educational system began with the cluster of New England colleges. The original purpose of these schools was religious in nature and the curriculum offered was comparable to the education for a gentleman. The schools were private and therefore catered to those who could pay the fees prescribed. Thus, the students who sought entry into these colleges came from families who were financially able to send them and who were dedicated to a specific religious persuasion. Young women did not make their appearance on the educational scene until some years later; therefore, these early schools enrolled only male students. As a response to the needs of a developing country for specialized human resources, these colleges and others that followed were forced to extend their offerings beyond the traditional liberal arts. The religious emphasis was diminished to make way for curriculum activities with occupational orientation. These changes in purpose and focus provided some diversification in the student population; however, American higher education was responsive to the needs of a relatively small segment of the growing population of this country.

The land-grant and state university movement extended educational opportunities to a larger portion of the population. Since the cost to the student of this education was minimal compared to the cost of private education, opportunities for preparation for some productive endeavors were made available to students who did not have the financial resources to attend a private school. In addition, preparation for a wide variety of occupations attracted students with varying interests and objectives. The state universities initiated the concept of democracy in education; however, at the beginning some limitations were imposed. Although some state universities admitted women from the outset, many universities continued to restrict education opportunities to young men. Employment opportunities in the work world were not extended to women except in a few occupations. Preparation for these could be obtained by apprenticeship, on-the-job training or in special institutions.

Education for women began in the separate, private, liberal arts colleges. Since the young women enrolling in college were not preparing for the world of work, these schools did not offer curriculums with occupational orientation. These women came primarily from wealthy families and their principle purpose in going to college was for personal and social development. As more occupations opened their doors to women, demands were made upon the universities to provide educational opportunities to women. Private and state universities established semi-independent women's colleges on their campuses and made provisions for limited curriculum opportunities other than the traditional liberal arts. Oberlin College in Ohio was established in the 1830's on the basis of sex equality for women and race equality for Negroes. Coeducation appeared in a few private colleges but principally in the state universities of the West.

Technical and professional education in universities expanded to include preparation for some of the newer occupational fields and attracted students mainly from the middle and upper classes who had definitive vocational goals and aspirations. The laboring groups had little opportunity for higher education of a practical sort. The preparatory education for college was in the private academy, which was not accessible to the working class. It was not until a system of public secondary education developed that the students from the lower socioeconomic groups could gain entry into higher education.

Because of inferior secondary school training and cultural issues in race relations, separate colleges and universities were established for Negroes under private and public control. These colleges traditionally enrolled greater numbers of female than male students. This was partly due to the high dropout rate of Negro boys attending high school, estimated to be between 50 and 75 percent of the total enrollment, at least one-and-a-half times as great as the rate for white boys [1]. Another factor was the tendency of Negro parents to send their daughters to a college when a choice had to be made. A study reported in 1965 indicated that there were more than 122 women to every 100 men in Negro educational institutions as opposed to 67 women to every 100 men in institutions of higher learning in general [2]. The curriculums of these schools emphasized training in professional and vocational areas and offered limited opportunities for study in the liberal arts disciplines. Perhaps the explanation for the vocational orientation of the curriculum in the typical Negro college was the traditional dependence of the Negro on employment in highly restricted occupations. The struggle that Negroes have waged for acceptance in trades and professions formerly closed to them has been long and arduous, and only a partial victory has been won so far.

The nineteenth century witnessed the beginning of the democratic experiment in higher education. No other country tried to establish so many institutions of higher education. Almost every religious denomination was active in founding colleges as a means of spreading their religious doctrines as well as providing a general education for the youth of the land. The state university movement accelerated to meet the democratic demands for public higher education and became a great force in American higher education by the end of the century. Private colleges and universities broadened their fields of study to attract the intellectually and financially elite. The individual institutions of higher education were thought of as possessing a particular climate or culture, probably because of the many common characteristics of the students attending a particular college. Among the various colleges and universities considerable diversity in student characteristics were noted.

The twentieth century is endeavoring to cope with the problems of how to educate everyone. The momentum is too great to attempt to avoid the issue. For centuries the test of admissibility to various levels of an educational system and the standard by which progress through the system was measured was set up by the system itself. The word of the system was taken about qualifications for entrance, about graduation, and about the curriculum.

Robert Hutchins has noted that "if everybody is to go to school, some school must welcome them. If everybody is to be educated, the school must in some manner hold on to and interest him. As the notion spreads that education is the key and the only one, to a useful and productive life, discrimination among students must break down, for who can be denied the chance to become useful and productive" [3].

THE CHANGING CHARACTER OF AMERICAN HIGHER EDUCATION

The brief review of the student in American higher education seems to indicate that education beyond the secondary school has been a privilege which has been accorded selected individuals. The conviction in former years that only the selected few could be educated must be attributed to social, political, and economic conditions, not to the incapacity of men of any color, race, nationality, social status, or background. It came to be taken for granted that education, like leisure, was the privilege of the few, and this was justified by arguing that only the few had the ability to profit by it.

Colleges and universities across the land established the machinery within these schools to insure that students possessing certain characteristics and qualities were admitted to certain schools. More frequently than not these characteristics and qualities had little to do with the student's ability or his motivation to learn. Family status, financial ability, racial, religious, and sex characteristics seemed to be, in many instances, major determinants of who went to what school. When the pressure for universal schooling began to be irresistible, bulwarks were thrown up against the incoming flood. Secondary schools participated in the screening process by utilizing a variety of procedures and devices to shunt off those who were regarded as "academically inferior" into occupationally oriented curriculums.

It is very likely that prospective students perceive the nature and purpose of higher education differently from those who manage or teach in these institutions. The pathways to becoming more useful and productive are many and varied and depend upon individual talents, motivations, and goals. What constitutes a better life for one individual may not be valued to the same degree by another. Those who believe that formal education will enable them to become more useful and productive should be entitled to receive the appropriate education. This does not mean that everybody must be educated in the same way, at the same rate, or to the same extent. It does mean, however, that education has become a right of every individual rather than a privilege for a few.

The concept of an equal educational opportunity for all has precipitated some changes in the character of American higher education. The implementation of this concept by institutions, steeped in the traditions of a culture, that have become ineffective and inefficient has caused confusion, frustration, and disillusionment among faculty, students, and administration. During the 1960's, when social and scientific innovations were touching the lives of practically all human and social endeavors, the tide of reform began to sweep away the structure of educational institutions that had been painfully erected over the centuries. These changes have had a direct impact upon the nature and characteristics of the student population in colleges and universities. The major focus of the changes have been directed toward curriculum offerings and patterns, policies pertaining to admission, enrollment, transfer, and graduation, and special institutional arrangements.

CURRICULUM OFFERINGS

Colleges and universities have extended their curriculum offerings to a wide array of scientific and professional fields that are demanded by society. These diversified curriculums have attracted students, graduate and undergraduate, with highly specialized career goals. At the same time, many institutions have attempted to strengthen the liberal arts studies to provide the balance needed in an environment of specialization. The attention to and extension of these curriculums provide opportunities for the student with cultural and social interests and abilities.

The responsibility of the university to assist those employed in technical, semiprofessional, and professional activities to keep abreast of new knowledge is manifest in the continuing and adult education programs offered by the universities. The student who seeks these opportunities is probably older, has had some years of work experience, and desires new knowledge in specialized areas.

The liberal arts colleges, which at one time enrolled students who had no definite career goals, have developed occupationally oriented curriculums. Among the many occupational areas included in the college offerings are teaching, nursing, business administration, and physical therapy. Some of these schools have also developed graduate programs in specialized areas. Concern has been expressed that these colleges are beginning to take on the characteristics of professional schools.

At the same time that the liberal arts colleges are becoming more professionally oriented, the independent professional school is becoming more liberal. Teachers' colleges, which were the outgrowth of the normal schools, are beginning to resemble in a limited fashion the undergraduate division of the university. The single professional focus of the teachers' colleges has given way to curriculums preparing for a variety of occupations and including substantial offerings in the liberal arts and sciences. Since both the liberal arts colleges and the successor to the teachers' colleges are multipurpose in nature, they attract students with a wide range of interests, abilities, and career aspirations.

Junior colleges are rapidly developing semiprofessional and technical curriculums in such fields as engineering, business, agriculture, teaching, and health. A president of a junior college in a large eastern city informed the writer that his college is offering curriculums for forty different health occupations. In addition to these terminal programs, the junior colleges offer the sequence of liberal arts and sciences comparable to the lower division studies in a four-year college.

In addition to the various formal educational programs that terminate with a degree being granted, almost all of these institutions offer opportunities to those not seeking organized study activities. Opportunities for personal and social enrichment for citizens in the community are frequently available in such areas as art, literature, music, drama, politics, and finance. These activities might be considered as leisure-time or intellectual hobbies for adults and frequently for those who have retired from gainful employment.

The expansion of curriculums and educational opportunities by colleges and universities have brought to all of the campuses students with diverse interests, abilities, and goals for a useful and productive life. At one time the institutions had single but different purposes and attracted students with compatible purposes. More recently the diverse offerings in all institutions has encouraged a heterogeneous student population in all colleges and universities.

ENROLLMENT, GRADUATION, AND TRANSFER POLICIES

The policies and practices pertaining to admission, transfer, and graduation of students that have been devised by the system of higher education and have become a part of that system are being subjected to serious review. The question raised is, Are these policies exercised for the good of the students or are they administered to perpetuate a system which may or may not be effective and efficient in contemporary society? The changes that have taken place lead one to believe that efforts are being directed to provide a learning climate and processes which are more compatible with the characteristics of present-day youth.

ADMISSION POLICIES. The environment of colleges and universities across the country is rapidly changing in relation to sex characteristics. Schools are abandoning or are considering the abandonment of the one-sex education system. The long tradition of male education at universities such as Harvard, Yale, and Princeton is being relegated to the history of higher education. There has been a steady and rapid development of coeducation in many of the formerly all-male schools. Likewise, women's colleges are beginning to open their campuses to men. Although the move toward coeducation has not been as rapid in the traditional women's colleges as in the men's schools, men are visible in the classrooms at Vassar, Bennington, and other formerly all-women schools.

Those observing this phenomenon, which is indeed changing the character of American higher education, see several reasons for this widespread shift to coeducation. The major causes for this activity can be grouped under two categories: (1) pressure from students, and (2) competition to get quality students. Students, faculty, and family believe the co-ed campus is a more natural environment for young people. They believe that coeducation is more full and meaningful and encourages healthier relationships in daily living. From the point of view of school administration, the possibility of a quality school losing its quality students is a real one. One college official indicated that any college remaining all male is working with a decreasing number of students. Although schools are not faced with a choice between coeducation or closing their doors, they do anticipate an economic bind. The successful adventures of the coordinate women's colleges in the male universities (Harvard-Radcliffe, Columbia-Barnard, Brown-Pembroke) in sharing faculty, curriculum, and extracurricular activities give support to the concept of coeducation. The need to attract quality students and the rather tardy realization that both sexes provide a natural educational climate are the direct forces in the movement for coeducation. In addition, an indirect force is the mood of young people today, an attitude that demands involvement in the activities of the school and society and that prohibits interference with individual codes of politics and sex. This activity has been virtually restricted to the Northeast because other areas of the country either had never started one-sex schools or had abandoned them as financial mistakes after the growth of the land-grant movement and state college.

ENROLLMENT POLICIES. Higher education began at a time when formal education at the secondary level did not exist, and college education was not necessary for most occupations. Young boys attending the early colleges received preparatory education in the private academies or through tutors. It was not at all uncommon for boys to be admitted to colleges at the ages of thirteen or fourteen. As all social endeavors became more complex, formal education at the secondary or postsecondary school levels was required for preparation for new and developing occupations. For those who had the necessary personal and financial resources, the usual educational progression was college enrollment immediately upon completion of high school. This is not to say that no students delayed college admission; the majority, however, continued their educational pursuits without a break in the educational years. Thus, students attending college have more typically fallen into the 17–21-year-old age group.

Students entering schools of nursing during the same era displayed somewhat different age characteristics. Records of students seem to indicate that women did not usually engage in this type of education until later in life. Social limitations of young women restricted their mobility from the family, and it was not unusual for these women to delay educational opportunities in nursing until they were approaching their late twenties. Changes in social norms of behavior of women and the rapid development of occupational and educational opportunities in nursing have brought students to schools of nursing at a much younger age.

The rapid technological innovations in this country became obvious to veterans of World War II when they returned to a world of work that was vastly different from the one they left upon entering military service. The retraining needs of the GI's in a variety of occupational fields made necessary the provision of educational programs for this purpose on all levels. This was true also for military nurses who returned to a civilian practice that was reflecting scientific and technological changes. Through the assistance of federal funds, veterans were offered the opportunity to attend colleges and universities to prepare for occupations of their choice. These young men and women had probably served three to four years in military service, and during this time many of them had acquired a spouse and in some instances had young children. Not only were the veterans older than the typical college students, but they also had family responsibilities. Initially colleges and universities viewed with much concern the assimilation of these men and women into school environments. Fears were expressed that because they were older and had major family responsibilities, these students would not have the necessary energy and motivation to complete their programs of study. Experience of schools enrolling the veterans has demonstrated positive outcomes. For the most part the GI's have been serious, conscientious, and highly motivated students. They have taken their share of honors at graduation, and their names have been conspicuous on the deans' lists. The veterans of military service continue to contribute to the variability of the characteristics of student populations in many schools and colleges.

The favorable experiences of veterans in higher education precipitated interest in and development of educational activities for adults. These have taken a variety of forms and include basic general college preparation for older students who have not previously had the time or money to engage in regular full-time educational programs. The opportunities for schooling offered in late afternoon and evening made it possible for the mature student to continue in his job and at the same time participate in formal education. Basic education has been extended to include specialized training for the adult student who wishes to gain new knowledge in his field of specialization or who wants to prepare himself for a different occupational endeavor. Finally, as a response to society's need to provide useful intellectual activities for persons who have retired from gainful employment, colleges and universities offer a vast array of educational opportunities for citizens of the community who have passed the age of sixty-five. The liberalization of admission policies that were at one time directed solely to the 17–21-year-old age group have brought to the college campus students of varying ages. Thus, students in higher education today form a heterogeneous age group, ranging from adolescence to advanced age.

Attention by schools to the interests, abilities, and motivations of young people has prompted the relaxation of the admission requirement of high school graduation. Academic acceleration of intellectually and socially able students has been formalized among some secondary schools and colleges to enable these students to enter college before completing all high school requirements. Through specially designed programs, many high school students who have completed their sophomore or junior year are admitted into the freshman class at a number of colleges and universities. Students who possess the necessary abilities to participate in these programs enter and graduate from college at a much earlier age. Surveys of the performance of these students while in college and after completing their programs of study seem to indicate that the majority are entirely successful in their academic achievements. Not only do they qualify for the honor awards in scholarship, but they also demonstrate leadership skills in organizational activities. In comparing these students with others within the same college, it appears these talented young people are equally successful in obtaining marriage partners and have assumed the responsibilities of parenthood. It is acknowledged, however, that advanced standing is planned for selected students.

GRADUATION POLICIES.   Institutions of higher education have not only endeavored to accelerate students' progression from high school to college but have also initiated policies directed toward expediting students' attainment of necessary educational requirements for graduation. The development of activities to implement these policies is based upon several assumptions which indicate that (1) people can and do acquire learning at the college level in nontraditional ways, (2) institutions of higher education must be concerned with what an individual knows, not with how many hours he has sat in class or the number of credits he has amassed, and (3) nontraditional learning can be measured and compared with learning acquired by traditional students [4].

Although there has been some reluctance to grant credit for a course on the basis of examinations that have been developed internally, institutions of higher education have accepted the concept of granting credit by examination. External examination programs have been used by collegiate institutions for awarding credit in a variety of fields. In institutions where these examinations have been used, the performance of certain groups of students and of armed forces personnel gives support for the validity of the tests as a measure of academic achievement. Positive experiences with the use of general achievement examinations led to the development and use of examinations in various specific subjects that are designed to assess a student's overall mastery of the subject and to compare his grasp of the information, ideas, and skills with those normally expected of students who successfully complete the course [5].

Nursing education has gained some experience in the use of examinations for the purpose of granting credit for nursing courses in the undergraduate curriculum. These examinations have been designed for the graduates of hospital diploma and associate degree programs in nursing who want to work for a baccalaureate degree in nursing. In the one instance the registered nurse attains her clinical education in a noneducational institution. The graduate of the associate degree program, however, attains her clinical education in an educational institution, but the placement of this instruction is on a lower collegiate level than that in a baccalaureate program. Clinical courses in nursing in community junior-colleges are offered during the freshman and sophomore years, and in the baccalaureate curriculum they are scheduled primarily during the junior and senior years.

When a practitioner wishes to move from one type of practice (technical) to another (professional), some assessment of her clinical knowledge must be made for the purpose of curriculum planning. To assess the knowledge of the student in certain clinical nursing courses, externally prepared examinations in specific nursing courses have been and are presently being used. The manner in which credit allocation is made varies among institutions. In some instances blanket credits are given for successful completion of the battery of tests. Or credit allocation may be made on the basis of satisfactory performance on individual tests within the battery and in line with the numbers of credits assigned to the comparable course in the curriculum. More recently schools of nursing began using internally developed tests in clinical nursing. Examinations of this nature are designed to measure the competencies of the student who has completed the specific nursing course in the undergraduate curriculum. Successful performance of the graduate nurse on the tests covering specific nursing courses enables her to obtain the credits that are assigned to these courses. These "challenge" examinations are usually scheduled when the registered nurse has acquired the appropriate prerequisite knowledge.

The use of achievement examinations in the general and specific subject areas enables students to meet the requirements of these academic programs in other ways than the traditional manner. In this way colleges may recognize that knowledge and skills can be attained in diverse activities. In responding to the needs of able and ambitious young people, colleges and universities enable young people to proceed through their educational program and accomplish their goals in considerably less time than the traditional educational pathways allow.

REMEDIAL ACTIVITIES. Institutions of higher education are presently endeavoring to make available educational opportunities to students who have not previously been admissible to college. One of the criteria for admission to colleges and universities is the requirement of satisfactory performance on certain scholastic aptitude tests. These tests include measures of verbal (qualitative) and mathematical (quantitative) skills. The level of performance considered to be satisfactory is determined by the individual school. The various tests used for this purpose are prepared by testing companies such as the American College Testing Service and the College Entrance Examination Board. Individual tests are developed by subject-matter specialists and psychologists. The language of these tests reflect what might be called the middle-class urban American culture. Psychologists have alerted test users that the tests do have a cultural orientation that might induce a handicap for some students.

Recently colleges and universities have become aware of the reality of this culture bias. Efforts to assist students from minority and low-income groups to engage in higher education activities have revealed the difficulty these students have in achieving passing scores on the tests. Responding to this problem, the College Entrance Examination Board has recommended to colleges and universities that these tests not be used for the selection of minority or low-income students. The Board indicates that the test scores tend to discriminate against these students, who have potential for achievement in higher education. The College Entrance Examination Board further indicates that when these tests are utilized, they should be used only after admission decisions are made, and then for research and diagnostic purposes only [6].

Students who are considered to be culturally deprived are being admitted to colleges and universities without the usual admission prerequisites. Efforts are exerted by the faculties to diagnose the areas of weakness or limitations in these students' academic backgrounds. Remedial programs are in effect to bring these students up to the level whereby they may profit by and enjoy ongoing curriculum activities. In past years these students would have been screened out during the admission review or would have been eliminated from the college because of their inability to tolerate the prescribed academic experiences [7]. Reports of a few systematic study projects in nursing education are providing some useful information for nurse educators. Success of students in the remedial programs and in the nursing curriculum are noted. By means of these policies and activities, students from minority and culturally deprived groups are now visible among the student population.

TRANSFER OPPORTUNITIES. The rapid growth of diverse occupational activities, the educational preparation for these activities, and the high degree of mobility of all persons has centered attention on the concept of the transfer student. The development of community junior-colleges has also increased the movement of students from one school to another. For some colleges, the transfer student creates discontinuities in an otherwise orderly process. But there is every reason to believe that the nature of our society will continue to support the migration of many students which generates many of the transfers among various educational institutions.

The philosophy of community junior-college education implies that these colleges will offer academic opportunities comparable to those offered in the first two years of a four-year college. Students who enroll in the transfer curriculum of the community junior-college will proceed to the senior college or university for specialized areas of study.

For many students career goals are not well crystallized when they enter college. During the initial college years, some students may change their occupational decisions or may become more certain of their educational goals. In some instances these students may find that the college they are attending does not offer the necessary preparation for a particular occupation. A transfer to a college that has the desired offerings is indicated.

The geographical mobility of people in this country is demonstrated vividly in the number of times the family changes its place of residence. When families move from one location to another, the college-bound children may be required to change colleges primarily for financial reasons. On occasion financial reverses in the family may force the offspring to transfer to a college less costly to the student.

Not all colleges encourage the transfer student. Although private institutions are not prone to reject transfer applicants, the percentage of matriculating students who are transfers is smaller in private than in public institutions. Even though many colleges do not have definite policies that discourage the transfer from one college to another, the nature and structure of the curriculum may present barriers to transfers. Curriculums that focus on specialized fields of study during the early college years (freshman and sophomore) make it difficult for students to proceed with their studies in other colleges without considerable time and effort spent in making up necessary requirements. Nursing curriculums at the baccalaureate level generally have not facilitated transfer of students into or out of the programs of study. Ideas relating to structure and sequence of learning opportunities as described in the curriculums, whereby considerable clinical education is offered on the lower division level, have direct influence on the possibility and desirability of transfer.

Responding to the needs of students who wish to transfer to other schools, some schools of nursing are making appropriate curriculum revisions. Placing the curriculum offerings for specialized occupational preparation on the upper division level allows students to make changes in career goals and appropriate schools to pursue these goals during their freshman and sophomore years with little academic hardship to them. In one particular school of nursing the enrollment in one division of the baccalaureate program is comprised of approximately 90 to 95 percent transfer students. The University of Maryland School of Nursing–Walter Reed Army Medical Center Division admits students into the junior year who transfer after two years of study in other colleges. The approximately 100 students who enter this program as juniors transfer from over eighty different colleges.

Recent surveys indicate that the percentage of transfers among new students at four-year colleges is increasing. Data from this sample of colleges indicate that newly enrolled transfers increased about 50 percent from 1961 to 1966. Colleges participating in this survey estimated that during the next four years transfers will increase by 75 percent [8]. The geographical mobility of the population in general is reflected in the movement of students from one college to another. It is likely that colleges which do not encourage or accept transfer students may be limiting their potential resources. It is obvious that transfer students are altering the once stable college environment to one which displays students on the move.

COOPERATIVE INSTITUTIONAL ARRANGEMENTS

The rapidly increasing college enrollments are placing heavy drains on all school facilities and resources. The need to maintain an adequate faculty in quantity and quality is ever present in all institutions. The demand for physical facilities is far greater than the ability to supply them. This is true no less in nursing where human and clinical resources are being taxed to the limits of tolerance.

In an effort to utilize all resources to a maximum without unnecessary duplication, schools of nursing have participated in cooperative instructional activities and continue to do so. This means that students from one school can enroll in another school of nursing for specific curricular activities. The duration of the student's experience is relatively short, and the students may be thought of at that time as transients. Because of the specific nature of this arrangement and the circumscribed time allotted for this experience, the participating students frequently do not truly become a part of the school environment. Opportunities for leadership and extracurricular activities are limited; however, these students do bring to the school environment a bit of another culture, which is frequently refreshing and stimulating.

The activities of the regional education groups through regional education associations (Southern Regional Educational Board and Western Interstate Commission on Higher Education) have facilitated the movement of students from one part of the country to another to pursue education of a specialized nature. The efforts of institutions of higher education within a region to make specialized education available to students within that region are directed toward minimizing duplication of resources, such as faculty and facilities, and reducing the costs of the education to the student. The initial activity of nursing in this endeavor was the project in graduate education sponsored by the Southern Regional Education Board. Graduate nurses in fourteen southern states were offered opportunities to enroll for graduate study in nursing in that region [9].

An additional effort on the part of institutions of higher education to serve a larger group of students is the formation of the consortium of universities. Students enrolled in any one of the member universities have access to courses offered by the other universities in the consortium with full credit and with little administrative regulations. This arrangement facilitates the student's progress through his program and contributes to the mobility of students from one institution to another.

The relaxation of some of the requirements of the religious orders makes it possible for members of these communities to attend schools other than those under religious auspices. It is not uncommon today to observe many nuns and priests pursuing programs of study in state universities. The cost of the education to the student or the religious community may be less, and the school may be more accessible than one under religious control. These students have become conspicuous among other students on the college campus.

The review and revision of administrative policies and curriculum offerings in colleges and universities reflects a changing orientation of higher education in this country. Although the concept is not fully attained, education is considered to be a right rather than a privilege. The purposes of formal education are focused to a greater degree on the individual needs of students in a changing society. The climate of many schools is reflecting the diverse characteristics of American people.

THE ASSESSMENT OF THE CHARACTERISTICS OF STUDENTS

A prevailing theory is that a relevant curriculum should give attention both to the growth of the person and to the building of a better society, neither of which can be sought in isolation from the other. In previous chapters mention has been made of the changing characteristics of twentieth-century America and of the resulting implication for the provision of health care to the people of this nation. Some direction for nursing practice can be inferred from the contribution of these practitioners to the improvement of society through more adequate health care. In response to society's needs for human resources to make this country a better place to live in, educational institutions have made some radical departures from their previous life styles. To accommodate society's demand for specialized manpower on the one hand and to adapt to the needs and desires of students' for educational opportunities on the other, schools on all levels of the educational ladder have altered their administrative procedures and curriculum offerings. As a result of these changes, we have within our colleges and universities populations of students displaying diverse characteristics. Since the major function of the curriculum is to facilitate the growth of the student in certain predetermined ways, assessment of the student in relation to selected characteristics seems desirable.

Assessment of the characteristics of students is done with specific purposes in mind. The data obtained provide teachers and others with useful information that can be utilized in the development of a school environment responsive to the needs of students. This pertains primarily to the nature of the curriculum offerings; however, attention to the personnel services to students is implied. The development and organization of student personnel services in relation to housing, finances, counseling, and social living appears to have been an outgrowth of the movement within higher education to make appropriate educational opportunities available to greater numbers of students. Gathering information about students in a systematic way is an integral part of doing a good job of teaching, developing curriculum, advising and counseling, and institutional planning. The content of the information obtained may reflect whatever is of local concern to students, teachers, and the institution in general. The range of student differences among colleges in almost any characteristic emphasizes the need for greater congruence between institutional planning and student potential for learning, growth, and achievement.

INSTITUTIONAL ASSESSMENT

The procedures and devices utilized for the assessment of student characteristics may vary among institutions. Whatever the procedure that is deemed appropriate for a particular school, the seriousness of intent will be a major factor in determining the usefulness of the information revealed. A description of the efforts of one large university to identify the demographic characteristics of students follows. There is no intent to suggest that theirs is the best or only way to proceed toward the goal. The activities of this university in gathering data about students has provided a means for identifying their characteristics and the instrument utilized is adaptable to changes in the environment of the college. The continued use of the instrument with modifications over a ten-year period of time has given the school a chronological perspective of student characteristics.

The original instrument, University Student Census, was developed by cooperative activities of faculty members, student personnel workers, and some academic deans. Each year, when freshman students come to the campus during the summer for orientation, the census is administered. For the older students who are returning to the University, the census is administered throughout registration week at the beginning of the fall term. As a result, approximately 95 percent of the full-time undergraduate students complete the census questionnaire.

The information obtained about students is used in several ways. Of major importance are the research studies that make use of the data. An example may be studies of the characteristics of students who encounter disciplinary difficulties. Another important use of the census material is in the counseling work with students in the counseling center. Information obtained by means of the census can give the counselor considerable information about the student, which may be useful in the counseling process. The teachers in the various schools and colleges can identify in what ways the students in a specific college may be like or different from the students in other colleges of the university. Certain questions on the census are directed to obtaining information that is useful in curriculum and instruction. Studies of the validity and reliability of the instrument have been made and, in instances where certain questions lend themselves to this type of analysis, they have been found to be reliable and valid.

The characteristics of the students in the school of nursing revealed by the census have implications for curriculum. A theory is held by many educators that, with more college experience, students gain broader and broader knowledge. There is some evidence, however, to suggest that many students become more deeply involved in specific behavior patterns and do not necessarily get more broadly knowledgeable over time. The data from this survey seemed to support the latter notion. The students responding to this questionnaire gave indication that they were not aware of the broad educational and cultural resources and opportunities which were available to them.

The relationship between the student and his advisor is an important one. The growth of the student in various educational directions—academic, social, cultural, and personal—may be dependent upon a skillful and interested advisor. The nursing students were among some 30,000 students enrolled on this campus, and one might wonder about the possibility and probability of an effective student-advisor relationship. The majority of these students indicated that their advisors were both knowledgeable and interested in them. This favorable response is surprising in view of recent concerns of students in higher education about the lack of adequate communication, and the negative responses warrant further analysis and exploration. The role of the teacher in guiding the instructional process is an essential one if effective learning is to take place. One would assume that in a university of this size the relationships between teachers and students would be casual if not distant. More than half of the nursing students indicated that they were well acquainted with two or more of their instructors. Although this response reflects favorably upon the educational climate, the lack of student-teacher relationships of other respondents is a major concern to the school in relation to its cause and its effect on the growth of the student.

The characteristics of the nursing students revealed by the census indicated that a large majority had serious concerns about academic survival. The preoccupation of these students with the issues òf competition relates to their adequacy of educational skills, such as reading and study skills. A large percentage of their learning was crammed rather than systematic. What we know about learning and the eventual loss of crammed knowledge suggests implications for curriculum planning in nursing. We do expect students to come to the clinical portion of the curriculum with some basic scientific concepts and principles. If these are lacking, and from this information it appears that they may be, some modification in curriculum activities and procedures is indicated.

Nursing students in this university appeared to have some unique characteristics in relation to students in other colleges. Nursing students indicated a clearly fixed vocational goal, and the goal was decided upon much earlier in the student's life. The educational career plans of nursing students appeared to have considerably longer history than did the career plans of their peers in other colleges of the university. Again, the most important factor in choice of a career was notably different between nursing students and other college students. Being of help to others was more important to nursing students than security, money, or working conditions, which were factors influencing career choices of other students [10].

The general implication of systematic data-gathering is that it produces powerful knowledge for the people who gather the data. This knowledge can be put to very constructive use in institutional planning, in research, and in counseling and advising services with students. The census-type procedure described is a means of better understanding students. It is also a tangible means by which an institution can indicate that it cares about students' attitudes and characteristics. Systematic understanding of students is relevant to curriculum development and instructional planning.

COMPREHENSIVE ASSESSMENT

The increasing interest in higher education, by the general public and by the prospective college student in particular, has emphasized the need for comprehensive information about the typical college student and about the variations between students of different institutions. The changing character of higher education and the results of studies of college students have indicated that American colleges attract extremely diverse groups. Earlier surveys and assessments reported great student differences in educational and vocational goals, interests, potential for academic work, attitudes, and values. A recent study attempted to obtain a more complete account of the typical American college student and the variations in characteristics among students from college to college. The American College Survey was a comprehensive assessment of 12,432 college freshmen in thirty-one institutions [11]. In addition to its descriptive value, the survey enabled participating institutions to receive extensive information about their freshman class, which could be utilized in reexamining admissions and educational programs. The American College Survey also provided basic information for coordinated scientific studies in the areas of achievement, careers and curriculums, student growth and development, institutional climates, and conservation of student potentials.

The thirty-one colleges in the survey included junior colleges, four-year undergraduate colleges, and universities. The geographic locations of these schools were representative of diverse regions of the country. Their enrollments varied from what might be considered a small college (272) to a relatively large institution (17,394). The majority of the colleges were coeducational. The American College Survey was administered to freshman students (6,289 men and 6,143 women) in 1964. The specific findings of the survey revealed the diversity in the various characteristics of college freshmen.

The student choices of careers indicated that men showed more diversity in their selections than women did. Whereas men chose engineering, education, and business fields, women demonstrated a preference for various careers in education. Economic aspirations of both sexes were high, but men expected to earn a higher income than women. The educational aspirations of the freshmen students implied that women have lower educational aspirations than men. In relation to the popular life goals and aspirations, the typical freshman was concerned with his interpersonal relations, his personal comfort, and his acquisition of a meaningful orientation to the world. Information pertaining to the marital or dating status of freshmen showed that there was a greater degree of pairing off than in earlier studies. Such a trend toward early psychosexual involvement might mean that the acquisition of the usual educational goals of intellectualism, breadth of interest, and experience and competency would be lessened because of the student's intense relationship with another person.

Students appeared to think of themselves as practical and realistic persons. They tended to prefer carefully organized assignments instead of independent reports and papers. Less than half of the students believed that the classroom or laboratory was the place where one was most likely to encounter important ideas. These students tended to reject one or more of our civil liberties and believed that it was necessary to restrict the freedom of certain political groups. The women students in this survey appeared to have a greater need for church affiliation than did men. The differences among special interests between men and women were noted. Women were characterized by social interests, creativity in the expressive arts, and homemaking competencies. Men were characterized by their interests in scientific and technical operations, scientific achievements, and athletic competencies.

The survey described the differences of student characteristics across colleges. The data obtained are useful because of their implications for admission practice, choice of a college, institutional planning, and evaluation of institutional impact. Some striking differences appeared in the attitudes of women students enrolled in junior- and four-year colleges about attending college. A far greater percent of women in junior colleges than of those in four-year institutions felt that going to college was important in preparing for a career. Following a formal religious code was considered essential for men in junior colleges; however, men in four-year colleges did not find this important to them. Developing a meaningful philosophy of life was consistently more important for women than men in the three types of institutions. It was of least importance for men in junior colleges, but it became greater in importance in four-year colleges and universities.

The economic aspirations of men and women in junior colleges were somewhat less than the aspirations of those in four-year colleges and universities. The men enrolled in all types of institutions indicated higher economic aspirations than did women. The educational aspirations of students demonstrated that a far greater percent of those enrolled in universities aspired to the highest educational preparation (doctoral degree). The differences between men and women in the various colleges revealed that women had lower educational aspirations than men, and the women in four-year colleges revealed less aspiration for completing doctoral study than did those in other types of educational institutions.

The American College Survey contains numerous scales to assess a student's interests, potential for various kinds of achievement, attitudes, and other orientations. The Vocational Preference Inventory was used here to interpret vocational interests. The Potential Achievement Scales were used for the prediction of extracurricular achievement, and the Extracurricular Achievement Record indicated the extracurricular accomplishments during the high-school years. The Preconscious Activity Scale was interpreted as an originality measure, especially in the fields of art, literature, and music. The Range of Competence Scale measured those activities in which the students could do well or competently within such areas of competency as scientific, technical, athletic, governmental, homemaking, and social areas. The Student Orientation Survey was interpreted to assess the student's orientation in matters academic (intellectual concerns), collegiate (social and extracurricular life), vocational (preparation for the world of work), and nonconformist (involvement in the world of art, literature, and politics). The utilization of these scales in the survey provided descriptive information portraying the differences between students in the junior college, the four-year college, and the university in these characteristics.

The Vocational Preference Inventory revealed the vocational interests of men in junior college as being primarily conventional (clerical occupations) and those of women as enterprising (supervising and sales occupations). The students enrolled in state universities displayed realistic vocational interests (technical and skilled trades) for women and conventional interests for men. Artistic (musical, artistic, and literary occupations) vocational interests characterize men and women in four-year colleges.

The scales used to determine the differences in achievement and originality revealed a high measure of musical potential among men and artistic potential among women in junior colleges. In state universities, men and women displayed high musical potential; however, women also demonstrated high musical achievement. Students in four-year colleges, men and women, revealed high literary achievement.

The scales used to determine competency, or those things the students could do well, also revealed some variations among the schools. Women enrolled in junior colleges displayed competencies in business and clerical activities, while men revealed competencies in government and social studies. In state universities women indicated competencies in technical work, and men recorded competencies in scientific endeavors. Both men and women in four-year colleges showed foreign language competencies.

On the scale to determine the student's orientation, men and women in junior colleges revealed a vocational orientation. In state universities men displayed a vocational orientation, and women, a collegiate orientation. Students in four-year colleges, male and female, exhibited the nonconformist type of orientation.

The results of the American College Survey extend our knowledge of the diversity among college students. The implications of this study seem to indicate that not only is there a college for almost any level of intellectual capacity but also there is a college for many configurations of attitudes, outlooks, personality traits, interests, and goals. The present information suggests that students differ relatively little from college to college in about half the variables and that colleges differ a great deal in the other half of the descriptive variables. The extreme variation for a limited number of variables may represent an outcome of current admission policies and practices. The descriptive scales showing little variation among colleges may represent the student qualities that are generally neglected in admissions, such as artistic accomplishments, interpersonal competency, and dramatic arts potential. Since students are different in almost any characteristic, the selection and rejection of applicants is a powerful and pervasive tool for shaping the character of a student body. Colleges by relatively simple methods can modify the nature of their entering classes. The admissions process is then not only a powerful process through which it is possible to raise or lower the intellectual level of a student body, but it is also a process through which a college can obtain various combinations of student values, personalities, interests, and goals.

Our knowledge of student characteristics may have its greatest value when it is applied to the teaching process and to the development and revision of curriculum. The diverse student groups have great differences in potentials, goals, interests, and values. Such differences imply great variations in response to teaching methods. Information about students can be employed to learn what student traits can be exploited to facilitate the student's learning and to establish some goals for his personal development. We have just begun to explore the potential applications of this new knowledge.

IMPACT OF COLLEGE UPON STUDENTS

Although it is sometimes asserted that attitudes and values are instilled early in life and are most easily modified in infancy and adolescence, curriculum planning in our colleges and universities assumes that attitudes and values are still modifiable at age 17–21 or older. If we defined education in its broadest sense, we might expect that there would be a change or reinforcement of certain ideals, beliefs, and interests of students from their freshman to senior year. Contradictory evidence has been presented regarding the impact of the college on student attitudes and values. College students have been described by those who have assembled great quantities of evidence about them as coming to college, performing the tasks required of them, and passing through and out into their individual lives, having little felt the impact of values and ideals of the liberal education they presumably came there to get. Students appear to create a private world that exists alongside and largely independent of the academic world of the college.

One of the reasons it is immensely difficult to know what makes education important to the life of a student is precisely that it is inseparably bound up with his personal needs and with the pressures of the world he lives in, either on or off the campus. One of the early studies that endeavored to determine change in students' basic values was done by Newcomb at Bennington College [12]. This study and similar ones which followed seemed to indicate that students' activities and values do indeed change.

During the past decade research concerning the impact of colleges on students focused attention on different aspects of the college environment. One of the most prominent works on the topic of changes in attitudes and values during college years has been Jacob's study of the changing values of college students. This investigator reported that students regarded vocational preparation, skills, and experience in social relations as the greatest benefits of college education. His study did not discern significant changes in student values that could be attributed directly to either the character of the curriculum or to the basic courses in social science, which students take as part of their general education. Jacob went on to report that there were few significant changes in values during the college years and that the changes among the few that could be noted were in the direction of greater conformity [13]. The results of this study seemed to indicate that expertise of the instructor or the particular teaching approaches or methods used appear to have little influence on the changes in the values of the student.

There is a theory expressed by some investigators that the change in values may be due to peer-group influences rather than to the college environment at large. As the student population becomes less homogeneous, it is likely that a student can find a group in which he can share his college experience. It is suggested that it is this group that contributes to the change or reinforcement of attitudes and values. At the time these studies were made, the students' living arrangements provided a single source of daily contact. Peer-group influence is almost certain to be enhanced, since there is considerable overlap between membership in formal college units and in living units.

Some theoretical formulations have been suggested by Newcomb, which are based upon research in the area of group behavior. Basic assumptions applicable here indicate that if people want and need other people, then their responses to educators are potentially rewarding or punishing. Group members develop sets of consensual expectations about each other. Such consensual expectations about each other's behavior are known as norms. Groups have power over their members because the same processes of interaction that result in members' feeling favorable toward each other also result simultaneously in their adapting to norms which enable them to aim at success rather than failure. The student peer groups, as a special case of a general phenomenon, are subject to the processes of social interaction [14]. Diagram 1 illustrates these interdependent influences upon final student characteristics.

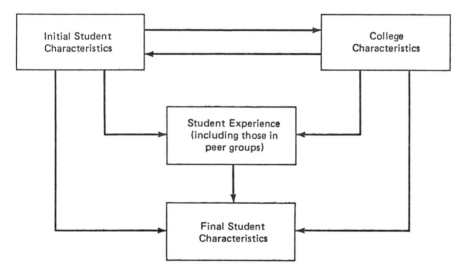

DIAGRAM 1.   An illustration of interdependent influences upon final student characteristics. (From T. M. Newcomb, Student Peer-Group Influences. In N. Sanford [Ed.], *The American College.* New York: Wiley, 1962, p. 472.)

Olesen and Whittaker, in their study of nursing students, demonstrated that a student should not be viewed as the passive recipient of formal academic influences. The study details the ways in which student culture contributes powerfully to the processes of socialization and professionalization [15].

Colleges in this country vary enormously in almost every conceivable respect. Peer groups of the most diverse form arise within all but the smallest college. In virtually all colleges, regardless of size and character, there are roommate pairs or triads, interest and activity groups, and informal circles of friends whose impact upon their members is often decisive. Newcomb has identified three factors contributing to the formation of particular peer groups. One of these factors is concerned with previous acquaintances of students, especially in secondary school. In cases where these friendships persist from high school to college, they form the basis of peer-group influence. The likelihood of frequent face-to-face contact of students is a major factor in group formation. The more intimate kinds of interpersonal relationships that characterize smaller rather than larger groups have a relatively great impact upon group members. Lastly, people are most likely to interact and thus to develop close relationships when shared interests in some aspect of their common environment bring them together. Contiguity and common interests would seem to account for the beginning of most group relationships [16].

There is at the moment little research evidence to indicate that intellectual outcomes vary, other things being equal, with frequency of student-teacher contact. It appears then that the teacher's influence, if it is to be effective, must be caught up in the norms of student groups, and the degree to which this occurs bears no necessary relationship to frequency of the teacher's direct contact with students. Teachers' influence can operate at a distance, mediated by some students so as to affect others; this can happen if the colleges are willing to supply the necessary conditions.

There is some evidence to indicate that colleges and teachers have an impact on certain career decisions of students. Students making the decision to seek graduate or professional training during college years attribute their decisions to the influence of college teachers. Thistlewaite obtained information on the relative holding power and attractiveness of different fields of study, the characteristics of faculty and students in these fields, the effects of intellectual and social atmosphere upon motivation to seek advanced training, and the traits of instructors that had the greatest influence upon talented students. The study revealed that college environments characterized by faculty affiliation, enthusiasm, or emphasis upon achievement, humanism, and independence were associated with increased student motivation to seek advanced degrees in the arts, humanities, and social sciences. College environments characterized by a lack of faculty emphasis upon student compliance were associated with increased motivation to seek advanced degrees in the natural and biological sciences. Faculties that students perceived as enthusiastic, warm, and informal in their relationships with students and as stressing achievement, humanism, and independence were associated with more frequent changes in students' plans to seek advanced training in the arts, humanities, and social sciences. Faculties that students perceived as enthusiastic and not exerting great pressure for compliance were associated with more frequent changes in students' plans to seek advanced training in the natural and biological sciences. Traits attributed to teachers who were most influential upon students varied from field to field [17].

Thistlewaite was also concerned with the development of motivation to seek advanced training among the various fields of study. The most important result of this study is the discovery that students who are treated one way during the educational process will have higher aspirations than comparable students who are treated in other ways. Teachers who are supportive appear to have the greatest influence upon students' aspirations. Such teachers are distinguished by the following attributes: willingness to discuss students' goals, willingness to help students discover their special talents, willingness to give special tutoring or to counsel students having difficulty, and willingness to take care to spare the students' feelings when giving negative evaluations [18].

Changes occurring in the students' critical thinking ability, attitudes, dogmatism, traditional value orientation, and religious, social, and political views was the focus of a study by Lehman. The findings of his study revealed that there were significant changes in critical thinking ability, attitudes, and values from freshman to senior years. Both males and females became less stereotyped in their beliefs. Both males and females became less traditional-value oriented from freshman to senior years. All students studied became more open-minded and more receptive to new ideas. For the most part, the greatest magnitude of change occurred during the freshman and sophomore years. A proportionately greater percentage of seniors said that the social life in college was not most important but was essential for one's development. It was evident that the informal, nonacademic experiences have a greater impact upon personality than do the formal, academic experiences, such as courses and instructors. It is only after the students entered their major field of study that any evidence of the impact of formal academic experiences appeared [19].

The monumental publication prepared by Sanford provides abundant research information of the influence of various aspects of the college environment on the values, attitudes, and achievements of students. The different personality characteristics of students appear to react with the dominant features of the environment of the college, which may reinforce the student's initial behavior or bring about some modification in that behavior [20].

THE IMPACT OF THE STUDENT UPON THE COLLEGE

The characteristics of students as revealed by the studies pertaining to the impact of college on their behavior seem to portray a mood of passivity. The student entered college and gained some information and skills which were useful to him in the work world. In many instances the college experience and environment did not seem to influence his attitudes, values, or general orientation to life. Although some schools had more success than others in the development of the student as an individual, the majority of schools studied provided little evidence of positive effects in this direction. At the time of these studies, students offered little resistance; they accepted the state of affairs of the college, seeking nourishment for individual growth through other than academic activities.

If the climate of the college during this era was described as peaceful and passive, it is likely that the pendulum has swung to the opposite extreme. The ongoing activities of student protests and revolt indicate that students desire more than a perfunctory academic involvement during their college experiences. On virtually every campus in the country, the very roots and fiber of college life are being torn from their historical and cultural moorings by the impact of student discontent and dissonance. Immediate diagnosis of the different maladies is probably not appropriate while the organism, the college, and the society in general is still in a state of shock.

The reactionary involvement of college students has been a repeated phenomenon in the development of higher education since the founding of Harvard College in 1636. In every instance colleges modified their environment in ways that were more in keeping with the characteristics, needs, and aspirations of the students. Problems of the past centered on issues of rigid discipline of personal and social living, regimented and dogmatic instructional procedures, irrelevant curriculum content, and the abdication of the teachers of the academic courses from activities associated with the development of the student as an individual. (The various student personnel workers in colleges have since then taken up the slack in the latter issue; this separation of the teaching from the counseling staff has in some instances created polarization of the development concerns of the student.)

Educators and behavioral scientists who are involved in or studying student activism are making some observations. The term *activism* does not lend itself to precise definition; however, Axelrod proposes a definition that permits classification by degree of participation. This definition of activism has four parts: (1) Activism is partly activeness in the psychological sense, as opposed to passivism; it is an orientation characterized by initiative and attempt at mastery of frustrating conditions instead of submission, conformity, and inhibitory self-blame. (2) Activism is also a social or environmental perspective that locates conditions of personal or group malfunctioning in institutional structures, and, instead of accepting these as given, attempts to change them. In most instances students involved devote themselves to constructive work in hospitals, inner-city and ghetto projects, and Peace Corps activities. They attempt to bring about changes in the social order within the existing framework of society. (3) The activist has a tendency to explore his inner life and assert his impulses, which help to free his potentialities and to overcome restrictions that inhibit the range and pleasure of his experience. This tendency is demonstrated in the greater freedom of expression of impulses, labeled by some as the "new morality." (4) The activist is willing to risk some future social or economic opportunities or to take personal risks, physical or psychological or both, in the service of the cause in which he believes [21]. Numerous studies of the characteristics of student activists reveal useful information. Contrary to the belief of many, student activists have experienced a closer, effective relationship with their parents. Their expression in activist movements reflects those of their parents, but in a purer or less compromising form. The large number of Jewish students in these activities reflects the sensitivity of this group to social injustices [22].

The personal characteristics of student activists and the circumstantial situations in their lives may account for their behavior. Katz has identified several factors that might contribute to activism among students. Positive determinants were economic affluence (after twenty years of affluence some members of the present generation are taking a more fundamental look at social institutions), the confidence students gained through their previous success experiences achieved during schooling, and the success of the civil rights movement, which gave students training in tactics of dissent and a new sense of power of individuals to influence the course of political and social events [23].

Students are asking the colleges and universities to rethink their roles, and they are asking these institutions to become active agents of change. Relevance has become a key word of the younger generation of students. They are concerned with questions pertaining to goals, purposes, and values. No longer are they satisfied with fragments of knowledge and skills as ends in themselves.

They are searching for greater articulation of the deep purposes of human society and the relationship of what they are learning to the attainment of this goal. They manifest deep concern for the problems of contemporary society rather than the acquisition of skills, which insure upward mobility [24]. The activities of young people in an effort to bring about changes in social institutions in the direction of democratic social values reveal the characteristics of this group. A study of about two dozen young people between the ages of nineteen and twenty-nine who worked in the National Office of Vietnam Summer reported their influence on the tone and direction of this summer project. This study, which was published by Keniston, revealed that these people held a strong belief in a set of basic moral principles: justice, decency, equality, nonviolence, responsibility, and fairness. Although academic life was a great temptation to them, academic life, as these young people saw it, at that time was a symbol of irrelevance and irresponsibility. They clearly rejected immersion in the conventional middle-class life, academic or political. Some observations reported by Keniston described what he calls "the tension between participation and power." This tension was related to the discomfort felt by many young radicals when they were in a position of control over another person, especially if the other person was expected to do routine, boring, or unenjoyable work. For many it was extremely difficult either to lead or to follow, especially when it entailed power, control, or domination. In their personal manner and values, these young people favored open, equal, and direct relationships with other people; they were psychologically and ideologically hostile to formally defined, inflexible roles and traditionally bureaucratic patterns of power [25].

Keniston saw the young radicals as psychological adults but sociological adolescents. Their major psychological energies were involved in an effort to define their basic relationship to the existing society, deciding how, where, and whether they will enter it [26]. This was a group earnestly seeking new values, looking for ways for people to remain people and to confront one another in trust and respect.

Another study gives support to some of Keniston's observations of the young radicals. Reisman's report of the activities of the student cooperative at the University of Toronto indicated that it was difficult to get students to take responsibility. Even where students obtained the power to control their own lives and their own education, they found it difficult to create the structures that would sustain an ongoing cooperative and an ongoing self-direction in the educational process. Their hesitancy to assume control of one another even when it seemed necessary to establish an effective group effort was similar to the characteristics of Keniston's young radicals. Reisman observed, however, that when adult control disappeared, the young's control of each other intensified [27].

The characteristics of the students in the studies reported by Keniston and Reisman portrayed these young people as deeply committed to democratic social values and goals and to working within the system to bring about changes in an effort to realize these goals. There appear to be other activists who present some different characteristics. Another group was characterized as alienated youth and was the subject of a longitudinal study supported in part by a grant from the National Institute of Mental Health. This study by Keniston endeavored to search for an explanation of the estrangement of youth from American society. Alienation, as defined by Keniston, was the explicit rejection of what his subjects saw as the dominant roles and institutions of American society. Central to alienation was a deep and pervasive mistrust of any and all commitments to people, to groups, to American culture, or even to the self. Pessimism and skepticism were common. Although the students in the study disliked their society and were pessimistic about its future, they seldom supported social reform or political action. Anger, scorn, and contempt were pervasive among them; few had clear positive values, but among their goals were honesty and direct confrontation with unpleasant truth [28].

The alienated students frequently attacked their college and despised any traces of college spirit. They disliked and distrusted institutional involvements and responsibilities; they were seldom happy when truly involved with a group. In an attempt to analyze the behavior of these young adults, Keniston stated that American society makes extraordinary demands on its members, demands resulting from chronic change, social fragmentation, and an intellectual climate that constantly undermines positive values. Chronic social change destroys one's sense of continuity with the past. Social fragmentation and specialization has lessened the meaningfulness of work. A sense of connection with a tangible accomplishment and a sense of personal responsibility for what one does are eventually vitiated in a highly organized society. Keniston makes the charge that "instrumental values have replaced virtuous character as standards of human values" [29].

Another type of student reactionary was identified by Lobenthal. For this student, participation in protests offered satisfactions that have nothing to do with explicit aims of The Movement, or of any movement. Although a few of these students may have been dissenters, probably the majority were experimenting for the first time with the profound experience of personal involvement in a mass movement of some kind. It appears that some psychological aggrandizement was insured for all participants when they suddenly found themselves projected into an exalted realm of ideas, activity, and publicity. Their new roles were a source of new status [30].

SUMMARY

Institutions of higher education are responding to the need for trained manpower for a rapidly changing scientific and technological society. At the same time a reinterpretation of democratic social values is indicating that education is a right of all persons rather than a privilege of a few. Colleges and universities have modified their administration policies and curriculum offerings to accommodate the needs of students with diverse characteristics, and at the same time they have provided society with specialized manpower. At one time the characteristics of students enrolled in a particular college were relatively homogeneous. More recently, however, these characteristics display wide heterogeneity. Similar characteristics of students, such as age, sex, race, religion, and marital status, are visible on all college campuses. In some aspects colleges are becoming more alike in terms of their curriculum offerings. A wide range of occupational and professional programs are offered among the various institutions of higher education.

There are some characteristics of students and of colleges that present considerable diversity. Studies of the personalities of students enrolled in specific colleges indicate that these colleges may attract and hold students with similar personality structures. Identification of the characteristics of these colleges in relation to the personality structures of attending students presents the notion of compatibility of the student and the college. The possibility of altering the environment of the college through the admission procedure is a challenging idea. The self-analysis of colleges and universities has revealed to faculty and administration that a vital component of the student's life appears to be influenced very little by college experiences. Although the student acquires useful information and skills for occupational endeavors, his values, ideals, and beliefs remain essentially unaltered throughout his college life. Most institutions of higher education proclaim that the modification and reinforcement of social values and goals are major institutional objectives. Students' lives appear to be untouched by the experiences that the school offers for this purpose. At the time of these studies, students offered little resistance; they accepted the occupational goals of the school and sought nourishment for their value orientation elsewhere.

The climate of the college and university is different today. Although the students recognize the necessity for specific information and skills to perform some useful work, they are asking that these be anchored in the social values of this country. They are witnessing the grave disparity of opportunity in all aspects of living among individuals and groups. They want to see the social goals of this country translated into action, and they want to be involved. Seriousness of purpose of today's college student is already, and will be increasingly, a major factor in shaping change both within and without the college or university. As more and more students have become more and more impatient with policies and attitudes that they feel deny expression of both their aims and their abilities, they have begun to seek new ways of expressing themselves and of finding means for direct participation in affairs of their concern. Never have young people had greater freedom to move about, to express themselves, and to make their own personal decisions. Earlier exposure to adult problems and experiences has produced a degree of youthful sophistication not prevalent in past generations. The greater awareness of themselves and their needs, and the better preparation for coping with the problems they identify mark this younger generation and have produced in them a deep disillusionment and a restless impatience. Eager for revolutionary change and the immediate correction of long-standing social ills and injustices, concerned young people have little tolerance for what they consider to be the failure of our traditional institutions to adapt to change.

Nursing students are among the ranks of those protesting the obvious neglect of society to remedy its ills. Their professed commitment to help others underlies their choice of a career. Their educational experiences bring them face to face with the problems of poverty, disease, urban decay, segregation, and minority groups. Change in positive directions comes too slowly for them and is impeded by the bureaucratic system. As nursing becomes more professional in nature, it is likely that nurses will affiliate more closely with the profession rather than with the employing institution. As this occurs, nursing students will voice louder protests against social institutions that tend to perpetuate substandard living for its citizens.

Administrators and teachers must address themselves to these questions: Do I know what I ought to know about the reservoir of young people into which nursing must dip in order to carry out the social role and obligations that the institutional forms we have developed to support such values? The answers to profession has assumed? What do I know about the quality of their commitment to social values, including health? How do they feel about the various these questions and other related ones become a vital source for curriculum decisions.

REFERENCES

1. Holland, J. H.   The Negro and higher education. *NEA J.* 54:23, 1965.
2. McGrath, E.   *The Predominantly Negro Colleges and Universities in Transition.* New York: Teachers College Bureau of Publications (Columbia University), 1965. P. 85.
3. Hutchins, R. M.   *The Learning Society.* New York: Mentor, 1968. P. 22. students. *Coll. Board News.* P. 1, 1970.
4. College Entrance Examination Board. *College Credit by Examination Through College Level Examination Programs.* Princeton: College Entrance Examination Board, 1970. P. 7.
5. Ibid., p. 23.
6. College Entrance Examination Board.   Board testing of minority/poverty
7. Jones, J. F.   *Upgrading Intellectually Deprived Students to Achieve Professional Success.* Baltimore: Helene Fuld School of Nursing, 1965.
8. Willingham, R. W., and Findikyan, N.   Transfer students: Who's moving from where to where, and what determines who's admitted. *Coll. Board Rev.* 72:4, 1969.
9. Bixler, G. K., and Simmons, L. W.   *The Regional Project in Graduate Education and Research in Nursing.* Atlanta: Southern Regional Education Board, 1960.
10. Magoon, T. M.   Demographic Characteristics of Nursing Students. In V. C. Conley (Ed.). *Curriculum and Instruction in Medical-Surgical and Psychiatric Nursing: Baccalaureate Programs.* Washington, D.C.: Catholic University of America Press, 1970. P. 79.
11. Abe, C., et al.   *A Description of American College Freshmen.* Iowa City: Research and Development Division, American College Testing Program, 1965.
12. Newcomb, T. M.   *Personality and Social Change.* New York: Dryden, 1943.
13. Jacob, P. E.   *Changing Values in College.* New York: Harper & Bros., 1957.
14. Newcomb, T. M.   Student Peer-Group Influences. In N. Sanford (Ed.), *The American College.* New York: Wiley, 1962. P. 469.
15. Olesen, V. and Whittaker, E. W.   *The Silent Dialogue: A Study in the Social Psychology of Professional Socialization.* San Francisco: Jossey-Bass, 1968.
16. Newcomb, op cit., p. 474.
17. Thistlewaite, D. L.   College press and changes in the study plans of talented students. *J. Educ. Psychol.* 51:222, 1960.

18. Thistlewaite, D. L. Fields of study and development of motivation to seek advanced training. *J. Educ. Psychol.* 53:53, 1962.
19. Lehman, I. Changes in critical thinking, attitudes and values from freshman to senior years. *J. Educ. Psychol.* 54:305, 1963.
20. Sanford, N. (Ed.). *The American College.* New York: Wiley, 1962.
21. Axelrod, J., et al. *Search for Relevance.* San Francisco: Jossey-Bass, 1969. P. 107.
22. Ibid., p. 109.
23. Katz, J. (Ed.). The Activist Revolution. In *No Time for Youth: Growth and Constraint in College Students.* San Francisco: Jossey-Bass, 1968. P. 392.
24. Cohen, N. E. The university and social change. *School and Society* 97:480, 1969.
25. Keniston, K. *Young Radicals: Notes on Committed Youth.* New York: Harcourt Brace & World, 1968.
26. Ibid., p. 267.
27. Reisman, D. The young are captive of each other: a conversation with David Reisman and T. George Harris. *Psychol. Today* 2:28, 63, 1969.
28. Keniston, K. *The Uncommitted: Alienated Youth in American Society.* New York: Dell, 1960.
29. Ibid., p. 422.
30. Lobenthal, J. S., Jr. The catabolism of a student revolt. *J. Higher Educ.* 40:717, 1969.

SUPPLEMENTARY READINGS

Allen, J. E., Jr. Campus activism and unrest. *School and Society* 96:357, 1968.
Dressel, P. L., Mayhew, L. B., and McGrath, E. J. *The Liberal Arts as Viewed by Faculty Members in Professional Schools.* New York: Teachers College Bureau of Publications (Columbia University), 1959.
Freedman, M. The passage through college. *J. Soc. Issues* 12:16, 1956.
Gordon, D. M. Rebellion in Context: A Student's View of Students. In R. S. Morison (Ed.), *The Contemporary University, U.S.A.* Boston: Houghton Mifflin, 1956.
Guisti, J. P. Students and the 1970's: Calm after the storm. *School and Society* 97:360, 1969.
Harrison, E. D. The Negro college in a changing economy. *J. Higher Educ.* 36:263, 1965.
Johnston, D. B. The student and his power. *J. Higher Educ.* 40:205, 1969.
Kelly, N. C. The student voice in curriculum planning—threat or promise? *Nurs. Outlook* 17:59, 1969.
Lehrer, S. Higher education and the disenchanted students. *School and Society* 97:427, 1969.
McGrath, E. J. *The Graduate School and the Decline of Liberal Education.* New York: Teachers College Bureau of Publications (Columbia University), 1959.
McGrath, E. J., and Russell, C. H. *Are Liberal Arts Colleges Becoming Professional Schools?* New York: Teachers College Bureau of Publications (Columbia University), 1958.

Muldrow, C.   Now it's students of nursing. *Amer. J. Nurs.* 69:1252, 1969.

National League for Nursing.   *Baccalaureate Education for the Registered Nurse Student.* New York: National League for Nursing, 1966.

Parker, G. G.   50 years of collegiate enrollment: 1919–20 to 1969–70. *School and Society* 98:282, 1970.

Parker, G. G.   Statistics of attendance in American universities and colleges, 1967–1968. *School and Society* 96:9, 1968.

Reed, R. D.   Curricular changes in colleges and universities for Negroes. *J. Higher Educ.* 98:153, 1967.

Roushenbush, E.   *The Student and His Studies.* Middletown: Wesleyan University Press, 1964.

Russell, C. H.   *Liberal Education and Nursing.* New York: Teachers College Bureau of Publications (Columbia University), 1959.

8 INFLUENCE OF PSYCHOLOGICAL AND LEARNING THEORIES ON CURRICULUM DEVELOPMENT

MANY psychologists have tried to understand how learning occurs, and some have tried to predict and control the course of learning. The aim of the scientific investigation of learning, as with other disciplines, is to arrive at fundamental laws or principles that describe the phenomenon. Educators have a vital interest in the development of laws of learning, since curriculum development revolves around selection of goals and methods of learning or instruction.

It may be helpful to review the major events in the development of behavior and learning theories. It should be remembered that research on the learning process requires selection of an appropriate unit of behavior to study and a methodology appropriate to both theoretical and practical interests. In the survey, the limitations and inadequacies of the available theories will become apparent, and the need for more practical approaches will be clear. Theories of instruction seem to be needed for more concrete solutions to the problems of teaching and learning in school environments.

HISTORICAL BACKGROUND

Beliefs about the learning process underwent a marked change in the nineteenth century, based on a pragmatic orientation in psychology to man and society, paralleling trends in the development of education. During the first half of the century, the traditional rationalism of Europe was manipulated by American writers into a psychology of human faculties that supported mental discipline as the basis of the learning process. The theory of rationalism proclaimed that man learns best through reason; that sense experience is limited to sensory knowledge of natural objects, whereas reason can achieve permanent and absolute knowledge of abstract concepts as well. This doctrine *considers* human reason superior to sense perception in acquiring the real knowledge that gives meaning to everyday experience. The reasoning mind is looked upon as a special spiritual creation, quite different from the physical body and found only in men, as distinguished from animals.

According to this *faculty psychology*, the mind consists of separate, independent, ready-made capacities or faculties, such as memory, judgment, reason, will, imagination, and taste. The faculties are considered to be merely potential until brought into actuality by training and practice. The development of the powers of the mind was the supreme aim of education. For the exercise of the faculties, the *form* of studies was considered more important than their content. The classics and mathematics were believed to have greater value for mental discipline than the so-called practical studies, the physical sciences, and modern languages.

As long as faculty psychology remained the dominant theory of learning, the defenders of mental discipline and of the traditional, prescribed studies held their position securely. But a new theory of *empiricism* began taking hold, and advocates of this theory attacked the extreme emphasis on the classics, mathematics, and traditional philosophy, maintaining they were not sufficiently adapted to the varying interests, capacities, and goals of the students. By the end of the nineteenth century, faculty psychology had ceased to be the dominant learning theory.

Experimental psychology grew out of the trend toward empiricism. As empiricism developed in this country, it emphasized the need for objective study of mental processes and recognized that sensory, motor, and physiological processes greatly affect mental development. Laboratory methods and experiments were based on the theory that mind, far from being an isolated entity or faculty, is really the entire functioning of the organism in adjusting its behavior to its environment. Experimental psychology drew support from studies of heredity conducted by scientists such as Wilhelm Wundt and John Galton. As faculty psychology became suspect in view of the new experimental psychology, it was replaced by a belief in the worth of the individual for his own sake. In addition, the individual was seen as a part of nature, living in constant interaction with his physical and social environment. In other words, life was viewed as a continual interactive adjustment between an active individual and an active environment. Experimental psychology defines behavior as response to one's immediate environment, modified by past experience.

Long before the development of experimental psychology, some notions were expressed by philosophers and scientists concerning the association of ideas and sensations. Thomas Hobbes (1588–1679) indicated that man learns about the external world through his senses [1]. Also supporting this doctrine of empiricism was John Locke (1632–1704), who stressed experience and environment as the sources of knowledge and learning. In Locke's view, the new-born baby possesses for a mind merely a "blank tablet," upon which perceptions from the outside world are accumulated. Ideas and values have their origins in experience of the external world, including other people [2]. To David Hartley (1705–1757) the basic law of learning was the association of ideas. Repeated sensations leave traces in the nervous system. When different sensations have occurred together often enough, the occurrence of one sensation will call up the memory of others. Simple ideas are built into complex ideas by such association [3].

James Mill (1733–1836) applied associative principles with thoroughness and detail. Frequently referred to as the "associationist par excellence," he made vigorous attempts to show that the associative processes are adequate for the highest complexities of mental life [4]. Learning by association was further developed by Alexander Bain (1818–1903), who stated two fundamental laws of association—contiguity and similarity. Contiguity is the recurrence of previous concurrences of actions or sensations; similarity accounts for constructive association. Bain is considered to be the forerunner of the connectionists (who will be discussed later) [5].

The developments in experimental psychology and the changing viewpoints concerning human nature made way for the scientific study of human behavior and learning. Vigorous attempts have been made by teachers on all levels to utilize the outcomes of laboratory learning research in classroom activities, but because learning research and teaching emphasize different variables, the application of learning research is not always obvious. Nevertheless, knowledge of some of the major learning theories may provide a springboard for further investigations of the classroom learning process. This review of representative learning theories includes a brief description of each theory and suggests its implications for education.

LEARNING THEORIES AND THEIR INFLUENCE ON EDUCATION

The learning theories considered here are classified into three major groups: (1) early learning theories, (2) gestalt psychology and field theories, and (3) recent or current learning theories. Where appropriate, the fundamental re-search approach used in the development of the theory is cited. While it is obvious that such a brief treatment hardly does justice to the psychology of learning, the summary is presented to direct the reader to the development of theories of learning and to note the application of this knowledge to educational practices. Although the early learning theories (the first group to be discussed) set the stage for ongoing investigations of the learning process, this presentation does not necessarily place all the theories in chronological order. Theoretical formulations by different theorists often took place concurrently and influenced one another. The dates of the life span of the major proponents indicate roughly the time period associated with each theory.

EARLY LEARNING THEORIES

Among the early learning theories that made outstanding, unique contributions to psychological thought at the time of their development were connectionism, formulated by Edward L. Thorndike, functionalism, described by John Dewey, and behaviorism, expressed by John Watson.

CONNECTIONISM

At the close of the nineteenth century, the United States had embarked upon an experiment in mass education. Connectionism, the name we give the theory developed by Edward L. Thorndike (1874–1949), was, in the United States, the starting point for the study of the human learning process and has greatly influenced the development of other learning theories. The most outstanding contribution of this theory was the hypothesis that human behavior can be modified. This theory and those that followed changed the focus of learning from mental discipline to the concept of associations or bonds between sense impressions and impulses to action.

Thorndike defined learning as the modification of associative bonds through behavior which seeks to maintain the organism's adjustment to its environment. Much of learned behavior begins with trial-and-error learning, or as Thorndike sometimes called it, selecting and connecting [6].

The basis of learning as described by Thorndike is the association between sense impressions and impulses to action, hence the name connectionism [7]. Thorndike postulated two central processes, some sort of internal connection between sensation and response, and the automatic effect of reward (food, hunger reduction) or punishment (lack of food, hunger) on those connections. Presumably the stimulus-response connection was strengthened if it led to a satisfying state of the organism. Thorndike, as a result of his experiments on animals, believed that animal behavior was influenced very little by ideas, that the bulk of animal learning could be explained by the cause-effect relationship between external stimuli and responses to those stimuli. He concluded that the same mechanical process occurred in humans. He acknowledged, however, that the reasoning power of man enabled him to change himself for the better and to act for the good of all men.

Three major laws of learning were formulated by Thorndike to explain the phenomenon of learning—the law of effect, the law of readiness, and the law of exercise. These are not laws in the same sense as Newton's law of gravitation, but are the rules according to which learning was believed to occur. The role of motivation in learning was identified very early; after some laboratory experiments, this phenomenon came to the forefront.

Thorndike's interest in the effects of rewards and punishments on animal learning had profound influence on his thinking about human learning. The *law of effect* describes the strengthening or weakening of a stimulus-response connection that occurs as a consequence of this connection. When a modifiable connection is made and produces a satisfying state within the organism, the strength of the connection is increased. If an annoying or nonsatisfying state of affairs follows the connection, its strength is decreased. Essentially, Thorndike maintained that rewards or successes reinforce the learning of rewarded behavior, while punishment reduces the tendency to repeat behavior leading to punishment. Thorndike later revised his law of effect, after observing that in laboratory experience the effects of rewards and punishments were not equal in strength and opposite in effect. Reward appeared to strengthen more dependably than punishment weakened [8].

The *law of readiness* describes the supposed physiological conditions under which the law of effect operates. Thorndike described three types of states of readiness: (1) When a "conduction unit" is ready to conduct, conduction by it is satisfying. (2) When a conduction unit is ready to conduct, not to conduct is disturbing. (3) When a conduction unit unready for conduction is forced to conduct, conduction by it is disturbing. He gave the term conduction unit no precise physiological meaning (he predated behaviorism). By readiness he seems to mean preparation for action. The preparatory adjustment suggests muscle activity, visual orientation, and accompanying attitudes. This concept should not be confused with maturational readiness, such as reading readiness, which came later [9].

The *law of exercise* applies to the strengthening of associative connections through practice or the weakening of connections due to absence of practice.

Strengthening here means an increase in the probability that the response will be made when the situation recurs. Thorndike held that when practice is discontinued, the connection is weakened and memory loss or forgetting occurs. The type of actions that are influenced by practice include repetitive tasks, rote memorizing, and acquiring muscular skills [10]. Later Thorndike found that practice brings improvements only because it permits other factors, such as knowledge of results, to be effective; practice itself does nothing. Repetition of situations produces no change in the strength of connections; connections are strengthened when the behavior is rewarded, not when the connection merely occurs [11].

Thorndike was interested in the transfer of school learning to real-life situations. It was his theory that this transfer depends upon the presence of identical elements in the original learning and in the new learning. If an activity is learned more easily following learning of another activity, it is because the two activities have common elements.

Thorndike saw intelligence as related to the transfer capacity of an individual. He believed that the more specific learned connections the individual has at his disposal, the more intelligent he is [12].

Thorndike's theory pertains to the strengthening of specific connections by reward (or punishment). He suggested that practice in a school setting should be based on careful analyses of the components of a good performance. If errors are correctly diagnosed and not rewarded, they will not be repeated. The theory stressed the importance of motivation as a system of external rewards and punishments. In actual use, the theory is more consistent with drill and habit formation than with learning involving insight, understanding, and meaning.

FUNCTIONALISM

The influence of John Dewey (1858–1952) on educational thinking is well known. According to Dewey, learning is gauged by problem-solving or intelligent action in which the person continually evaluates his experience in the light of its foreseen and experienced consequences. Learning in this sense is not simply an acquisition or achievement but a continuing interaction with the environment [13].

The main argument of Dewey's theory is that an activity should be thought of as a "reflex circuit": between stimulus and response, between one movement and another, between organism and environment, there are no real breaks. Teachers may introduce breaks for convenience in thinking of the activity, but the distinctions they use are of their own making, they are not in the nature of things.

Dewey addressed himself to the classroom learning situation more directly than any other learning psychologist considered in this chapter. He even founded an experimental elementary school at the University of Chicago. He emphasized the child's interests and his motivation to solve his own problems, a dynamic innovation in psychology. Interest serves as the basic motivational construct in Dewey's system. Interest is the critical link between the pupil's stage of growth and where the teacher hopes he will be. Interest is what sustains the effort of trying out various solutions on the way to one's goal [14].

In contrast to Thorndike's concern for specificity, Dewey proclaimed the fallaciousness of the notion that a person learns only the particular thing he is studying at the time. The concomitant formation of attitudes, of likes and dislikes, may be more important than the particular lesson. These attitudes are what count in the future. The desire to go on learning is the most important thing learned [15].

The goal of learning should always be made as definite and clear as possible and should be constantly clarified as the learning process continues. Learning becomes the process of adapting means to ends. Educational activities capitalize on the directing and energizing influence of goals. A goal is, in Dewey's words, a felt difficulty. Experience is most likely to be meaningfully integrated or reorganized when the discovery of new relationships is instrumental in the attainment of the individual's objectives [16].

Dewey's innovative emphasis on the functional needs of the individual as the basis for structuring classroom learning stimulated various group efforts collectively referred to as the progressive education movement. The ideal sought by all of these educators was the growth of the individual toward independence and self-control through directed exposure to an environment suitably scaled to the child's developing needs. Not the least important in this process was the child's own selection and adaptation of materials and methods appropriate to goals which he sets for himself. The problems or goals were social as well as individual, for education was envisaged as a preparation for life in a democracy through democratic living. Dewey believed that schools often failed to stimulate understanding, because they imposed routine tasks instead of presenting problems and because they neglected to set up conditions for active use of what was being learned [17].

Dewey's ideas appealed to a generation committed to making the world safe for democracy. Democratic education, viewed as the instrument of social reform, was the hope of all classes. Dewey's philosophy of education and his psychology of learning were seen as a means to this end.

BEHAVIORISM

The founder of behaviorism, John B. Watson (1878–1958), proclaimed that psychology must break with the past, discard the concept of consciousness, and begin at the beginning to construct a new science following the example of the physical sciences: it must become materialistic, mechanistic, deterministic, and objective. For Watson, mental processes and consciousness are not fit subjects for scientific study, since consciousness cannot be seen, touched, or exhibited in a test tube [18].

For the behaviorist, learning is a matter of bringing about automatic reactions through conditioning. According to Watson, it is necessary first to find out what reactions are possible in the human infant through its native constitution, and then to discover, bit by bit, how other reactions are added. Reactions already present become conditioned, and through further conditioning more complex forms of behavior are built up. Watson indicated that the newborn infant inherits neither intelligence nor special abilities. He maintained that conditioning is the simplest form of learning, the elementary process to which all learning is reducible. All the complex behavior patterns that an adult displays grow out of the few simple responses that the infant has in its repertoire, largely through learning or conditioning, but also through growth or maturation. In this process the social environment is of prime importance [19].

In 1913, when behaviorism was officially inaugurated, animal psychology had attained a respectable position. Methods of studying animal behavior had gained precision and permitted experimental control. There are several obvious advantages to using animals for psychological research. (1) More complete control of the conditions of the experiment is possible. (2) It is possible to study the entire life span of many animals and, in some short-lived species, to study the same process over several generations. (3) Animal research enables the scientist to use certain procedures that cannot be used on human beings, such as removing parts of the brain or impairing sense organs. Watson started the animal laboratory at the University of Chicago, where he developed methods of studying animal behavior.

The main tenet of Watson's theory was that all human activities can be explained by reference to the stimulus-response paradigm. The subject matter of behaviorism is observable, measurable behavior. Observation of behavior is fundamental to all the investigative procedures of behaviorism, and scientific observations may be made either with or without instruments. The conditioned reflex technique developed by Pavlov is of prime importance in Watson's behaviorism [20].

Under the influence of behaviorism, the trend toward studying psychological processes in relation to physiological processes was strengthened in American psychology. The importance of studying the organism as a whole in its environment became increasingly apparent. Behaviorism constantly demanded that only objective knowledge (observable, measurable behavior) be accepted as scientific, and thereby Watson achieved the final separation of psychology from traditional philosophy. In American psychology generally, behaviorism has increased the emphasis on objective methods of observation and on quantitative and experimental research.

Behaviorism recognizes the importance of early childhood development. Watson believed that in the first six years of life a person is made or marred. It is during these years that the child learns to meet the world with fear or confidence, with hostility or friendliness, and to succumb to difficulties or to master them [21].

This summary of some of the major theories of learning cannot be considered to be a comprehensive review. It is acknowledged that other philosophers, psychologists, and scientists contributed to the body of knowledge on human behavior and learning, and no doubt influenced the theories discussed.

The approaches to the study and analysis of learning made by Thorndike, Dewey, and Watson are quite varied, yet each made significant contributions. Thorndike's law of effect inspired many investigative approaches which in general validate his original idea. Dewey's radical departure from the generally accepted approach to learning, the mental discipline view, led to misinterpretation at the time. However, the impact of his psychology of learning eventually brought about major reforms in school practices. Although many of Watson's theories about learning have been refuted, his stringent demands for precise, orderly methods of research contributed to the development of psychology as a science. These theorists provided fertile ideas for the ongoing investigation and analysis of human learning.

GESTALT AND FIELD THEORIES

A group of German psychologists who were more affected by philosophical traditions than by the mechanical models of physical science challenged the concepts identified with Thorndike and Watson. The men associated with this psychological theory are Wertheimer, Koffka, and Köhler, and the theory was labeled gestalt psychology. The German word *Gestalt* may be translated as a pattern or configuration. The basic concern of this psychology is perception—its patterns, its presumed dynamic organization, and its holistic nature. As compared with the theorists already surveyed, the gestaltist tends to be more concerned with complex relationships, central processes, and dynamic interactions than with specific movements or units of association. To the gestaltist, perception is primary, and behavior is a product of the organization of the perceptual field.

The generalized notion of a field within which all events occur is common in modern physics and astronomy. More recently it has been found enlightening in approaches to the study of biology, psychology, and sociology. All events in nature, including psychological and educational, occur within some field the structure of which determines and controls the events. The inherent properties of an object are said to be ultimately traceable to forces impinging upon it from the surrounding field. The field is construed as the effective whole, determining the attributes and behavior of the parts coming within its influence. Some examples of part-whole phenomena which can be described in relation to a physical field are the effect of the solar system on the ebb and flow of tides, the individual as a member of the family, the family as a component of a larger social system, and the classroom situation composed of interacting individuals and events [22].

Gestalt psychology maintains that psychological analysis is concerned with a more extended behavior system than the sensation, the reflex, or the associative bond. The field as a whole must be understood before any detail of it can be properly interpreted. Two major gestalt theories are presented here—the classic gestalt theory formulated by Max Wertheimer in 1912 and the field theory described by Kurt Lewin.

CLASSIC GESTALT THEORY

Gestalt psychology began with the recognition of visual perception as a psychological problem. The figure-ground characteristic was the first defined property of the visual field. It illustrated the importance of organization and relationships in perception. Not only is organization seen as important, but there is believed to be a congruence of organization in brain processes that makes the relationship more fundamental than discrete sensations.

Gestalt psychology rested upon the assumption that there is an essential unity in nature. Learning is a matter of grasping the relationships assumed to exist among physical, psychological, and biological events in the external world. Learning occurs through insight rather than by trial and error, and insight is possible only if all necessary elements are visible. Insight will occur more readily if the aspects to be brought into relationship can be seen in close proximity. To some extent, insight depends on past experience. From the gestalt psychologist's point of view, learning involves a problem situation that tends to disturb the equilibrium of the organism. In seeking to restore equilibrium by solving a problem, the organism follows certain laws of perceptual organization [23].

The *law of closure* indicates that in a perceptual pattern closed areas hang together better than unclosed areas and thus are more readily seen as figures. In a problem situation, the organism sees an incomplete whole, and internal tension results, providing the impetus toward completion of the whole. Achieving "closure" or completion is satisfying to the learner—it restores equilibrium. The law of closure may be considered to be the gestalt psychologist's alternative to Thorndike's law of effect.

A second gestalt law, the *law of proximity*, asserts that discrete elements will be seen in grouped arrangements according to the nearness of the parts. Whatever favors organization will also favor learning, retention, and recall. The equivalent of the law of proximity in stimulus-response theories is association by contiguity.

The *law of similarity* suggests that items similar in form or in color tend to be grouped perceptually. The law of similarity is based on the idea of interaction, whereby like things together produce a unitary object or event rather than a connection between similar items.

The *law of good continuation* is related to closure in the organization of perception. Lines will be seen as continuing, so as to form objects or satisfying patterns—for example, a part of a circle might be seen as a circle [24].

One aspect of gestalt psychology should be mentioned, although it will not be elaborated here. Some theorists believed that any experience leaves a remnant or *trace* in the nervous system. This trace changes or decays over time, with a corresponding change in memory reported. A new experience always takes place against a background of previously formed traces. Thus, the trace system is continually undergoing transformation. In particular, since the trace may stabilize in the absence of practice, distributed practice appears to be more effective for long-term learning than massed practice. The details of this *trace theory* were largely speculative since it predated any accurate knowledge of the functioning of the human nervous system. Much energy was spent in controversy over the exact nature of unobservable, unverifiable traces, and this aspect of the more general gestalt theory did not bring credit to its parent.

The gestaltists define intelligence as the capacity for insight, and learning as the process of gaining insight. Intelligence is equated with innate capacity for the higher forms of learning requiring structuring and restructuring of the field. The usefulness of practice is that it enables the learner to restructure the field as a result of new relationships acquired during practice.

Motivation in learning is described in relation to the concept of problem-solving in which the problem produces disequilibrium in the learner, and the tension created by the disequilibrium is the source of motivation to solve the problem.

Interest in thinking, problem-solving, and creativity led the gestaltists to formulate views on the influence of the organization of material on learning. Katona theorized that the inherent organization of materials would affect both ease of learning, retention, and transfer to new materials [25].

Gestalt psychology made significant contributions to education through its attention to the relationship between perception and learning. The emphasis placed on organization, meaningfulness, and perception had considerable impact upon the educational environment. The gestalt emphasis on problem-solving also altered considerably the nature and types of learning activities in the schools.

FIELD THEORY OF KURT LEWIN

Field theory, formulated by Kurt Lewin (1890–1947), developed from classic gestalt psychology. Lewin's theory is not specifically a psychology of learning, but it is relevant to learning. The basic characteristic of field theory is its concentration upon the individual's perception of the field rather than the objective, physical field only. Lewin insisted on studying what he termed the *life space* of the individual, which consisted partly of the state of that individual as a product of his history and partly of his physical and social surroundings.

The concept of life space as described by Lewin includes the environment, the person, and the interaction between the individual and the objective environment. The objective environment is the stimulus situation that acts upon the individual's perceptual apparatus and upon which his motor apparatus acts. The psychological environment is the environment as it exists for the individual and is determined by the objective environment and the characteristics of the person. The properties of the individual—his needs, beliefs, and values, and his perceptual and motive systems interact with the objective environment to produce the life space.

Learning, in this instance, takes several forms, since it involves a variety of changes in the structure of one's knowledge. Changes in cognitive structure come about through perceptual patterning according to the needs of the individual. Learning effects changes in the interests and values of the learner, namely, changes in the attractiveness of one goal over another. Goal attractiveness Lewin called *valence* and changes in goal attractiveness, *valence changes*. Goals may lose attractiveness when the associated activities are repeated to the point of monotony. Goals that were initially unattractive may become attractive through a change in the meaning of the goal-related activity. The individual's choice of goals at any time is influenced by previous experiences of success and failure [26].

Lewin believed that the existence of an association does not in any way guarantee reproduction of the association; the reproduction must be motivated. The concept of tension as the source of this motivation plays a central role in Lewin's theory as it does in the classic gestalt theory. A state of tension exists within the individual whenever a psychological need or an intention exists, and the tension is released when the need or intention is fulfilled. According to Lewin, a definite relation exists between tension systems of the person and certain properties of the psychological environment [27].

The problems of insight, of acquiring knowledge, and of other kinds of changes in cognitive structure seem to be closely related to the laws that govern perception. After insight is gained, the structure of the life space is changed. In an unstructured or new situation the person may feel insecure because the psychological directions are not defined; in other words, he does not know what actions will lead to what results. Learning is essentially structuring the life space to the extent that problem solution is possible.

Lewin delved into numerous problems relating to learning broadly conceived as any change in the person that produces a change in his psychological environment. Considerable attention was given to levels of aspiration as shown in the goals toward which a person strives. Another fruitful area of research was Lewin's exploration of the influence of group characteristics upon the behavior of a member of the group.

Although field theory was not intended to be a theory of learning, some applications to education can be drawn. According to Lewin, the life space of an intelligent person is more highly structured than that of a less intelligent person. Practice may facilitate learning because the change in cognitive structure or in motivation may require repetition. Motivation of the learner is central to this theory and relates to tension systems, levels of aspiration, and goal achievement. The process of change in cognitive structure is directly related to understanding and becomes the primary focus of learning. Forgetting of once-learned materials appears to be due to a lack of ego-involvement on the part of the learner and to the repression of too difficult, or undesirable, tasks [28].

Gestalt psychology and field theory were initially oriented to the study and explanation of perception and its influence on human behavior. Learning, although an important aspect of human behavior, was not the major focus of these theories. The theories are holistic in nature and give consideration to the total life situation. While the learning environment of the individual has direct impact upon the learner, the characteristics and behavior of the learner in turn also affect the situation. Gestalt psychology and field theory offered a sharp departure from the early stimulus-response theories, which were somewhat mechanistic. Whereas the stimulus-response theories focused attention on parts of behavior, gestalt psychology and field theory gave primary consideration to the more complex psychological processes, such as insight learning and problem-solving. Lewin endeavored to fit his theory into a mathematical system. Because of the complexity of the theory, with its numerous interacting variables, it has been difficult to assess its applicability to the practical problems of curriculum and instruction.

RECENT OR CURRENT LEARNING THEORIES

Several relatively recent or current learning theories have a stimulus-response orientation; others appear to be diametrically opposed to the S-R approach. Although research techniques within stimulus-response psychology have shown considerable refinement since the time of Thorndike and Watson, other factors have also facilitated the theory's increasing acceptance and application. One major strength of stimulus-response psychology has been the availability and reproducibility of its research findings and of the conditions under which learning occurs. It provides a research orientation appropriate for experimental study and practical application in that it deals with observable, measurable events. Its approach is considered more compatible with objective research because it attempts to empirically support or reject its hypothesis. Secondly, the stimulus-response analysis of learning appeared to be more consistent with available knowledge of human physiology than were the interpretations of the field theorists.

More recent stimulus-response theories do reflect the influence of the gestalt and field theories. Stimulus-response theories have begun to accept and utilize interpretations of learning that are both cognitive and purposive. Two of the major interests of contemporary stimulus-response theorists are the role of cognitive processes, such as thinking, reasoning, and problem-solving, and the purposive nature of drive and reinforcement. Although these are not new developments in the psychology of learning, the emphasis on the broadening of stimulus-response theories to include cognitive and purposive processes is a distinctive feature of current learning theories. Theories of learning are becoming more eclectic. Four of these recent approaches will be described. Although in each instance the individual credited with the specific theory is mentioned, other psychologists have been identified with the theories. These theories, although they attempt to explain a wide variety of behavior, focus primarily on learning and motivation with specific attention to the connections between physical stimuli and observable responses. The theorists have endeavored to find principles underlying complex behavior in man and higher animals [29].

THEORY OF CONTIGUOUS CONDITIONING

Following Watson in both time and approach, Edwin R. Guthrie (1886–1959) developed his basic principles of learning in the 1930's. The basic premise underlying the theory of contiguous conditioning was that a combination of stimuli which has accompanied a movement will on its recurrence tend to be followed by that movement. Of central importance is the principle of association by contiguity. Emphasis is placed upon association of stimuli (the activation of sense organs) and responses (the contraction of muscles and secretion of glands) [30].

According to Guthrie, responses, which are the answers to stimuli, are limited to the contraction of muscles or the secretion of glands. He separates responses into two types: movements, which refer to motor and glandular activities, and acts, consisting of a class of movements, the total result of all the movements in the class being the goal of the act. When we observe the behavior of an individual that results from a stimulus situation, we usually select some outstanding detail of an infinitely more complicated total response. The total response, however, always includes a set of internal events—heart beat, breathing, endocrine secretion, vasomotor changes, and changes in musculature [31].

The principle of association described by Guthrie states that a stimulus pattern that is present at the time of a response will, if it recurs, tend to produce the same response. The stimulus and the response—a stimulation of sense organs and a corresponding response of muscular contraction or glandular secretion—are associated. The stimulation becomes the occasion for the response because of a past association of the two. Both stimulus and response are observable. If the original stimulus occurs but fails to elicit the response, there has been no association. A stimulus pattern gains its full associative strength on the occasion of its first pairing with a response. Learning takes place in one trial—the first successful trial [32].

Forgetting is a case of failure to give a response to a cue. Forgetting is generally attributed to a lapse of time in which new associations are formed and replace the old. Forgetting requires active unlearning, that is, learning to give a new response to an old cue. If there were no interference with old learning, there would be no forgetting [33].

The repeated pairing of cue and response is found to increase the certainty and energy of the response. The effect of practice depends not on mere repetition but on the conditions of repetition, and these conditions vary enormously in different learning situations. Practice should elicit the response from a variety of situations. Effective practice is conducted in the general situation in which we desire the future performance to occur. In learning any skill one must acquire not just one association or even a series of associations but many thousands of associations that will connect specific movements with specific situations.

The motivational state of an organism—its hunger, thirst, or state of comfort or discomfort—has no place in Guthrie's theory. The motive is important for what it causes the organism to do and in keeping the organism active until a goal is reached. Reward preserves the behavior from disintegrating rather than strengthening it directly. The act leading to the reward, the last act in the problem situation, is the one favored when the situation recurs [34].

Guthrie indicates that an activity to be learned must be broken down into the movements required. By learning many separate movements, the learner develops a repertoire of movement responses. Likewise the teacher must select curriculum materials so that the component movements can be learned. Once the student has learned certain responses, the learning will be permanent unless it is interfered with by new learnings. To prevent such interference, Guthrie advocates distributed practice and drill.

SYSTEMATIC THEORY OF LEARNING

A comprehensive theory of behavior utilizing the methodology of the physical sciences was developed by Clark L. Hull (1884–1952). Hull indicated that a theory of behavior is a systematic, deductive derivation of the principles of behavior from a relatively small number of primary principles or postulates. Hull attempted to use equations and mathematical procedures in his systematic theory of learning [35].

According to Hull, learning is a means by which the organism comes to perceive its world through stimuli impinging upon its neurological structure and the acquisition and strengthening of habits that insure its survival.

The systematic theory of learning rests upon some fundamental assumptions about the organism and its environment. At birth there begins a dynamic relationship between the organism and its environment—the environment acting on the organism and the organism acting and reacting upon the environment throughout life. The individual's environment has two aspects—the internal environment and the external environment. The external environment is further divided into (1) the inanimate environment (which follows the laws of the physical sciences), and (2) the organismic environment (the laws of which are or would be those of the behavioral sciences) [36].

The physiological study of vertebrates shows that survival requires a variety of optimal conditions, such as air, water, food, temperature, and intactness of body tissue. When conditions for survival deviate from the optimum, a state of need is said to arise. The survival of the organism can be insured only if the deviation in its external environment is corrected. The particular combination of muscular contractions necessary to satisfy a need depends on the nature of the need, on the exact state of the environment at the time, and on the state of the environment following the organism's activity. The first requirement for survival under these conditions is that both the need and feedback on the state of the environment must be brought to bear upon the effectors (muscles and glands), which will participate in terminating the need [37].

Neural impulses, which are set in motion by stimuli from the internal and external environments, are routed from sensory receptors to the muscles and glands to produce the action needed for survival. If the first action or reflex reaction does not terminate the flow of impulses triggered by the need, other portions of the body become active, and the resulting movements evoked by the need effect the termination of the need. Continued survival of the organism will be facilitated if, as the result of this success, the random act or combination of acts that eliminated the need should on subsequent occasions acquire tendency to predominate over other acts that did not lead to a reduction of the need. If reinforcement occurs during this process, there will result from this conjunction of events an increment to habit formation.

Habit, according to Hull, is an unobservable entity. It is, however, anchored in observable antecedent conditions or stimuli and observable behavior. The concept of the habit family hierarchy indicates that there are several possible routes from a starting point to a goal, where need satisfaction can be found. The alternatives constitute a habit family, a set of alternative behavior patterns arranged in a preferred order reflecting the organism's reinforcement history. Reinforcement increments the strength of a habit [38].

The unique mathematical system devised by Hull gives operational definitions for all the variables considered and expresses the relationships among the variables in mathematical terms. Here at last was a system that generated testable hypotheses. From certain known conditions one could deduce the state of an unknown variable, and the means for verifying the deduction were implied by the theory. For example: hunger drive in an animal such as a rat can be roughly equated with number of hours of food deprivation. It is not difficult to measure the strength of a rat's pull on a restraining harness as it runs to food. It can be readily assumed that running will be closely related (proportional) to hunger. Suppose the rat is being trained to run to food along a certain path, and we want to know how the habit is developing. The habit is really internal and can only be inferred, but we assume that speed of running will be closely related (proportional) to the strength of the habit. As stated above, running, an observable response, is proportional to hunger (defined as hours of food deprivation, hence a measurable, specifiable stimulus condition) and to habit strength, and we can easily find the unknown, habit strength.

Hull said, in fact, that the effects of drive (hunger) and habit strength are multiplied to give the observable response tendency (running), which he called reaction potential. The important thing for the educator studying learning theories is not the exact relations posited but the fact that such a thorough-going attempt was made to set up a concrete deductive system giving rise to eminently testable hypotheses. Perhaps its greatest contribution has been in showing the way to gauging and controlling inferred processes by defining them operationally. Hull's system could be considered a refinement of Watson's behaviorism.

Although Hull was not primarily interested in the application of his theory to practical learning situations, some inferences can be made. The theory recognizes individual differences in the capacity to learn. The concepts of distributed and massed practice are incorporated in this theory. Distributed practice appears to facilitate effective learning. All improvements due to practice depend on reinforcement. The selection of appropriate educational stimuli and specification of the desired responses will determine the success or failure of the curriculum. Content materials should be selected carefully on the basis of their potential contribution to educational goals. Since learning is thought to occur by stimulus-response association, curriculum material that requires practice and repetition should be presented in such a way as to build up desired habits relating to the subject.

OPERANT CONDITIONING

The greatest break with conventional stimulus-response psychology is the system developed by B. F. Skinner (1904– . . .). Skinner's operant conditioning is a theory developed along the lines of Thorndike's law of effect. Learning as defined by Skinner is not a question of individual characteristics but a matter of the reinforcement of behavior to a desired level of performance. The learner is studied not in terms of abstract concepts like personality and insight, but as an organism whose observable behavior can be manipulated through reinforcement [39].

Operant conditioning deals with voluntary responses that an organism emits to produce the stimuli, as distinguished from classic conditioning, in which the stimuli precede and elicit the response. Responses that are not correlated with any known stimuli are *emitted* responses, called *operants*. Responses that are *elicited* by known stimuli are called *respondents*. Skinner indicates that most human behavior is operant in nature [40].

The two types of responses Skinner identifies correspond to two types of conditioning. The conditioning of respondent behavior, or classic conditioning, called Type S because reinforcement is correlated with the stimulus. Classic or Type S conditioning requires the approximate simultaneity of two stimuli to elicit the response. The conditioning of operant behavior or operant conditioning, is called Type R because of the association of the response with reinforcement. In operant conditioning, reinforcement cannot occur unless the conditioned response is emitted. Skinner has essentially changed the usual S-R formula into an R-S formula; in other words, when the desired response is emitted, a reinforcing stimulus is presented. This tends to condition the response, or to cause it to be repeated. Similarly, failure to reinforce will result in the extinction or nonperformance of the response.

Skinner refuses to consider or study motivation in learning or internal mental processes, because he feels psychology should be strictly scientific and study only observable, measurable behavior. The conditions for reinforcement of behavior appear to be assumed in a commonsense way. Food is reinforcing to a rat or a pigeon. Being told he has given a correct answer is reinforcing to a learner in school. The circumstances that result in conditioning are reinforcing by definition. According to Skinner, both Type R and Type S conditioning describe learning as a function of the conditions that influence the organism in its adaptation to the demands of the environment [41].

A reinforcer is defined by its effect. Any stimulus is a reinforcer if it increases the probability of a response. A positive reinforcer is any stimulus the presentation of which strengthens the behavior upon which it is made contingent—such as food, water, or good grades. A negative reinforcer is defined as any stimulus the withdrawal of which strengthens the behavior upon which it is made contingent—for example, loud noise, bright lights, or electric shock. The effect of reinforcement in either case is essentially the same: the probability of the desired response is increased.

The fundamental premise of operant conditioning is that the response must occur before it can be reinforced. A specific form of a response may be obtained by reinforcing successive approximations—a process called *shaping* the behavior. Operant responses are emitted with an original form or intensity. When only the specific form is reinforced, the higher form may be obtained. The shaping process permits the finally learned behavior to be very different from that originally emitted.

An important variable for Skinner is the *schedule of reinforcement*. Skinner observed that a conditioned response may be retained longer if an occasional performance of the response during conditioning is not reinforced, that is, if the response is given *intermittent reinforcement*. One can reinforce only every third response or one response per minute, for example. Skinner and others have amassed large amounts of data showing the relative efficacy of different schedules for training different types of response in the laboratory and in simple social settings. Practical examples are not hard to find, since probably most of human learning is by intermittent reinforcement. Gamblers persevere on the basis of only the rarest reinforcements—the fact that anyone has ever won the game seems to be all that is needed to keep them going. The child who persists in a certain annoying habit probably does so, in part, because his mother or his teacher was unable to punish him *every* time he did it—"getting away with it" a few times seems to strengthen the response in spite of the occasional punishments for engaging in it.

The central theme of Skinner's system is his belief in the objective methods of science. He acknowledges the complex nature of behavior and the problems in studying it. He believes it is the obligation of psychology to predict and control behavior and that there is nothing essentially insoluble about the problems which arise in doing so.

Skinner has a deep concern for the improvement of human conditions and endeavors to attack practical problems. In describing human learning, Skinner considers differences in capacity of minor importance. He has little use for describing various traits in studying individual differences.

The concern for reinforcement of responses implies that the teacher must provide reinforcement according to a planned schedule. Since operant responses presumably are strengthened through actual work with concrete materials, subject matter that necessitates "doing" is essential in any curriculum. The selection of stimuli becomes the dominant function in the learning situation. The course of instruction depends upon the student's rate of development.

The formation of habits is virtually guaranteed by the proper arrangement of stimuli leading to the reinforcement of desired responses. This implies the need for appropriate sequencing of subject matter units and skills in the learning program. The notion of sequence of stimuli in learning probably has been most useful in the development of programmed instruction, pioneered by Skinner.

Gagné's Hierarchy of Learning Sets

Robert M. Gagné (1916–   ) asserts that there are no general rules of learning known at present that can be used as guides in designing instruction. There are, however, a number of useful generalizations which can be made about several distinguishable classes of performance change, or learning. The purpose of a curriculum, according to Gagné, is to organize the educational situation in such a way that students who are at a certain stage incapable of exhibiting certain kinds of behavior, become capable of exhibiting those kinds of behavior [42].

Gagné defines learning as a change in human disposition or capability, which can be retained, and which is not due to growth or maturation. Learning shows itself as a change in behavior, and is inferred from a comparison of behavior before the individual was placed in the learning situation with his behavior after such treatment. The change may be an increased capability for some type of performance or an altered disposition of the sort called attitude, interest, or value [43].

Gagné recognizes eight types or categories of learning, each with its own rules, and arranges them in a hierarchy from simple to complex. He assumes that each higher order of learning in the hierarchy builds upon the one below it. The eight types can be summarized as follows:

1. Signal learning, or learning to make a general diffuse response to a signal, as in Pavlovian conditioning.
2. Stimulus-response learning, or learning of a connection between a precise response and a discriminated stimulus.
3. Chaining of two or more stimulus-response connections.
4. Chaining of verbal associations.
5. Discrimination of similar but different stimuli.
6. Concept learning.
7. Principle learning.
8. Problem solving [44].

Gagné defines knowledge as that inferred capability which makes possible the successful performance of a class of tasks that could not be performed before the learning was undertaken.

Gagné identifies several factors which influence change in behavior. There is the matter of individual differences. A curriculum which sets out to change behavior must take account of the fact that changes occur differently in different individuals. There is also the matter of motivation. This becomes a problem of identifying what kinds of motivation will bring about the particular kinds of learning contemplated by curriculum builders and how these motivations may be established in the human being. In addition, the content and sequence of material in a curriculum affect the ease with which knowledge is acquired or new behavior learned. Finally, there are many different types of human performances to be learned, each with its own peculiar set of variables.

Gagné's theory gives direct attention to the planning of sequences of instruction within content areas. He indicates, for example, that to do problem solving in physical science, the scientific principles to be used must have been previously learned. And before these principles can be learned, one must be sure there has been previous acquisition of relevant concepts. A strong emphasis in Gagné's analysis is upon the structure of knowledge, an important supplement to principles of learning whenever a practical instructional task is under consideration.

For each of the eight types of learning Gagné describes some of the required conditions of learning. Once the conditions of learning have been set forth, the instructional situation can be designed. Gagné explores the resources which may be utilized to accomplish the various instructional functions, including media of instruction and modes of teacher-student interaction. Gagné's theory offers a practical approach to the problems of curriculum and instruction in any subject matter.

The current learning theories appear to be attempting to resolve the major points of difference between the stimulus-response and the field theories. Although there is some agreement that the laws of learning are basically the same in the laboratory and the classroom, applications of laboratory research findings to classroom settings have not been extensive. The classroom presents complex problems which usually are not present in the laboratory. Thus, although a knowledge of existing learning theories provides worthwhile information, this knowledge is incomplete for the problems of curriculum and instruction.

THE NATURE OF LEARNING

Each of the learning theories described has offered some notions about learning that provide a frame of reference for investigative activities. The various theorists focus their attention upon the components and processes of learning that are compatible with their ideas as points of departure for study and analysis. The research designs are constructed to validate the role of the selected variables. The operational definition of learning for the purpose of experimental research must be limited to those variables the researcher is considering. Thus it is very likely that most of the definitions of learning included in research reports will not be useful to the teacher and curriculum worker. The definition of learning for research purposes may be too narrow in scope for application to the practical affairs of teaching.

But somehow teachers must arrive at a definition of learning that will be meaningful and useful to them in their professional activities. Once the definition has been formulated and agreed upon, they must translate the definition into concrete aspects of curriculum and instruction. The author has formulated a definition of learning which is compatible with her beliefs. Following this, certain generalizations drawn from the theories of learning discussed earlier are listed. It should not be considered an exhaustive list, however.

LEARNING DEFINED.   Learning is a psychological process involving both psychological and psychomotor activities. The process of learning cannot be observed but can be inferred from changes in the behavior of individuals. These changes take place through practice and experience directed toward the satisfaction of needs. Behavior changes include acquisition of knowledge, skills, interests, appreciations, and attitudes. Needs are considered to be intellectual, social, emotional, and physiological.

GENERALIZATIONS FROM THE LITERATURE ON LEARNING THEORIES

1. *Learning requires perceiving.* The learner is the key to perception, and the important thing in learning is how the learner perceives the situation. Dewey interpreted learning as a transaction between the organism and the environment. Gestalt psychology, field theories, and other cognitive theories place great emphasis on the role of perception in learning. Experiments with humans and animals give primary attention to the role of perception in problem-solving and insight learning.

2. *The extent of learning depends upon the individual characteristics of the learner.* The learner brings to the learning situation a vast array of characteristics determined by his heredity and environment. Learning takes place within the structural and functional limits that characterize the individual. The role of individual differences in learning was early identified by Thorndike. Gestalt psychology gave attention to the past experiences of the individual in the learning process. Field theories describe the various forces within the individual that influence learning, such as goals, desires, and aspirations. Personality theories emphasize the role of past experience, direct and vicarious, and the force of individual needs on learning. Research indicates that the learning of certain activities is dependent upon growth and maturational factors.

3. *Environment influences the extent of learning.* Many aspects of the environment affect the individual as he learns. Dewey refers to education as growth of the individual toward independence and self-control through interaction with his environment. Watson indicated that the individual cannot be seen apart from his environment—the environment determines his growth and development. Field theories describe the interaction of the learner and his environment in structuring his life space. In Hull's system, particularly, an at-

tempt is made to quantify and control all the salient aspects of the current learning environment.

4. *Learning is dependent upon the activity of the learner.* This activity is goal-directed, purposeful, and meaningful for the learner. Dewey emphasized the importance of experience and activity—we learn to do by doing. Stimulus-response theories imply the need for activity of the learner in performing the appropriate response. For gestalt psychologists the activity of the learner is problem-solving by means of restructuring his environment. In field theories the activity of the learner consists of acts necessary for maintaining equilibrium among tensions. And according to Hull, the learner is constantly seeking means of need reduction for survival.

5. *The motivation of the learner influences learning.* A student usually learns what he wants to learn and has difficulty learning material that does not interest him. Drives and incentives have played an important role in several theories of learning. Motives are difficult to specify and to measure, for they depend on such a variety of factors; often the individual himself is not fully aware of his motives. Motives may be intrinsic, such as achievement, recognition, and security, or extrinsic, such as material gains, grades, and promotions. Studies seem to indicate that the amount of interest cannot always be equated with the amount of material learned as measured by the usual testing procedures.

6. *Reinforcing a desired behavior tends to increase the probability that the behavior will be repeated in a similar situation.* Reinforcing includes both the idea of rewarding and of confirming. Practically all learning theories give attention to the role of reinforcement in learning. Stimulus-response and behaviorist theories place major emphasis upon reinforcement. "Right" or a nod of the head by the teacher or a high grade may be reinforcing as well as confirmation of desired behavior. Punishing inappropriate behavior may not decrease its probability; continuing the activity may be more attractive to the individual than the punishment is offensive to him, or the person may have no other response available. The effects of reinforcement on learning are well documented.

7. *Positive transfer of learning from one situation to another can be facilitated when certain conditions are present.* Transfer of learning usually takes place because a new situation is similar to an earlier learning environment. Thorndike's theory explained transfer of learning as due to the presence of identical elements in the old and new situations. Guthrie indicated that the only way to be sure to obtain a specific behavior in a new situation is to prac-

tice that particular behavior in the situation. Gestalt psychology suggests that for transfer to take place, certain relationships of elements should be learned. Studies suggest that positive transfer from one situation to another—from in school to out of school, from one subject to another, from one grade level to another—can be facilitated by making certain that the learning task is meaningful and not too difficult, by emphasizing the principles and methods of problem-solving rather than specific solutions, and by giving help to the learner as needed.

8. *Practice determines the effectiveness and efficiency of learning.* Practice facilitates learning if the learner has knowledge of the results of his practice. Thorndike indicated that practice brings improvement only because it permits other factors to be effective; practice alone does nothing. Guthrie stated that practice brings improvement because improvement refers to outcomes of learning rather than to movements. Gestalt psychology describes practice as successive exposure bringing out new relationships. Skinner indicates that conditioning is dependent upon repeated reinforcements, not practice alone. There is still controversy over the management of practice in the learning of skills. Some general notions seem to be applicable to the learning of a variety of skills: (1) guide responses carefully in the early stages of skill development, (2) provide appropriate practice tasks, (3) space out practice periods, and (4) provide the learner with knowledge of results.

INSTRUCTIONAL THEORIES

The amount of research on learning is vast. Yet, when a college teacher asks what findings from these researches will be of direct value to her as she plans a course or as she faces a class, the answer is usually "nothing." Carefully controlled laboratory explorations of learning simply do not mirror real-life academic or classroom situations, where influences that might be ruled out in the laboratory must be accepted.

Behavioral scientists more recently have endeavored to distinguish between behavioral science learning theory and instructional theory. They indicate that if a theory does not serve the purpose for which it is planned, either the theory or the use should be changed. The distinction between behavioral science learning theories and instructional theories, reflects the different needs of the laboratory and the classroom. Behavioral science learning theory is used to describe and explain recurring patterns of human behavior. Instructional theory is used to predict the effects of socially permissible teachers' activities on students.

This implies that instructional theories are a special case of behavioral science learning theories. The major emphasis in behavioral science learning theory is on developing propositions that are general enough to apply to broad classes of situations. This may make them too broad to apply to a particular practice situation. On the other hand the focus of instructional theories may be too narrow for generalization to a variety of learning events. It appears that very little of instructional theory can be deduced from existing learning theories in the behavioral sciences [45]. Psychologists and educators are crying out for usable instructional theories, theories to guide the teacher in selecting the most effective means for manipulating teacher, student, and situation variables to produce desired outcomes. The classroom teacher does not have this information available to her at present. Until such time as research yields an appropriate body of knowledge about the instructional process, teachers must rely upon information from general learning theories.

SUMMARY

The efforts of psychologists to analyze the learning process have resulted in a variety of learning theories. The study of learning has been influenced markedly by developments in other disciplines, such as philosophy, physics, and physiology. The theories described here fall in three groups, early learning theories, gestalt and field theories, and current learning theories.

The early learning theories are represented by connectionism, formulated by Edward L. Thorndike, functionalism, described by John Dewey, and behaviorism, developed by John B. Watson. Although these theories approach the study of learning from different angles, each made a significant contribution to the development of learning theory. This necessitated a break with the traditional psychology, which was deeply rooted in philosophy. Thorndike's belief that human behavior could be modified initiated a change in the focus of learning away from the concept of mental discipline. Dewey's concept of learning involved the total individual, his needs, interests, and activities, thus offering a theory of learning that was serviceable in the classroom. And even though the rigid physiological orientation of Watson has been refuted, his demands for strict scientific methodology set up American psychology in the business of science.

Gestalt psychology and field theory, although not initially proposed as learning theories, offered a counter influence to the early mechanistic stimulus-response theories. These theories developed from the field of perception and, with concern for the total situation of the learner, gave consideration to the more complex psychological problems of insight learning and problem-solving.

More recent or current learning theories display a stimulus-response orientation, although they reflect the influence of gestalt and field theories. The systematic theory of learning developed by Hull has a physiological foundation, but it includes as intervening variables such processes as drives, incentives, and inhibitions. The system is built upon a set of postulates that relate the intervening variables to observable stimuli and responses. The association of stimulus-response events by contiguity—making repetition the primary condition for learning—is the underlying notion of Guthrie's theory of contiguous conditioning. The learning system developed by Skinner is an attempt to describe rather than explain behavior. Skinner introduces the notion of operant conditioning, or the conditioning of operants—responses that are emitted, voluntary, and not triggered by any identifiable stimuli. This contrasts with classic (or Pavlovian) conditioning, in which a respondent or an elicited response is conditioned to a specific stimulus. In either case, reinforcement is given, contingent upon the desired response, to modify behavior. Skinner espouses a science of behavior that will enable us to predict and control behavior.

The learning theories that have been presented are general in nature and offer no specific guidelines for the teacher in classroom situations. Some generalizations about the nature of learning drawn from the theories are suggested. These too are general and allow for interpretation by teachers and curriculum workers.

It appears that learning theories developed in controlled laboratory situations are not directly applicable to the classroom situation. In most instances these theories were not developed for direct application to the practical teaching-learning environment. Psychologists and educators are presently voicing the need for instructional theories to guide the teacher in selecting effective means for obtaining the appropriate educational goals. Since instructional theories are not yet available, the general learning theories may offer a source of information for some curriculum decisions.

REFERENCES

1. Butts, R. F. A *Cultural History of Education.* New York: McGraw-Hill, 1947. P. 251.
2. Ibid., p. 321.

3. Ibid., p. 322.
4. Heidbreder, E. *Seven Psychologies*. New York: Appleton-Century-Crofts, 1933. P. 55.
5. Sandiford, P. Connectionism: Its Origin and Major Feature. In *The Psychology of Learning*. Forty-first Yearbook of the National Society for the Study of Education, Part II. Chicago: University of Chicago Press, 1942. P. 107.
6. Hilgard, E. R. *Theories of Learning*. New York: Appleton-Century-Crofts, 1948. P. 19.
7. Ibid.
8. Hilgard, E. R. *Theories of Learning*, 2d ed. New York: Appleton-Century-Crofts, 1956. P. 27.
9. Ibid., p. 18.
10. Ibid., p. 19.
11. Ibid., p. 26.
12. Ibid., p. 25.
13. McDonald, F. J. The Influence of Learning Theories on Education. In *Theories of Learning and Instruction*. Sixty-third Yearbook of the National Society for the Study of Education, Part II. Chicago: University of Chicago Press, 1964. P. 13.
14. Dewey, J. *Democracy and Education*. New York: Macmillan, 1961. P. 127.
15. Dewey, J. *Experience and Education*. New York: Macmillan, 1938. P. 48.
16. Dewey, J. *How We Think*. Boston: D. C. Heath, 1910. P. 146.
17. Ibid.
18. Heidbreder, op. cit., p. 235.
19. Heidbreder, op. cit., p. 243.
20. Watson, J. B. The Place of the Conditioned Reflex in Psychology. *Psychol. Rev.* 23:89, 1916.
21. Watson, J. B. *Psychological Care of Infant and Child*. New York: W. W. Norton, 1928.
22. Hartman, G. The Field Theory of Learning and Its Educational Consequences. In *The Psychology of Learning*. Forty-first Yearbook of the National Society for the Study of Education, Part II. Chicago: University of Chicago Press, 1942. P. 166.
23. Wertheimer, M. *Productive Thinking*. New York: Harper & Brothers, 1945.
24. Hilgard (1948), op. cit., p. 183.
25. Katona, G. *Organizing and Memorizing*. New York: Columbia University Press, 1940. P. 83.
26. Hilgard (1956), op. cit., p. 279.
27. Lewin, K. *Principles of Topological Psychology*. New York: McGraw-Hill, 1935.
28. Hilgard (1956), op. cit., p. 284.
29. Hill, W. F. Contemporary Development Within Stimulus-Response Learning Theory. In *Theories of Learning and Instruction*. Sixty-third Yearbook of the National Society for the Study of Education, Part I. Chicago: University of Chicago Press, 1969. P. 270.
30. Guthrie, E. R. *The Psychology of Learning*. New York: Harper & Row, 1952.
31. Guthrie, E. R. Conditioning: A Theory of Learning in Terms of Stimulus, Response and Association. In *The Psychology of Learning*. Forty-first Year-

book of the National Society for the Study of Education, Part II. Chicago: University of Chicago Press, 1942. P. 18.

32. Ibid., p. 30.
33. Ibid., p. 28.
34. Hilgard (1956), op. cit., p. 57.
35. Hull, C. L.   Conditioning: Outline of a Systematic Theory of Learning. In *The Psychology of Learning*. Forty-first Yearbook of the National Society for the Study of Education, Part II. Chicago: University of Chicago Press, 1942. P. 61.
36. Ibid., p. 62.
37. Ibid., p. 44.
38. Ibid., p. 43.
39. Skinner, B. F.   *The Technology of Teaching*. New York: Meredith, 1968. P. 240.
40. Skinner, B. F.   *Science and Human Behavior*. New York: Free Press, 1953. P. 65.
41. Ibid., p. 54.
42. Gagné, R. M.   A psychologist's counsel on curriculum design. *J. Res. Sci. Teaching* 1:27, 1963.
43. Gagné, R. M.   *The Conditions of Learning*. New York: Holt, Rinehart & Winston, 1965. P. 5.
44. Ibid., p. 58.
45. Woolridge, P. J., Skipper, J. K., Jr., and Leonard, R. C.   *Behavioral Science, Social Practice and the Nursing Profession*. Cleveland: Press of Case Western Reserve University, 1968. P. 32.

SUPPLEMENTARY READINGS

Bruner, J. S.   *On Knowing*. Cambridge: Harvard University Press, 1962.
Bruner, J. S.   *Toward a Theory of Instruction*. Cambridge: Harvard University Press, 1962.
Dewey, J.   *Human Nature and Conduct*. New York: Hall, 1922.
Dewey, J.   *Experience and Education*. New York: Macmillan, 1938.
Engelman, S.   *Conceptual Learning*. San Rafael: Dimensions, 1969.
Estes, W., et al.   *Modern Learning Theory*. New York: Appleton-Century-Crofts, 1954.
Hunt, E.   *Concept Learning—An Information-Processing Problem*. New York: Wiley, 1962.
Katona, G.   *Organizing and Memorizing*. New York: Columbia University Press, 1940.
Mowrer, O. H.   *Learning Theory and Behavior*. New York: Wiley, 1960.
Skinner, B. F.   Are theories of learning necessary? *Psychol. Rev.* 57:193, 1950.
Skinner, B. F.   *Verbal Behavior*. New York: Appleton-Century-Crofts, 1951.
Skinner, B. F.   The science of learning and the art of teaching. *Harvard Educ. Rev.* 24:86, 1954.
Waetjen, W. B. [Ed.].   *New Dimensions in Learning: A Multidisciplinary Approach*. Washington, D.C.: Association for Supervision and Curriculum Development, 1962.
Wertheimer, M.   *Productive Thinking*. New York: Harper & Bros., 1945.

III PROCESS OF CURRICULUM DEVELOPMENT

9 OBJECTIVES FOR CURRICULUM AND INSTRUCTION

THE development of a curriculum and instruction is dependent upon a definition or concept of nursing practice that is agreed upon by the faculty. The definition of nursing should enable the faculty to describe with some precision what the graduate of a particular program (professional or technical) knows and does in the practice of nursing. The conceptualization of nursing and nursing functions provides a frame of reference for the identification of objectives for the specific nursing curriculum.

An important first consideration in curriculum development is the identification of behaviors that the student should demonstrate at the end of the school program. These behaviors are considered to be the objectives of the curriculum and are known as terminal behaviors. The objectives of the curriculum may be thought of as the bridge between what the student knows when she enters school and what she knows when she completes the educational program.

INITIAL CONCERN FOR EDUCATIONAL OBJECTIVES

The importance of defining instructional objectives as an initial step in the planning of instruction was emphasized a number of years ago by Ralph Tyler. There can be little doubt that the activity stimulated by this initial formulation has been tremendously productive in the design of achievement tests, in the conduct of evaluation programs, and in the broader enterprises of course and curriculum planning. Interest in the measurement of achievement in education precipitated activity among psychologists in the development of examinations. The responsibility for developing university-wide examinations in a variety of subjects forced the examiners, together with faculty, to face squarely the fact that achievement measures cannot be sensibly designed until the course instructor states the objectives of her course. Such statements need to be made in terms of specific types of observable behavior if measures of achievement are to be constructed [1].

There are two special types of instruction in which the importance of specifying objectives has been explicitly recognized. The first of these is technical training in the military service, which is evident in the reviews of research oriented to the training of military personnel. The terms *task description* and *task analysis* used by the military reflect a recognition of the importance of specifying what the outcomes of training need to be before the training is planned. There is little formal difference between a task description and a set of instructional objectives. The specification of training objectives is considered to be accomplished by means of a technique that has broad usefulness in the development of personnel subsystems for man-machine systems, namely, task analysis. By using this technique, training objectives can be stated in behavioral terms. The second type of instruction is programmed instruction. Scarcely any writer in this field has failed to state that the specifying of objectives is an important first step in planning the instructional program and in making the assessment that will follow it.

The continuing efforts of the psychologists who were interested in the development of achievement tests stimulated enthusiasm for the possibilities of securing a common terminology for describing the behavioral characteristics they were trying to appraise in the various schools—the types of responses to content, subject matter, problems, or areas of human experience. These responses embraced a range of human behaviors, including knowing about something, solving problems of various kinds, evincing an interest in some types of human experience, having an attitude toward some object or process, or expressing feelings and views on a variety of phenomena. Objectives relating to these responses specify in operational terms the actions, feelings, and thoughts students are expected to develop as a result of the instructional process. It seemed to the psychologists that some way of classifying and ordering the types of responses specified as desired educational outcomes might be useful to teachers and others interested in assessing achievement. Bloom and his colleagues considered two distinct processes that would give meaning to educational objectives. One process was defining the objective in behavioral terms and then seeking the evidence that is relevant in determining whether the students have achieved the objective. This process has been a part of curriculum development and performance evaluation for a number of years. The second process was that of attempting to classify an objective so as to give specific information about what is intended by the objective. The rationale for the development of a taxonomy of objectives indicated that if educational objectives are to give direction to the learning process and to determine the nature of the evidence to be used in appraising the efforts of learning experiences, the terminology must be clear and meaningful [2].

Bloom and his colleagues began their study of educational objectives by identifying three types of objectives: cognitive, affective, and psychomotor. The *cognitive* objectives were those that emphasized remembering or reproducing something which had been learned. These objectives vary from simple recall of material learned to highly original and creative ways of combining and synthesizing new ideas and materials. The *affective* objectives, they felt, emphasize feeling tones and emotions. These objectives are expressed as interests, attitudes, appreciation, values, and emotional sets or biases. Those objectives concerned with muscular or motor skill, manipulation of materials and objectives, or acts which require neuromuscular coordination were classified as *psychomotor* objectives [3].

The study group acknowledged that these three types of objectives are not independent one from the others. They recognized, however, that attainment of objectives in one area, such as cognition, does not necessarily indicate the attainment of objectives in another area, such as psychomotor learning. Once it became obvious to the psychologists that most of the objectives stated by teachers within their own institutions fell into these three categories, their initial efforts were directed to the development of a taxonomy of educational objectives in the cognitive domain [4]. The frame of reference for this endeavor is implied by the equation formulated by this group: "objective = behaviors = evaluation technique = test problems" [5]. An objective has come to mean a particular set of behaviors; a specific set of evaluation techniques was accepted as the appropriate way of appraising these behaviors, and a particular set of test problems was recognized as a valid indicator of the particular objective and its behaviors. As the group proceeded with its task, it became apparent to them that the various objectives in the cognitive domain varied in complexity. Objectives calling for synthesis of ideas required different mental activities than did the objectives demanding simple recall of information. The principle of complexity was used as a basis for ordering the objectives in the cognitive domain.

The development of objectives in the affective domain proceeded with less assurance. The psychologists found a lack of clarity in the statements of affective objectives that appeared in the literature. Also it appeared that complexity, used as the basis for ordering the cognitive objectives, was not useful with the affective objectives. Over the years it seemed teachers had given less attention to these objectives than to those in the cognitive domain and had shown little concern for evaluating the affective behaviors.

The hesitancy of teachers to use affective measures for evaluation purposes stems partially from the inadequacy of appraisal techniques. Frequently, behaviors in the affective domain must be inferred from overt behaviors, which may or may not be valid, such as judging an interest in art by the number of visits to art displays and museums. Certain attitudes and values may be considered to be private matters and not open to public scrutiny. The degree of attainment of affective objectives within a school or grade level is difficult to determine without raising the question of indoctrination. Where it is possible to identify acceptable behaviors in the affective domain and to specify the appropriate level of attainment, these behaviors may not undergo a process of change like that noted in the cognitive area. Some affective behaviors show a rapid transformation in a relatively short period of time, whereas others develop slowly, requiring a long period of time.

The Bloom study group were motivated to work toward developing a classification of affective objectives with full knowledge of the inherent problems. Research findings reporting the insignificant influence of college education on the values of students stimulated efforts to prepare a taxonomy of objectives in the affective domain. The analysis of objectives dealing with affective behavior yielded a wide range of behaviors—from the awareness of a phenomenon by the individual to a state in which the phenomenon is the individual's life outlook. Thus, the ordering principle for the affective objectives became the degree of internalization. A handbook of affective behaviors appeared in 1964 as companion to the 1956 handbook of cognitive behaviors [5].

EDUCATIONAL OBJECTIVES AND THE LEARNING PROCESS

Previous descriptions of learning and the learning process suggest that learning is a matter of acquiring new behaviors. The individual can do something at the end of the instructional program that she could not do before engaging in that program. The learner will be different in some ways than she was at the onset of the program. The graduate of a basic professional program in nursing will care for an acutely ill patient in a different manner than would a high school graduate entering the nursing school. The graduate of the nursing curriculum demonstrates that she has acquired knowledge about the patient and his illness; she has attained skills in assessing the patient's needs, in making judgments concerning the appropriate nursing care, in establishing relationships with the patient and his family, and in performing certain techniques and procedures that are a part of the plan of care. Although these nursing behaviors are only a few of the many that the student acquires, it appears that the general categories of behavioral changes which take place include attaining knowledge, skills, attitudes, appreciations, and interests. Thus, the terminal behaviors (the objectives of the curriculum) are expressions of the behavior changes that the student acquires as a result of curriculum and instruction. In other words, curriculum and instruction are means by which the learner acquires the appropriate behavior that will enable her to perform the activities of her occupational role.

Modifying behavior has always been the goal of educational programs. Modification or change of behavior as a result of experience or training is a widely accepted and familiar definition of learning. The essential innovation in behavior modification is the emphasis on evaluation and measurement techniques, more specifically those techniques of determining how effectively behavior is actually modified in the direction identified by the educator. Consideration is given to the educator's professional obligation and implicit commitment to the scientific ideal of repeatability of results. Such a commitment implies that there is no contradiction between setting appropriate goals and evaluating these goals with precision and accuracy. The three aspects of behavior modification in the achievement of behaviorally stated educational goals include (1) the evalution or diagnosis of the student, (2) the analysis (or sequence) of the functions—task to be learned, and (3) the procedural methods and management techniques of the teacher.

Ideally, the teacher bases her decisions as to what to teach and how to teach on the individual characteristics of the learners. This implies that the teacher gains information about the student's learning repertoire—the knowledge, skills, and attitudes that she brings with her to the learning situation. These initial behaviors of the student in the specified area of learning are what the teacher builds upon. The sequence or analysis of functions and tasks in terms of observable behaviors is a second aspect of behavior modification. Precise learning abilities and disabilities can be identified only when sequences of required behaviors have been stated in terms of what initial capabilities the student must possess and what the student is expected to be capable of doing following a particular period of learning. Such curriculum planning must also include the constraints under which the curriculum is taught: space, time, available materials, and resource persons.

The procedural methods and management techniques of the teacher may be classified into two major categories, which include verbal interaction and stimulus-response techniques. Interaction techniques involve the effect of specific teacher behaviors on student behavior. The teacher's behavior, usually verbal, is quantitatively classified according to several behaviorally specified measures, for example, accepting, praising, clarifying, giving information or directions, criticizing, and asking questions. This quantitative classification is examined in terms of what type of student verbal behavior it elicits. Classification records of this type enable the teacher to view the consequences of her own behavior objectively. Using this approach the teacher may set objectives for quantitative and qualitative verbal behavior for students as well as herself. Various stimulus-response techniques provide means of evaluating or measuring the effectiveness of reinforcement techniques. Three requirements in the use of such techniques are (1) identifying and measuring the frequency of the behavior to be acquired, reinforced, or eliminated, (2) identifying the conditions that lead to the development and maintenance of the behavior, and (3) delineating the behavior the teacher will exhibit in order to establish the conditions for change.

REASONS FOR SPECIFYING OBJECTIVES

The broad goals of education have been formulated by a number of national groups and commissions as well as by outstanding educational scholars. There appears to be agreement among these groups and individuals on three broadly stated goals: (1) the purpose of making it possible for the individual to participate in and to share with other people a variety of aesthetic experiences, (2) the development of responsible citizenship, and (3) the development of individual talents to achieve satisfaction in a life work or vocation [6].

Although there appears to be no real argument about the appropriateness of these goals, there is considerable debate about the degree of attainment required and about the particular ways in which the goals will be reached (involving both content and method of education). Before such debates can be resolved, we need to define what is actually meant by participating in and sharing with others a variety of aesthetic experiences, what is meant by responsible citizenship, and finally, what is implied by achieving satisfaction in a life work or vocation. In other words, what will the individuals be like who have achieved these goals? Secondly, we need to analyze, or break down into smaller components and stages, the progression toward these goals.

Gagné distinguishes between human behavior and performance. Performance, he indicates, relates to observable human accomplishment. Behavior is what brings about performance; performance is an outcome of behavior. The fundamental reason why human performance is related to education is that it must be used to define what happens or what is supposed to happen in the educational process. Education is for learning; yet it is of great importance to keep in mind just what learning means and how we know when it has taken place. We infer that learning has occurred when there is a change in the performance of the student from a given time to some later period which is not solely due to the maturation of the student. The change in performance is what provides evidence of learning. Performance is the fundamental class of data one must have in order to infer learning. Since observable human performance is the basis on which the inference of learning is made, it would seem to follow that these same performances should constitute the objectives of education [7].

The fundamental reasons for specifying objectives of education are addressed to those who are trying to understand education, to study it as a process, and to improve its quality. Definitions of objectives are necessary to guide the behavior of the teacher. Specifying the nature of the terminal behavior that is aimed for indicates to the teacher and the student what must be learned. Describing the objectives of the educational program provides the teacher with some guidelines for the design of the program of instruction. There will be no proof of learning unless the instructor and the student agree on what the learner will be able to do after she has completed the instruction. Designation of terminal behavior will provide a basis from which inferences can be made by the instructor about the kinds of behavior modification required throughout the program.

The aim of an educational program is the establishment of the capability for certain kinds of behavior; the learner must be able to do something after completing the instruction that she could not do beforehand. To know whether a program has fulfilled such an aim, it must be possible to observe or measure this post-learning behavior. This is why the objectives of education must be specified in terms that allow reliable observation. A capability of the learner that cannot be so specified cannot be measured. It is not possible to construct or use a valid achievement test without clarifying the objectives that the test is supposed to measure. One cannot measure the outcomes of a course in English, or chemistry, or nursing without knowing what particular changes in behavior are sought in the English or chemistry or nursing course, since the test is a device for determining whether these changes have actually occurred. It is necessary to have objectives clearly formulated, that is, stated in specific terms, if one is to measure any change brought about by a program of education.

The formulation of a statement of objectives is nothing less than the definition of certain classes of terminal behaviors, each of which, regardless of its specific content, implies a particular set of conditions of learning required for its establishment. The behaviors may relate to overall thinking (cognitive), feeling (affective), and doing (psychomotor) behaviors, or they may be behaviors within any one of these major categories. Within the cognitive category, more specific behaviors might include those pertaining to memorizing facts, defining terms, making comparisons, and discriminating between and among similar events, episodes, or phenomena. In the psychomotor behaviors, varieties of behaviors could include tactile and kinesthetic skills, hand-eye coordination, and using the hands and body with ease and dexterity.

Defining objectives and making them known to the learner enables the learner to program her own activities. Giving the learner prior knowledge about the variety of responses that are expected of her may have the effect of controlling the reinforcement and therefore improving the efficiency of her learning. Most investigators of learning agree that a set of conditions that either follows or accompanies the newly acquired behavior serves the function of raising the probability that this behavior will occur again when the situation calls for it. This set of conditions is known as *reinforcement*. Unless the student knows what the objectives are, she is likely to resort to memorizing information or mechanically completing workbook tasks rather than carrying out relevant learning activities. Objectives provide the student with a goal about which she herself can organize her own learning activities.

Unless objectives are known, it is impossible to know what the student's capabilities are at any given moment, hence whether she has been learning. It is impossible to carry on the enterprise of education without assessing each student's attainments from time to time. It makes no sense to try to teach something that the student either knows already or cannot possibly learn because she does not have the prerequisite knowledge. We must know what the student is capable of doing at any given moment in her educational development—that is, the level at which she is currently performing. Thus, the major reasons for specifying educational objectives are those concerned with (1) describing the nature of the terminal behavior, (2) measuring the post-learning behavior, (3) defining the various classes of terminal behavior, and (4) defining the conditions of learning and reinforcement of the learner [8].

PROCESS OF DEFINING OBJECTIVES

Since it is possible to bring about a great many changes in behavior through curriculum and instruction, some of which would be quite undesirable, and since the time that the school can devote to the attainment of all the possible objectives is limited, it would seem evident that every school and every instructor must decide what objectives should be aimed at and select the several objectives that can be attained with some degree of success. Although this argument for a careful selection of objectives seems obvious, a great many schools and teachers carry on the process of instruction without having a clear conception of the ends to be reached. It is true that in schools and colleges the materials and procedures become traditional and are passed on from one generation to another without a clear realization of the ends they are expected to achieve. Many teachers find themselves using particular books and carrying on particular kinds of instructional procedures, not so much because they have certain ends in mind, but because these materials and these procedures have been used for many years and are accepted as having value without any clear perception of their underlying purposes. Teachers may carry on instruction without having clearly formulated objectives. Yet, if instruction is to be rationally planned and choices made among various possible materials and procedures of instruction, there must be a clear understanding of the ends to be sought.

It should be clear that the end goals in a particular school or course should be those not already attained by the student; those that can build upon her previous background of skills, abilities, knowledges, attitudes, and interests; and those that to some degree help the student to deal with her own problems, to satisfy her own interests, and to meet her own needs. It is also clear that the goals of education in a particular school or course should be to some degree those knowledges, skills, abilities, and interests that have significance in contemporary society and that can help the student carry out her occupational roles. Some of these objectives may be conflicting, and it will be necessary to make a choice among them. The school or instructor will wish to emphasize objectives that are most in harmony with its philosophy of education. Likewise, the selection of objectives may be facilitated by giving consideration to the psychology of learning. Although this information may not give precise direction, some guidelines presently are available which indicate that certain objectives may not be attainable at a particular developmental stage of the learner. These objectives may be more appropriately attained at some other stage in the student's education.

LEVELS OF OBJECTIVES

Central to establishing a relevant curriculum is identifying the goals that the curriculum is designed to achieve. Statements of desired general outcomes serve as a starting point for more specific objectives. But if these goals are defined *only* in broad general terms, the possibility is great that such curriculum development efforts will have little effect on students' classroom performance. Each of generally stated outcomes probably suggests several student abilities to the person who formulated it. If the statements were left in this vague, generalized form, they would give no practical guidance to the many persons expected to put the curriculum into effect. So the first step is to identify specific objectives of curriculum goals. To accomplish this, one must look at each of the generally stated outcomes and ask, What would we expect the student to be able to do after she has achieved this goal? It should be noted that the objectives developed here are not as detailed as those on which a test or other evaluation procedure would be based. The listing of such detailed objectives could result in an unwieldy curriculum document. Specificity can result in triviality. This can be overcome by relating any behaviorally stated objective to its more broadly stated nonbehavioral goal and giving the student a rationale for achieving the objective.

Burns suggests that behavioral objectives start with an identification of the type or category of behavior expected, followed by a behavioral description [9]. The nonbehavioral objectives, which typically appear in course curriculum guides, include types of behavior illustrated by words such as knowledge, understanding, or skill.

Burns offers a combination of nonbehavioral and behavioral objectives which may be stated as follows: The student has knowledge of the nursing process so that when given a situation describing nursing intervention in the care of a patient, she identifies without error the steps in the nursing process. Objectives stated in this manner reveal to the student (1) the action required ("identifies"), (2) the context or content ("the steps in the nursing process"), and (3) the criterion ("without error").

The most important function of behavioral objectives is in the direct use of these objectives by the student to learn the expected behavior and to evaluate her own progress in learning the behavior. The statement of an objective and an accompanying statement describing the behaviors of those who have achieved this objective at varying levels of performance provides a means for evaluating progress.

Tyler indicates that the most useful degree of specificity of objectives is the level of generality of behavior that one is seeking to help the student acquire [10]. One indication of a high level of generality is that the description identifies a performance that can be valued in and of itself as being of effective use in the individual's life. Another level of generality or specificity relates to the probable effectiveness in teaching the student to generalize the learning to the desired level. In other words, the objectives should express a purpose that makes sense within the larger context of the person's life goals, and this purpose should be distinguishable from others.

ANALYSIS OF HUMAN PERFORMANCE.   Objective statements of performance provide empirically observable foundations to which all speculations, hypotheses, and innovative hunches about educational improvement must be referred. In designing a curriculum, it becomes very evident that certain objectives depend on others. There are such things as subordinate objectives; there are performances that are prerequisite to other performances. Practically all educational objectives have prerequisites, and such an analysis of objectives must be done if an effective sequence of instruction is to be designed. When one conducts such an analysis, she begins with a task, a statement of an objective having a distinct purpose. But the statement of performances that result from the analysis are considerably more detailed than this. Their purposes cannot usually be understood alone; they can be understood only as a prerequisite to the more generally stated objectives with which the analysis began.

Closely related to this reason for breaking down educational objectives into finer units is the need for assessing student progress. To do it properly, it is necessary not only to state objectives but also to analyze them. Tests that are based on such detailed performance statements can be truly diagnostic of students' progress within the framework of a curriculum. One of the important reasons for analyzing objectives is to determine some important facts about the conditions for learning them. To clarify what is needed for learning, the original objective must be broken down into more specific statements of performance.

Gagné defines productive learning as the kind of change in behavior that permits the individual to perform successfully an entire class of specific tasks rather than simply one member of the class [11]. Beginning with the final task, or terminal behavior, the question is asked, What kind of capability should an individual have to possess if she were able to perform this task successfully? The answer to this question identifies a new class of tasks, which appear to have several important characteristics. It appears that what we have defined by this procedure is an entity of subordinate knowledge that is essential to the performance of the more specific final task [12]. In developing objectives, it is necessary to take into consideration the initial, intermediate, and terminal behaviors of the student. Initial behavior consists of the behavioral repertoire that the student brings to the instructional situation. Terminal behavior comprises the specific final set of accomplishments the student is to have at the end of the instructional course. The specification of objectives must be made in terms of behavioral end products, that is, in terms of what the student must be able to do when she has completed the program of instruction. Intermediate behaviors are the many and varied behaviors that are acquired during the process of attaining the terminal behaviors. These are identified and described on a continuum of increasing specificity and decreasing complexity.

In the course of the instructional sequence, between the initial repertoire and the terminal behavior, the student performs activities that would enable her to reach the terminal behavior or degree of subject matter competence specified by a particular curriculum component. The student activity that the teacher encourages and uses for this purpose can be called *intermediate behavior*. The instructional process seeks to use the intermediate behaviors to reach desired educational objectives. The process is greatly helped by the detailed specification of the behaviors that the student will perform toward the approximation of the final or terminal behavior.

The concept of terminal and intermediate behaviors is somewhat fluid in relation to the curriculum as a whole or to an aspect of curriculum. The terminal behavior of the curriculum as a whole may indicate that the graduate nurse practices professional nursing at the degree of competence described by the faculty. In this instance the intermediate behaviors become the objectives of the major components of the curriculum:

The student
1. Describes the cultural and socioeconomic influences on health and illness
2. Develops and initiates plans for nursing action in health maintenance of aging and aged persons
3. Develops and initiates plans for nursing care to the pregnant woman and her family during the child-bearing experience
4. Develops and initiates plans for nursing care to children and adults who are experiencing some acute pathophysiological aberration

These are a few of the intermediate behaviors that must be acquired before the terminal or final behavior "practices professional nursing at a designated level of competence" can be attained.

Each one of the intermediate behaviors becomes a terminal behavior at the next level of curriculum planning. The behavior "develops and initiates plans for nursing action in health maintenance of aging and aged persons" becomes a terminal behavior for that area or phase of the curriculum. The behaviors that the student will acquire in order to approximate the terminal behavior for this aspect of the curriculum might include the following:

The student
1. Specifies the indicators of health of older pesons
2. Describes the assessment of health status of older persons
3. Describes the physiological and psychosocial changes that take place in aging persons
4. Develops and initiates plans of nursing intervention in an effort to alleviate the health problems of older persons

These behaviors become the means whereby the terminal behavior for this curriculum component may be attained. They are thus considered to be intermediate behaviors at this level of the curriculum.

Proceeding to the next level of instructional planning, each of the intermediate behaviors may become a terminal behavior for specific learning opportunities. Each behavior can be analyzed to identity the activities that will be encountered in the effort to acquire the more specific terminal behavior. Analysis of what the student will need to know "to describe the physiological and psychosocial changes that take place in aging persons" yields the following:

The student
1. Specifies the general characteristics of the aging process in terms of causes and consequences
2. Specifies the anatomic and physiologic changes that take place in aging
3. Specifies the bodily changes in aging that affect appearance
4. Specifies the basic psychological changes in older persons
5. Specifies the changes in social behavior of older persons

The degree of specificity and simplicity of behaviors to be attained in this area of the curriculum depends upon the initial behaviors or the learning repertoire that the student brings to this phase of the curriculum. This can be determined by examination of curriculum events preceding this learning opportunity and by performance evaluation of the students (pretesting). If further specificity is indicated, each of the aforementioned intermediate behaviors may become a terminal behavior for a specific learning episode. The behavior "specifies the changes in social behavior of older persons" becomes a terminal behavior that can be subjected to analysis for the identification of subbehaviors or intermediate behaviors which are required for the attainment of this terminal behavior. This analysis reveals what the student needs to know in order to approximate the behavior and includes the following:

The student
1. Specifies the factors that affect the socialization of older persons
2. Specifies the behavior manifestations of older persons when social needs are not met
3. Specifies the relationships between health, retirement, and adjustment in old age
4. Identifies the characteristics of good adjustment in aging persons
5. Specifies the roles of voluntary associations in the adjustment of aging persons
6. Specifies the role of federal and state legislation in the adjustment of older people

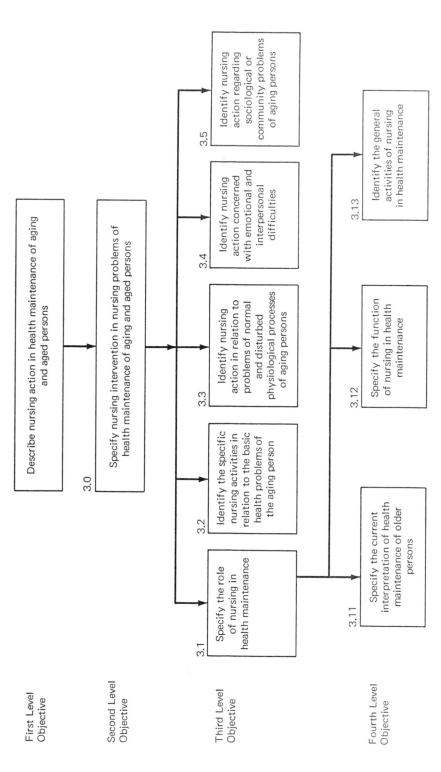

First Level
Objective

Describe nursing action in health maintenance of aging and aged persons

3.0

Second Level
Objective

Specify nursing intervention in nursing problems of health maintenance of aging and aged persons

Third Level
Objective

3.1

Specify the role of nursing in health maintenance

3.2

Identify the specific nursing activities in relation to the basic health problems of the aging person

3.3

Identify nursing action in relation to problems of normal and disturbed physiological processes of aging persons

3.4

Identify nursing action concerned with emotional and interpersonal difficulties

3.5

Identify nursing action regarding sociological or community problems of aging persons

Fourth Level
Objective

3.11

Specify the current interpretation of health maintenance of older persons

3.12

Specify the function of nursing in health maintenance

3.13

Identify the general activities of nursing in health maintenance

DIAGRAM 2. Behavioral components and subject matter subtopics in relation to nursing action in health maintenance of aging and aged persons. (Continued on pages 236–237.)

(Diagram 2 continued)

First Level
Objective

Describe nursing action in health maintenance of aging and aged persons

3.0

Second Level
Objective

Specify nursing intervention in nursing problems of health maintenance of aging and aged persons

3.2

Third Level
Objective

Identify the specific nursing activities in relation to the basic health problems of the aging and aged persons

3.21

Specify nursing action to maintain good hygiene and physical comfort

3.22

Specify nursing action to promote optimal activity, exercise, rest, and sleep

3.23

Specify nursing action to promote safety through prevention of accidents or injury

3.24

Specify nursing action to maintain good body mechanics and to prevent deformities

Fourth Level
Objective

3.3

Third Level
Objective

Identify nursing action in relation to problems of normal and disturbed physiological processes of aging and aged persons

3.31

Specify nursing action necessary to facilitate the maintenance of a supply of oxygen to all body cells

3.32

Specify nursing action necessary to facilitate the maintenance of nutrition to all body cells

3.33

Specify nursing action necessary to facilitate the maintenance of elimination

3.34

Specify nursing action necessary to maintain fluid and electrolyte balance

3.35

Specify nursing action in relation to the physiological responses of the body to certain drugs

3.36

Specify nursing action necessary to facilitate the maintenance of regulatory mechanisms and functions

3.37

Specify nursing action necessary to facilitate the maintenance of sensory functions

Fourth Level
Objective

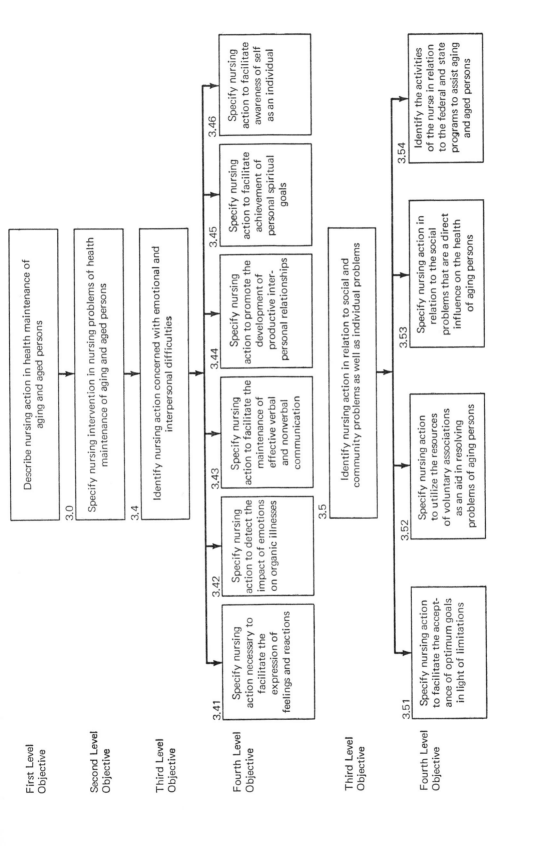

First Level Objective

Describe nursing action in health maintenance of aging and aged persons

Second Level Objective

3.0 Specify nursing intervention in nursing problems of health maintenance of aging and aged persons

Third Level Objective

3.4 Identify nursing action concerned with emotional and interpersonal difficulties

Fourth Level Objective

3.41 Specify nursing action necessary to facilitate the expression of feelings and reactions

3.42 Specify nursing action to detect the impact of emotions on organic illnesses

3.43 Specify nursing action to facilitate the maintenance of effective verbal and nonverbal communication

3.44 Specify nursing action to promote the development of productive inter-personal relationships

3.45 Specify nursing action to facilitate achievement of personal spiritual goals

3.46 Specify nursing action to facilitate awareness of self as an individual

Third Level Objective

3.5 Identify nursing action in relation to social and community problems as well as individual problems

Fourth Level Objective

3.51 Specify nursing action to facilitate the accept-ance of optimum goals in light of limitations

3.52 Specify nursing action to utilize the resources of voluntary associations as an aid in resolving problems of aging persons

3.53 Specify nursing action in relation to the social problems that are a direct influence on the health of aging persons

3.54 Identify the activities of the nurse in relation to the federal and state programs to assist aging and aged persons

The analysis of human performance in relation to the curriculum as a whole reveals the terminal behavior to be attained by the student. A step-by-step breakdown of the terminal behaviors into the tasks and activities required to attain these behaviors provides evidence of the means by which the behaviors at different levels can be acquired. This analysis of performance gives evidence of the intermediate behaviors, which bridge the gap between the student's initial behavioral repertoire and the attainment of the final behaviors.

The objectives pertaining to nursing action in health maintenance of aging and aged persons is presented in Diagram 2, which indicates the levels of behavioral components and subject matter subtopics.

PROCESS OF BEHAVIORAL ANALYSIS

Once it is known what nurses will do in a specific type of practice (technical, professional), efforts must then be directed to determining what human capabilities are necessary. This is the process of behavioral analysis or task analysis. The curriculum worker makes inferences, based on knowledge of the nature of human functioning, concerning what kinds of abilities, skills, and knowledge are required for the nurse to carry out the specific function. The results of task analysis provide immediate definitions of the various human performances required and suggest the measures which will have to be applied in the assessment of these performances.

It is apparent that the technologies of task description and task analysis have been markedly advanced in technique and objectivity because they occurred within the framework of systems development. The contrast between these techniques and those of traditional "job analysis," with its unsystematic procedures and poorly defined terminology, is quite striking. The techniques of task description and analysis have been remarkably successful on the whole in forecasting human performances required by newly developed systems as well as in determining the human capabilities that need to be selected, trained, and supported on the job [13]. Although there are gaps in scientific knowledge about human behavior and in the conceptualizations of nursing practice, information about the dimensions of human functions and how these dimensions are affected by the process of learning is available.

The techniques and procedures of task analysis and task description may be applied in the identification of the behavior expectations and behavior descriptions of the nurse who is engaged in the functions of nursing. If a curriculum of instruction is to assist the nursing student to acquire designated behaviors (behavior expectations) in the manner in which they are described by the faculty (behavior descriptions), these must be identified and made known to students and teachers. If the professional or technical nurse is expected to give nursing care to a patient and his family, specific behavior expectations must be identified and described. One faculty group at the University of Maryland devoted considerable time and effort to analyzing the behavioral expectations of a graduate of a baccalaureate program in the area of community health nursing. These instructors developed behavior descriptions of the practicing nurse in community health nursing. The description identified four major behavior expectations:

The nurse
1. Establishes, maintains, and promotes effective relationships with individuals, families, and health personnel.
2. Establishes, maintains, and promotes effective communication with individuals, families, and health personnel.
3. Applies clinical science information in the performance of nursing activities.
4. Performs certain nursing procedures in the care of individuals and families within the framework of a community health agency.

These behavior expectations were considered to be the major focus of nursing in this area of practice. Each of these behavior expectations was subjected to an analysis that revealed activities and tasks in an increasing degree of specificity, moving toward the basic and fundamental units of the activity. These are described in relation to the expectations of the terminal behavior and the subknowledges or capabilities, which may be the basic units of the activity (see Table 2). It is obvious that the subknowledges do not operate independently; they are identified, however, for the purpose of analysis and description.

The analysis of the behavior expectations of a professional nurse in this particular phase of nursing is not the only or most inclusive analysis that might be made. It is included to describe the way in which a group of teachers carried out the process of behavioral analysis for the purpose of identifying the subknowledges or capabilities that provide direction for curriculum and instruction. These subknowledges give attention to the learning tasks and processes in a specific area of nursing practice.

To illustrate the process of behavioral analysis in another aspect of nursing

TABLE 2. Terminal Behavior and Behavior Description for Student Providing Professional Nursing Care to a Patient and Family Within the Framework of a Community Health Agency

Behavior Expectations	Subknowledge or Capabilities
1. Establishes, maintains, and promotes effective relationships with individuals, families, and health personnel	
2. Establishes, maintains, and promotes effective communication with individuals, families, and health personnel	a. Utilizes and interprets different modes of communication (verbal, symbolic, gestures, body movements, somatic signals) b. Utilizes and interprets the mode of communication appropriate for the developmental stage of the individual c. Interprets communication with attention to the social, emotional, and cultural environment of the individual and family d. Is sensitive to the purpose and process of therapeutic communication e. Creates an environment in which there is a useful balance between control and permissiveness f. Is skillful in selective listening and in reflecting upon communication g. Gives instructions that are clear, realistic, mutually acceptable, and understood by the individual and family h. Times messages so that the listener has sufficient time to perceive and evaluate them i. Addresses individual(s) by name using a modulated voice and indicating a concern for his (their) welfare j. Makes relevant contribution to group thought based on analyses of the situation k. Prepares written reports that provide relevant information for continuity of care l. Uses language which is clear, appropriate, and easily understood by the family
3. Applies clinical science information in the performance of nursing activities	a. Perceives new clues in the situation that may alter nursing judgments b. Utilizes objective devices whereby observations may be made more accurate c. Makes careful recordings of observations d. Identifies the influence of bias and prejudice in observations, and makes an effort to overcome or prevent these influences.

Behavior Expectations	Subknowledge or Capabilities
	e. Makes nursing judgments based on the physiological status or problems of the patient
	f. Is sensitive to the impact of body changes upon the individual's self-concept
	g. Makes nursing judgments based on knowledge of the individual's psychological mechanisms and defenses
	h. Is sensitive to the influences of socioeconomic and cultural environment on patterns of living
	i. Makes differential nursing judgments based on individual's age, sex, marital status, income, educational background, and family responsibilities and relationships
	j. Makes nursing judgments in relation to the environmental conditions that may precipitate disease or prevent recovery from illness
4. Performs certain nursing procedures in the care of individuals and families within the framework of a community health agency	a. Performs activity with coordinated muscle movements and visual perception
	b. Is able to devote the major portion of her attention to the individual
	c. Performs activity with minimum of lost motion or wasted energy and with apparent ease, grace, and pleasing appearance
	d. Performs activity with attention to individual needs and scientific principles
	e. Performs activity with appropriate imagination and creativity
	f. Perceives new clues; analyzes them selectively for refinement of activity
	g. Organizes necessary equipment and arranges materials for the most expeditious care
	h. Uses care in the handling of equipment to prolong their useful lifetimes

TABLE 3. Terminal Behavior and Behavioral Description for Student Providing Professional Nursing Care to a Patient (and Family) Who Is Experiencing Difficulty Maintaining Adequate Oxygen Intake

Behavior Expectations	Subknowledge or Capabilities
1. Describes factors that influence the prevention and control of tuberculosis	a. Consults authentic sources of information concerning the incidence, trends, and characteristics of tuberculosis
	b. Relates to appropriate persons regarding problems involved in the occurrence of tuberculosis for the community, city, state, nation, world

(Continued on pages 242–243)

(Table 3 continued)

Behavior Expectations	Subknowledge or Capabilities
	c. Obtains pertinent information about patient's home, family, education, employment, socio-economic status, and favorite pastimes
	d. Consults available sources in an effort to discover means of identifying persons contacted by the patient
	e. Participates in the overall tuberculosis control program by assisting in epidemiological investigations, case findings, and diagnostic and follow-up programs
	f. Is alert to the existing policies relating to the protection of personnel, patients, families, and other contacts, and to the prevention of environmental contamination
	g. Describes pertinent scientific information concerning the mode of attack of the tubercle bacillus and the subsequent infectious process
2. Specifies the attitudes and emotional reactions of patients and families toward tuberculosis	a. Provides an environment that allows patient and family to express their feelings
	b. Interprets the behavior of the patient and family in relation to its effect on the treatment regimen
	c. Assists patient and family to retain their self-respect and control their own lives
	d. Provides opportunities for patient and family to make choices in the arrangements of daily living within the framework of the patient's illness and prescribed treatment
	e. Protects patient and family from stress-producing situations whenever possible
	f. Gives support and assists family to meet stress-producing situations when stress cannot be avoided
	g. Demonstrates her respect for the individual's right to his feelings as expressed by his behavior
3. Provides nursing care to the individual patient and his family	a. Communicates with patient and family to identify their problems as they see them, to identify their concerns in the situation, and to assess their nursing needs and goals
	b. Obtains information from patient and family about their knowledge of protection of self and others, their need and desire for assistance in learning more about the illness, and other unmet health needs of the family

Behavior Expectations	Subknowledge or Capabilities
	c. Prepares a flexible realistic nursing care plan for patient and family based on the total plan of care
	d. Administers medications and treatments, and performs nursing procedures safely and skillfully
	e. Helps patient and family to understand the reason for and implications of each procedure
	f. Assists patient to understand the medical therapy regimen
	g. Is alert to the significance of behavior on the part of the patient and family that may affect their response to care
	h. Modifies nursing goals according to the responses of the patient and family to care and progress toward recovery
	i. Understands the emergency nature of the situation in view of known condition, treatment, and behavior of patient and family
	j. Prepares the patient and family for emergency measures that may need to be taken
	k. Participates in planning with family for continued care of patient after discharge from hospital
	l. Helps patient and family understand the communicability of tuberculosis, and teaches them how to protect themselves and others against tuberculosis through personal and environmental hygiene measures
4. Participates as a member of the health team in providing care to patient and family	a. Specifies the roles of the various health workers contributing to the care of the patient
	b. Participates in clinical conferences to plan patient and family care and to share experiences with other group members
	c. Arranges with appropriate health services for health education of the patient and family
	d. Obtains relevant information from other professional workers who have contributed to patient and family care
	e. Investigates facilities and resources for services needed by the tuberculosis patient and family
	f. Helps patient and family to recognize their needs, and encourages them to avail themselves of the services
	g. Participates in nursing and interdisciplinary research in the care of the tuberculosis patient and his family

practice, the work of another group of instructors is recorded (see Table 3). In this instance the faculty were concerned with the practice of professional nursing in the care of patients experiencing difficulty in maintaining adequate oxygen intake. A model was derived utilizing a patient with an infectious disease (tuberculosis) which presented a number of variables that would influence the plan of care. These variables included the prevention and control of the infectious process; the emotional reactions of patient, family, and community to this illness; the concern for interdisciplinary and community planning; and the implications of long-term nursing and health care planning involving interagency cooperation. The major behavior expectations were identified and then were subjected to further behavioral analysis.

The major purposes of identifying the more specific behavior expectations of a nursing function are that (1) it assists in collection information about the activities and tasks used to decide what to teach, and (2) it allows for more detailed analysis of activities and tasks which specifies the knowledges and skills required of the nurse to perform her function. Usually, the identification of the expectations of a particular behavior are made by a review of the current and projected role functions of the nurse practitioner. Information can also be obtained through communication with professional colleagues in nursing service activities. Some issues may arise when nursing service personnel and nursing educators have different views in relation to the expected behaviors of the beginning practitioner in nursing. These issues are real, since frequently the educator is more concerned with preparing the student for a changing society than are nursing service administrators, who must deal with the overwhelming practical problems of today.

The literature reveals the problems of the beginning nurse practitioner who finds herself in a situation where others have different role expectations of her. Formal and informal efforts have been directed to determining the role expectations of the technical and the professional nurse that are held by faculty members and by nursing service personnel. In a recent survey of faculty members representing five baccalaureate nursing programs and supervisors from nine community health agencies, it was reported that differences were found to exist between role expectations held by nursing educators and nursing supervisors concerning the beginning community health nurse practitioner. The most salient difference was that nursing educators consistently anticipated a higher level of competent functioning in the beginning practitioner than did the nursing supervisor [14]. A similar survey of faculty members within one associate degree program in nursing revealed considerable confusion among the teachers as to the functions of the technical nurse [15]. If curriculum development and instructional planning are to utilize some rational and systematic approach, the faculty must agree upon the behavior expectations of the graduate of the educational program. Behavior descriptions of these expectations specify the knowledges and skills needed to perform the functions inherent in the particular role. More detailed analysis of these knowledges and skills indicates the tasks to be performed in the cognitive, affective, and psychomotor components of the behavior expectations.

COGNITIVE BEHAVIORS

Psychologists, particularly in the area of operant conditioning, indicate that the behavior analyst must specify the behavior desired and the conditions under which it will occur and be reinforced. Given a simple response such as a key peck and a simple reinforcer such as a pellet, an animal such as a pigeon readily acquires key-pecking behavior. The laboratory psychologist has a relatively easy time learning how to teach because deciding what to teach is relatively easy.

The problems of education are not always so simple. In the cognitive domain, that of acquiring knowledge and understanding, the concerns of instructors about what to teach, how much, where, and when are issues that are not easily managed. Bruner has described knowledge as a model constructed to give meaning and structure to regularities in experience [16]. This definition, when applied to nursing, indicates that nursing knowledge is the representation of the regularities occurring in a specific aspect of experience. Early techniques of analyzing subject matter to determine what to teach emphasized the analysis of the verbal repertoire of a subject matter expert. A chemist will give a verbal answer if asked a verbal question. A nurse will give a verbal answer to a verbal question. Yet the answers they give may not differentiate the chemist from the nonchemist or the nurse from the nonnurse. A reader of science or nursing journals could, if given sufficient time, appear learned in a particular field by memorizing passages from the publications. Educators are fearful that much of the activity in some of our schools may resemble this model of learning. They might agree with Whitehead, who said, "a merely well-informed man is the most useless bore on God's earth" [17].

Discerning educators are not convinced that many students truly "understand" the subject matter. What do educators mean when they indicate that the desired outcome of a learning opportunity is that the student understand the idea, event, or phenomenon under consideration? What is a nursing student like who understands the impact of a technological culture on the health and illness of a family of low income? What behavior of the student would educators agree upon as indication of understanding? The objective "the student understands the impact of a technological culture on the health and illness of a family of low income" is the place to start an analysis of what she will be required to do. This analysis gives direction to the teacher and the student in determining the course of learning.

A person who understands chemistry behaves like a chemist under certain conditions. Similarly, a person who understands nursing behaves like a nurse under certain conditions. Some part of the action may be verbalizing–naming or giving a formula, but the understanding shown by this verbal repertoire is a strong function of the situation in which it occurs. Each subject matter is a way of looking at reality in terms of certain classes (concepts), hierarchies of classes (conceptual structures), and stated relations between classes (principles) [18]. Psychologists studying concept learning agree on what they mean by "concept." A concept is a class or category consisting of many members that differ in some ways but are alike in certain key ways, causing us to treat them alike. Common examples in the literature are "dog" and "chair," which obviously demonstrate that members of a class of objects or animals may vary in many observable ways and still remain a dog or a chair. The attainment of a concept calls for the perception of a relationship between concept instances; for example, in the concept or category "dog," there exist poodles, collies, German shepherds, and Great Danes. The perception of this relationship is in large measure dependent on the probability of occurrence of the relevant associative responses to the concept instances [19]. People respond to the instances of the concept "dog" in some common and relevant ways. Also, it is very likely that people's responses to instances of the concept "chair" differ in ways from their responses to instances of the concept "dog." The instructor does not make up the concepts she wishes to teach. She must tease these out of the subject matter, which consists of aspects of real experience.

The learner really understands a concept when she can correctly classify previously unmet bits of reality into examples and nonexamples. To really understand a concept is to be able to discriminate real instances in an array of new items from noninstances, especially those that bear a strong resemblance to the members of the concept class. Psychologists use the terms *generalization* and *discrimination*. These are the key behaviors that distinguish an expert from nonexperts. When educators expect a student to generalize to completely new instances of a concept as a result of instruction, the instructional process must be designed to accommodate this learning. Similarly, in testing for discrimination, the ability to see small differences should be a function of the instruction that teaches the student how to discriminate.

Good definitions can assist a student in looking carefully at the right aspects of reality. But although a definition may play a role in the learning of discriminations and generalizations, being able to state a definition—precisely, or in one's own words—is not evidence of understanding. The greatest oversight in most texts or teaching situations is the selection of only one illustrative example. By its nature, no concept can be learned from a single example. A single example is never consistent with only one concept. For example, the concept "role" as "the expected behaviors of one within a social group" must be illustrated by relating the concept to a variety of reality situations, such as the family group, the work group, the church group, the school group, and to other examples of social roles. The concept "mobility," which has been found useful in nursing curriculums, can be related to the situations in life that interfere with mobility, such as episodes of bed rest, or pregnancy, to situations that temporarily restrict mobility, such as fractures of long bones and vertebrae, and to situations in which mobility is permanently restricted, such as instances of spinal cord injuries, or the degenerative diseases of old age. The concept "mobility" is concerned with infringements upon one's social as well as physical life space.

The key to producing the kind of generalization and discrimination that educators want lies in the selection of a rational set of examples and nonexamples, based on the analyses of the concepts in the real world by subject matter experts [20]. The purpose of locating all these relevant and irrelevant properties of an aspect of reality is to select a rational set of examples that lead the student to generalize across the total set of instances, events, or episodes of reality. A set of examples is rational to the extent that it covers all the possibilities. When a student is mastering the full range of examples that fall within a class, she must simultaneously master the fine discriminations between aspects of the real world that resemble each other in many ways but which are members of different classes. The search for nonexamples or for close approximations to them is the test of the analyst's grasp of her subject matter. The analyst is required to select as test items a completely new set of examples and nonexamples, the examples representing the same fine discriminations taught in the instructional sequence. The manner in which the student performs on the test indicates how she sees the world in comparison to the way in which the expert does—what the student really understands. The problem the instructional designer must solve is the thorough analysis of the real-world situations (the universe) in which these behaviors occur. The expert, be she a biologist, chemist, historian, or nurse, responds to a complex world that she, as an expert, sees in a special way. Instruction that leads the student to see the world in the same way the expert does leads her to this understanding.

The process of behavioral analysis in the cognitive domain of learning is concerned with the identification of those behaviors that will lead the student to understand the specific concept, event, or phenomenon. The arrangement of these behaviors in a hierarchical form directs the learning on a continuum ranging from relatively simple mental activities to those of a complex nature, including understanding. The *definition* of terms at the beginning of the continuum deals with behaviors requiring simple recall and may be dependent upon memorization of facts. Proceeding upward in the hierarchy, other behaviors may require *identification* of the concept among other unrelated areas. A behavior requiring *specification* or telling about the concept in the learner's own words demands higher order mental activities. In the process of *comparing* and *contrasting*, the learner is expected to indicate the likenesses and similarities of concepts within a class of concepts. To *distinguish* or *differentiate* requires the learner to report the specific differences of concepts within a class and between classes of concepts. Finally, the *application* of the concept to new and novel situations may give an indication of the learner's understanding of that concept.

The identification of cognitive behaviors through behavioral analysis in the area of nursing of the aging is presented in Table 4. One phase of this instruc-

TABLE 4. A Behavioral Analysis of Nursing of the Aging Showing Cognitive Behaviors

Behavior	Subject Matter Biological and Psychosocial Changes in Aging
Defines or states the meaning of	Adaptation Homeostasis Character Socialization Stress Equilibrium Aging, aged Senility, senescence
Identifies	Conditions within living matter that influence adaptation Conditions within the internal and external environments that influence homeostasis

Behavior	Subject Matter Biological and Psychosocial Changes in Aging
	Changes in peripheral circulation during aging Changes in hair during the aging process Characteristics and function of the skin during aging Changes in the mouth and teeth of aging persons Changes in muscular activity in aging persons Changes in patterns of sleep and rest in aging persons Changes in bowel and bladder functions in aging persons
Specifies	General characteristics of the aging process Bodily changes in aging that affect appearance Sensory and perceptual changes that occur in aging Fundamental psychological changes in older persons Changes in social behavior of older people Agents that place strain on the adaptive capacity of the individual Changes in the reactions of aging persons to certain drugs Changes in the individual's ability to withstand temperature changes
Compares or contrasts	Basic needs of older persons with those of other age groups Developmental processes of older persons with those of other age groups Incidence and duration of disabling illness in older persons with that of the total population Incidence and duration of acute illness in older persons with that of the total population Basic health needs of older persons with those of other age groups
Distinguishes or differentiates	Characteristics and processes of senility and senescence Characteristics and processes of aging in normal human development Characteristics of health of an aging person in current concepts of health Concepts of aging and aged Concepts of disabling illness and chronic illness Concepts of mortality, morbidity, life expectancy, and age-specific mortality

Applies	Information found by research on the aging process in the biological and behavioral sciences in developing a plan of nursing care, giving consideration to:
	  a. Basic needs of the individual
	  b. Health problems of the older person
	  c. Problems of normal and disturbed physiological processes
	  d. Problems of emotional and interpersonal difficulties
	  e. Problems of socialization or disturbed social behavior

tional sequence, dealing with the biological and psychosocial changes in aging, is utilized for the presentation. This program of instruction is directed to students enrolled in a technical nursing curriculum. This illustration is not intended to represent the only approach to curriculum development in this phase of nursing, nor does it include all appropriate subject matter. It is presented to describe a process of behavioral analysis in cognitive learning.

At the moment, one of the difficulties inherent in subject matter analysis in nursing is the lack of well-defined concepts. That is to say, among nurse educators and practitioners there is a lack of agreement on the aspects of reality (concepts) within the area of experience called nursing. Considerable efforts have been made, and are being made, to identify nursing concepts that can give substance and structure to the subject matter. This is obviously a long and arduous task and is accomplished by research in nursing care. Since curriculum workers cannot wait for this to take place, another frame of reference must be selected. Nursing problems that are considered to be the primary focus of nursing have been identified by practitioners and educators and in some instances have become the fundamental ideas in the curriculum. The introduction of these ideas in their most basic form is followed by restatement of the ideas, exploring them in terms of interacting and intervening variables and in a variety of nursing situations. It is hoped that this process will increase the learner's ability to grasp, transform, transfer, and "really understand" the major ideas of the curriculum.

AFFECTIVE BEHAVIORS

Much emphasis is being placed on the importance of constructing educational objectives in terms of the performance to be expected from the student. This is indeed an effective means of providing for continuous evaluation of the student's proficiency in each component in an instructional system. Although the use of instructional objectives, stated in terms of behaviors to be displayed, does provide a device for assessing the effectiveness of instruction, this practice may not always guarantee that the quality and quantity of education will improve.

It seems relatively easy to select instructional objectives in the teaching of skills and processes. However, the objectives in science education are largely in the cognitive and psychomotor domains. Many educators are not convinced that the behavior of an educated person can be described and learned in terms so specific as to be measurable by assessment tasks. If we describe an educated person as one who has a well-defined value system that he lives by and is willing to defend, an appreciation of the arts, a concern for the future of mankind, and the ability to live in harmony with his fellow man, then educational objectives must be formulated in the affective domain as well as in the cognitive domain.

Educational goals such as these have been in existence for a long time, but they are usually stated in some obscure document such as a school philosophy, and they are frequently forgotten when the actual instructional sequences are planned. Teachers do not often consciously teach or test for affective objectives. Educators assume that people will develop a value complex as they continue to learn. If educators are to guarantee quality in education, they cannot afford to make such assumptions and then fail to measure actual outcomes.

If behavior in the affective domain is to be measured so that we can assess the effectiveness of instruction, it seems necessary that educators produce a test of action words and behavior descriptions to be used. It appears that the affective behaviors are dependent on other behaviors: cognitive and psychomotor. Harbeck has indicated that a rigid list of desirable behaviors in the affective domain may not be possible. She makes the following observations in relation to the formulation of these objectives: (1) it is likely that the affective overtones may be written into performance objectives in the cognitive and psychomotor domains; (2) objectives in the affective domain may have to be more open, specifying acceptable types of behavior to be expected in a given situation rather than insisting on a specific behavior for which an instructional sequence can be designed; (3) if less restrictive objectives are prepared, the evaluation items will be less precise [21]. Any attempt to assess students' willingness and ability to make value judgments and defend them will be some improvement over the present dearth in this area. Harbeck proclaims that if learning to make value judgments and building a value system are important parts of becoming educated, then this should be reflected in some way in the evaluation system.

Behaviors in the affective domain cannot be ignored, regardless of the difficulties encountered. Teachers do show values, and students do develop values. Sensitivity to and awareness of the environment initiates learning. Willingness to respond to situations is the basis for psychomotor responses, and value systems provide the motivation for continued learning and doing of what is considered to be of value to the student.

ATTEMPTS TO IDENTIFY AFFECTIVE BEHAVIORS. There has been little written in the professional education literature about the problem of educating the emotions. Daniel Prescott published a book entitled *Emotion and the Educative Process* in 1938, in which he demonstrates clearly that research evidence supports the idea that feelings and emotions play a critical role in blocking and enhancing learning. Emotions are a major determinant of what will be learned in any situation. More recently, Beatty and Clark have attempted to integrate personality theory, learning, and motivation into a single theory to explain the development of complex behavior and behavior change [22]. The authors of the self-concept theory of learning recognize some inadequacies of the theory, but they believe that the approach is a productive one. Beatty has extended this theory by relating it to feelings and emotions and their impact on behavior [23]. Self-concept, according to Beatty, is an organization of images that each person has about himself in the world. These images develop over time from the reflected appraisal of others around him. The images the individual is building are reinforced and become satisfying. If new and divergent appraisals continue to impinge upon him, and if there is insufficient reinforcement for his former image of self, then he will slowly change and integrate the new appraisals into his self-concept. As the individual grows and comes into contact with larger segments of the world, there is gradual and continuing change. A child experiences appraisals of what he is like and what he could or should be like. The concept of adequacy describes the way the child perceives what he should be if he really would be adequate and effective in the world.

As the individual is aware of discrepancies between the perceived self and his picture of adequacy, he formulates his goals or those things he could do in the world that would decrease the discrepancies. He tries to attain the goals in whatever situations he encounters. Consistent responses that tell him he is becoming more adequate strengthen the new behavior and lead to a change in the perceived self. He becomes more like his concept of adequate self, and this change is what we call learning.

A further breakdown of self-concept is described by Beatty. He indicates that every human being, regardless of his culture, organizes his experiences and learning around these four areas: worth, coping, expressing, and autonomy. Beatty describes the four areas of self-concept in the following manner.

Worth is the experience of love, of being included, of being given priority as a person over other things. One experiences others who are also loved and are included and are given priority. In instances when the other's needs receive greater priority, the individual develops a picture of even greater worth, which he may achieve in time. This provides the motivation to become more like the others receiving greater priority and thus becoming more worthy.

Coping is the experience of overcoming the inability to do something. This builds an individual's picture of himself as a coping person. Models that the individuals sees, such as mother, father, or a professional, are so much more capable that he develops a picture of coping ability he would like to achieve so that he can be like his models. Schools assist the individual to acquire this coping ability through their educational programs. Worth and coping become interwoven, and the concept that worth depends upon what others wish may be engendered. Schools, by their use of grades as a kind of global evaluation of the individual, contribute to the fusing of worth and coping.

Expressing sensation is reacting to experiences either pleasant or unpleasant. The pleasant ones are sought after and become the basis of participating in the arts. Many of the things of which we are aware stir up feelings and emotions, both pleasant and unpleasant. Our culture generally discourages the expression of strong emotions. This makes expression difficult and prevents learning of effective ways of expressing emotion.

Autonomy grows as an individual grows and develops feelings of worth, ability to cope, and ability to express, for he finds that every situation provides opportunities for making alternative decisions. As he discovers the alternatives that give him greater feelings of satisfaction, he becomes more autonomous, more capable of making choices and controlling his own future.

Beatty extends this interpretation of self-concept to feelings and emotions. In these terms feelings arise as a result of a comparison between incoming data and the self-concept. If the data (verbal and/or symbolic) are irrelevant to worth, coping, expressing, or autonomy, the reaction is neutral. The individual is not interested in the communication or may be even bored. If the data are relevant but are somewhat inconsistent with the self-concept, then either a pleasant or an unpleasant feeling is experienced. If the inconsistency is in the direction of telling a person he is more adequate than he had perceived himself to be, the feelings are pleasant. If the data indicate that he is less adequate, an unpleasant feeling arises.

In contrast to feelings, emotions arise when the inputs from the outside world are widely discrepant from the perceived self, and some outside situation or person is assessed as the source that is impeding or enhancing the self. Emotion is directed toward this situation or person and arouses the organism to action. The fact that an emotion calls for action takes on an added significance in our culture, which disapproves of strong emotion and its display. If an individual were able to express joy or anger physically and verbally, the discrepancy between the self-concept and the inputs could be resolved. This action uses the energy that has been mobilized by the emotions, and as the energy is dissipated, the people involved can explore new grounds for understanding.

An environment that allows and encourages the individual to express his emotions appropriately provides learning experiences for the development of a mature individual. Similarly, when an environment permits full expression of feelings, the individual stops intellectualizing and pays more attention to what is happening to him, and gains or regains the ability to feel. Feelings and emotions may be inhibitors or facilitators of learning. Educational horizons may be restricted or widened by feelings and emotional reactions to situations and persons.

There is considerable literature available that provides empirical and experimental data indicating direct relationships between an individual's self-concept, his manifest behavior, his perception, and his academic performance. Several studies have demonstrated that a person's self-concept has direct bearing on his intellectual efficiency. Other studies have demonstrated that there is a positive correlation between acceptance of self and respect for others. Also, when a person's feelings about himself change, his attitudes toward others change in the same direction. Experienced teachers have observed instances in which students' conceptions of their abilities severely restricted their achievement, even though their real abilities were probably superior to those demonstrated. Efforts to improve methods of measurement and evaluation have focused attention on the fact that the personalities of teacher and student influence the evaluation process.

Self-concept appears to be a factor that affects behavior patterns and adjustments. Social psychologists indicate that a person's self-concept is learned through interpersonal encounters with significant others. Teachers and others in the school environment become those significant others who can facilitate or inhibit the development of the self-concept. Nursing as an interpersonal process is dependent in part upon the self-concept of the nurse and her concern for the development of the self-concept of others in the nursing situation. The nurse's ability to love and be loved and her perception of herself as being worthy and becoming more worthy influences her ability to see others as worthy individuals. The ability of the nurse to express her emotions and feelings in constructive ways and her ability to allow others to express their emotions without becoming uncomfortable provides an environment for the exploration of mutual problems and needs. The ability to cope with unfamiliar situations is a measure of a mature individual. Satisfying professional experiences in varied situations offer resources that can be called forth when new and different decisions must be made. Lastly, the ability of the nurse to identify alternative courses of action and her ability to make choices appropriate at the particular time contribute to the development of the self-concept of the nurse. It is obvious that these abilities do not function independent of the attainment of necessary professional knowledge and skill. The self-concept is a dimension of professional practice and as such is a vehicle for utilizing the knowledge and skills of the profession in a meaningful way.

The major problem in the analysis of affective behavior, referred to here as self-concept, is the difficulty in defining precisely the construct, self-concept. There is little agreement among psychologists and educators as to the specific observable behaviors that express self-concept. The current definitions are vague and abstract, leading to considerable variation in interpretation. Since specific behaviors within the realm of self-concept are not identifiable, measurement and evaluation procedures tend to be subjective. The evaluation of self-concept as interpreted by one teacher may not be consistent with the evaluation by another teacher who defines the construct from a different point of view. The student whose self-concept is being evaluated may perceive herself in the situation from still another frame of reference. Inconsistencies in behavior evaluation may result and interfere with the goals of the educational process. A number of instruments have been developed in an effort to measure self-concept as the researcher defines it. These instruments are presently in the research and development stage, and caution should be exercised in using these devices to evaluate behavior for purposes of curriculum and instruction [24].

Whether the teacher of nursing uses self-concept for describing and analyzing affective behaviors or uses another approach for identifying and evaluating the feelings and emotions of the student, she should pursue these with as much objectivity and disciplined judgment as is humanly possible. Objectivity and disciplined judgment are essential, and continued effort should be exerted by teachers in consultation with psychologists to develop techniques for establishing conditions for learning and for evaluating the affective behaviors. Our age has glorified the technician and is the worse for it. But man has begun to realize that although he needs more and more persons with technical or specialized skills, these skills will spell doom for all unless they are controlled by people whose work is well-anchored in a positive view of humanity.

PSYCHOMOTOR BEHAVIORS

All professional and technical activities include some skills that are part of the practice of the particular endeavor. The attention to and degree of competence in the designated skills is determined by the nature and demands of a specific type of service to society. Kinsinger's theory-skill spectrum (Table 1) provides a general orientation to the emphasis placed upon skill activities by the various levels of workers within health occupations. Since all workers are concerned with skill performance, the analysis of behaviors in skill development is appropriate for the purposes of curriculum and instruction.

A skill is defined as an action that has special requirements for speed, accuracy, and coordination [25]. The performance of a skill involves visual and auditory perception and discrimination, recall of specific or general principles, decision-making abilities, and manual skills and operations. The combination and coordination of all these activities is classified as psychomotor behavior. These psychomotor behaviors can be divided into the subbehaviors or subtasks included in the skill activity on differential levels of complexity and performance requirements. Task analyses and task descriptions are the processes that are essential to behavioral analyses in this domain of learning.

DECIDING WHAT TO TEACH. It is generally considered inefficient—and is sometimes impossible in a formal educational program—to teach students to perform all tasks at the level of proficiency required on the job. The only tasks that instructors should analyze are those which are selected to be taught in the program of instruction. It is necessary to make two kinds of decisions about the tasks identified in the practice field: (1) Should the tasks be taught at all in formal training, and (2) if they are taught, what should be the level of proficiency to be attained by the student in a specific program of study? These decisions should be based on a predetermined set of rationales for making the decisions.

One consideration in deciding what to teach is what tasks the student can already perform. Even if she cannot perform a complete task, she may possess some of the skills and knowledges required for its performance. It frequently happens that one cannot perform a task because she has not mastered one of its components, even though she may have already learned most of them. The best way to determine whether a student can already perform the task is to test her. A second consideration is the importance of the task to the designated activity. The more crucial the task is, the more important it is to include it in formal training. Another consideration is the suitability of the situation for learning the task. Some tasks can be taught more easily on the job. And finally, the frequency with which the task is to be performed should be considered. The more often a task is performed, the greater the opportunity for development of further skill through practice. A task that is seldom performed but is highly important will require a high level of initial training.

TASK ANALYSIS AND TASK DESCRIPTION. The identification and analysis of psychomotor behaviors proceeds in two stages. The first stage is task derivation, and it consists of identifying discrete groups of behaviors directed toward a specifiable outcome. The second stage is task analysis in which tasks may be broken down into subtasks or groups of behaviors with specifiable outcomes of smaller scope. These are analyzed further into the physical and psychological requirements they impose on the individual performing the subtasks.

The analysis of the tasks involved in the administration of a hypodermic injection reveals subtasks directed toward specifiable outcomes:

A. Prepares equipment for hypodermic injection
   1. Washes hands
   2. Secures sterile syringe-needle units (2½ cc. syringe with #25 × ⅝-inch needle attached)
   3. Removes wrapper; secures needle hub to syringe tip; maintains sterility of syringe and needle
   4. Replaces needle sheath
   5. Calculates exact amount of correct medication
   6. Cleanses vial top with 70% alcohol saturated cotton ball (uses circular motion)

B. Prepares medication in syringe
   1. Draws exact amount of medication into syringe using aseptic technique
     a. Removes needle sheath
     b. Places needle sheath upright to avoid contaminating the rim of the sheath
     c. Draws calculated amount of air into syringe barrel
     d. Inserts needle into vial; inverts vial
     e. Ejects air
     f. Keeps needle tip below fluid level
     g. Draws exact amount of medication into barrel
     h. Observes barrel for presence of air
     i. Removes needle shaft from vial
   2. Draws plunger back in the barrel (approximately 5 minims of air)
   3. Replaces needle sheath
   4. Places syringe, medication card, 70% alcohol saturated cotton ball in clean cup on carrying tray

C. Prepares patient for administration of hypodermic injection
  1. Identifies patient
    a. Checks wrist band
    b. Asks patient to repeat name
  2. Explains nursing care
  3. Places patient in appropriate position
  4. Selects correct site for hypodermic injection
    a. Lateral aspect of upper arm 3 to 5 inches above elbow
    b. Lateral aspect of the thigh

D. Administers hypodermic injection
  1. Removes needle sheath
  2. Expels all air from barrel to check accuracy of amount of medication
  3. Draws a quantity of air into barrel (size of a small pea)
  4. Cleanses site for injection (uses circular motion)
  5. Holds 70% alcohol saturated cotton ball in right hand between fourth and fifth fingers
  6. Draws skin surface firm over site of injection
    a. Flattens tissue against underlying bone
    b. Elevates tissue between thumb and index finger
  7. Inserts needle shaft quickly
    a. Inserts at 30- to 60-degree angle
    b. Withdraws shaft so ⅛ inch of shaft can be seen
    c. Releases support on tissue
    d. Transfers syringe barrel to left hand
    e. Aspirates syringe
    f. Withdraws needle shaft if blood appears in barrel
  8. Injects medication slowly
  9. Places cotton ball over site of injection, withdraws needle shaft quickly
  10. Massages area slowly

Task analysis has shown the need for including information pertaining to the psychological characteristics of the tasks. In subtask derivation, information pertinent to the entire subtask is obtained, including the location at which the subtask is performed and its relationship to existing tasks. Analysis of the skills and knowledges required is concerned with the examination of the various steps or parts of the subtasks. This analysis results in a statement of the psychological requirements of the task, including the kinds of discrimination that must be made, the decision-making activities implied, and the motor responses required. Some of the psychological requirements pertaining to the subtasks of "prepares equipment for hypodermic injections" are identified in Table 5.

TABLE 5. Analysis of Tasks and Related Psychological Requirements

Subtasks	Psychological Requirements
A. Prepares equipment for hypodermic injection	Discrimination between subcutaneous, intramuscular, and hypodermic injection
1. Washes hands	Specifies purpose of hand washing
2. Secures sterile syringe-needle unit (2½ cc. syringe with #25 x ⅝-inch needle attached)	Identifies equipment and materials needed to give a hypodermic injection
	Differentiates disposable and nondisposable syringes and hypodermic needles
	Identifies the parts of a 2½ cc. syringe and states the purpose of each part
	Identifies the parts of a hypodermic needle and states the purpose of each part
	Differentiates a 2½ cc. syringe from other syringes
	Differentiates a hypodermic needle from other needles
3. Removes wrapper; secures needle hub to syringe tip; maintains sterility of syringe and needle	Specifies why equipment and medication is handled using aseptic techniques
4. Replaces needle sheath	Specifies arithmetical procedure for calculating medication dosage for hypodermic injection
5. Calculates exact amount of correct medication	
6. Cleanses vial top with 70% alcohol saturated cotton ball (uses circular motion)	Specifies the purpose for cleansing the vial top
	Specifies the purpose for using circular motion to cleanse a surface
	Identifies medication vial and ampule

The derivation of subtasks is made with attention to the goal of the activity. A task is never initiated in a psychological vacuum. There are a number of features about the psychological task setting that are of obvious importance. One of these is the clarity with which the individual has in mind the goal or outcome of the activity. Secondly, the motivational context of the situation influences the emphasis on certain aspects of task performance, whether concern is for speed, accuracy, or some other criterion. Lastly, the stimulus events in the situation indicate that the task should be performed, that is, there is a timeliness of task performance. The statement of the task as derived from the nursing function should contain an action verb and indicate the purpose in terms of a goal or a subgoal. The location in which the task is performed should be identified. The task may be discontinuous, or procedural. These tasks are readily divisible into discrete subtasks, and they frequently encompass a standard procedure. Or the task may be a continuous one in which a more or less continuous control action responds to a more or less continuously varying stimulus. Each task should be identified as one of these two types, since the learning requirements differ for each. An example of a discontinuous task is the preparation and administration of a hypodermic injection. A hot foot-soak may be considered to be a continuous task. In this instance the ongoing responses of the patient to the hot foot-soak determine action taken by the nurse in modifying task performance. Such responses may include the patient's tolerance for heat, the changes in appearance and condition of the skin, and changes in vital signs that may indicate some adverse reaction to the treatment.

The time required for the performance should be roughly estimated. Since the speed of performance is a significant factor in executing nursing care, a predetermined standard for task performance should be established. This estimate may be revised after the task is observed under simulation, prototype, or operational conditions. The frequency of task occurrence should be similarly estimated if the task is periodic, that is, if it occurs only under very unusual circumstances. The familiarity with the task to the person required to perform it should also be estimated. Related to the familiarity with the task is the familiarity with the equipment used in performing the task. In some instances the equipment is standard to the hospital and requires no new skill or knowledge to perform. The task requires no formal training, only familiarization with the location and/or installation of the equipment. The utilization of an oxygen tent for providing additional oxygen supply to a patient may be an instance of standard hospital equipment that requires reorientation in relation to installation and use in another location. In an effort to modernize hospital equipment and procedures, some of the standard equipment has been reconstructed or repackaged. When new pieces of equipment have been included, special training may be required. The use of the new parts may require the learning of new skills. Finally, entirely new equipment may call for new skills and knowledges. New principles or new applications of existing principles may be involved. Special training and possibly fundamental training may be required.

Task description is concerned with describing the tasks in sufficient detail to provide a basis for determining the items of knowledge to be imparted and the skills that must be taught. The determination of skills and required knowledge involves judgment, and a sound basis for this judgment should be laid. A detailed description of tasks must be prepared. It has been discovered that the description of tasks reveals a number of gaps in technical and training manuals. Steps may have been left out, descriptions of procedures may be vague and inadequate, and in some instances errors may have been identified. Some principles of task description include (1) ordering the tasks according to sequence of performance or procedure, (2) beginning each task with an active behavioral verb, and indicating the object of the behavior and its immediate results, (3) including the purpose of the task behavior in terms of the subgoals involved, and (4) including as much equipment data as are available, such as probability of malfunction or error [26]. Detailed task descriptions will be helpful in evaluating training devices and methods and may result in improved task performance.

IDENTIFICATION OF SKILL AND KNOWLEDGE REQUIREMENTS.   Task analysis information includes detailed descriptions of performance requirements. The descriptions are most effective if they are comprehensive, without too much emphasis on any one part of performance. The total skill requirements include sensing or perceiving cues or signals from the environment, information processing, which may include recalling information or interpreting the cues, and providing an output, which may be some action taken with hands or feet. To get at this information, the subtasks must be described in considerable detail, and then the details must be analyzed.

The aim of the instructional process is to teach the student to perform a task at the proper level. If the student is simply told to practice tasks, many of which are quite complex, without any clear guidance on how to proceed, she may spend a great deal of time in trial-and-error behavior. It is therefore important to identify all the components of the task so that they may be taught.

The word *knowledge* refers to a set of mental processes that enable a person to use symbols. A person knows something when he shows that he can use the symbols associated with it. Knowledge is presented to a student partly in symbolic form. People can use symbols just as they might use the objects represented by symbols. Symbolic cues may act as substitutes for actual cues, and symbolic responses may act as substitutes for actual responses. If a student learns the symbols (knowledge) appropriate to the task, they will assist her in performing the task. One of the reasons for describing the task in detail is to identify the specific items of knowledge to be used in the performance of the task because the knowledges required to support task performance are tied closely to cues, action, and indicators of correct action.

The theory of a discipline deals with a broad range of problems and provides a basis for action in numerous specific situations. Theory can be quite useful in preparing students to handle a variety of specific situations in which individual training might be impractical. If theory is to assist a student to perform a task, the principle derived from the theory must be related to both the cues and the actions of the task. Three elements must be learned if the knowledge is to assist effectively in task performance: (1) the knowledge content in the form of an idea or statement, (2) the cues that require the knowledge— situations calling for the knowledge must be identifiable by the student, and (3) the proper action indicated by the knowledge.

Certain physiological principles are utilized in determining nursing action in the performance of tasks involved in preparing and administering a hot foot-soak to a patient. Most basic of these principles is that which indicates that the blood serves as a means of transport for substances to and from the cells and that the volume and pressure of circulating blood must be maintained within certain limits to provide for changing demands of the organs. Directly related to this general principle are more specific ones which indicate the knowledge content and cues that identify the knowledge and determine the action to the knowledge and cues. Some of these specific principles include the following:

1. Patients should be observed for signs and symptoms of circulatory problems, particularly when the patient has a relatively large amount of blood in the periphery after a hot bath.
   a. Reportable signs and symptoms of circulatory problems may include changes in skin color, abnormal pulse rhythm, rate, or character, progressive drop in blood pressure, pounding heart or palpitations, numbness or tingling of extremities.
   b. When local application of heat or cold is made, the skin should be observed for color change. Treatment should be discontinued if color change is unusual (bright red, white, or cyanotic).

   c. Particular attention should be paid to controlling the external temperature and/or supplying or avoiding external warmth when the patient has impaired peripheral circulation, skin destruction, and decreased sensory perception of temperature.

2. There is a definite temperature range required for efficient cellular functioning.
   a. Heat can be defined as the kinetic energy of molecules.
   b. Heat travels from a point of higher temperature to one of lower temperature.
   c. Conduction is the transmission of heat through any substance.

3. Unbroken healthy skin and mucous membranes serve as a defense against harmful agents.
   a. Patients should be observed for signs and symptoms of injury to skin, particularly when the patient has peripheral circulatory disease or decreased sensitivity to pain and temperature, during application of physical and/or chemical agents to the skin.
   b. Signs and symptoms of injury may include color changes, lesions, and macerations.
   c. The skin should be protected from physical injury when administering treatments involving heat, by accurate measurement of temperature of hot water and avoidance of drying of the skin when hot soaks are used for a prolonged time.

It is likely that other principles could be identified which apply to this nursing task. More specific principles, ideas, or statements reveal the knowledge requirements and determine the action to the knowledge and the cues. The analyst must identify the knowledges and value of the skill level associated with the subtask. Knowledge requirements may be either specific items to be recalled or general principles from which may be derived many items of knowledge or solutions to problems. Jones and Fairman have developed rating scales for determining knowledge requirements and skill levels that are useful in the analyses of psychomotor behaviors. The following is a rating scale for knowledges:

0 — Requires no formal training and no more than a basic introduction to work

1 — Requires ability to read, write, and follow simple instructions; slight

need for using simple arithmetic; little training and adjustment to the work

2 — Requires moderate ability to comprehend reading material and instructions and to perform mathematical computation, with limited formal or on-the-job training and adjustment

3 — Requires intermediate technical knowledge, with considerable training prior to and during adjustment to work

4 — Requires high degree of technical knowledge, with extended formal and informal training for full adjustment to the work

5 — Requires a very high degree of complex and varied knowledge, with very extended time spent on both formal and informal training for full capability in the work [27]

The rating scale these authors have developed to estimate the skill level includes the following categories with the appropriate rating:

0 — Requires no dexterity, precision of movement, muscular coordination, or appreciable response to sensory cues

1 — Requires little dexterity, precision and coordination of movement, only slight muscular coordination, and slow response to sensory cues

2 — Requires limited dexterity, precision, and coordination of movement, with moderate response to sensory cues

3 — Requires considerable dexterity, precision, and coordination of movement, with steady responses to sensory cues

4 — Requires a high degree of dexterity, precision, and coordination of movement, with quick response to sensory cues

5 — Requires a very high degree of dexterity, precision, and coordination of motion, with complex and varied responses to sensory cues [28]

The rating scales for knowledge requirements and skill levels may be useful in determining the psychomotor behaviors desired for a particular type of practice in nursing. Starting with the task itself, the following question should be asked: What must a nurse know or be able to do if she has been told to perform a task but has been given no specific training in that task? The answer to this question will be a small list of major items of knowledge and/or skill. The same question will then be asked for these items, and so on, until each item of knowledge and skill derived from the task description has been added to the structure of the task.

In addition to the precise statements of what the student should be able to do when she completes a task, it is necessary to state the conditions under which the student's behavior will be observed. In considering the applicability of different kinds of conditions to a given objective, the major question to be answered is, Does it affect task performance? Only the particular conditions that are to be taught should be specified: conditions that restrict or broaden the amount of material the student must learn, conditions that determine whether the task is performed differently under different circumstances, or conditions that make task performance easier or more difficult.

TASK PERFORMANCE CRITERIA.   Since task description is virtually a statement of performance requirements, the description serves as a statement of task criteria. The task description should include the situational variables that should be sampled for presentation to the individual. The selection of these variables is determined by the importance of the event and the frequency of its occurrence in the type of nursing practice under consideration. In other words, decisions must be made regarding the selection of nursing skills and conditions and events for instruction.

The proficiency of task performance must also be considered in relation to the stage of development of the student within a specific instructional program. The descriptions of the levels of proficiency provide useful criteria for the evaluation of task performance.

SUMMARY

Interest in formulating objectives for curriculum and instruction received impetus from the activities of measurement and evaluation. The development of evaluation programs by colleges and universities made clear the need for instruments to measure achievement. The construction of achievement tests in turn pointed to the need for course objectives in the subject matter fields. The development of educational objectives was also stimulated by the efforts of the military in designing training programs for the various types of personnel. The specification of training objectives came about through the processes of task description and task analysis. Stating the objectives of instruction precisely in terms of student behavior was also considered to be the first step in the preparation of programmed instruction.

Psychologists and educators who were interested in the development of achievement tests stimulated enthusiasm in securing a common terminology for describing the behavioral characteristics that they were trying to appraise in the various schools, that is, types of responses to content, subject matter, problems, or areas of human experience. Objectives should specify the actions, feelings, and thoughts students are expected to develop as a result of the instructional process. The development of a classification scheme or taxonomy was considered to be useful to teachers for the activities of teaching and examination of achievement. A group of psychologists led by Bloom identified three types of objectives, involving cognitive, affective, and psychomotor behavior of students. Taxonomies of educational objectives in the cognitive and affective domains have been prepared by psychologists utilizing schemes appropriate for the behaviors implied.

The ongoing work of many psychologists and educators supported the notion that the statement of objectives clarifies the behavior changes considered desirable by a teacher in a specific phase of instruction. This also implied that the processes of curriculum development and instruction are directed to assisting students to modify their behavior. The concomitant activities of evaluation are concerned with the determination of the degree to which the behavior of the student has been modified or changed. Behavior modification focuses upon three major tasks of the teacher: (1) the evaluation of student prior to instruction, (2) the analysis and sequence of the task to be learned, and (3) the procedural methods and management techniques to be used.

Broad goals of education have been formulated by various educational study groups and commissions. Frequently these goals or objectives are stated in general terms, leaving considerable room for interpretation. Some statements are so very general that more definitive goals cannot be identified. More recently, attention has been directed to formulating objectives of education in terms of observable human behavior or performance. Differences in performance suggest that learning has taken place which is not solely the outcome of maturation. Specifying objectives in definitive terms clarifies the nature of the terminal behavior that is desired. It is likely that if this capability cannot be specified, it cannot be taught or learned or observed or measured. The statement of objectives in terms of definite behaviors is a requirement of a sound testing program.

The objectives of a particular school or course should be goals not already attained by the student, goals that can be based on her previous background of skills, abilities, knowledges, and interests. Formulating a statement of objectives requires the teacher to give attention to these knowledges, skills, and interests in relation to the issues of contemporary society. The philosophy of education of the teacher serves as a guide in selecting objectives that are appropriate at the particular time and place. The terminal behavior, the objectives of the curriculum, indicate what knowledge, skills, and attitudes the student will have at the end of the instructional program. The behavioral objective includes the behavior or action implied and the content or context of the behavior. The analysis of this behavior reveals that there are performances that are prerequisite to other performances. Breaking down educational objectives into finer units provides necessary information for the purpose of teaching and testing. Each of these finer tasks contributes to the attainment of the larger goal of learning. These subtasks, or subknowledges are considered to be intermediate behaviors in the teaching-learning process. Eventually the intermediate behaviors must approximate the initial behaviors of the student to assure that no gaps in learning occur.

The process of identifying objectives in a particular type or phase of practice requires an analysis of the behavior requirements of that practice. In the case of the curriculum worker, this implies describing what kinds of abilities, skills, and knowledges are required for the nurse to carry out the specific function. The result of behavior analysis provides definitions of the various human performances required. If a curriculum of instruction is to assist the nursing student to acquire the designated behaviors, these must be identified and made known to student and teachers. Behavioral descriptions of these expectations specify the knowledge and skills which are needed to perform the functions inherent in the role expectations. More detailed analysis of these knowledges and skills indicates the learning requirements in the cognitive, affective, and psychomotor components of the behavior.

REFERENCES

1. Tyler, R. W.   Achievement Testing and Curriculum Construction. In E. G. Williamson [Ed.], *Trends in Student Personnel Work.* Minneapolis: University of Minnesota Press, 1949. P. 391.
2. Krathwohl, D. R., Bloom, B. S., and Masea, B. B.   *Taxonomy of Educational Objectives. Handbook II: Affective Domain.* New York: McKay, 1964. P. 3.
3. Ibid., p. 6.
4. Bloom, B. S. [Ed.].   *Taxonomy of Educational Objectives. Handbook I: Cognitive Domain.* New York: Longmans, Green, 1956.
5. Krathwohl, Bloom, and Masea, op. cit., p. 9.
6. Gagné, R. M.   Educational Objectives and Human Performances. In J. D. Krumboltz [Ed.], *Learning and the Educational Process.* Chicago: Rand McNally, 1965. P. 1.

7. Ibid., p. 1.
8. Gagné, R. M. The Analysis of Instruction Objectives for the Design of Instruction. In R. Glaser [Ed.], *Teaching Machines and Programmed Learning, II.* Washington, D.C.: National Education Association, 1965. P. 21.
9. Burns, R. W. The theory of expressing objectives. *Educ. Techn.* 7:1, 1967.
10. Tyler, R. W. Some Persistent Questions on the Defining of Objectives. In C. M. Lindvall [Ed.], *Defining Educational Objectives.* Pittsburgh: University of Pittsburgh Press, 1964. P. 77.
11. Gagné, R. M. The acquisition of knowledge. *Psychol. Rev.* 69:355, 1962.
12. Ibid., p. 355.
13. Gagné, R. M. *Psychological Principles in System Development.* New York: Holt, Rinehart & Winston, 1966. P. 186.
14. Hines, P., et al. Role Expectations of Nursing Educators and Nursing Supervisors Regarding Beginning Community Health Nurse Practitioners. Unpublished Research Project, School of Nursing, The Catholic University of America, 1970. P. 50.
15. Burke, Sr. M. M., et al. Functions of Beginning Technical Practitioners as Identified by Nursing Faculty in an Associate Degree Program. Unpublished Research Project, School of Nursing, The Catholic University of America, 1970. P. 44.
16. Bruner, J. S. *On Knowing.* Cambridge: Harvard University Press, 1962.
17. Whitehead, A. N. *The Aims of Education.* New York: Mentor Books, 1929. P. 13.
18. Gagné, R. M. *The Conditions of Learning.* New York: Holt, Rinehart & Winston, 1965. P. 141.
19. Mednick, S. A., and Freedman, J. L. Facilitation of concept formation through mediated generalization. *J. Exper. Psychol.* 60:278, 1960.
20. Bruner, J. S., Goodnow, J. J., and Austin, G. A. *A Study of Thinking.* New York: Wiley, 1956.
21. Harbeck, M. B. Instructional objectives in the affective domain. *Educ. Techn.* 10:49, 1970.
22. Beatty, W. H., and Clark, R. A. A Self-Concept Theory of Learning. In H. C. Lindgren [Ed.], *Readings in Educational Psychology.* New York: Wiley, 1938.
23. Beatty, W. H. Emotion: The Missing Link in Education. In W. H. Beatty [Ed.], *Improving Educational Assessment and An Inventory of Measures of Affective Behavior.* Washington, D.C.: Association for Supervision and Curriculum Development, National Education Association, 1969. P. 74.
24. Beatty, W. H. [Ed.]. *Improving Educational Assessment and an Inventory of Measures of Affective Behaviors.* Washington, D.C.: Association for Supervision and Curriculum Development, National Education Association, 1969.
25. Smith, R. G., Jr. *The Development of Training Objectives.* Alexandria: Human Resources Research Office, George Washington University, 1964. P. 56.
26. Jones, E. M., and Fairman, J. B. Identification and Analyses of Human Performance Requirements. In J. D. Folley, Jr. [Ed.], *Human Factors Methods for System Design.* Pittsburgh: American Institute for Research, 1960. P. 49.
27. Ibid., p. 56.
28. Ibid., p. 55.

SUPPLEMENTARY READINGS

Aastereed, M., and Guntherie, K. What can be expected of the graduate with an associate degree? *Nurs. Outlook* 12:52, 1964.

Benne, K. D., and Bennes, W. Role confusion and conflict in nursing—What is real nursing? *Amer. J. Nurs.* 59:382, 1959.

Berkowitz, J. E., and Berkowitz, N. H. Nursing education and role conception. *Nurs. Res.* 9:218, 1960.

Brodt, D. The neophyte nurse: A role expectation study. *Nurs. Res.* 13:255, 1964.

Canfield, A. A. A rationale for performance objectives. *Audiovisual Instruction* 13:127, 1968.

Coe, C. R. The relative importance of selected educational objectives in nursing. *Nurs. Res.* 16:141, 1967.

Corwin, R. G. The professional employee: A study of conflict in nursing roles. *Amer. J. Sociol.* 66:604, 1961.

Eess, A. F., and Harbeck, M. B. *Behavioral Objectives in the Affective Domain.* Washington, D.C.: National Science Supervisors Association, 1969.

Gagné, R. M. [Ed.]. Human Functions in Systems. In *Psychological Principles in Systems Development.* New York: Holt, Rinehart & Winston, 1962.

Gagné, R. M. The Implications of Instructional Objectives for Learning. In C. M. Lindvall [Ed.], *Defining Educational Objectives.* Pittsburgh: University of Pittsburgh Press, 1964.

Gagné, R. M., and Bolles, R. C. A Review of Factors in Learning Efficiency. In E. Galanter [Ed.], *Automatic Teaching: The State of the Art.* New York: Wiley, 1959.

Gardner, J. W. *National Goals in Education in Goals for Americans.* The Report of the President's Commission on National Goals. Englewood Cliffs: Prentice Hall, 1960.

Geitgey, D., and Crowley, D. Preparing objectives. *Amer. J. Nurs.* 65:95, 1965.

Green, E. J. *The Learning Process and Programmed Instruction.* New York: Holt, Rinehart & Winston, 1962.

Harbeck, M. B. Instructional objectives in the affective domain. *Educ. Techn.* 10:49, 1970.

Kapfer, P. G. Behavioral objectives in the cognitive and affective domain. *Educ. Techn.* 8:11, 1968.

Krathwohl, D. R., et al. *Taxonomy of Educational Objectives. Handbook II: Affective Domain.* New York: McKay, 1964.

Krumboltz, J. D. *Learning and the Educational Process.* Chicago: Rand McNally, 1965.

Lindvall, C. M. *Defining Educational Objectives.* Pittsburgh: University of Pittsburgh Press, 1964.

Mager, R. J. *Preparing Objectives for Programmed Instruction.* San Francisco: Fearon, 1962.

Markle, S. M., and Tiemann, P. W. Behavioral analyses of cognitive content. *Educ. Techn.* 10:41, 1970.

Maxwell, M. The preparation of teachers of nursing. *Nurs. Forum* 7:365, 1968.

Mechner, F. Behavioral Analysis and Instructional Sequencing. In P. Lange

[Ed.], *Programmed Instruction*. Sixty-sixth Yearbook of the National Society for the Study of Education, Part II. Chicago: University of Chicago Press, 1967.

Rockefeller Brothers Fund. *The Pursuit of Excellence: Education and the Future of America*. Panel Report V of the Special Studies Project. Garden City: Doubleday, 1958.

Taber, J. I., Glaser, R., and Schaefer, H. H. *Learning and Programmed Instruction*. Reading: Addison-Wesley, 1965.

10 APPROACHES TO IDENTIFYING CONTENT IN NURSING

SUBJECT *matter* or its synonym, content, is a common term in educational theory and practice. It is used in textbooks on education, particularly in relation to curriculum and instruction. The term subject matter has not been defined precisely, probably because it is such a familiar one that its meaning is presumed to be clear and known to all. For the concept of subject matter to be fruitful, it should assist the teacher in at least three important tasks: (1) selecting subject matter for consideration in her courses, (2) organizing the subject matter so that there is some relation among its composite elements, and (3) evaluating the students' acquisition of the subject matter. Points of view on the nature and uses of subject matter are explored, and approaches to the identification of content for the curriculum are described.

THE NATURE OF SUBJECT MATTER

Smith, Stanley, and Shores describe subject matter by identifying the activities in which members of a social group participate. One type of activity involves hunting, selling, farming, and manufacturing, etc., which result in the procurement of food, clothing, shelter, or other necessities of life. The second type of activity involves the common life of the group, such as voting, discussing social issues, appreciating music, and obeying a system of law. From these activities evolve sets of skills, facts, rules of conduct, and aesthetic principles comprising what the social group has learned about the world—about the ways of using the world and improving its beauty, about man himself, and about how to live together. Such knowledge, values, and skills constitute the subject matter of the group. These authors indicate that subject matter is only a part of the total culture. Subject matter includes what men know and believe and their ideals and loyalties, but not everything they have produced. An institution such as the family is not subject matter, but what is known and believed about the family and the ideals for family life are subject matter. Tools and machines are not subject matter, but knowledge about tools and machines, how they are made and their operation and uses, is subject matter [1].

From this description one would assume that as a society develops, specialized social groups are formed. As each of these groups takes on differentiated roles and activities, the ideas, modes of operation, and relationships within the group and between group members become more highly specialized. Each group, family, church, or industry seeks to discover new knowledge about the group and its contribution to society. As society advances in the amount and diversity of accumulated knowledge, related areas of knowledge are organized and structured for communication and use by members of special groups.

In Western culture knowledge is organized in a number of disciplines, such as philosophy, history, and mathematics. Each discipline is both a kind of knowledge and a kind of knowing; it is both a system of ideas (facts and theories) and a means of acquiring them. Knowing is a human activity, and human determinations enter into the formulation of knowledge. Disciplines encompass the discovered patterns of possible development in knowledge. The history of thought makes it evident that new species of knowledge emerge from time to time. As knowledge evolves, new fields open for investigation, and where existing methods of inquiry could not be extended, new disciplines were defined, such as biochemistry, social psychology, and biomedical engineering. Some disciplines are primarily devoted to understanding, apart from the service of practical needs. Others are concerned mainly with application. The disciplines do not represent permanent ways of thought.

The rapid growth of knowledge has sent scientists, psychologists, and educators scurrying to define and classify the various disciplines. Schwab points out the existence of at least three great genera of disciplines: the investigative (natural sciences), the appreciative (arts), and the decisive (social sciences) [2]. Broudy arrives at five groupings by classifying disciplines with respect to the role played in the totality of knowledge:

1. Bodies of knowledge that serve as symbolic tools of thinking, communication, and learning.
2. Bodies of knowledge that systematize basic facts and their relations (the basic sciences), to give us a way of speaking and thinking about the world.
3. Bodies of knowledge that organize information along the routes of cultural development, as do history, biography, and evolutionary studies.
4. Bodies of knowledge that project future problems and attempt to regulate the activities of the social order, such as agriculture, medicine, and political science.
5. The integrative and inspirational disciplines that synthesize values in the form of philosophy, theology, and art [3].

Phenix defines a discipline as knowledge organized for instruction, which seems to equate a discipline with a school or college subject. This seems to be a practical definition for the purposes of curriculum development [4].

Teachers may speak of a subject as the name given to any body of knowledge, whether that body be large or small, highly organized or not, additional or new. It is generally assumed that subject matter is the middle term in a three-term relationship. Someone (the teacher) teaches something (history, biology, nursing) to someone (the student). We cannot just teach students, nor just teach subject matter. We must teach students something (subject matter), and we must teach subject matter to someone (students).

There are different points of view on the specific nature of knowledge that is appropriate for consideration as subject matter. Henderson has indicated that cognitive knowledge is the only proper substitute for subject matter in the statement "the teacher teaches subject matter to students" [5]. Considering cognitive knowledge as subject matter, we know what to select from the various types of knowledge. What knowledge to select for the curriculum and how to organize this subject matter into its most teachable and learnable form is the crucial, practical—and often puzzling—question in teaching.

Another pertinent question is whether the concept of subject matter should be limited only to cognitive knowledge. Surely it is as reasonable to speak of the teacher teaching the student how to read, or the teacher teaching the student how to operate the suction apparatus for gastric lavage, as it does to speak of the teacher teaching the student the history of medieval Europe, or the structure and functions of the respiratory system. Soltis finds it useful to consider both facts and skills as part of subject matter [6]. There is another generally recognized area of things which are neither cognitive knowledge nor skill knowledge but which seem to be a legitimate part of subject matter. Educators may speak of the teacher teaching the student to appreciate music or to appreciate the dignity and worth of all individuals. We mean by this that it is our intent as teachers to see that students develop a disposition to appreciate music or to appreciate and value human life. The notion that facts, skills, and dispositions are the concerns of teaching and learning suggests that they may be considered to be proper subject matter.

THE USES OF SUBJECT MATTER

The uses of subject matter have also been viewed in somewhat different ways. When we teach, we are trying to get someone to learn something, usually for a reason. When we teach pathophysiology to nursing students, we do so because we assume that knowledge of this subject matter will contribute to their giving or learning how to give nursing care to certain patients. The intent in teaching pathophysiology goes beyond the mere learning of particular aspects of pathophysiology. Mastering pathophysiology becomes a means of achieving the broader concerns of the subject matter of nursing. Soltis refers to this use of subject matter as a vehicle for carrying a person to a goal [7].

Henderson implies the same use of subject matter in his discussion of "knowing that" and "knowing how" [8]. These two kinds of knowledge are distinct; neither can be reduced to the other. To determine whether a person knows how to nurse a patient with a myocardial infarction, teachers think that observing what she does is more valid evidence than listening to what she says. The subject matter of "knowing that" requires one to give evidence of the existence of the knowledge. Knowing that the patient has had a myocardial infarction means that one has observed the signs and symptoms of the patient and has validated hunches by making various diagnostic tests and procedures. *Knowing that* a patient has this physiological aberration does not necessarily mean that the nurse *knows how* to care for this patient.

Henderson takes the position that knowledge about a subject is subject matter, that is, the cognitive knowledge. He further indicates that while "knowing that" is not the same as "knowing how," it is a means through which "knowing how" is approached. Henderson classifies cognitive knowledge into three categories: (1) statements of truth ("the excessive loss of fluids from the body disturbs the fluid and electrolyte balance"); (2) prescriptions, such as an order, directive, or command ("nurses should not judge the patient's behavior"); and (3) value statements, or words used to rate something ("she is an effective nurse") [9].

Martin has delineated the "knowing that" and "knowing how" into subcategories. The distinction that has been made implies that "knowing how" refers to skills or operations while "knowing that" refers to knowledge of factual propositions. Martin suggests two kinds of "knowing how": knowing how to perform a task, and knowing how to investigate a problem. The feature that distinguishes these two kinds of capacities is *practice* [10]. Knowing how to operate a suction apparatus implies having learned certain skills through practice. Knowing how to investigate a nursing problem does not necessarily imply the need to practice investigating problems. The term practice is vague, and probably many skills included in the practice are related. Practice for one skill may also serve as practice for another. For example, the repeated handling of certain instruments in changing surgical dressings provides practice in skills that are also necessary in handling instruments while assisting the surgeon in an operative procedure. Knowing the uses of the different instruments and developing tactile and kinesthetic sensitivity contributes to knowing how to handle instruments in other situations.

Martin explores the "knowing that" classification, which she divides into two types of dispositions: One type pertains to knowing how to investigate a problem and the other is concerned with knowing how to behave (as a nurse) in an ethical manner. Knowing that "this is how you investigate a problem" is regarded as different from the ability to perform a specific operation through frequent, regular practice. It does not suggest any specific details of knowledge, but rather, involves factual propositions of a general nature. The second type of "knowing that" refers to knowing a system of moral judgments or rules of conduct. Knowing that one should behave in a certain way refers to knowing rules of conduct. Martin believes there is a difference between "knowing that" sentences that refer to factual propositions and "knowing that" sentences that refer to moral judgments. She suggests that "knowing that this is how" may be considered to be a capacity, whereas "knowing that one should" may be subsumed under the category of dispositions.

The nature and uses of subject matter are viewed in a variety of ways by persons from the various disciplines. From the point of view of the health professional, knowledge or subject matter includes not only "knowing that" but also "knowing how." In addition, the value orientation of the particular society in relation to modes of professional behavior become a substantial aspect of knowledge. Subject matter may be considered broadly as including the principles, techniques, facts, values, processes, and modes of response that man has learned about himself and the world in which he lives. What teachers and others select from the subject matter becomes the content of a curriculum and instruction in the selected subject matter a means for attaining the objectives of the curriculum.

SUBJECT MATTER AND THE CURRICULUM

During the current period of curriculum reform, most of the debate within education hinges on an old and familiar question: What should the schools teach? This is a perpetual question, one that apparently every generation has to solve over again in light of changing conditions and changing needs. It can be answered only by reference to one's view of the nature of knowledge and of the teaching-learning process.

The almost incredible explosion of knowledge during the past several decades threatens to overwhelm teachers in every area of education, including nursing. It has been estimated that the useful information which we have available to us doubles every eight years. A noted educator suggested that if a biologist today were to go into outer space and stay there for four years, he would have a desperate time catching up with his fellow biologists when he returned. After eight years of absence, he would hardly be able to communicate with them.

What knowledge to select and how to organize this knowledge for learning are two problems that require constant attention. Since about 1955 a vivid awareness of this problem has led some scholars and researchers to explore ways of selecting, organizing, and teaching available information to make it more intelligible and more usable. Committees of physicists, chemists, mathematicians, biologists, social scientists, linguists, and specialists in English have worked devotedly and imaginatively in the development of elementary and secondary school courses. Making reference to these activities, Sand indicates that these studies have shifted the balance in learning from inventory to transaction [11]. An inventory of learning may result in an accumulation of inert knowledge. A transaction in learning occurs when students do something to the facts and the facts do something to the student by rendering experience more intelligible, by pointing the way to problems and making them felt, or by helping the student increase her ability to control some part of her environment [12].

The problems in nursing are especially complex. Since the subject matter called nursing is derived from many disciplines, the task of delineating what, how much, for whom, and for what purposes to teach is bewildering. Because of the lack of scientifically verified knowledge in nursing, the subject matter is ill-defined. Although some useful knowledge about nursing is being revealed by research activities, this is not yet sufficient for generating theories and principles about nursing. Within nursing the category of knowledge containing statements of truths, facts, and propositions may be called *descriptive* knowledge, since it provides the ways of thinking and speaking about nursing and its components and processes. It appears the major focus of the knowledge of nursing today may be categorized as *prescriptive*, since much of the information deals with directives based on what one thinks is good for the patient.

For the purposes of rational and systematic curriculum planning, teachers are faced with the task of determining what it is that the nurse (professional, technical) does for, to, with, and on behalf of individuals and their families to improve the patient's health and well-being in a way no one else does or can do. A conceptual frame of reference of the object and process of nursing is needed to provide a guide for the selection of content, which in turn gives direction to the formulation of the objectives of the curriculum. The specification of objectives in terms of behavioral end products, that is, what the student does at the end of the instructional program, is made in relation to the predetermined conceptual framework of nursing practice. As this task is undertaken, several problems come into focus. At the moment there is hardly any consensus within the profession regarding nomenclature and definition for the activities performed by professional and technical nurses. Nursing does not have a technical vocabulary that describes its purposes and functions and that clearly identifies and communicates the nature of nursing. The state of nursing knowledge makes it difficult to agree on appropriate intermediate and terminal behaviors for nursing students. In spite of these difficulties, some approaches to identifying and selecting content in nursing are being tried in attempts to develop a curriculum of instruction.

APPROACHES TO IDENTIFYING CONTENT IN NURSING

Six major types of approaches are being utilized to identify nursing content. These may be labeled: (1) designing "the nursing core," (2) defining and describing concepts, (3) utilizing the nursing process, (4) analyzing case studies,

(5) constructing models, and (6) utilizing a science theory. Analysis of curriculums that have been developed using one or another approach reveals that the above categories are not mutually exclusive. In some instances a curriculum may be developed using a combination of two or more approaches.

DESIGNING THE NURSING CORE

Literature in the field of curriculum development has suggested that in a given curriculum it is important to identify the particular content elements that will be used. This approach implies that once these common elements are identified, curriculum activities can be designed in which the elements become integrated according to some predetermined theme. The nature of a clinical nursing core developed as a response to the concept of core curriculum utilized in secondary education. The initial efforts of secondary school teachers and curriculum workers in the late 1940's were directed toward designing curriculum activities consistent with the needs and interests of students. Douglas indicates that "core" includes all of the common experiences that pupils ought to have in the curriculum or the required subjects. The term *common learnings* more accurately designates those experiences in the high school curriculum that all pupils should have, that is, the general education essential for all [13]. The core curriculum in this instance was a way of organizing some of the important common learnings within the high school curriculum, using the problem-solving approach to study questions of importance to youth in order to develop behavior essential in a democratic society. According to Douglas, the idea of an experience-centered, problem-solving approach is a concept basic to the core [14]. In addition, other characteristics of the core indicate that the subject matter in the core cuts across subject boundaries and draws upon any content needed to solve problems in general education. Also, the concept of a core necessitates cooperative planning by the teachers concerned. If the core is considered to be the heart of the common experiences, then core teachers need to work with teachers of other classes to provide for as much unification as possible.

Alberty describes core as that part of the total curriculum which is basic for all students and which consists of learning activities that are organized without reference to conventional subject lines [15]. He classifies interpretations of the core curriculum into six types, ranging from the concept of required subjects taught in a logically organized manner to the idea of activities planned by teachers and pupils without reference to any formal structure [16]. In most instances the major purpose of a core in a high school curriculum focuses on assisting adolescent boys and girls to cope with their developmental needs and tasks.

Colleges and universities have accepted the philosophical notion of some common learnings for all undergraduate students. The concept "general education" is perceived as a sequence of learning opportunities that is similar for all students regardless of their specific area of specialization. The application of this concept in curriculum development shows considerable diversity, which suggests that faculty are not in complete agreement as to what constitutes the common learnings [17].

The interpretation of core as required subjects taught in a logically organized manner was utilized by one baccalaureate nursing program for the purposes of general education as well as of foundation learnings for professional specialization. Kempf reports the activities of the faculty that identified the common learnings for nursing students, which were also shared with students in other professional education programs in the college [18]. The common core that was designed for all undergraduate students was based on the premise that a broad educational foundation is essential for all students regardless of their special occupational field of interest. The courses and their contents were planned with the recognition of the existing need for a common base on which to build an intelligent interest in personal, family, vocational, social, and civic interactions. Four comprehensive core courses—communications skills, natural sciences, social sciences, and humanities—serve as a foundation for living. For the nursing student they provide a base for courses in nursing. Specific objectives were developed for each core course, which gave direction to the selection of content for the courses.

More recently the concept of core has been considered by medical educators. Under consideration at the Johns Hopkins University School of Medicine is the possibility of creating a college of medical sciences that would admit all those interested in the health services. It is suggested that a "core base of varying complexity and subsequent multiple-track options would allow final differentiation of nurses, radiobiologists, research scientists and physicians" [19].

The need for a core program for the preparation of health technicians was identified by a study group of the Community College Health Careers Project, New York State Education Department. This group endeavored to identify the knowledge and skills considered common to a variety of health technologies. Some of the advantages they saw in the core program were: (1) utilizing faculty more effectively by offering all students entering these fields courses that cover material common to all of the occupations; (2) recruiting students for the health field in general and deferring for at least a semester a decision on which field best fits the student's interests and aptitudes; (3) relieving high school counselors of the need to keep abreast of the details in newly developing fields by enabling them to counsel broadly regarding opportunities in the general field of health service technology; (4) providing an opportunity for the college faculty to observe, evaluate, and counsel students before they choose a specific health field; and (5) providing students with a better perspective on the several health fields so that they make their career decisions with greater certainty and awareness. The comprehensive core program that was developed for health service technicians combines general education with courses essential to the various occupational goals. The courses in this program include human anatomy and physiology, psychology or sociology, language arts, mathematics or electives from general education, and basic health technology. Individualization of program planning is possible in relation to the students' previous education background.

The course Basic Health Technology is designed to introduce students to a broad spectrum of career opportunities and to assist them in selecting a specific career for which they have demonstrated interest, ability, personality, and character. The content of this core course has been identified and serves as a base from which special technologies depart. More specific objectives have been formulated which indicate that the course has been developed to enable students to (1) become oriented to health service resources, (2) gain experience with team relationships, (3) become acquainted with health field ethics, (4) gain knowledge of pathophysiology and pathopsychology, (5) learn how diseases are treated, and (6) develop the necessary skills in maintaining an environment conducive to the well-being of patients. These objectives give direction to the identification of content, which is useful for the various health service technicians [20].

A rationale for this core concept has been stated by Kissick, who sees a broader implication possibly extending into professional education:

It is suggested that the curriculums in the various clusters of health manpower . . . could be examined both for the common elements within each cluster and the relationships among the hierarchy of clusters. A determination of the portion of each curriculum devoted to generalizable knowledge and to technical skill could assist and enable an individual completing a program in one cluster to receive advanced standing in a curriculum in another cluster located above it in the hierarchy [21].

Another approach to the core concept is described by Allen, who defines core content as those major elements of content that are incorporated throughout the nursing curriculum and that permeate all learning experiences in varying degrees. Allen further indicates that core content flows through the courses to the learning experiences in clinical services where it is to be applied. Eight major areas of core content have been identified, which aid more specific delineation of content in each area. These areas are (1) social and health aspects of nursing, (2) specific nursing knowledge, (3) growth and development, (4) logic, (5) principles of body mechanics and posture, (6) interpersonal relations, (7) communication, and (8) sciences. The process of core content flow is described by the author to indicate how the content becomes the subject matter of the various nursing courses in the curriculum [22].

Within baccalaureate and graduate programs in nursing, some attention has been given to bringing together two or more courses with related content for the purpose of identifying some common elements that permeate the various courses. More recently faculties in these programs have tried to determine the common elements of maternity and pediatric nursing. The experience of instructors in the graduate program in maternal-child health at Boston University demonstrates their efforts to determine the core of the program without a loss of identity of either nursing specialty. The major focus of the core content in this program appears to be parent-child relationships within the framework of family care. The faculty believe that using this core as a point of departure for clinical knowledge in maternity and pediatric nursing enables the graduate student to perceive her role in family care with an increased commitment to the child and parents in times of crises, whether in the hospital, school, or home [23].

The book *Patient-Centered Approaches to Nursing*, published in 1960, stimulated interest among faculties of some schools of nursing to develop core courses dealing with common nursing problems [24]. These courses offered content focusing on the problems of patients that fall within the domain of nursing practice and emphasized the use of problem-solving approaches to the study of these problems. The identification of problems common to all patients, such as the need for food, oxygen, elimination, and maintaining a fluid and electrolyte balance, provides a means by which content can be selected and appropriate learning experiences offered to illuminate and implement the specific content. Faculties using this approach to core believe that it directs attention away from the medical diagnosis by clarifying and emphasizing the ultimate goal of nursing care—helping patients to solve their health problems.

This approach also tends to reduce the amount of unnecessary repetition of content and learning experiences in the courses in medical-surgical nursing and maternal-child nursing, which follow the core courses.

Another approach to the nursing core is the utilization of the common nursing problems as a frame of reference for developing content in the traditional courses, such as medical-surgical, pediatric, and maternal-infant nursing. In this instance, content and learning activities pertaining to the common nursing problems are dispersed throughout all nursing courses, with appropriate emphasis on specific problems in the various courses.

Other efforts to develop a core in nursing curriculums have utilized a unifying theme. One theme that appears to be useful and manageable in developing curriculum activities involves a sequence of developmental tasks. The plan for selection and organization of nursing content proposes using the major health problems and the developmental tasks from conception to senescence. The content of the nursing courses is selected on the basis of the major health problems and the developmental tasks of children, adolescents, adults, and aged persons.

Teachers in schools of nursing have endeavored to utilize a physiological or behavioral process as an approach to developing core courses and/or core content. Attempts have been made to develop curriculum activities using the process of homeostasis and stress-reduction as organizing themes.

Recent revisions of a baccalaureate curriculum include a clinical nursing core consisting of four courses. The content of the core utilizes the notion and processes of homeokinesis. The faculty has formulated a rationale for using homeokinesis which indicates that one may describe the individual (patient) as a world within a world comprised of multiple energy forces necessary for the crucial transactions that promote life and fulfillment of needs. These energy forces are in constant (kinetic) motion, and, when acting in harmony, serve to supply and support the human organism. This state of harmony of energy is referred to as "homeokinetic maintenance of life."

Homeokinesis presupposes the gratification of certain needs, the two most essential of which are nutrition and defense. An individual's homeokinetic state may be influenced in several ways. A threat or disruption to need satisfaction is a good example. When such threat or disruption occurs in the case of illness, the organism seeks to maintain homeokinesis or to compensate for its loss. Four types of action can readily be identified: (1) preventive, (2) preservative, (3) curative, and (4) promotive. When the above actions do not result in appropriate response regardless of the organism's efforts, homeokinesis is not maintained and decompensation occurs.

Since the goal of nursing is to assist the individual in maintenance of activities of which he is capable, the nurse functions within a role compatible with the individual's, a role that can fall anywhere along a continuum from homeokinesis to decompensation. The nurse's response differs in no way from that which the organism itself employs to maintain homeokinesis, that is, the nursing response also is of a preventive, preservative, curative, or promotive nature.

In this point of view, it becomes impossible to study man separately from his environment; it becomes essential for the nurse to individualize her approach to each patient as he responds to the environment and to be perceptive with regard to changes which are constantly occurring within the same patient.

It appears that designing a core in nursing curriculums takes several directions depending on the interpretation of core. The interpretation of core courses and core content influences the development of curriculum content and the organization of curriculum material. The purposes of core also vary; they include providing for career guidance, eliminating repetitive content, and studying a physiological or behavioral process that has relevance to nursing.

DEFINING AND DESCRIBING CONCEPTS

The concepts approach to the development of content in nursing has probably been influenced by the recent activities of psychologists, scientists, and educators directed toward identification of the structure of knowledge within a discipline. Bruner describes knowledge as a model constructed to give meaning and structure to regularities in experience. He also states that the organizing ideas of a body of knowledge are inventions for rendering experience economical and connected. Curriculum in the subject should be determined by a fundamental understanding of the underlying principles that give structure to that subject. Bruner indicates that teaching specific topics or skills without making clear their context in the broader structure of a field of knowledge is uneconomical, since they are likely to be forgotten [25]. Considerable attention has been given to the systematic analysis of various disciplines in an effort to identify the major ideas, concepts, and principles, and to structure these elements for efficient and effective learning.

The development and identification of concepts is no small task. Efforts to identify concepts in nursing and other disciplines are beginning to be felt in nursing practice and in the content of curriculums. Hofling and Leininger identify some psychiatric concepts which should become a part of all nursing practice. These concepts, although labeled psychiatric concepts, are derived from human development and behavior, in particular, human relations. The concepts of personality development and adjustment and those of disturbed psychological processes are described in relation to nursing action [26].

One of the clearest statements concerning the development and use of concepts in teaching came from a seminar group in psychiatric nursing that worked together over a three-year period with Dr. Loretta Zderad as consultant and program director. Their publication, *Developing Behavioral Concepts in Nursing*, contains considerable detail concerning process, which is not usually found in the literature [27]. Since the term *concept* had several meanings for the seminar members, they decided to adapt the dictionary definition, in which a concept referred to a thought or notion, an abstract idea generalized from particular instances. The twelve seminar members, all experienced teachers in psychiatric nursing, came from different schools of nursing. As a beginning they submitted lists of concepts which had meaning to them. A list of 144 different concepts was assembled. Criteria for selection of concepts to be described were formulated by the group. It was agreed that a variety of types of concepts should be studied and that each one should be of interest not only to the individual but to the entire group. Other criteria were the prevalence of the concept, its capacity for broad development, and the state of its description in the literature [28]. Each educator selected a concept that met the criteria and developed a working paper describing the concept. Each working paper gave consideration to an operational definition of the concept, application of the concept to nursing situations, and clinical nursing examples and descriptions. The sources used by the group included personal experiences with patients, notes on interpersonal relations, process recordings, tape-recorded nursing-care conferences, and interpretations of filmed portrayals of patient behavior. Data were sought from patients, other seminar members, nursing instructors, staff nurses, aides, nursing students, and nursing-school teachers.

The approach taken by the seminar members was to first study and describe the concepts in terms of their general significance and then to specify them in relation to nursing practice. The group members focused upon different factors, such as the nature, characteristics, development, function, and forms of the concepts. Regardless of individual emphasis, all members of the group experienced difficulty in distinguishing either related concepts or forms of one concept, and in defining their concepts. One of the problems encountered in describing some concepts was the need to differentiate them from related, similar, or overlapping concepts. Occasionally a concept appeared so broad and open to so many interpretations that distinguishing its type was a major problem. The concepts "acceptance," "hostility," and "hope" were considered to be multidimensional and nebulous concepts. Limiting the dimensions of the concepts to those that had relevance for nursing made possible a clearer and more precise definition and description of the concept. The seminar members found that writing operational definitions required identification and analysis of the behaviors or operations involved in the concepts and arranging them in serial order as they emerged. The development of the operational definitions of the concepts was thought to provide a good source of clues to nursing intervention [29].

The activities of the seminar members resulted in a description of the selected psychiatric nursing concepts that they found useful in teaching baccalaureate students. Although it was recognized by the group members that these concepts needed to be developed in relation to nursing applications, the utilization of these concepts throughout the curriculum seemed desirable. Questions were raised as to whether these concepts would require further exploration and description for use in clinical areas other than psychiatric nursing. The seminar members agreed that appropriate approaches and techniques for teaching in baccalaureate programs must be developed and used to help students learn how to conceptualize [30].

The process of identifying concepts in any discipline is a laborious one. Much sophisticated literature makes available the results of research in the areas of concept identification and development and the teaching of concepts. The issues and problems experienced by the seminar participants in developing behavioral concepts can be understood by reviewing the nature and characteristics of concepts. Henderson indicates that the act of conceptualizing involves forming a relation between terms, persons, contexts, and meanings [31]. Each member of the relation is also a concept. Henderson states that a concept cannot exist without persons to have them; however, the number of persons involved makes no difference. If only one person is involved, the concept is a personal concept. Although concepts may be held by more than one person, the size of the set of persons may vary. A group may have a concept of democracy shared by each of its members but not shared by the general public. It is very likely that there are few if any concepts held by every member of a particular society, but somewhere on the continuum between the singleton set (one person) and the universal set (all persons) is a set of sufficient number that a concept held by all its members can be regarded as a common, general, or conventional concept.

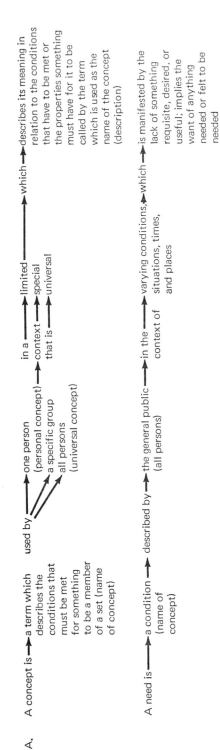

A.

A concept is → a term which describes the conditions that must be met for something to be a member of a set (name of concept) → used by →
- one person (personal concept)
- a specific group (universal concept)
- all persons (universal concept)

→ in a → context that is →
- limited
- special
- universal

→ which → describes its meaning in relation to the conditions that have to be met or the properties something must have for it to be called by the term which is used as the name of the concept (description)

A need is → a condition (name of concept) → described by → the general public (all persons) → in the context of → varying conditions, times, situations, and places → which → is manifested by the lack of something requisite, desired, or useful; implies the want of anything needed or felt to be needed

B.

A need is → a construct → described by → psychologists (specific group) → in the context of → personality theory (special context) → which → stands for a force that organizes perception, apperception, intellection, conation, and action to transform an unsatisfying situation that is provoked directly by internal processes or by environmental forces. It leads the organism to search for or to avoid or, when encountered, to respond to certain kinds of press. Each need is characteristically accompanied by a feeling or emotion. It gives rise to behavior which changes the initiating circumstances to bring about an end situation which stills the organism (description)

C. A need is ⟶ a requirement ⟶ described by ⟶ a group of professional nurses (special group) ⟶ in the context of ⟶ the practice of nursing (special context) ⟶ which ⟶ holds the nurse primarily responsible for assisting the individual to meet or cope with a situation or condition. Nursing needs vary in relation to the individual's biophysical and psychosocial background, medical diagnosis, physician's orders, and persons involved in his care. Nursing needs are physical, environmental, instructional and informational, emotional, and coordinative. Individuals have several types of needs (description)

(name of concept)

DIAGRAM 3. Definition and development of concepts: A. According to Merriam-Webster (*Webster's Seventh New Collegiate Dictionary*. Springfield: Merriam-Webster, 1956, p. 981);B. According to H. A. Murray (*Explorations in Personality*. New York: Oxford, 1938, p. 123); C. According to C. Coe et al. (*The Report of One Approach to the Identification of Essential Content in Baccalaureate Programs in Nursing*. Boulder: Western Interstate Commission on Higher Education, 1967, p. 10); D. According to D. Schwartz (Nursing needs of chronically ill ambulatory patients. *Nurs. Res.* 9:185, 1960); and E. According to B. Meyer (Development of a method for determining estimates of professional nurse needs. *Nurs. Res.* 6:24, 1957). (Continued on pages 288–289).

287

(Diagram 3 continued)

D. A need is → a requirement → described by → a nurse researcher → in the → a study of → which → implies specific action
for nursing care (personal concept) context of chronically ill on the part of the nurse
(name of ambulatory in an effort to
concept) patients (special individualize nursing
context) care. Needs include
physical nursing care,
administration and
understanding of
medicine and treatment,
health education, and
those human needs not
now routinely given
attention in the patient's
record, such as those
stemming from the
patient's daily activities,
his work and recreational
habits, eating and sleeping
patterns, state of loneliness
or companionship, range
of interest and knowledge,
and use of available
community resources
(description)

E. A need is → a requirement for professional personnel (name of concept) → described by → researchers (special group) → in the context of → nurse manpower (special context) → which → indicates the number of professional nurses required to maintain the the rate of 258 professional nurses per 100,000 population. This estimate takes into consideration loss due to attrition. Two kinds of needs are implied: recruitment needs—the number of new graduates needed, and school expansion needs—need for schools to expand their present capacity (description)

289

The context within which the concept is used indicates which meanings are appropriate. The meanings of the concept "acid" would imply different characteristics when used in the context of the chemistry laboratory than when used in the context of the hippie culture. The learning of concepts requires students to ascribe certain meanings to a particular term. These meanings may be the statements of the conditions that have to be met or the properties something must have to be called a concept. The identification and development of concepts requires that all persons within a special group, such as nursing, associate the same meanings with the term that is designated as the name of the concept. An illustration of the definition and development of a concept is given in Diagram 3.

Defining and developing concepts in nursing requires attention to this process. This type of activity seems appropriate for faculty to engage in, for curriculum development requires the study in depth if teachers are to come to real understanding of the content of the curriculum. This is indeed an essential step prior to sharing it with students. Even after three years of intermittent work, the psychiatric nursing seminar members stated that the concepts "need to be developed more, especially in regard to nursing applications. This would entail not only more theorizing but also more testing of the ideas under various conditions" [32]. The subject matter of nursing does not have a precise technical or scientific vocabulary, which fact makes for difficulty in describing the conditions that must be met or the properties that nursing as an activity of nursing must have to be called by a certain term. In addition to the problems of concept definition and development there are those pertaining to concept teaching and learning. Some attention will be given to these processes in a later chapter.

UTILIZING THE NURSING PROCESS

A third approach to the identification of content in nursing is called the nursing process by some faculties and problem-solving or the analytic process by other groups of teachers. Problem-solving implies that there is a problem to be solved. What are the distinctive problems in nursing to be solved? The nursing process, as defined in the literature, indicates that these problems are assessment of the needs of the patient, development of a plan of care to meet his needs, implementation of the plan of care, and evaluation of the care provided in relation to the patient's needs. In this instance, what are the specific nursing situations that give focus and direction to the nursing process? Since it is likely that not all patients or potential patients need the services of nurses, in what situations or under what conditions do nurses intervene in the health care regimen of the person?

The elements of the nursing process have been explored by Yura and Walsh. As a frame of reference for determining patients' needs for the purpose of nursing assessment, the hierarchy of needs developed by Maslow is used. These needs, arranged in an order of importance or potency include (1) physiological needs, (2) safety or security needs, (3) needs for love or belongingness, (4) esteem needs, and (5) self-actualization needs. The impact of health and illness of the individual on his ability to meet his needs becomes the focus of nursing assessment and intervention. Without disregarding the past history of the individual, the existential view of man is suggested to add substance and meaning to other aspects of nursing assessment and care. Yura and Walsh describe nursing assessment as the continuous, systematic, critical, orderly, and precise method of collecting, validating, analyzing, interpreting information about the physical, psychological, and social needs of a patient, the nature of his self-care deficits, and other factors influencing his condition and care [33].

In an endeavor to make a nursing diagnosis for the individual, the typology of nursing problems developed by Abdellah is utilized [34]. Knowledges from the natural, behavioral, and medical sciences are identified which are useful in understanding the problems and appropriate courses of action for alleviating the patients' problems. The approach that is made by the nurse in assisting the patient with his problem and the response of the patient to this approach becomes the content of nursing. This approach to the identification of content in nursing implies the dynamic, fluid nature of the subject matter of nursing. As we gain more knowledge about people and their problems and health needs, the content of nursing takes on new dimensions.

The nursing process is described by another group of teachers at Wayne State University as including (1) data collection, (2) validation of data, (3) interpretation of data, (4) validation of interpretation, (5) formulation of a plan of care, (6) implementation of a plan of care, and (7) validation of the plan of care. The attention to the need for validation throughout the nursing process seems to imply that the subject matter of nursing is fluid and unstable and must be continuously reassessed, reversed, and developed in relation to nursing practice.

A group of instructors in graduate programs in medical-surgical nursing defined the nursing process as "that which goes on between the patient and the nurse in a given setting." It incorporates the behaviors of both the patient and the nurse and the resulting interaction. It is comprised of the following steps: (1) perception, (2) communication, (3) interpretation (assessment), (4) intervention (nursing action), and (5) evaluation [35]. In this instance the specific characteristics of the patients give direction to the identification of the content of nursing. The common characteristics of the patients included in this phase of nursing include some alteration in body functions and in the situational environment of the patient—the hospital. This concept of the nursing process implies that the content of nursing is developed not only by data from the patient but also by means of interaction between patient and nurse.

The faculty at the University of California at San Francisco has incorporated the concept of the analytic process in their review and revisions of the baccalaureate curriculum. This approach to problem-solving categorizes the various types of decisions to be made and includes (1) identification decisions, (2) planning decisions, (3) execution decisions, and (4) evaluation decisions.

Identification decisions are required when an event occurs that causes disequilibrium in one of the patient's systems and the coping strategies of the patient are insufficient to restore the equilibrium. The event or interruption to equilibrium is viewed in relation to its antecedents or the factors directly or indirectly producing the interruption and in relation to the effects or the immediate consequences of the interruption. Internal and external resources available to the patient for coping with the event are identified. All possible manifestations that result from altered functioning of the system(s) are explored, and the patient and family manifestations are identified. The alternative ways of carrying out nursing intervention are identified, with attention given to the consequences and probable effectiveness of each action. Identification decisions are made in relation to the priority given to specific patient problems. Setting priorities is usually a function of the problems that present the greatest threat to the patient.

Planning decisions are made in relation to the selection of a nursing intervention which may satisfy the needs of some patient system that is in disequilibrium. These decisions necessitate the analysis of alternative nursing interventions to relieve problems arising in the proximal (directly observable features and actions) and distal (set of relations to objects, events, or systems outside the proximal system) systems. Possible nursing actions are those that might reduce the threats to the patient revolving around fluid requirements, aeration of body cells, nutrition, communication, activity, and pain.

Execution decisions are those that pertain to determining which action is most appropriate based on the probability of the effectiveness of each alternative. Lastly, evaluation decisions are made to determine whether the action achieved the intended purpose. Evaluation of the action taken is made, and necessary revisions are made.

The analytic process as described by this group of teachers seems to imply that the content of nursing evolves through decision-making by nurses as they review the causes and the manifestations of events producing disruption in the equilibrium of the body systems: the nurse identifies possible nursing interventions in relation to the problem priority, designs nursing actions to relieve the specific problems, and evaluates the effectiveness of the nursing interventions [36].

Regardless of the interpretation of problem-solving or nursing process approach, there is implied both a nursing object or goal to be attained and a systematic procedure for attaining the goal. Abdellah and her colleagues have offered a set of problems that appear to be within the framework of nursing responsibilities [37]. More recently other nurse educators and practitioners have given deliberate attention to identification of the major components of nursing practice. It is the belief of these nurses that "it is the establishment of the unique contribution of the profession that guides the development of the body of knowledge and the design of the systematic programs of professional education" [38]. Without a definite focus of nursing, we can become involved in collecting a plethora of information about patients that may or may not make a difference in nursing care, simply because the specific nursing problem has not been identified.

Another interpretation of problem-solving as an approach to identifying content within a discipline is suggested by Bruner. In developing the concept of structure of subject matter, Bruner indicated that the subject matter of a discipline should include not only the major ideas or the basic and underlying principles of a field, it should also include the modes of inquiry used by a specific discipline in developing the body of knowledge. Bruner states that "mastery of the fundamental ideas of a field involves not only the grasping of general principles but also the development of an attitude toward learning and inquiry, toward guessing and hunches, toward the possibility of solving problems of one's own" [39]. Although much of the knowledge that is called nursing has not been developed through scientific investigation, nursing research is becoming visible. Opportunities are available to teachers to focus attention on the modes of inquiry into the practice of nursing from which the content of nursing is developed.

ANALYZING CASE STUDIES

The case-study approach to developing content has been used by several professions. Law and medicine have utilized this method to assist practitioners in making professional decisions and to aid the researcher in scientific investigations. Nursing has found the clinical case or care study to be an effective method of teaching. More recently, nursing case studies have been developed and analyzed in an effort to identify the content in nursing.

A formal, large-scale endeavor utilizing case studies to identify content in nursing was the study conducted by the Western Council on Higher Education in Nursing [40]. Participants in this study selected 750 patients receiving nursing care through health agencies used for nursing clinical experience by the thirty-four baccalaureate nursing programs in the West. An assumption was made that it should be possible to infer knowledge essential to nursing from a study of the nursing needs of a representative sample of patients. Nursing faculty members tried to identify and list in order of priority the nursing needs of these patients at the time of the observation. In this study a nursing need was defined as "a requirement for assistance, for provision of which the nurse is primarily responsible, of an individual in meeting (coping with) any situation and/or condition with which the individual is faced" [41].

One difficulty observed by the faculty in collecting the data on patients was the variety of different interpretations of the concept "nursing need" in specific settings by the faculty members making the observations. These faculty members, however, were considered to be expert nurses who were qualified to identify the nursing needs of the patient and to assign priority to the needs.

As a result of the observations five categories of nursing needs were identified: (1) physical, (2) environmental, (3) instructional, (4) emotional, and (5) coordination of services. Efforts were also directed to determining the priority of these needs in relation to certain patient characteristics, such as age, sex, income, size of family, value conflicts, communication barriers, availability of physical, emotional, and financial assistance, and medical diagnosis. The relationships between these variables and the nursing needs of the patients in the sample gave direction to the identification of essential content in baccalaureate programs in nursing.

This approach has been used by individual schools perhaps in a less formal manner. One school that participated in the project, published by the Western Interstate Commission for Higher Education, used the case-study approach in determining the focus of nursing content. The faculty of the University of California at San Francisco collected actual patient case histories over a period of one year. The analysis of these histories assisted the teachers in identifying the wide range of factors (physiological, social, personal, cultural, psychological) and their interrelationships regardless of the nature of the interruption in the health process. The problem situation of each patient was viewed in relation to the phases of the health maintenance-restoration cycle and indicated the specific nursing problems. The information from the case-study analyses enabled the faculty to develop problem models that present clusters of variables in typical patient situations to which the nurse must respond with problem-solving activities.

Identification of the components of nursing care through case-study analysis is a practical means for determining the content of the curriculum. The recordings of clinical care of patients by faculty, nurse practitioners, and students can provide cumulative evidence of the primary focus of nursing. From this information, teachers can infer the substantive knowledge and skills needed to provide appropriate professional or technical care. The efforts of one nurse were directed toward identifying through case-study analysis the nursing-care of a fourteen-month-old child with a medical diagnosis of hydrocephalus. The nurse cared for this child during the pre- and post-operative periods. The surgical procedures involved a right arachnoid-peritoneal shunt with a laminectomy of the second and third lumbar vertebrae. After providing continuous nursing care for the child over a three-week period, the nurse terminated her relationship. The summary of her recordings of the daily nursing care given in Table 6 indicates the primary focus of nursing. Eight categories of nursing activities and the approaches used in implementing the nursing care were identified. Decisions for determining the approaches to be used were based on specific patient data, such as age, family relationships, socioeconomic, and developmental status.

The careful analysis of nursing care given to patients presenting varying personal, social-psychological, and medical problems can provide useful information from which one may infer the focus of nursing care and the different approaches in implementing nursing-care activities. The content of nursing can be developed by giving attention to the knowledge and skills needed by the nurse to provide the necessary care. This approach is, indeed, a very useful one. Replication of these analyses of nursing care can provide substantial information about and direction of nursing care.

TABLE 6.   Summary of Nursing Care of a Fourteen-Month-Old Child with Hydrocephalus

Categories	Approaches
1. Preventing pressure areas on skin	a. Turn every two hours b. Hold in arms c. Cleanse and powder body skin folds, particularly under chin d. Apply special skin cream e. Use foam rubber pillow
2. Maintaining nutritional status	a. Encourage eating by cuddling, caressing, and singing b. Feed slowly, giving small amounts at frequent intervals c. Offer glucose d. Observe and record amount of sustenance and intravenous fluids absorbed e. Give prescribed vitamins
3. Observing for elimination	a. Observe for and record bowel movements and urinary output b. Give enema when needed c. Take appropriate measures to prevent the need to strain when passing stool
4. Providing for safety and comfort	a. Prevent additional increase in intracranial pressure by preventing vomiting, straining at stool, comforting by walking and talking, caressing and providing for physical comfort to avoid long periods of crying b. Prevent infections by bathing and by handwashing and gowning of those giving care c. Keep surgical dressing clean d. Keep crib sides up and secure e. Restrain infant's arms when he is receiving intravenous fluids. Remove restraints at intervals to allow some freedom and activity f. Control physical environment by keeping room warm and clean, dimming lights, preventing unnecessary and loud noise
5. Promoting development of body muscles and bones	a. Encourage holding of bottle and rattle b. Keep body in proper alignment c. Encourage activity of arms and legs d. Provide passive exercise of arms and legs
6. Promoting social and emotional development	a. Provide continuous and pleasant contacts between nurse and infant by caressing, humming, and playing b. Respond to needs in a firm but gentle manner c. Change position frequently to extend social space d. Walk with infant to provide for more social contacts e. Hold tenderly after a painful experience

Categories	Approaches
7. Observing for and preventing complications	a. Observe vital signs b. Give alcohol sponge to reduce fever c. Turn every 2 hours to prevent respiratory difficulties d. Observe for signs of hemorrhage and excessive drainage e. Maintain proper body alignment to prevent dislodging of shunt tube f. Observe anterior fontanelle for fullness or depression g. Change position to increase or decrease intracranial pressure
8. Providing health teaching to parents	a. Discuss care of infant b. Demonstrate care c. Engage parents in care of infant: bathing, feeding, changing d. Provide supervision with reassurance, encouragement, and understanding
9. Assisting the physician	a. Assist with examinations and diagnostic procedures b. Assist with treatments and medications c. Communicate appropriate data to physician about infant's responses and reactions

CONSTRUCTING MODELS

Models are analogies, which are ways of representing a given phenomenon. They are used to represent events and event interactions in a highly compact and illustrative manner. When utilized for this purpose, they help to explain facts or events that are puzzling. A model is a structure of symbols interpreted in certain ways, and it represents the subject matter specified by the interpretation. Relations among the symbols are presumed to correspond to relations among the elements of the subject matter. Kaplan distinguishes five different interpretations associated with the term *model*. The first is any theory presented with some degree of mathematical exactness and logical rigor. The second presents a conceptual analogue to some subject matter. The third interpretation is a nonlinguistic or a physical model analogous to some other being studied. The fourth is a formal model of a theory. The fifth is an interpretive model, which provides an interpretation for a formal theory [42]. It appears, however, that regardless of the type of model or the purpose for which it is used, a model is either a replica of a set of laws or events, or it represents the set of laws or events symbolically.

Model building is an accepted practice for those who are engaged in the development of theory within a discipline. Since models may be used to describe or explain simple and complex phenomena that occur within the context of a circumscribed area of human activity and may be used at any level of that activity, models may be constructed to illustrate the components and interrelationships of nursing within the system of health care. Also, models may be constructed to demonstrate the interrelationship of the components of nursing-care activities within the system of nursing. In many disciplines models are constructed for the purpose of hypothesizing the nature and impact of the relationship of two or more components of the model. Research efforts directed toward testing the hypotheses contributes to the development of theory within the discipline.

There is some evidence that nurse researchers are constructing models for the purpose of hypothesis testing. This is indeed fundamental to theory development, which is a requirement of a scientific discipline. Models are the analogies that help one to think about problems. Theories are more than analogies, for they must have some degree of empirical verification. A model is a convenient way of looking at things, but a theory has to reflect knowledge and, to be accepted, must have demonstrated its ability to predict events.

Models have been constructed by nursing faculty to describe the relationship of nursing and the patient to situational variables. The University of California school makes use of "problem models," which have been developed by the faculty from information obtained from patient histories. The objectives for use of the models were stated as (1) to involve the student as completely and rapidly as possible in the decision-making and problem-solving processes, (2) to expose her to a diversity of patient problems in a variety of settings, (3) to provide opportunity for her to view the health maintenance-restoration cycle in its entirety, (4) to bring about a heightened awareness of the complexity of patient problems, (5) to provide opportunity for her to make decisions and critical evaluations, and (6) to provide opportunity for her to learn technical skills at the time needed. Students study representative problem models rather than a great number of specific problems. Examples of the problem models selected and developed by this faculty include a child with an acute problem of immobility, an aged patient in a nursing home, a family with small children and pregnant mother, and a multiproblem family [43]. These models are presented as actual problems in an effort to induce analytic thought processes and decision-making. The development of the models indicates the kind and placement of theory and skill instruction and the patients selected for clinical experience.

UTILIZING A SCIENCE THEORY

Mention was made earlier that some teachers have found it useful to utilize a physiological or social concept as a theme in developing core courses or core content. Concepts such as homeostasis, equilibrium, and stress-reduction have been considered by instructors in schools of nursing as desirable focuses of nursing care. The utilization of these concepts in curriculum planning requires the faculty to come to some agreement about the meaning of these concepts within the domain of nursing and about the appropriate nursing activities that describe the focus of nursing care.

A deliberate and conscientious effort was made by a group of nurses to utilize a social theory as a frame of reference for defining clinical content in community health nursing. The project was developed and undertaken by the Western Council on Higher Education in Nursing, a constituent of the Western Interstate Commission for Higher Education. The activities of this group gave attention to graduate education in community health nursing, which "prepares a specialist to function in the changing field of public health which affects and is affected by society's constantly evolving forces" [44]. This group further indicated:

Critical analysis of old, and evolving of new, theoretical bases for community health nursing, a rationale for the selected theoretical framework, consideration of new approaches with subsequent opportunities to test and evaluate these approaches, and the expanded role of the community health nurse as professional health worker and health team member are all necessary adjuncts to the identification of the scientific basis required for community health nursing practice [45].

The social theory selected as a frame of reference for the curriculum project was the social action theory of Talcott Parsons. The project group found it necessary to formulate some statements of beliefs about community health nursing that would direct their search for and development of a conceptual framework. Exploration was made of the major focus and elements of Parsons's theory of action and the relevance of the theory for community health nursing practice. Concepts and roles of the community health nurse were selected and discussed within the broad framework of the theory for action in an attempt to make the theory operational. The concepts selected included (1) high-level wellness, (2) stress, (3) socialization and interstitial role, (4) communication, and (5) problem-solving and decision-making. Each of these concepts was explored in relation to the nurse's role and responsibilities in community health nursing. The information and materials developed during the discussions were considered to be appropriate content for the graduate curriculum in this area of nursing.

As a result of considerable deliberation in an effort to define the content of community health nursing utilizing Parsons's theory of action, the participating faculty members agreed that the theory was too abstract and illusive to be useful in curriculum development. Efforts on the part of the group to test the theory were not productive. The teachers felt that the general orientation of the theory did provide a structure for defining and explaining the phenomenon of community health nursing practice. This group also indicated that other theories, perhaps those which may be categorized as middle-range theories, might be explored for their contribution to identifying content in nursing. Theories of communication and decision-making may be more manageable for the purpose of studying community health nursing practice and the concomitant activities of curriculum development.

Behavioral scientists have validated the findings of this faculty group by indicating that theories such as the theory of action and others are too global for direct test or application. This indeed is not the purpose of such theories. Their contribution to knowledge is the way in which they describe and explain certain phenomena that occur within society.

SUMMARY

The rapid development of knowledge in all of the disciplines has precipitated problems for teachers on all levels of education and in various types of curriculums. Deciding upon what to teach in a particular instructional program requires the teacher to explore the nature and uses of knowledge for the purposes of teaching and learning. What is selected from the particular area of knowledge or discipline becomes the subject matter of the curriculum.

Various points of view about the nature of subject matter have been expressed. A somewhat restrictive viewpoint indicates that cognitive knowledge —that dealing with facts, theories, and propositions—is the only proper subject matter. More encompassing descriptions of subject matter include not only facts, theories, and propositions but also skills needed to perform certain tasks and operations. Also included in some descriptions are the "dispositions" or "tendencies," which deal primarily with the emotional or feeling aspects of the subject matter. Subject matter is expressed in an operational manner by the statement: someone (the teacher) teaches something (subject matter) to someone (student) for some purpose (objectives of instruction). The subject matter selected to assist in attaining the objectives is appropriate for a curriculum of instruction.

The term subject matter has been used to refer to different kinds of knowing. "Knowing that" is concerned with statements of truth—facts and theories. "Knowing that" may also refer to rules of behavior or conduct. Knowing that the nurse should behave in a particular way directs attention to the concerns of ethical professional conduct. "Knowing how" pertains to learning how to perform certain tasks that are specific in nature. Another type of "knowing how" is concerned with such processes as investigating problems where the subject matter may be general. A difference noted in the requirements of the types of "knowing how" is the need for practice. Practice is required for the development of skills and operations; however, it is not necessarily a requirement for activities such as problem investigation. One's view of the nature of subject matter and its contribution to the teaching-learning process will provide a frame of reference for defining content for the curriculum.

Nurse instructors have the same concerns of subject matter selection as do other teachers. The ill-defined nature of nursing knowledge presents additional problems. Since there is not complete agreement within the profession as to the object and processes of nursing, the subject matter appears to be fluid and unstable. Efforts have been made by individual nurses and groups of teachers to identify content in nursing. Six types of approaches have been utilized, sometimes singly, sometimes in combination with other approaches. These include (1) designing a nursing core, (2) defining and describing concepts, (3) utilizing the nursing process, (4) analyzing case studies, (5) constructing models, and (6) utilizing a science theory.

Designing the core in nursing curriculums takes several forms, depending upon the interpretation of core. How one interprets core courses and core content determines how content will be developed and organized. In most instances the concept of core relates to the bringing together of fundamental ideas about nursing in some type of meaningful relationship. The purposes for developing core, whether it be a springboard for further exploration of ideas or a theme that permeates the curriculum, determine the way in which core is presented.

Efforts to define and describe concepts in nursing have been ongoing in both formal and informal activities. Although some concepts have been described by faculty members in the area of psychiatric nursing, questions are raised as to whether these concepts can be generalized to other phases of nursing. The teachers who have engaged in this process have found it to be useful for the purposes of curriculum and instruction.

The nursing process and other problem-solving approaches have been utilized for content development. This approach implies both an object and a process of nursing. Engaging in problem-solving activities presupposes a problem to be solved. Those who have endeavored to use this approach have found it necessary to develop a conceptual framework of nursing practice in relation to the primary focus of nursing. Using this approach focuses attention on the modes of inquiry into the practice of nursing from which the content of nursing is developed.

Constructing models directs attention to the various components and variables within the activity of nursing and the relationships of these components and variables to each other. A model is usually conceived as a structure of symbols interpreted in certain ways, and what it is a model of is the subject matter specified by the interpretation. Models are used for the purpose of explaining facts and events. Researchers utilize models for formulating hypotheses concerning the nature and impact of, or the relationships of two or more components of the model. Models have been constructed by nursing faculty to describe the relationship among the events in nursing.

Utilization of a science theory as a means of defining the content of community health nursing was attempted by a group of teachers. Talcott Parsons's theory of action became the frame of reference for this curriculum activity. The group also considered a formal testing of the theory, but these efforts were not productive. While this group of teachers acknowledged that the theory was much too general for this purpose, they did feel it was useful for identifying concepts about community health and roles of the community health nurse for curriculum and instruction.

REFERENCES

1. Smith, B. O., Stanley, W. O., and Shores, J. H. *Fundamentals of Curriculum Development.* New York: Harcourt, Brace, and World, 1957. P. 127.
2. Schwab, J. J. Structure of the Disciplines: Meanings and Significances. In G. W. Ford and L. Pugno [Eds.], *The Structure of Knowledge and the Curriculum.* Chicago: Rand McNally, 1964. P. 6.
3. Broudy, H. S. To regain educational leadership. *Studies Philos. Educ.* 2:132, 1962.

4. Phenix, P. H.   The Disciplines as Curriculum Content. In A. H. Passou [Ed.], *Curriculum Crossroads*. New York: Teachers College Bureau of Publications (Columbia University), 1962. P. 58.
5. Henderson, K. B.   Uses of Subject Matter. In B. O. Smith and R. H. Ennis [Eds.], *Language and Concepts in Education*. Chicago: Rand McNally, 1961. P. 43.
6. Soltis, J. F.   *An Introduction to the Analysis of Educational Concepts*. Reading: Addison-Wesley, 1968. P. 31.
7. Ibid., p. 33.
8. Henderson, op. cit., p. 43.
9. Ibid., p. 43.
10. Martin, J. R.   On the Reduction of Knowing That to Knowing How. In B. O. Smith and R. H. Ennis [Eds.], *Language and Concepts in Education*. Chicago: Rand McNally, 1961. P. 59.
11. Sand, O.   Basis for Decisions. In R. Leeper [Ed.], *Role of Supervisor and Curriculum Director in a Climate of Change*. Washington, D.C.: Association for Supervision and Curriculum Development, National Education Association, 1965. P. 3.
12. Ibid., p. 3.
13. Douglas, H. B.   *The High School Curriculum*. New York: Ronald, 1956. P. 236.
14. Ibid.
15. Alberty, H.   *Reorganizing the High School Curriculum*. New York: Macmillan, 1948. P. 154.
16. Alberty, H.   *Reorganizing the High School Curriculum*, rev. ed. New York: Macmillan, 1953. P. 167.
17. Thomas, R.   *The Search for A Common Learning*. New York: McGraw-Hill, 1962.
18. Kempf, F. C.   A common core of learnings for all. *Nurs. Outlook* 3:132, 1955.
19. The Carnegie Commission on Higher Education.   *Higher Education and the Nation's Health*. New York: McGraw-Hill, 1970. P. 51.
20. Kinsinger, R. E.   A core curriculum for the health field. *Nurs. Outlook* 15:28, 1967.
21. Kissick, W. L.   *Health Manpower in Transition*. Mimeographed. Washington, D. C.: U.S. Public Health Service, 1966.
22. Allen, D. E.   Core content in the basic curriculum. *Nurs. Outlook* 1:286, 1953.
23. Bruce, S. J., and Hall, E. J.   Maternity and pediatric nurses study and work together. *Amer. J. Nurs.* 63:105, 1963.
24. Abdellah, F. G., et al.   *Patient-Centered Approaches to Nursing*. New York: Macmillan, 1960.
25. Bruner, J. S.   *The Process of Education*. Cambridge: Harvard University Press, 1966. P. 17.
26. Hofling, C. K., and Leininger, M. M.   *Basic Psychiatric Concepts of Nursing*. Philadelphia: Lippincott, 1960.
27. Zderad, L. T., and Belcher, H. C.   *Developing Behavioral Concepts in Nursing*. Atlanta: Southern Regional Education Board, 1968. P. 111.
28. Ibid., p. 7.

29. Ibid., p. 29.
30. Ibid., p. 111.
31. Henderson, K. B. A Logical Model for Conceptualizing and Other Related Activities. In B. P. Komisar and C. B. J. Macmillan [Eds.], *Psychological Concepts in Education.* Chicago: Rand McNally, 1967. P. 97.
32. Zderad and Belcher, op. cit., p. 111.
33. Yura, H., and Walsh, M. *The Nursing Process.* Washington, D.C.: Catholic University of America Press, 1967.
34. Abdellah et al., op. cit., p. 24.
35. Lewis, L., et al. *Defining Clinical Content, Graduate Nursing Programs: Medical-Surgical Nursing.* Boulder: Western Interstate Commission for Higher Education, 1967. P. 6.
36. McDonald, F. J., and Harms, M. T. A theoretical model for an experimental curriculum. *Nurs. Outlook* 14:48, 1966.
37. Abdellah et al., op. cit., p. 16.
38. Department of Baccalaureate and Higher Degree Programs. *The Shifting Scene: Directions for Practice.* New York: National League for Nursing, 1967. P. 4.
39. Bruner, op. cit., p. 20.
40. Coe, C., et al. *One Approach to the Identification of Essential Content in Baccalaureate Programs in Nursing.* Boulder: Western Interstate Commission for Higher Education, 1967.
41. Ibid., p. 10.
42. Kaplan, A. *The Conduct of Inquiry.* San Francisco: Chandler, 1964. P. 267.
43. Harms, M. T., and McDonald, F. J. A new curriculum design. *Nurs. Outlook* 14:52, 1966.
44. Ford, L. C., et al. Preface to *Defining Clinical Content, Graduate Nursing Programs, Community Health Nursing.* Boulder: Western Interstate Commission for Higher Education, 1967.
45. Ibid., p. 1.

SUPPLEMENTARY READINGS

Belth, M. *Education as a Discipline.* Boston: Allyn and Bacon, 1965.
Broudy, H. S. Mastery. In B. O. Smith and R. H. Ennis [Eds.], *Language and Concepts in Education.* Chicago: Rand McNally, 1961.
Bruner, J. S., Goodman, J. J., and Austin, G. A. *A Study of Thinking.* New York: Wiley, 1956.
Engleman, S. *Conceptual Learning.* San Rafael: Dimensions, 1969.
Gagné, R. M. *The Conditions of Learning.* New York: Holt, Rinehart & Winston, 1965.
Hunt, E. B. *Concept Learning.* New York: Wiley, 1962.
Parker, J. C., and Rubin, L. J. *Process a Content: Curriculum Design and the Application of Knowledge.* Chicago: Rand McNally, 1966.
Woodruff, A. D. Cognitive Models of Learning and Instruction. In L. Siegel [Ed.], *Instruction: Some Contemporary Viewpoints.* San Francisco: Chandler, 1967.

11 DESIGN AND STRUCTURE OF THE CURRICULUM

THE concept of curriculum design brings into focus the various theoretical and practical issues concerned with curriculum development. It is the design characteristics that makes one curriculum similar to or different from another. Any adequate curriculum design defines the important components or aspects of the curriculum and determines their relationship to each other and to the tasks to be undertaken. A curriculum pattern provides a consistent framework of values and priorities for dealing with the operational decisions of teaching-learning situations. A curriculum design has the quality of an organic unity in which the dimensions and domains of the educational endeavor are coherent and identifiable. The curriculum design should: (1) identify the factors involved in curriculum; (2) define the relation between these factors and other activities; and (3) predict and control the educational behavior of the learner.

It is likely that the problems of an individual teaching plan, an organizational plan for a subject area, an approach to the overall curriculum, and an overall plan for education in general are merely various descriptions of the same problem: curriculum design. All of the components of curriculum design are present in some degree at these various levels of planning and organizing.

THE NATURE OF CURRICULUM DESIGN

Curriculum design is a statement of the relationships that exist among the elements of a curriculum as they are used to make decisions about instruction.

The role of curriculum design in the improvement of educational programs can best be seen as having the following functions: (1) defining the elements of the curriculum and their relationships in curriculum development, (2) stating the means used for selecting and organizing learning opportunities, and (3) indicating the role of teachers and students in curriculum planning and development.

A curriculum design must provide answers for the following questions that teachers ask:

1. What do I know about the student, and how can I prepare and manage an environment that will promote optimum learning?
2. How can I identify, define, and use instructional objectives to determine the scope, direction, and emphasis of the student's learning opportunities?
3. How can I select and organize these opportunities so as to aid the student to achieve worthwhile educational ends?
4. How can I develop instructional strategies so that these opportunities are most efficiently utilized by the student to achieve these ends?
5. How can I evaluate performance to determine the extent and quality of the student's development toward these ends?

Since every learning situation must include a learner, a purpose, a content, and a process, curriculum design must also recognize and account for the part these factors play in the learning experiences of students. Learning does not take place in a vacuum; it is essentially social in nature and in context. Every learning experience involves all four of the above-mentioned elements in some degree. All curriculum activities have content and purpose; developing the curriculum is not a process of deciding either-or but of deciding what will produce effective development of students. Most people recognize that both students and content must be considered.

The task of the curriculum planner is to establish an environment in which the learner may learn. The curriculum planner can only approximately anticipate the conditions under which learners may have learning experiences; however, opportunities are identified and selected that will produce the appropriate environment for learning. The specific nature of the learning environment and the types of opportunities selected depend upon a variety of factors inherent in the educational process.

All social institutions, including schools, may be justified in terms of the goals or purposes they claim to serve. Once the goals are recognized and accepted, means must be selected for the attainment of the goals. In the case of the school, the curriculum is the means to achieve the goals, and the instructional process provides for the implementation of curriculum opportunities. The process of evaluation helps us to determine the adequacy of the means in producing the desired result—the achievement of the goals. The results of evaluation help us to redefine the goals and to revise if necessary the means for achieving them. The objectives of the curriculum state the behaviors that the student is expected to acquire. Curriculum strategies within a subject matter deal with the selection of opportunities for learning. Instructional strategies are the plans by which the events and opportunities are arranged to bring about the desired behavior of the student. These strategies involve the utilization of various resources for instruction, giving attention to the specific characteristics of the learners and the nature of the learning process. Research in the subject matter area and in teaching and learning strategies provides information for continuous review and revision of curriculum content and processes.

Variations in curriculum design have been identified with the ways of organizing subject matter. Some common schemes of organization include: the broad fields of curriculum, the core curriculum, the activity curriculum, the problems curriculum, and the experience or needs curriculum. Each of these calls for a different design, since each requires some different questions to be answered. When the curriculum has as its major focus the needs and interests of students, information must be sought that enables the curriculum worker to utilize the needs and interests of students in relation to the subject matter area. When the major emphasis of the curriculum is on the subject matter, the arrangement of the curriculum is dependent upon the inherent organization of the subject matter under consideration. Recent attention to the structure of the disciplines stresses the organizational features of the individual disciplines and the need for careful programming of each discipline according to its own characteristics and rules.

The activities of psychologists and subject matter specialists have restored to some degree the issues pertaining to content versus process. There has been much discussion about the content of the disciplines and the modes of inquiry associated with them. Process is interpreted as content, where the chemistry student learns not only the subject matter of chemistry but also how to behave like a chemist, or the nursing student learns both the subject matter of nursing and the behavior patterns of the nurse practitioner. The modes of inquiry into the field of chemistry by the chemist are different from those used by the nurse in the course of nursing. Each discipline has an organized body of knowledge and appropriate processes; these should be considered inseparable in designating curriculum content.

School organization has considerable influence upon the design of the curriculum. Curriculum workers usually must fit the curriculum to an already fixed organizational structure. Theoretically, administrative units are developed to facilitate curriculum development; however, all too often they present obstacles in designing new curriculums or revising established ones.

FUNCTIONS OF CURRICULUM DESIGN

The curriculum design defines for the curriculum worker what the faculty group considers to be the important elements in the curriculum. It also includes how the elements are to be combined to produce a well-balanced curriculum. The following elements have priority in the initial stages of curriculum development:

1. The curriculum is based on the educational beliefs and convictions of the teachers who are responsible for its development.
2. The purpose of the curriculum provides the means for selecting and giving direction to the needs of students.
3. The individual needs of students must be considered in relation to the needs of society and the capacity of the school to meet them.

To be useful to curriculum workers, a curriculum design must make clear the basis upon which the curriculum decisions are made. What is to be done? What subject matter is to be used? What classroom procedures are to be followed? How are the results to be appraised? The design points out these questions and indicates the relationships among them. The objectives serve as a basis for determining subject matter, learning opportunities, teaching approaches, and evaluation procedures.

The overall design of the curriculum must be viewed on several dimensions and on different operational levels. The dimensions of the curriculum are the direction and scope, and breadth and depth of curriculum activities. By operational levels are meant, for example, the translation of the overall goals of the curriculum into those goals at the course level and then to the level of day-by-day instruction. A suggested outline of a design of a nursing curriculum is presented in Diagram 4, which includes the important elements and questions.

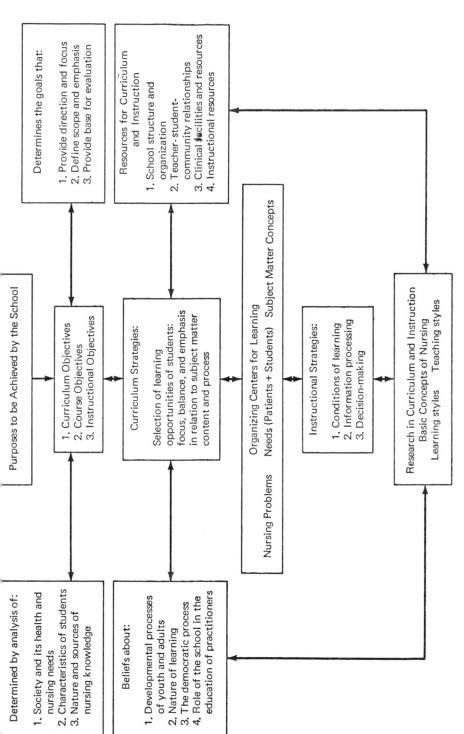

DIAGRAM 4. A design of a nursing curriculum.

309

To permit appropriate curriculum decisions, the design must make explicit the nature and function of the components of the curriculum. A fundamental concern is the nature of the learning opportunities for students providing the appropriate focus, balance, and emphasis in relation to the objectives of the curriculum. The developmental status and other characteristics of the students determines the types of opportunities to be selected to assist the student in reaching the objectives. These learning opportunities are selected, organized, and developed to help the student acquire the behavior patterns indicated by the objectives. Other bases for determining what learning oportunities should be considered and how they should be organized include faculty beliefs concerning the nature of the society in which the student lives and the role of the school in that society.

The curriculum design will be more functional if it has as its central focus the specific organization of curriculum opportunities. Attention is directed to the use of organizing centers in selecting and organizing activities, content, and processes in ways that are meaningful to students. The use of organizing centers also permits development of curriculum components in a sequence that contributes to the overall goals. The more common organizing centers include nursing problems, patient and student needs, and subject matter concepts. Identification of the approach to be used determines the objectives at the instructional level. Other factors in the selection of learning opportunities include the interests of students, the plan for continuity, the ability of the student to utilize the opportunity, and the resources of the teacher, the school, and the community. Approaches differ primarily in what they consider most important as a basis for selection.

The curriculum design indicates the factors to be considered in curriculum development but does not prescribe a specific approach by which to study and analyze the factors. As long as all factors are considered in a sequence that is useful to the teachers, the particular approach makes little difference. All curriculum designs have essentially the same concerns: students, subject matter, and educational processes. Curriculum patterns differ in the way in which these elements are combined and the degree to which each is used to make decisions.

The relationship of students to teachers, to other instructional personnel, and to the community are vital issues in curriculum development. The particular approach being used will determine in some measure the types of relationships that are necessary to make curriculum decisions. The subject matter approach will probably involve teachers to a greater extent than the needs approach. Utilizing needs, particularly student needs, as a curriculum approach suggests the combined efforts of teachers and student in making curriculum decisions. Nursing problems as an approach implies the involvement of teachers, students, other instructional personnel, and the community in curriculum decisions. The curriculum design must indicate the roles and responsibilities of teachers, students, and others in making major curriculum decisions.

A good curriculum design, one incorporating the information and processes that have been described, will provide adequate orientation to the issues of curriculum development. The design indicates the tasks to be undertaken in planning and organizing the instructional program. These tasks are continuous in nature, since any changes in the major concerns of the curriculum—students, teachers, and subject matter—will require review of other components and dimensions of the curriculum.

OBJECTIVES AND CURRICULUM DESIGN

The central focus of curriculum design relates to the derivation, specification, selection, mediation, and assessment of objectives. Attention to and skills in these areas are essential if the curriculum worker is to prepare behaviorally oriented learning opportunities and materials for use by students and others in the school environment.

One of the major determinants of the objectives of the curriculum and of the instructional process is the nature of the society in which the school exists. The society must be viewed in relation to technological and scientific changes, cultural expectations, changing sentiments, values, mores, and other things that society approves or disapproves. Since schools have the obligation to preserve and transmit changes in the ways of thinking, feeling, and doing that are sanctioned by society, the objectives of the curriculum must reflect the desires and aspirations of that larger group. Obviously schools are not responsible for all aspects of social change but select those which are appropriate to their primary missions.

Another source that we draw upon in the formulation of objectives is the nature of the individual (the student). Information about the personal ability, achievement, hopes, aspirations, and intellectual and social development of the individual is required in selecting objectives that are feasible and reasonable.

A third source of information that is important in determining objectives of the curriculum is the nature of knowledge, or the discipline, or the subject matter of the curriculum. Recently considerable attention has been directed to the structure of knowledge in relation to the fundamental ideas of a particular body of knowledge. Although these basic sources of information provide a theoretical and practical approach to determining the objectives for curriculum and instruction, it appears that inevitably one source becomes predominant. The priority that the school places on the factors which influence the selection of learning opportunities determines the *direction and focus* of the objectives of the curriculum.

If we conceptualize a curriculum in which the disciplines (subject matter) receive primary consideration, with the nature of society and the needs of the individual secondary, the objectives we formulate will reflect the primary role of knowledge in the curriculum. The departmental structure according to the major disciplines that is prevalent in many universities reflects this emphasis on knowledge in the various curriculums.

If the nature of society is ranked as the most important concern in curriculum building, and the nature of knowledge and the needs of the students are placed in secondary roles, different kinds of objectives are selected and an entirely different kind of curriculum develops. Elementary school curriculums have reflected this philosophy, in which social concerns are primary. In this instance, group concerns, social expectations, learning to fit into the group, functioning as a member of the group, and learning to live by the rules of the group are of paramount importance in the design of the curriculum.

The third order of priority presumes that student needs are primary, while the nature of society and the body of knowledge are secondary. This represents an entirely different assumption, which leads to different kinds of objectives and a different curriculum design. Students today seem to be asking the schools to be attentive to their individual needs and interests. They seem to be pleading with the schools to give consideration to their growth and development, their motivations and ambitions as a focus in directing education. One's choice of a primary concern in the formulation of objectives will cause her to look at curriculum design in different ways. The different primary purposes or objectives of the curriculum will dictate selection of different content, learning opportunities, organizational strategies, and evaluation procedures.

The statement of objectives included in the curriculum design indicate the *scope and emphasis* of the curriculum. Determining the number of different important elements to be considered at a given time in an educational program pertains to the *scope* of the curriculum. It refers to the breadth and variety of opportunities that the school provides and essentially means the "what" of the curriculum, or the range of the subject matter. Formerly, the term scope related to the coverage of subject matter by the teacher; however, a more appropriate interpretation describes scope as the varieties of ways of behaving or the range of behaviors to be developed by the student.

The objectives of the curriculum, course, or lesson form one of the important definitions of the scope of the curriculum, course, or lesson. The statement of objectives on the various levels also suggests the essential behavior to be acquired during particular times in the learning sequence. It is obvious that no one school program, course, or lesson can include all desirable objectives that might be suggested. Selection must be made in terms of significant and essential objectives that are considered appropriate at a given time and place. The statement of objectives is a concrete and realistic definition of what the program or learning opportunity is trying to achieve.

If the statement of objectives provides a definition of the number and types of different aspects of learning that are included in the curriculum, the evaluation of that curriculum, course, or lesson should consider all of these aspects in judging the adequacy of the program. Too often a nursing curriculum is judged primarily on the basis of the graduates' competencies in technical or manipulatory skills without giving comparable attention to other facets of learning, such as human relations and problem-solving behaviors.

Most learning opportunities that are selected will contribute to more than one objective. For efficiency of learning, consideration should be given to ways in which the essential elements can be utilized to assist students to attain more than one objective of the course or curriculum. This implies that the scope of any learning opportunity may be extended to include the development of facts, concepts, skills and abilities, and changes in attitudes. Attention should be given to the appropriateness of extending the learning opportunity to the attainment of more than one objective in relation to the focus of learning at the particular time and the ability of the student to accommodate the various aspects of learning.

The behavior modifications described in the objectives for a course or a lesson suggest the scope of the various behavior changes required. This ensures that the behavioral aspects relate to more than acquiring information. The scope of behaviors required in a specific phase of the curriculum may suggest mental operations requiring comparing, discriminating, describing, and applying knowledge in problem-solving activities.

Similarly, the objectives specify the content or subject matter area in which the behavior will be developed. An objective stating that the student "establishes effective communication" means very little to the student or teachers unless it also specifies with whom and under what circumstances the student establishes effective communication. The objective "establishes effective communication with the mother of a mentally retarded child," provides the content area in which the behavior operates. The diversity of nursing episodes in which the behaviors will occur is indicated by the scope of the curriculum objectives.

In addition to indicating the scope of the curriculum, the statement of objectives also suggests the emphasis to be made in the educational program. The objectives of technical nursing programs will probably give greater attention to the application of scientific principles in the nursing care of the patient with a specific health problem. The emphasis in the objectives of the baccalaureate curriculum is on concern for preventive aspects of health in the nursing activities of health teaching and guidance. Likewise, the objectives of the technical nursing curriculum emphasize the role of the nurse as a team member in the cooperative activities of providing nursing care, whereas the objectives of the baccalaureate curriculum emphasize the leadership role of this nurse in delegating, directing, supervising, and evaluating the nursing care given by others.

Within a specific curriculum, different emphasis may be placed on the utilization of the various sciences in nursing at different times. At one time the emphasis in nursing curriculums focused on the natural sciences. More recently the emphasis has been more in the direction of the behavioral sciences.

The objectives of the curriculum also reflect the emphasis placed on the various behavioral changes desired. Baccalaureate and graduate level curriculums place greater emphasis on process objectives, such as analysis, synthesis, and problem-solving. The technical nursing curriculums focus attention on the application of knowledge to nursing care activities. The particular behavioral emphases found in the curriculum objectives must also be dealt with in the course objectives and in the instructional objectives. The emphases must be compatible with the subject matter curriculum under consideration.

The statement of objectives within the curriculum design define what is important, what the major focus should be, what the scope of the curriculum is in relation to the range of behaviors and content areas, and what the specific emphasis of the curriculum is. They also form the basis for evaluation of the outcomes of the curriculum in terms of performance.

IDENTIFYING AND ORGANIZING CURRICULUM OPPORTUNITIES

The objectives of the curriculum provide the curriculum worker with a description of the finished product of the school. This description indicates the capabilities that the student has acquired during the educational process. The curriculum worker must then work backwards, using her own intuition and inventiveness to identify a set of events and opportunities that is most likely to produce the required set of behaviors. The process of identifying and organizing curriculum opportunities is a vital function of curriculum design. It begins with the analysis of objectives.

ANALYSIS OF OBJECTIVES

In analyzing objectives the curriculum worker identifies the demands of the social and professional environment, the implied subject matter, and the interests and capabilities of the learners. This description provides an outline of the activities to be performed and the functional context in which the learner is intended to perform the activities. It includes the human, material, and institutional capabilities required to produce the designated product or graduate. From this the curriculum worker can infer, with some degree of probability, a set of opportunities for instruction. This inference is dependent upon a clear, unambiguous, and comprehensive description of the functional characteristics of the completed product of the school, the graduate.

An objective of a nursing curriculum describes the graduate nurse as one who gives nursing care to an individual and his family within the context of the American society. Human capabilities that are inferred from this activity may include the following activities:

1. Identifies the needs of the individual and his family for nursing care, assesses patient's and family's resources for helping themselves, and diagnoses the nursing problems
2. Applies knowledge about nursing and related science information in developing a plan of nursing care
3. Utilizes the particular resources observed in the patient and family in administering the plan of care
4. Observes the responses of the patient and family to the nursing care and modifies the plan of care as necessary to assist patient and family to attain their health goals

5. Provides for continuous evaluation of nursing care in relation to the ever-changing variables within the patient-family-nurse physical and social interaction and modifies nursing care accordingly

The activity implied in this curriculum objective also describes the necessary material capabilities. These capabilities include the delineation of subject matter areas at the appropriate levels of generality. Some of these areas that appear to serve this purpose include: human development and behavior, normal physiological and psychological functioning, aberrations of normal functioning, and therapeutic programs and services designed to assist the individual and his family with their health problems. In addition, certain psychosociological mechanisms of patients, family, and nurses relevant to health is indicated. Availability of health care services and the characteristics of social and health agencies in the community are considered to be material capabilities. Within this category of capabilities are the characteristics of the students in relation to their needs, interests, and abilities. Finally, the commitment of the profession to the continuous upgrading of the practice of nursing by scholarly and scientific endeavors are necessary material capabilities.

The third classification of capabilities that pertain to the designated activity is that provided by the institution (school). These capabilities include the human and physical resources—competent teachers and appropriate clinical resources—libraries, various types of instructional materials, and resource persons, such as physicians, social workers, nutritionists, and public health and other community workers.

The description of the various capabilities relates to an activity of nursing implied in one curriculum objective. Other activities are identified through the analysis of other objectives, and the desired human, material, and institutional capabilities are described.

It appears obvious that the activity "gives nursing care to a patient (or potential patient) and his family within the context of an American community" is much too general for the purpose of identifying and organizing curriculum opportunities. Further analysis of the activity of nursing must be made to delineate more specifically the functional context and the implied subject matter. The nursing activity "gives care to an aged man with multiple health problems in a nursing home . . ." indicates a more specific aspect of the general activity "gives nursing care to a patient. . . ." The more specific nursing activity permits identification of human, material, and institutional capabilities required for this activity. These capabilities are the opportunities or events for

TABLE 7. Analysis of a General Nursing Activity in Relation to Human, Material, and Institutional Capabilities: Giving nursing care to a patient or potential patient and his family within the context of an American community

Human	Material	Institutional
Identifies the needs of the individual and his family for nursing care—assesses patient's and family's resources for helping themselves—diagnoses the nursing problems	Description of subject matter at the appropriate level of generality (what is known about):	*Human and Physical Resources*
	Human development and behavior	Competent teachers
	Normal physiological and psychological functioning	Appropriate clinical resources:
Applies knowledge about nursing and related science information in developing a plan of nursing care	Aberrations of normal functioning—and appropriate medical treatment regimens	Hospitals Homes Extended care facilities Industry Clinics Physicians' offices Social-educational agencies
Utilizes the particular clues, cues, and resources observed in the patient and family in administering the plan of care	Perception of individuals and families of their need for nursing care	*Libraries*
Observes the responses of patient and family to the nursing care and modifies the plan of care as necessary to assist patient and family to attain their health goals	Perception of nurses and other health workers of patient's and family's need for care	Nursing, allied professional, social, and natural science
		Instructional Materials
	Characteristics of social agencies and institutions available for health	Audiovisual media Skill laboratories Programmed instruction Computer-assisted instruction
Provides for continuous evaluation of nursing care in relation to the ever-changing variables within the patient-family-nurse physical and social interaction and modifies nursing care accordingly	Availability of health care services	
	Nursing approaches to help patient and families meet their health needs	*Resource Persons*
	Description of the characteristics of students in terms of their initial capabilities, attitudes, and interests	Physicians Social workers Nutritionists Public health workers (official voluntary agencies)
	Description of the status of nursing profession in relation to nursing practice and the commitment of the profession to improve practice by means of scholarly and scientific endeavors	

learning that are required to meet the individual, social, and professional demands of the specific activities within a specific functional context. These in turn contribute to attainment of the requirements implied in the general activity or the objective of the curriculum. The descriptions contained in Tables 7 and 8 present the analyses of a general and a specific nursing activity in relation to the human, material, and institutional capabilities inherent in each activity. The purpose of presenting these analyses is to demonstrate a method for the identification of curriculum opportunities that will produce the behaviors indicated in the objectives of the curriculum.

TABLE 8.   Analysis of a Specific Nursing Activity in Relation to Human, Material, and Institutional Capabilities: Giving nursing care to an aged man with multiple health problems in a nursing home in the context of an American community

Human	Material	Institutional
Identifies the specific nursing problems in relation to the care of aging and aged persons: 1. Personal hygiene and physical comfort 2. Optimal activity, exercise, rest, and sleep 3. Prevention of accidents and injury 4. Maintain good body mechanics Identifies nursing action in relation to problems of normal and disturbed physiological processes: 1. Maintenance of a supply of oxygen to the body 2. Maintenance of nutrition 3. Maintenance of fluid and electrolyte balance Responses of body to certain drugs	Description of subject matter at the appropriate level of generality: Physiological and psychological changes in aging and aged persons General characteristics of the aging process Role of heredity and environment in relation to biological and psychosocial changes in aging Sensory and perceptual changes in aging Psychological changes in aging Changes in social behavior of older persons Characteristics of the health status of aging persons: Causes of illness and death in persons 65 years of age and older	*Human and Physical Resources* Competent teachers of geriatric nursing Appropriate clinical resources: Nursing homes Extended care facilities Retirement residences Voluntary associations (senior citizens) *Library Resources* Publications Geriatrics Gerontology Geriatric nursing Bibliographic materials Journals Nursing Sociology Public health Medicine

Human	Material	Institutional
Maintenance of sensory functions	Health differentials in relation to sex, marital status, race, economic status, and occupation	Research reports Nursing Behavioral science Statistical reports
Identifies nursing action concerned with emotional and interpersonal difficulties	Characteristics of senescence	*Instructional Materials*
		Films
Facilitates expression of feelings and reactions of aging persons	Response of society to the needs of aging citizens—available health services: Home care	Tapes Slides Programmed instruction
Detects the possible interrelatedness of emotions and organic illness	Hospital Extended care facilities Nursing homes Retirement residences	*Resource Persons* Physicians
Facilitates the maintenance of effective verbal and nonverbal communication	Homes for the aged Response of community to the social needs of aging	Specialists in geriatrics Social workers Nutritionists
Facilitates patient's awareness of self as an individual with varying physical, emotional, and developmental needs	citizens—personal services: Meals-on-wheels Housekeeping Senior citizen groups Part-time employment Housing for elderly	Clergy Public health workers
Identifies nursing action regarding sociological or community problems as well as those of the individual:	Nursing approaches to assist elderly persons to meet their health needs	
Facilitates acceptance of optimal goals in light of physical and emotional limitations	Description of the learners in relation to their initial capabilities, attitudes, and interests in the nursing care of aging and aged persons	
Utilizes resources of government as well as voluntary agencies to aid in resolving problems of aged	Description of the status of nursing in relation to nursing care of aging persons, and the commitment of the profession to improve practice by means of organized efforts to interest nurses in this area of practice and by scholarly and scientific investigations in this area	
Develops plan of nursing care, administers, evaluates, and modifies care in relation to the individual response to care		

ORGANIZING CENTERS

The organization of curriculum opportur ies can best be approached in terms of organizing centers. An organizing center is whatever the teacher has used to relate the learning opportunities of the student in some type of meaningful organization. The function of organizing centers is perhaps more vital at the present time because of the rapid growth of the various fields of knowledge. At the same time that new knowledge is appearing, some aspects of available knowledge (facts and skills) become outmoded.

Learning has a purpose, which may be an immediate concern but which may also extend into the future. The most profitable and economical learning is that which can be applied to a variety of problems in different contexts. The notions expressed recently by psychologists and subject matter specialists about the structure of a discipline attempt to identify the major ideas, concepts, principles, or problems of the discipline. Whereas much factual detail may be of a temporary character and usage, the major ideas are relatively stable and will endure over long periods of time. The major ideas of the discipline become the organizing centers for learning experiences in the curriculum. Common centers include an interest, a fact or skill to be learned, a job to be accomplished, a problem to be solved, or a question to be answered.

In order to achieve specific educational goals, the instructor must make decisions in selecting content, materials, and methods. The end product, that is, the total situation to which the student is called upon to respond, is the organizing center for learning. The organizing center should be broad enough to provide a number of places where students can "catch hold of a problem, idea, concept or principle and move it somewhere in time and space" [1]. The intent of the organizing center is to confront the student with a situation calling for a response or series of responses. Since the organizing center should cause the student to practice the behavior that is sought, the teacher must have clearly in mind what this behavior is and recognize it when it occurs.

Organizing centers should have the following characteristics if they are to be useful for instruction:

1. Significance for learning. The organizing center has potential for developing in the student those behaviors that result from deepening and broadening certain understandings, skills, and values that underlie the curriculum. This means that the center suggests activities that are of interest to the students that they recognize as worthwhile.

2. Accessibility. Ideas that are considered desirable for organizing centers must be available in publications (books, journals) as well as in the clinical problems of patients and families. The elucidation and implementation of the ideas contained in the organizing centers must be possible through human and material resources, which can serve as curricular activities and learning opportunities.

3. Breadth and scope. The organizing center must lend itself to the demands of many interests and capabilities represented in a group of students. The center must provide opportunity for moving several related curriculum elements along together—cognitive, problem-solving, and operational skills.

4. Thematic organization. The organizing center lends itself easily to learnings that have gone before and that are likely to lie ahead. It enables students to "tie things together" and perceive related wholes rather than a series of fragmented learnings.

5. Developmental potential. The organizing center encourages students to seek new avenues for learning. Initial explorations should stimulate productive study.

The concept that the center of attention is a learning opportunity which may activate behavior does not disregard other elements or aspects of learning; it does, however, focus attention on what is significant in educational learning, namely, the goal and its role in the control and direction of learning. If an organizing center can be approached in more than one way by the learner, its power to provide for individual differences is increased. The centers that have narrow limits for knowing and learning (such as the learning of a specific skill) restrict their usefulness in accommodating the individual differences among students.

EXAMPLES OF ORGANIZING CENTERS

The faculty of a baccalaureate nursing program utilized nursing problems as the focus of curriculum content. Certain problems for which the nurse has chief responsibility were chosen as organizing centers for learning. In adopting this subject matter approach, the following assumptions were made by the curriculum workers:

1. The specific nursing problem becomes an integral part of the instructional program.

Fun, Form, and Figure (Physical Activities)

Fitness and physical potential; developing physical potential through movement; factors influencing potential—sleep, rest, nutrition, relaxation, inheritance; inventory of physical potential; basic skills in work; basic skills in play; basic principles of exercise; figure development; increase in vitality; improved body control

Structure and Function of the Body

Anatomical structure and physiological processes of the body; muscular and skeletal systems provide a means for locomotion, support for body structures, and protection for soft tissues; all the movements of the body are brought about through the action of muscles; muscle tissue performs mechanical work by contracting—muscle contraction is under nervous control; peripheral nerves are subject to injury through trauma, stretching, or pressure; if traumatized, the part they supply is paralyzed and rendered insensitive; good posture means good anatomical relationships of the body parts to each other when the body is in different positions; concepts of force, torque, equilibrium

Care of Patients with Minimal Limitation of Movement

Concepts of static postures—lying, half-lying, sitting, standing; concepts of dynamic postures—lifting, carrying, holding, pushing, pulling, walking, climbing; basic postural patterns in work; use of body in performing work; efficient use of body—work, rest, relaxation, fatigue, position, environmental factors, optimum work heights, shoes, and clothing

Assisting the patient to become more efficient through rest, ease, comfort; body alignment, rest, and change; kinds of support; methods of giving support; measures to protect skin; measures to maintain normal range of movement; environmental factors that may influence patient care—bed, chair, clothing; detection of postural deviations, self-help procedures.

Care of Patients with Temporary Limitation of Movement

Care of patients with a medical or surgical problem that causes discomfort and interferes with self-care; changes of position should be made slowly and smoothly; appropriate use of active or passive exercise; adjustments of position to provide for as near normal body alignment as possible; rest and exercise in the care of the patient who has undergone surgery—loss of muscle and muscle weakness; effect of exercise on the psychological status; exercise promotes relaxation and reduces pain; exercises essential to the protection of respiratory, circulatory, and joint function; devices used to increase mobility of patients in bed; range of motion exercises; exercise of arm and shoulder on the affected side of radical mastectomy patient

Care of patients who have loss of or change in function of a part of the muscular or skeletal system—immobilization of fractured bone; use of traction to align a part and to stretch contracted muscles; injured part maintained in good alignment; observation for signs and symptoms of interference with circulation and peripheral nerve damage; care of patients who have inflammation of a joint (e.g., rheumatoid arthritis)—body parts maintained in as normal alignment as possible; exercises involving the affected joint should be done as ordered—moved through complete range of motion; care of pregnant woman—encouraged to maintain the closest approach to normal body alignment; the body should be balanced over a firm base of support in standing, walking, squatting, or rising; the pelvis and lower extremities should provide a firm support for the vertebral column; patients should be encouraged to use proper wearing apparel (e.g., brassiere, foundation garment, shoes, hosiery); patients should have normal or physiologically possible active exercise of the major

Care of youth and adults with traumatic injuries resulting in amputation of limb(s); use of braces or prosthetic devices; planning for rehabilitation; social and emotional response of patient and family; motivation of patient and revision of self-concept; vocational rehabilitation. Care of patients with spinal cord injuries; prevention of contractures and foot drop; care of skin; movement of joints and muscles; frequent change in position; rehabilitation program in extended care facilities or home; continuity of care to promote optimal progress. Care of patients who have experienced a cerebral vascular accident—maintaining body alignment; active or passive range of motion as indicated by physician, providing support for affected limb; prevention of contractures and decubitus; retraining of bowel, bladder, and speech; modification of environment to permit patient to care for himself

Care of patients with degenerative diseases and progressive deterioration of the skeletal system; anatomical and physiologic changes in aging that affect mobility—gradual loss in elasticity of connective tissue, causing some rigidity of body structures; bones become rarified and fractures occur easily; lessened elasticity of blood vessels impedes circulation, which makes it difficult for patient to tolerate changes in position; gradual deterioration and atrophy of nervous system leads to lessened nerve acuity and to impaired sensation; muscular activity is less adequate; attention to preventive posture is essential because of the inability to exert required muscular effort to remain in erect position; increments in body weight in trunk area affect mobility (physical and psychological); changes take place in perception of the body—perception of movement of body parts; loss of visual efficiency restricts movement. Psychological changes may result in mild depression and isolation; effects of compulsory retirement and declining health and mobility; efforts of community organizations and agencies to promote physical and social mobility of aging persons

DIAGRAM 5. Use of a nursing problem, promoting mobility, as an organizing center.

2. The learning opportunities planned around the nursing problem are built upon the student's previous knowledge, understandings, experiences, and skills.
3. The concepts and principles related to the nursing problem are best learned when the instructional approach is personalized.
4. The presentation of the nursing problem in a variety of clinical situations provides for breadth of learning.
5. The presentation of the nursing problem in clinical situations of increasing complexity provides for depth of learning.

One of the problems that the instructors selected as an organizing center was that of maintaining and promoting optimal mobility of the patient or potential patient. The justification for the selection of this problem was based on the need of all individuals to maintain physical and social mobility to perform the activities of daily living and to engage in occupational and/or social activities. The concept of maintenance was viewed as a continuum that included preventive, therapeutic, and restorative aspects of nursing care.

Since good health implies that an individual has the physical potential necessary for daily living with ease and grace, it seems appropriate to expect those who are responsible for health teaching and care to understand the basic principles of efficient and effective movement of the body. Nursing care should assist individuals in the development and use of their physical potential through movement, rest, and relaxation. Nursing care should prevent disabilities, shorten convalescent care, and assist the patient in regaining optimal mobility after certain limitations have been experienced. Also, nursing should help the person to make full use of existing capabilities when a permanent limitation is imposed. Knowledge of principles and concepts pertaining to mobility and how to apply them in nursing practice is important not only to the patient but also to the nurse for the efficiency of her movements and the protection and development of her physical potential.

In this instance, a specific problem, promoting mobility, becomes an integrative thread that runs through the whole curriculum. The introduction of the problem to the student is personalized in that the student herself and her problems are the focus of attention. The learning progresses in identifiable stages, each stage built upon the previous one through focusing on student-patient, student-patient-family, student-patient-family-community relationships. This sequence may be considered as proceeding from simple to complex learning opportunities, since each stage requires the student to attend to more and different variables in problem-solving activities in nursing. Promoting mobility is inherent in a variety of nursing situations, and the various situations provide breadth of learning. The increasing complexity of nursing situations in which promoting mobility is a problem enhances depth of learning. A description of some components of curriculum content is offered in Diagram 5. This is not to be considered complete or comprehensive; however, these ideas are presented to illustrate the concept of an organizing center for learning in relation to horizontal and vertical continuity of curriculum elements.

The same faculty also used another nursing problem, preventing infections, as an organizing center. The instructors believed that this was a nursing problem which permeated the total curriculum. Protecting the defenses of the patient or potential patient was viewed as a major concern of nursing, and preventing infections is a means to this end. The instructional approach could be personalized, since it is vital that the student learn to protect her own defenses as well as those of others. The sequences in learning followed a pattern similar to that of promoting mobility: progressing from the focus on the student, to student-patient, to student-patient-family, to student-patient-family-community relationships. The variety of nursing situations that are concerned with preventing infections facilitates breadth of learning, while the increasing complexity of these situations requires depth of learning.

CONTINUITY OF CURRICULUM OPPORTUNITIES

One of the most important problems in curriculum planning is assuring continuity in the student's learning. All teachers want one curriculum episode to contribute to the next one, one phase or course in the curriculum to build upon the previous one. Teachers want to help students transfer knowledge gained in the school to events in their life's work beyond the school. Continuity of curriculum episodes is concerned with the identification of appropriate organizing centers that are accessible, comprehensive, and movable. This means that the major ideas reappear in the curriculum according to a plan developed by the faculty, with the goal of gradual development of the ideas in depth and breadth over the length of the curriculum. The continuity of the student's learning is facilitated if the following occur:

1. The organizing centers suggest instructional activities at several levels of the curriculum.
2. There is agreement between teachers and students about what they are trying to accomplish.

3. The planned sequences that are worked out, such as progressing from simple to complex, from proximal to distal, or from concrete to abstract activities, reflect the perceived continuities needed in the student's learning experiences.

4. Performance skills are developed in situations where applications are made and seen by the student as having significance for educational goals.

5. A consistent effort is made to use the student's present and past experience as a basis for moving to the next learning opportunity and to new organizing centers.

Continuity of the elements of the organizing centers is seen as a major factor in the identification and organization of curriculum opportunities. To achieve continuity between successive learnings, the student must be assisted by a planned curriculum that encourages cumulative learnings.

Changes in ways of thinking, acting, and feeling develop slowly. No one learning experience may have an immediate and marked influence upon the learner. It may take several years to see the behavior implied in the objectives actually taking shape in the student. It is by means of the accumulation of the many learning opportunities that these changes take place in the learner. Continuity through reiteration of curriculum elements means taking the student from where he is to a situation in which his social and psychological environment call for different modes and patterns of behavior.

SEQUENCE OF CURRICULUM OPPORTUNITIES

It should be obvious from the preceding discussion that repeating certain elements in the curriculum is not all bad. On the contrary, repetition of curriculum elements is desirable if it takes the student closer to her educational goals. However, if the elements simply recur at various points in the curriculum with no progress toward understanding of the knowledge or proficiency in a skill, this is not desirable. It is hoped that each successive experience builds upon the preceding one but goes more deeply into the elements involved. In a proper sequential development of a concept, idea, or problem, each time it is presented it is viewed in a new situation that introduces different variables, and the student is required to develop new behaviors in the context of different content.

Obviously, everything cannot be taught or learned at the same time; some things have to come before others. Some rational plan is necessary for developing a curriculum that reflects a sequential pattern. Psychological factors determine the optimal time for learning a specific concept, principle, or skill. Ausubel makes a distinction between the formal organization of the subject matter content of a given discpline as set forth in authoritative statements in generally accepted textbooks and the internalized representation of the knowledge in the memory of particular individuals [2]. It is reasonable to assume that the psychological and logical structures differ with respect to the sequential ordering of component elements. The processes involved in the psychological organization of knowledge imply a hierarchical structure that is progressively differentiated in terms of degree of generality and inclusiveness. Ausubel further states that when subject matter is programmed in accordance with the principle of progressive differentiation, the most general and inclusive ideas of the discipline are presented first and these are later progressively differentiated in detail and specificity. This order of presentation recognizes that new ideas and information can be learned and retained only to the extent that more inclusive concepts are already in the cognitive structure [3].

The development of programmed instruction and the research studies in this area seem to indicate that continuity or sequence is found in the learning of the individual and that it is sequence of learning rather than of content which counts. When material is arranged in sequential order and the student learns one small step before going on to the next, even slow learners can go much further in learning various concepts and skills. The operant behavior theory of B. F. Skinner suggests that through a gradual advance from simple to complex responses or a series of successive approximations, a teacher may shape the terminal behavior of the student in whatever way she wishes. The whole process of becoming competent in any field is divided into a great number of small steps, with reinforcement contingent upon the accomplishment of each step [4]. According to Skinner, the subject matter itself contains the means for effecting behavior change. Use of this method to present carefully planned content sequences could increase learning efficiency [5].

Continuity is expressed in the curriculum by specifying what experiences and content are to be placed at each grade level. Some organizing principles that have been used are: moving from the concrete to the abstract; going from experiences close to the student's life to those in the larger community; moving from the simple to the complex; using chronological order; and following the logic of a subject. Smith, Stanley, and Shores, for example, report that the order of discovery is different from the order of telling about discovery. How things are found out or worked out—or learned—is ordinarily referred to as the psychological order. How these things are systematically arranged for communication constitutes the logical organization [6]. The authors indicate that the sequence appropriate to the problems of the research specialist is not necessarily the sequence appropriate to the doer. The scholar's problem is primarily intellectual—the discovery and verification of further knowledge. The problems of the man and the citizen are practical problems. There is a difference between the organization of material appropriate to the development of a systematic body of theoretical knowledge and that appropriate to the application of knowledge in some practical human enterprise.

The sequence of curriculum events as it pertains to the acquisition of knowledge is suggested by Taba [7]. This author describes levels of knowledge as a useful way to view sequence. The levels she describes include: specific facts and descriptive ideas at a low level of abstraction; basic ideas and principles; concepts, which are complex systems of highly abstract ideas; and finally, thought systems and methods of inquiry.

Systematic planning of a curriculum sequence is accepted as a rational and logical concern of curriculum development. It is evident, however, that several approaches may be taken. The selection of a sequence to be followed is dependent upon the objectives of the curriculum, the organizing centers used, and the emphasis upon these in the overall curriculum plan.

INTEGRATION OF CURRICULUM OPPORTUNITIES

Educators and schools have been criticized for establishing an environment in which students are expected to accumulate quantities of precise knowledge. The mental activities of memorization are used for the purposes of recitation and examination. Many years ago Whitehead indicted university education because of its emphasis on "inert ideas," ideas that bear little relationship to the students' needs, interests, or goals [8].

The teaching and learning of ideas are a means to an end rather than an end in itself. The ideas about a phenomenon are not isolated and independent but are part of a larger whole which describes or explains the phenomenon. Providing the opportunities and the environment in which the ideas can be seen in relation to other ideas and as a part of the whole is the concern of integration of curriculum opportunities.

The term *integration* has been used to indicate the relationships among elements that are the concern of a discipline.

Integration assumes the existence of parts that relate to each other to make a larger whole. It involves an appropriate adjustment of the parts to the parts, the parts to the whole, and the whole to the parts, in such a way that the whole becomes more closely knit. The integration of curriculum opportunities is a process that considers the curriculum as a series of parts interrelated in a special educational pattern.

Without integration in the curriculum, learning results in a series of discrete episodes unrelated to each other. There is evidence to indicate that information can be retained for longer periods of time if the material is organized in some meaningful way. Interest in thinking, problem-solving, and creativity led Max Wertheimer to formulate views concerning the influence of the organization of materials on learning and problem-solving [9]. Pursuing the views of Wertheimer, Katona indicated that the inherent organization of meaningful material would affect both ease of learning, retention, and transfer to new materials [10]. Later studies demonstrated that organization of materials into meaningful patterns facilitated retention of the learned materials. It seems that if one can connect many ideas, there is greater depth of meaning and greater economy in recall. Thus, it follows that the more organized the material, the better the retention. To achieve integration in school learning experiences (that is, a unity of understandings, skills, and knowledge), those experiences need to be planned so that they enhance rather than diminish opportunities for relating various bodies of knowledge. Bloom describes this process as a function served by integrative threads [11]. An integrative thread is any idea, problem, method, or device by which separate learning experiences may be related. The relationship may be perceived by the student or the instructor. An ultimate goal of education should be training the student to seek her own relationships among ideas, problems, or skills. Bloom suggests the following criteria for the selection, development, and use of integrative threads in the curriculum:

1. Integrative threads must have continuing usefulness in relation to a great variety of problems and questions. This implies attention must be given to problems identified by students in addition to those formulated by teachers.

2. Integrative threads should be chosen to allow for extension of meaning with time and future experience. This implies that integrative threads may take on different meanings and understandings by different persons.

3. Integrative threads should add new meaning to experiences, enabling the student to compare and contrast experiences that initially may have appeared unrelated.

4. Integrative threads should be sufficiently comprehensive to extend over the range of subject matter or experiences in the field of endeavor.

5. Integrative threads should have meaning and value for the student [12].

The major ideas, concepts, or problems that have been identified as the substance of the discipline provide useful integrative threads. The concerns of concept development and problem-solving are related to the ability of the student to use a wide range of subject matter, different ways of viewing phenomena, and various methods of approaching problems. The ultimate outcome of the use of integrative threads is the possibility that the student will continue to seek meaningful relations between new ideas and those already encountered.

BALANCE IN CURRICULUM OPPORTUNITY

A balanced curriculum is a curriculum that offers opportunities for mastery of knowledge and for internalizing and utilizing the knowledge in ways appropriate to one's personal and occupational endeavors. Beyond this general concept of balance, many variations in specific description may occur. Since curriculum is viewed from different frames of reference—subject matter, student needs, experience or activity, values—the curriculum components that are to be maintained in balance will take different forms and dimensions. Students, teachers, administrators, and prospective employers may place importance on different educational opportunities. In some instances emphasis may be assigned to the acquisition of proficiency in skill learning rather than to thinking, reasoning, and other aspects of intellectual development. Some employers may place greater value on the abilities of practitioners to be innovative in styles of practice. Some curriculum workers may place greatest importance on certain subject matter fields. These differences in emphasis do not preclude the possibility of a balanced curriculum.

At times in our history social change has been so rapid that adaptations in educational purposes and programs have been accelerated. World War I, the depression years of the 1930's, and World War II were occasions for startling shifts in educational philosophy and curriculum, in contrast to the more stable intervening years in our history. A marked change in the orientation of curriculums on all levels of education was precipitated by the need of this country to compete with other nations in the concerns of national defense. Increased emphasis was placed upon training in the natural sciences. Financial resources from both private and public agencies made possible the development of extensive curriculum opportunities in these fields. It could be said that the curriculum balance favored the natural sciences and mathematics. More recently, curriculum has stressed the behavioral sciences. The increasing complexity of our technological society has precipitated issues and problems in human relations, namely, relationships among individuals, groups, and the community. The behavioral sciences provide information by which these problems can be studied and approaches designed to resolve or alleviate them. If one projects what the curriculum emphasis will be in the immediate future, it appears there is increasing concern about our value orientation and structure. Values and other feeling behaviors have been a concern of curriculum but only in an indirect way. It is frequently assumed that if appropriate learning opportunities in the cognitive or skill areas of learning were made available, the desired affective behaviors would develop. More direct attention to this phase of the curriculum is urgently needed. The internalization of values, attitudes, and appreciations compatible with our democratic culture is a vital process in humanizing knowledge and skills.

From this point of view it can be seen that curriculum development has a significant relationship to the society which supports the school and to the relative stability or fluidity of the culture. In times of cultural stability the curriculum of the school remains constant and may be in balance. However, in periods or rapid social change, the lag in incorporating scientific findings into school practices is slow, and at such times imbalances in curriculum are very noticeable. Perfect curriculum balance is probably impossible to achieve because institutions of all kinds are almost always slow in adapting to new needs and demands of the culture.

The curriculum of American schools is a constant battleground of conflicting demands. Pressures for curriculum change come from within and from outside the school. Curriculum imbalance may occur because faculty with vested interests in certain subject matter fields exert pressure to emphasize these subjects in the curriculum. The basic curriculum in nursing is planned to prepare a generalist in nursing practice. This curriculum is usually developed by a group of specialists in nursing—those who have had extensive preparation in specialized areas of nursing practice. The interest and efforts of a nursing specialist in her particular field may create some dislocation in the curriculum by directing the attention of the student away from the generalist orientation. Another source of pressure that may produce imbalance within the curriculum is the faculty member who perceives her role as a guardian or protector of students. This faculty member places major importance on those teacher activities which pertain to telling, demonstrating, providing detailed guidelines for practice, directing, and preventing mistakes. Although these activities may be entirely appropriate in the initial stages of learning, undue emphasis on them may do a disservice to the student's self-development. In this instance there is an imbalance between passive or teacher-directed learning and active, student-discovery learning. Pressures from teachers within the curriculum environment can produce imbalances in the content of the curriculum as well as in the learning styles of students.

Forces within the learning situation may also precipitate imbalances in curriculum opportunities. This pertains primarily to the clinical environment in which learning experiences take place. In some instances distortions in curriculum activities occur because these clinical environments are focused on meeting the needs of other persons. Clinical facilities of hospitals located in the inner city are utilized by residents of the inner city, and these people frequently exhibit gross social problems as well as medical pathology. Problems relating to poverty, malnutrition, illegitimate pregnancy, birth defects, tuberculosis, and other infectious diseases are widespread. Attention to the extremely abnormal conditions diminishes the opportunity to learn about the care of people who may be considered to be more "normal" in their health needs and social behavior. These clinical facilities may also be utilized by a medical school for teaching and research. A hospital unit may have a high proportion of patients with a similar disease or health problem who are undergoing specialized treatment for study purposes. The use of public facilities for clinical learning opportunities for nursing students may place undue attention on specific disease manifestations and obscure the broader goals of nursing.

Pressures from outside the school can also produce imbalance in curriculum opportunities. These pressures may come from various voluntary organizations and special interest groups. The goals of these groups may be highly commendable in terms of their social values; however, their impact on curriculum activities may serve the best interests of the students. These groups are dedicated to the alleviation of specific health or social problems and desire to transmit their knowledge and skills to the public. Since the services of these groups are available without charge, instructors in schools of nursing utilize them in their curriculum activities. The participation of these groups need not produce any detrimental effects if care is taken to preserve a balance between generalized knowledge and a narrow, specialized orientation.

Value judgments serve their best function when they take into account all available facts. In selecting and organizing learning opportunities for the nursing curriculum that will provide an appropriate balance of content as well as behavior, teachers, administrators, and community representatives assume the responsibility of reviewing the relevant facts and information before making value judgments about the goals of the curriculum.

STUDENT-TEACHER-COMMUNITY RELATIONSHIPS

The roles of students, teachers, and community participants in curriculum development have been controversial issues from the beginning of formal education. Student unrest on college campuses, which has resulted in protests and demonstrations, is not a twentieth-century invention. History records instances in which curriculums were not in tune with the needs, interests, and goals of students, and efforts were exerted by students and others to bring about change. Peddiwell's satirical description of the reluctance of education to face the issues of means and ends is a thoughtful, if humorous, attack. He states that "in addition to having a strictly magical purpose, the paleolithic university also had magical subjects. From the very beginning of the university, the value of education it gave was determined by reference to the magical properties of various subjects rather than by any attempts to discover real changes in students. Thus one subject was considered to give a double dose of magic, while another might give only one-tenth of a dose. Indeed, there were certain subjects which were thought to be antimagical in their effect" [13].

The institutional goals of American higher education include (1) the discovery of new knowledge, which involves "basic" or "pure" research, (2) the synthesis of knowledge, which is concerned with the assimilation of new knowledge to the total body of knowledge and provides for a reinterpretation of the total body of knowledge, (3) the transmission of knowledge, or teaching, and (4) the application of knowledge to problems in the community or society in general.

Probably no one, including our most reactionary students, disputes the desirability of perpetuating these institutional goals. But fervor is generated when one or more of these goals is neglected in favor of others. Dedicated and conscientious students are reminding educators that in many instances the teaching goal of higher education is being neglected in the overindulgence of the research goal. Similarly, various groups in society have voiced concern about the activities of colleges and universities in the application of knowledge to problems that exist in the community outside the school campus. In this instance the issue is not neglect but the appropriateness of the activities and projects the institutions support. Today the question has a new focus: What is the responsibility of the college or university for helping the nation and the world solve difficult social and technological problems, such as the deterioration of our cities, the population explosion, inequities in health care available to various segments of society, dysfunction in the biosphere, increased life span, and the war effort? The controversial issue appears to be the extent to which application in the social sphere, particularly a narrow social sphere, is a college or university's responsibility. No one seriously questions the fact that this is a matter of enduring importance.

It is primarily in these areas—transmission of knowledge and application of knowledge to social problems—that continuous participation of teachers, students, and community representatives is of paramount importance. The curriculum decisions involved in the attainment of these goals have compelling influence on students and others in relation to short-term and long-term effects. These decisions should not be the sole responsibility of one segment of the school community—the teachers. Any teacher who is to be at all intelligent in selecting, organizing, and offering the learning opportunities must be able to see clearly her responsibilities in this process and the degree of freedom she has for carrying them out. Analyses of student unrest in the literature give some indication of students' expectations when they come to college: "intimate contact with faculty and peers, a sense of community, the hope for deep interpersonal communication, true intellectual stimulation" [14].

TEACHER-COMMUNITY RELATIONSHIPS

Students of nursing have opportunities to experience face-to-face contact with community health and nursing problems and want to become involved in problem-solving activities. Since nursing practice takes place in the community, learning opportunities in the practice of nursing must be obtained in community agencies. If these learning opportunities are to be meaningful to the student, they must present nursing as it is. Our tendencies to "dress-up" nursing or to create artificial situations to provide "good" learning experiences are not in the best interests of the students or the community agencies involved. Students are quick to sense an artificial learning experience, and they then search for reality through other kinds of nursing activities.

The objectives of the curriculum and the faculty's conceptualization of nursing practice give some indication of the types of community agencies that may provide appropriate learning opportunities. In the past, one type of agency, the general hospital, has provided the major practice area for nursing schools. With the acceptance and implementation of the concept of distributive nursing practice, some faculties will find it necessary to utilize a variety of community agencies and organizations to offer the necessary learning opportunities. Arrangements for the use of these agencies by the school require cooperative planning by agency and school personnel. The fundamental issue in such planning is developing approaches whereby both groups of professionals, practitioners and teachers, contribute to the goals of nursing with sensitivity to the problems encountered by each group in attaining the goals. Agencies are frequently overwhelmed by the numbers of students from a variety of nursing programs seeking practice experience during the same time period. Not only do these arrangements dilute the quality of the learning experience for students, they also create distortions in the quantity and quality of nursing care available to the patients.

A third factor in teacher-community relationships is the teacher's involvement in the practice of nursing in an agency. It was once a common practice in nursing, for the head nurse and supervisor in the hospital to be also clinical instructors for nursing students. More frequently than not, the head nurse's and supervisor's activities in hospital management were so demanding that their responsibilities as instructors were neglected. In an effort to protect the educational programs, schools of nursing employed faculty who had no nursing service responsibilities, thus separating the practitioner and instructor roles. More recently, consideration is being given to the merger of these roles in a different way, in which the clinical professor assumes responsibility for the care of selected patients. Then the clinical professor performs the practitioner as well as the teacher role. This appears to be feasible in situations where agency management and operational activities are delegated to other personnel. The literature reports some interesting cooperative endeavors in university schools of nursing and community health agencies. The major purpose of these endeavors is to provide quality nursing care and at the same time to offer relevant learning opportunities to students.

STUDENT-TEACHER RELATIONSHIPS

The subject matter of the curriculum determines the responsibilities of students and teachers in the transmission of the knowledge. In well-developed disciplines, the logical arrangement of the subject matter reveals the theorems, postulates, principles, or concepts that should be imparted to assist the learner in understanding the particular phenomenon. The subject matter defines what should be taught and learned. In the less well-developed disciplines, the problems approach may be utilized in the transmission of knowledge to students. In this instance the identification of the problems (health, nursing, patient, student) is the joint responsibility of teachers and students. Problem identification by the instructor alone probably will not excite the curiosity, imagination, or problem-solving activity of the student. The curriculum approach utilizing student needs as its focus obviously engages the learner in planning and selecting learning opportunities. The responsibility for identifying needs gives the student a primary role in curriculum activities. Identification of student needs by the teacher alone is risky business. Continuous validation of these needs by the student is imperative if the curriculum is to have meaning for the student.

There are a variety of approaches to selecting the subject matter of the curriculum. The learning opportunities selected should enable the student to receive and assimilate the subject matter of the curriculum. In this instance teachers and students are involved in the identification of appropriate learning opportunities. Since more than one type of experience may facilitate the attainment of a particular objective, it seems desirable to offer several alternative opportunities from which the student may select those that are most useful to her. Although the subject matter may suggest the principles or concepts to be learned, the student and teacher cooperate in planning appropriate learning opportunities. Involving the student in selecting her own learning experiences provides for growth in decision-making behavior.

SUMMARY

Curriculum design is concerned with the identification of the elements of the curriculum and how these relate to each other in a pattern of organization. The curriculum design deals with the optimal environment for learning and with the necessary resources for instruction.

The major focus of the curriculum design is the statement of objectives that have been developed through careful analysis of the health and nursing needs of society, the characteristics of contemporary students, and the nature and sources of knowledge utilized in nursing practice. Using the statement of objectives as a frame of reference, strategies for the selection of learning opportunities can be formulated. The subject matter of the curriculum must be designed to be compatible with the general orientation of the professional or technical nursing curriculum. The concerns of focus, emphasis, and balance are inherent in the processes of identification and delineation of the subject matter called nursing.

The organization of subject matter for instruction requires teachers to select an approach that is acceptable to them. This becomes the focal point for curriculum development and improvement. Some approaches that have been used by nursing faculties include nursing problems, student and patient needs, and subject matter concepts. The approach selected suggests the organizational scheme of the curriculum. Organizing centers for learning consistent with the specific approach are selected, and these become the integrative threads of the curriculum. Reiteration of the organizing centers in different nursing contexts provides for breadth of learning opportunities, while increasing the complexity with each repeated exposure provides for depth of learning. The notion of sequence of learning opportunities refers to the progression from relatively simple learning activities to those that are more complex. This implies that the learning opportunities selected deal with increasing numbers of the variables involved in the problem-solving activities of nursing care. The efforts of teachers in one school of nursing using nursing problems as organizing centers were described. The problems "promoting mobility" and "preventing infections" were developed as integrative threads that provided for breadth and scope of learning. Sequence of curriculum opportunities progressed from rather fundamental learning experiences, which focused on the student and her health needs, to those of a complex nature, which involved the patient, family, and community.

The roles of students, teachers, and community participants are determined by the curriculum. A curriculum such as nursing, which has as its major purpose the preparation of practitioners who will assist in alleviating the problems of men, must be deeply rooted in the issues and concerns of contemporary life. The relevance of the curriculum is determined by the degree to which the subject matter focuses upon the current social and health issues. This frame of reference demands that teachers, students, and community participants develop and maintain relationships that facilitate the ongoing development of the curriculum. This implies thoughtful consideration to changes, however small, that may improve health and nursing conditions. The vitality of the curriculum is dependent upon community relationships that are oriented to the ever-changing needs of society.

REFERENCES

1. Goodlad, J. I.   The organizing center in curriculum theory and practice. *Theory Into Practice* 1:215, 1962.
2. Ausubel, D. P.   Some Psychological Aspects of the Structure of Knowledge. In S. Elam [Ed.], *Education and the Structure of Knowledge*. Chicago: Rand McNally, 1964. P. 222.
3. Ibid., p. 241.
4. Skinner, B. F.   The science of learning and the art of teaching. *Harvard Educ. Rev.* 24:86, 1954.
5. Skinner, B. F.   Why we need teaching machines. *Harvard Educ. Rev.* 31: 396, 1961.
6. Smith, B. O., Stanley, W. O., and Shores, J. H.   *Fundamentals of Curriculum Development*. New York: Harcourt, Brace & World, 1957. P. 246.
7. Taba, H.   *Curriculum Development: Theory and Practice*. New York: Harcourt, Brace & World, 1962. P. 175.
8. Whitehead, A. N.   *The Aims of Education*. New York: Macmillan, 1929. P. 58.
9. Hilgard, E. R. [Ed.].   The Place of Gestalt Psychology and Field Theories in Contemporary Learning Theory. In *Theories of Learning and Instruction*. Chicago: National Society for the Study of Education, 1964. P. 62.
10. Katona, G.   *Organizing and Memorizing*. New York: Columbia University Press, 1940. P. 83.
11. Bloom, B. S.   Ideas, Problems and Methods of Inquiry. In N. B. Henry [Ed.], *The Integration of Educational Experiences*. Fifty-seventh Yearbook of the National Society for the Study of Education. Chicago: National Society for the Study of Education, 1958. P. 91.
12. Ibid., p. 95.
13. Peddiwell, J. A.   *The Saber-Tooth Curriculum*. New York: McGraw-Hill, 1939. P. 78.
14. Brown, D. R.   Student stress and the institutional environment. *J. Soc. Issues* 13:92, 1967.

SUPPLEMENTARY READINGS

Anderson, V.   *Principles and Procedures of Curriculum Improvement*, 2d ed. New York: Ronald, 1965.

Association for Supervision and Curriculum Development.   *Balance in the Curriculum*. Washington, D.C.: National Education Association, 1961.

Beauchamp, G. A.   *Curriculum Theory*. Wilmette: Ragg, 1968.

Brown, E. L.   *Nursing Reconsidered: Part I*. Philadelphia: Lippincott, 1970.

Bruner, J. S.   *The Process of Education*. Cambridge: Harvard University Press, 1961.

Burns, R. W., and Brooks, G. D. [Eds.].   *Curriculum Design in a Changing Society*. Englewood Cliffs: Educational Technology, 1970.

Elam, S. [Ed.].   *Education and the Structure of Knowledge*. Chicago: Rand McNally, 1964.

Ford, G. W., and Pugno, L. [Eds.]. *The Structure of Knowledge and the Curriculum*. Chicago: Rand McNally, 1964.

Hughes, P.   Decision and curriculum design. *Educ. Theory* 12:187, 1962.

McDonald, J. B., Anderson, D. W., and May, F. B. *Strategies of Curriculum Development*. Columbus: Merrill, 1965.

Oliver, A. I. *Curriculum Improvement*. New York: Dodd, Mead, 1965.

Parker, C. J., and Rubin, L. J. *Process as Content: Curriculum Design and the Application of Knowledge*. Chicago: Rand McNally, 1966.

Pilder, W.   Curriculum design and the knowledge situation. *Educ. Leadership* 26:593, 1969.

Schlotfeldt, R., and Macphail, J.   An experiment in nursing: Rationale and characteristics. *Amer. J. Nurs.* 69:1018, 1969.

Smith, B. O., Stanley, W. O., and Shores, J. H. *Fundamentals of Curriculum Development*. New York: Harcourt, Brace & World, 1957.

Tyler, R. W.   Curriculum Organization. In N. B. Henry [Ed.], *The Integration of Educational Experiences*. Fifty-seventh Yearbook of the National Society for the Study of Education. Chicago: National Society for the Study of Education, 1958. P. 105.

12 EVALUATION OF CURRICULUM AND INSTRUCTION

THE purpose of the curriculum of a school is to bring about changes in the students and to move them in specified directions. This implies that education is a rational activity and that professional educators can, by looking at the expressed needs of their students and the expressed and implied needs of society, determine what sorts of people the society wants and needs. The curriculum is, or should be, one of the important devices by which this comes about.

Evaluation becomes a process for finding out to what extent the curriculum as developed and organized is producing the desired results. The process of evaluation also involves identifying the strengths and weaknesses of the curriculum plans. This provides a means for checking the validity of the hypotheses upon which the instructional program is based and checks the effectiveness of the particular instruments, that is, the teacher and other conditions, that are being used to carry forth the instructional program. As a result of evaluation it is possible to observe in what ways the curriculum is effective and in what ways it needs improvement. This chapter will explore the evaluation process, the purposes and methodology of evaluation, issues and problems pertaining to evaluation, and some general notions relating to curriculum research and evaluation.

THE EVALUATION PROCESS

The importance of evaluation cannot be overemphasized. Probably no other single phase of the teaching-learning process is more important. The extent to which the teacher is successful in evaluation may determine success or failure in teaching.

Evaluation may be defined as the process used in determining the value or worth of something; educational evaluation is the process used in determining the effectiveness of teaching and/or the value of a learning opportunity in assisting students to achieve the goals of education. The degree of teaching effectiveness and learning is measured by utilizing the various tools and techniques available to teachers for gathering information that will contribute to intelligent evaluation. The evaluation of the degree to which the educational objectives have been achieved requires the selection or construction of *valid*, *reliable*, and *practical* instruments and techniques for appraising specific phases of student behavior.

Establishing appropriate goals and objectives is basic to the educational process and a necessary prerequisite to effective teaching and evaluation. If teachers are to make their maximum contribution to the growth and development of students, they must understand and succeed in translating general objectives into classroom and clinical instructional objectives and activities. Instructors must guard against a tendency to include only those types of learnings that can be taught and tested most easily, such as knowledge of facts. Effective teaching is concerned with the physical, emotional, social, and mental development of students. Attention must be focused on the development of skills, understandings, interests, attitudes, and values in all areas. Designing appropriate means for assessing all types of behavior changes is of paramount importance in the evaluation process.

In the evaluation process two key ideas need to be kept in mind: the concept of a *goal, norm, value,* or *standard* of adequacy of progress toward the goal. Evaluation is different from measurement in that measurement provides information while evaluation makes value judgments about the measurements made.

Evaluation requires appraisals of student behavior, since it is the change in these behaviors that is sought in education. It is implied that evaluation must involve more than a single appraisal, in fact, it is necessary to make an appraisal at an early point and other appraisals at later periods to identify changes that may be occurring. Without knowing where the students were at the beginning, it is impossible to tell what changes have taken place. Some students may have achieved some of the objectives before they begin the instructional program. In other cases, almost all of the changes noted at the end will have taken place during the time the instruction went on. It is clear that an educational evaluation involves at least two appraisals: one in the early part of the educational program, and the other at some later point, so that the change may be observed and measured.

Since evaluation involves gathering evidence about behavior changes in the students, any valid evidence about the behaviors desired as educational objectives provides an appropriate method of evaluation. This is important to recognize because many people think of evaluation as synonymous with giving paper-and-pencil tests. While paper-and-pencil tests provide a practicable procedure for getting evidence about several kinds of student behavior, there are many other kinds of desired behaviors that are not easily appraised by these procedures. Several kinds of *evaluation devices* are needed.

Evaluation assumes that it is possible to estimate the typical reactions of a student by sampling her reactions. We do not ask the student all possible questions about the facts, principles, and concepts that may be involved in her education. We choose a sample of these things to question her about, and we infer from her reactions to this sample how she will react to the total set of items involved. This holds for all types of human behavior: attitudes, interests, and intellectual and psychomotor skills. It is assumed that it is possible to infer the person's characteristic performance by appraising her reactions in a sample of situations in which this reaction is involved.

EVALUATING THE INFLUENCE OF THE LEARNING ENVIRONMENT

The evaluation of the effectiveness of the learning environment entails analysis of the various aspects of the environment and the evaluation of these in relation to the contributions they offer to the learning environment as a whole. These aspects include: the physical plant and space, equipment available, and size in relation to numbers of students. More specifically: lighting, ventilation, general attractiveness, necessary utilities (water, electricity, gas) for instructional activities, and the general standards of housekeeping. Instructional equipment and materials might include: library resources and teaching devices such as audiovisual equipment, multimedia instruction equipment, learning laboratories, and other kinds of instructional hardware.

Stake suggests the development of a matrix of evaluation information. This matrix should include the many characteristics of the instructional program to be evaluated. The evaluator must choose the specific variables to be described and judged. The matrix should also include sources of information about the variables to be evaluated, such as teachers and administrators. A principle task of the evaluator is to concentrate on variables related to the

TABLE 9. Variables in Curriculum and Instruction to be Evaluated Utilizing a Specific Instructional Device—Programmed Instruction

Variables	Examples
Antecedents	
Student characteristics	Background, aptitude, previous experience with programmed instruction
Teacher characteristics	Experience, teaching style, personality, attitude
Type of school	Physical plant, climate for innovation
Curriculum content	Subject matter coverage, concepts, terminology, focus, emphasis
Instructional aids	Library materials, visual aids, equipment
Concomitant course work	Sequence of course, time allotment, field work for application
Transactions	
Teaching strategies	Relationship of discourse, inquiry, assignments to programmed text
Student-teacher interaction	Conference for interpretation, explanation, implementation
Student-student interaction	Discussions, demonstrations
Time allocation	Student time in using text, teacher time in conferences, evaluation of learning outcomes, demonstrations
Outcomes	
Gain in student competence	
Knowledge	Facts, understanding application
Skill	Perceptual-motor, application of science principles and concepts
Attitudes, interests	Relationship of knowledge and skill
Effects on staff; teacher changes	Insight, knowledge, skill in teaching approaches
Administrative changes	Effective use of instructional media to conserve human and material resources
Community effects	Relationship with school in the effort to identify necessary skill level for safe professional practice

goals of her audience (students), variables leading to curriculum decisions (content, instructional materials), and variables that are available from the appropriate sources (budget, facilities, human resources). Stake identifies the sources of information according to four categories:

Intents: What different goals people (teachers, students) have

Observation: Perceptions of what actually happens

Standards: Statements by certain experts as to what should happen in a situation like ours

Judgments: Data on how people feel about aspects of our situation (administrators' judgments pertaining to the efficient use of human and material resources and costs) [1]

Characteristics of the instructional program to be evaluated are classified by Stake as antecedents, transactions, and outcomes. The use of this evaluation matrix is described as it may be applied to an instructional variable in nursing. If a published programmed text is being used to teach the knowledge and skills needed to carry out "bag technique" in community health nursing, the variables may be identified and organized according to antecedents, transactions, and outcomes. The specific instances of the antecedents, transactions, and outcomes are described as they apply to teaching by programmed instruction in Table 9. A method for collecting data about the utilization of this teaching approach in relation to the characteristics of the instructional program to be evaluated is presented in Table 10.

Stake uses two approaches to describe the utilization of the data collected. One approach is to find the *contingencies* among the antecedents, transactions, and outcomes. In this instance, contingencies refer to the relationships among the variables in these categories. The search for contingency is the search for causal relationships, or what caused what to happen. Do certain teacher characteristics precipitate a specific type of student-teacher interaction that brings about changes in student attitudes about specific kinds of patients? Knowledge of what causes what obviously facilitates the improvement of instruction. The task of the evaluator is to identify outcomes (gain in student's knowledge) that are contingent upon particular antecedent conditions (student characteristics, and particular instructional transactions (student-student interaction).

Every day the teacher arranges her presentations and the learning environment in a way that, according to the logic of the instructor, leads to the at-

TABLE 10. Matrix of Evaluation Information Utilizing an Instructional Device—Programmed Text in Nursing*

Program Rationale	Data for Evaluation			
	Intent Sources	Observation Sources	Standard Sources	Judgment Sources
Antecedents				
Student characteristics				
Teacher characteristics				
Curricular content				
Curriculum context				
Instructional materials	A			
Physical plant				
School organization				
Community context				
Transactions				
Communication flow				
Time allocation				D
Sequence of events				
Reinforcement schedule				
Social climate				
Outcomes				
Student achievement		B	C	
Student attitudes				
Student skills				
Effect on teachers				
Instructional effects				

Interpretation:

Example A (Instructional materials): Specifications of a published programmed text—intent source

Example B (Student achievement): Teacher description of behavior outcomes of student—observation source

Example C (Student achievement): Expert opinion of knowledge and skills needed for adequate performance—standard sources

Example D (Time allocation): Administrator's judgment of feasibility of use of programmed text—appropriate use of human and material resources—judgment sources

* Adapted from R. E. Stake, The countenance of educational evaluation, *Teacher's Coll. Rec.* 68:529, 1967.

tainment of the instructional goals. The instructor's contingencies are likely to be logical, supported by satisfactory previous experience. However, the teacher, even the master teacher, needs to examine the logical and empirical

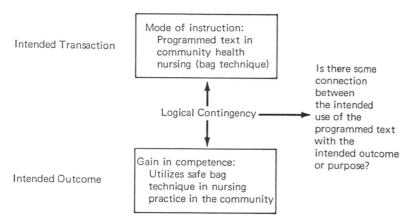

DIAGRAM 6.   Evaluation of contingency between intended transaction and intended outcome.

bases for their contingencies. One of the first steps in evaluation is to record the contingency between an intended transaction and a purpose or an intended outcome (see Diagram 6). To do this the teacher might ask herself, Is there a logical connection between the use of programmed instruction in bag technique (intended transaction) and the intended outcome or purpose—does the student demonstrate safe bag technique in nursing practice in the community? If a relationship exists between the two intents, a logical contingency exists between them.

The evaluation of intents involves the search for logical contingency, and the teachers rely on previous experience and perhaps some research activity with similar observables. The immediate observation of the variables is not ncessary to determine the contingencies among intents.

The second approach in processing the evaluation data is the search for *congruence* between intents and observations. In this instance intents (descriptive data of goals) and observations (what actually happens) are congruent if what was intended to happen does in fact happen. To be fully congruent, the intended antecedents, transactions, and outcomes must be identical with the observed antecedents, transactions, and outcomes. Most curriculum evaluation focuses primarily on the congruence of intended and observed outcomes. Evaluation can serve a more useful purpose in curriculum review and revision if more is learned about the congruence of antecedents and transactions. The evaluator can compare the intent information with the observation informa-

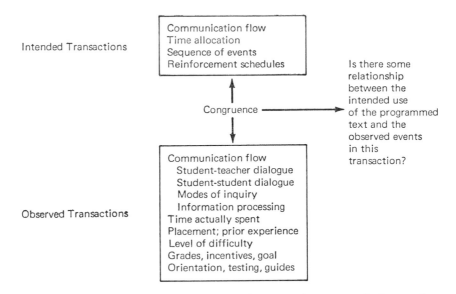

DIAGRAM 7. Evaluation for congruence between intents and observations.

tion, note the discrepancies, and describe the amount of congruence as illustrated in Diagram 7.

So that the data obtained from this comparison will be meaningful to the evaluator, a common language is used to describe the goals and the actual operations. A language that is meaningful to educational personnel is the focus on teacher, student, and administrator behavior.

The evaluation of observed contingencies depends upon empirical evidence. To say "the nursing student progressed rapidly in the acquisition of understanding and skill in bag technique because a published programmed text was used" demands empirical evidence. The usual evaluation of a single program alone will not provide the data necessary for contingency statement. Relationship requires variation in the independent variable to answer, What happens with *various modes* of instruction of bag techniques? This is illustrated in Diagram 8.

PURPOSES OF EVALUATION

The general purpose of evaluation is to determine whether the expected has happened or is happening. This purpose provides a general framework for

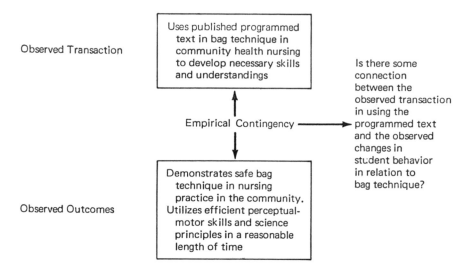

DIAGRAM 8.   Evaluation of observed contingencies, using empirical data.

evaluation, which accommodates all empirical questions regarding the effectiveness of a given program designed to accomplish specified objectives. A distinction is made between empirical questions, the answers to which are based on empirical data, and value questions, the answers to which require judgments of desirability. Value questions must be dealt with in deciding on program objectives and procedures; empirical questions deal with what actually happened, whether desired or not.

EVALUATION OF INSTRUCTION

Some possible purposes of evaluation at the instructional level are identified:

1. Clarification and possible redefinition of the objectives of the curriculum
2. Development of more adequate and reliable means of measurement
3. Appraisal of the development of students
4. Adaptation of sources and programs to the individual student
5. Motivation of student learning through continual self-evaluation
6. Improvement of instruction

The clarification of the objectives of the curriculum may appear to be an inappropriate purpose of evaluation, since evaluation is presumed to begin with a previously determined set of objectives. However, such an objective as "attainment of satisfactory relationships with patients" is so general that the attempt to define it and to evaluate student attainment of it brings greater insight into the objective and modifies some of the preconceptions about it.

The lack of reliable techniques of measurement has greatly impeded the placing of suitable emphasis on some goals of the curriculum. In part, this may be a result of the common pattern that things not tested for are apt to be ignored. It may also be that the inability to measure some behaviors reflects a lack of understanding of just what it is that is wanted.

The third purpose—appraisal of the development of students—is one often talked about in education but seldom dealt with adequately. The question of how and how much students change as a result of their educational experiences requires an extensive program of pre- and post-testing over a period of time. Such appraisals of progress are difficult because they must involve very careful experimental designs in which extraneous factors are controlled so that conclusions can be drawn. They also involve technical problems in the proper interpretation of test scores.

The fourth purpose—adaptation of courses to the individual student, at the simplest level—involves the pretesting of students for appropriate placement in courses. At a more complex level, it may involve assignment of students to special services (counseling, reading, study skills) or the development of individualized courses and assignments.

The motivation of student learning through self-evaluation is a purpose based on one of the accepted principles of learning. As objectives become understandable and important to students, and as information regarding achievement is available to them, the desire for further improvement increases. The realization that some improvement has taken place is a source of satisfaction to the student. Self-evaluation is a potent learning incentive and a procedure too seldom exploited.

The improvement of instruction is seen as a major purpose of evaluation. This purpose may disturb some instructors, for it seems to imply that instruction is poor. It really implies only that instruction can be improved through study of the instructional process and through determination of its effects on students. Evaluation becomes a technique highly significant in modifying and improving instructional practice through relating it more directly to previously stated outcomes.

EVALUATION OF CURRICULUM OR PROGRAM

At the program or curriculum level of evaluation, Stufflebeam has classified the functions of decision situations in education as planning, programming, implementing, and recycling. *Planning* decisions are those that focus on needed improvements by specifying the domain, major goals, and specific objectives to be served. *Programming* decisions specify procedures, personnel, facilities, budget, and time requirements for implementing planned activities. *Implementing* decisions are those directing programmed activities. And *recycling* decisions include terminating, continuing, evolving, or modifying activities [2]. The different kinds of evaluation decisions give attention to the purposes these decisions will serve.

Four phases or processes of curriculum or program activity are identified, which indicate the focus and purpose of evaluation. These are described as context, input, process, and product evaluation. *Context* evaluation is used when a curriculum is first being planned. The major objective is to define the environment in which change is to occur, the environment's unmet needs, and the problems underlying those needs. For example, context evaluation would determine the need to establish a nursing program in a specific locality, the population the school would serve, and the availability of potential students for the program. The method of context evaluation begins with a conceptual analysis to identify and define the limits of the domain to be served (county, state, region, or nation) and the major constituents, such as youth-adults, high school students-high school graduates, or religious-nonreligious. The analysis attempts to identify the discrepancies among the intended and actual situations for each of the subparts of the domain of interest (that is, availability of teachers, physical and clinical resources, interest and support of the community) and to identify needs. Context evaluation involves both empirical and conceptual analysis as well as reference to theory and authoritative opinion, to assist in making judgments regarding the basic problems underlying each need. Decisions served by context evaluation include deciding upon the setting to be served, the goals associated with meeting needs, and the objectives associated with solving problems.

Input evaluation is used after context evaluation to determine how to utilize resources to meet program goals and objectives. The purpose of this evaluation is to identify and assess relevant capabilities of the institution that is developing the program, strategies which may be appropriate for meeting program goals, such as arrangements for clinical resources, acquisition of library resources and other instructional materials, recruitment of teachers and students, and designs that may be appropriate for achieving objectives associated with each program goal. The end product of input evaluation is an analysis of alternative procedural designs in terms of costs and benefits. Alternative designs are assessed in terms of their resources, time and budget requirements, potential stumbling blocks and the consequences of not overcoming them, relevance of the designs to program objectives, and overall potential of the design to meet program goals. The usual practices in education for input evaluation include committee deliberations, surveys of the professional literature, and employment of consultants. The decisions based on input evaluation usually result in the specification of procedures, materials, facilities, schedules, staff requirements, and budgets. Recent activities in curriculum revisions that orient the student to the nursing problems of patients or potential patients as opposed to disease manifestations suggest different arrangements for clinical practice. The assignment of students to a particular clinical unit of the hospital is giving way to greater flexibility and freedom of selecting patients who present specific nursing problems regardless of their geographical location in the hospital. Although this pattern of clinical practice appears to some instructors to be more compatible with the subject matter of nursing, careful analysis and evaluation of this approach by nursing faculty must be made in relation to the necessary human and material resources for sound planning.

After the designated course of action has been approved and implementation of the design has begun, *process* evaluation is necessary to provide periodic feedback to those responsible for continuous review and refinement of curriculum plans and procedures. The objective of process evaluation is to detect or predict defects in the procedural design or its implementation. The strategy is to identify the potential sources of failure in a curriculum project. These may include interpersonal relationships between staff and students, communication channels, understanding and agreement with the intent of the program by persons affected by it, and adequacy of the resources, physical facilities, staff, and time schedules. The development of techniques of team teaching are visible in nursing curriculums. Continuous evaluation is needed to determine whether team teaching is in fact in process or whether students are being subjected to a parade of personalities, which may precipitate problems in interpersonal relations between students and teachers and problems in communication. The purpose of process evaluation is to help the staff make their decisions a bit more rational in their continual effort to improve the quality of the program.

Product evaluation is used to determine the effectiveness of the curriculum activity after it has been implemented and has had a tryout. The objective of product evaluation is to relate outcomes to objectives and to context, input and process. By measuring and interpreting outcomes of instruction and by comparing these with predetermined standards, information is made available for deciding whether to continue, terminate, or modify the activity. The method is to define operationally and measure criteria associated with the objectives of the activity, to compare these measures with predetermined absolute or relative standards, and to make rational interpretations of the outcomes, using the recorded context, input, and process information.

EVALUATION OF THE SYSTEM OF EDUCATION

Evaluation of curriculum and instruction may have purposes that extend beyond the immediate teaching situation or specific curriculum. Evaluation is important in the broader education enterprise. In this context five purposes are identified:

1. To add to the substantive knowledge of the educational process
2. To provide information in order to adjust, discard, or otherwise change the application of an ongoing educational process
3. To provide justification for a political-social-economic action relating to education (funding)
4. To create a document (usually a report or a paper) that can be passed through the educational system and thus contribute to the efficient operation of the system
5. To provide means of informing the educational community about the success of an endeavor

Measurements and evaluations of well-defined curriculum projects that are conducted through systematic procedures may provide material and information for the body of educational research and would add to the substantive understanding of instructional processes. The results of such projects may not always be directly applicable to the problems of instruction, but they do provide a basis for forming hypotheses for further investigations. The organization of specific learning opportunities may be studied systematically by a school faculty, and certain conclusions drawn may suggest a different arrangement for more effective learning. The findings of the study may not be applicable to other school situations until those situations are studied to identify the characteristics and variables operating there that may influence curricular patterns.

The second purpose is considered to be most important when examining ongoing programs or projects in curriculum and instruction. The decision-maker receives feedback which tells her how well the process is going and what changes need to be made. The evaluation is open to criticism, since it is assumed that the decision-making process in a given school is rational. It may not always be, and the following questions must be asked: Who are the decision-makers, and what are their motivations and models for decision-making? There is room in the educational enterprise for a variety of persons to participate in decision-making. The kinds of decisions expected must be appropriate to the decision-making ability of the particular faculty member. This indicates that the decision-maker has sufficient data for making a decision, is aware of the various alternatives, and possesses insight into the possible consequences of her decisions. Vested interests in certain educational activities and threats to personal or professional security may be motivations that influence the objectivity of the teacher's decision-making.

The third purpose of evaluation in a broader context is the purpose of providing information for justification of action by certain groups, internal and external to the school. This action may be appropriating funds, hiring additional teachers, and acquiring instructional devices. For example, a decision by the faculty to develop and utilize multimedia instruction requires evaluation of the instructional program to justify the purchase and installation of equipment and the reorientation of staff to insure appropriate use of the materials of instruction. Unless the faculty can project, on the basis of evidence, more effective learning by students and conservation of instructors' resources, the project may not receive the necessary attention for funding purposes.

Evaluation reports are necessary for the proper conduct of the enterprise. Reports to various officials, such as the college or university president, keep them informed as to how the various parts of the institution are functioning. Evaluation reports from various segments of the college or university provide the top level decision-makers with pertinent information which enables them to take actions to maintain the equilibrium of the total organization.

Finally, the evaluation process is undertaken to provide data on new developments so that these data may be disseminated throughout the educational community, enabling similar schools to take advantage of the findings. It is very helpful for those who want to try out an innovative approach to know the results of similar attempts. For example, recent efforts of faculty to utilize the clinical specialist employed by the service agency for clinical instruction of students are being reviewed by other faculties for possible changes in their instructional programs. Likewise, the impact upon the instructional environment of the professional who assumes dual nursing care and teaching roles is attracting the attention of faculties of nursing schools. Care should be taken to determine the similarities and differences in the situations under review to be sure that the approach is an appropriate one for the new situation.

METHODOLOGY OF EVALUATION

Curriculum evaluation requires collecting, processing, and interpreting data pertaining to the use of an educational program. For a complete evaluation, two kinds of data are collected: (1) objective descriptions of goals, environments, personnel, methods and content, and outcomes, and (2) personal judgments as to the quality and appropriateness of those goals, environments, personnel, methods and content, and outcomes. These evaluative efforts should lead to better decision-making, better development, better selection, and better use of curriculum.

GOALS AND ROLES OF EVALUATION

Scriven has described the function of evaluation in two ways. At the methodological level, he refers to the *goals* of evaluation. In relation to a particular sociological or pedagogical context, he distinguishes the several possible *roles* of evaluation [3].

Evaluation as a methodological activity is essentially the same whether one is trying to evaluate a new computer, a teaching machine, plans for a house, or plans for a curriculum. The activity consists of (1) gathering data about performance and combining them with a weighted set of goal scales to yield either comparative or numerical ratings and (2) justification of the data-gathering instruments, the weightings, and the selection of goals.

The *roles* of evaluation in particular contexts vary enormously. It may be a part of the curriculum development of a field experiment on the improvement of some instructional strategy, a data-gathering activity to support the purchase of some educational materials, or data-gathering to support a request for research funding for a specific project. One role that has often been assigned to evaluation is the assessment of curriculum changes. This role does not preclude evaluation of the final product for other purposes. Evaluation can and usually should play several roles. Not only can it have several roles with respect to one educational enterprise, but it may have several specific goals with respect to each of these. It may have a role in the ongoing improvement of the curriculum, or it may serve to enable administrators to decide whether the entire finished curriculum represents a sufficient advance over the available alternatives to justify the expense of adoption by the school.

Any curriculum builder is engaged in *formative* evaluation. She is presumably doing what she is doing because she judges the material being presented in the existing curriculum as unsatisfactory. She believes her own new material is better than that which is in use currently. She is probably engaged in field testing the new material while it is being developed, and from this she gets feedback on which to base further revisions. Information is collected on two questions: (1) Are the students showing signs of responding and changing in the direction of program objectives? (2) Have the intended program procedures been implemented? If the field testing is elaborate, it may amount to *summative* evaluation of the early forms of the new curriculum.

The purpose of summative evaluation is to determine to what extent a program has fulfilled its intended product goals (did the students enrolled in the program change as hoped for?). Summative evaluation is a form of *product* evaluation. A second form of product evaluation is *comparative* evaluation, in which two or more programs are contrasted in terms of their effects on students.

Regardless of the role of evaluation, the opinions of the subject matter expert should be given serious consideration. Sometimes it will be almost all one has to go on, and it will suffice for some decisions. Participants may have the uneasy feeling that evaluation necessitates value judgments and that value judgments are essentially subjective and not scientific. Some value judgments are essentially assertions about fundamental personal preferences and as such they are factual claims. Making such a claim does not show that it is right or wrong for everyone to hold these values; it only shows that somebody does or does not hold them. Another kind of value judgment is the claim that the performance of some entity in a clearly defined context is as good as or better than another's. It is possible to find out not only whether such assertions are believed by the individuals who assert them but also whether it is right or wrong for anyone to believe them. Finally, there are value judgments in which the criteria themselves are debatable. In such issues, the debates turn out to be mainly disputes about what is to count as "good" rather than arguments about the straightforward facts of the situation, that is, what is in fact "good."

It is sometimes thought that in dealing with people, one is necessarily involved in moral value judgments and that at least these are essentially subjective. Value judgments about people are by no means necessarily moral, since they may refer to their health, intelligence, and achievements. These judgments may be made by referring to a predetermined set of criteria.

ROLES ENACTED IN EVALUATION

The numbers of types of participants in evaluation depend to a great extent upon the nature of the evaluation activity. Four major roles that people can assume in the evaluation process have been identified as follows:

1. The doer: the student, the teacher, the practitioner whose behavior is being evaluated
2. The observer: the person who is looking at what the doer is doing
3. The judger: the person who is taking the results of the observations and judging their value and adequacy
4. The actor: the individual who acts on the results of the evaluation [4]

It is obvious that these roles are not always played by different persons. Most frequently, the student is the doer and the actor, while the teacher is the observer and the judger. In the instructional process, if the evaluations are to become as educative as possible, the actors and doers must work together with the observers and judges, and the teacher must have an important part in or an understanding of these four roles in evaluating her own development. Agreement must be reached on two points: at the goals to be achieved, and the definition of the norms to be used.

DEFINING GOALS

The goals of a specific area of instruction, curriculum, or program emerge out of the goals of the educational enterprise. These have been prescribed in a general way by the society in which the school exists. The professionals who assume responsibility for the conduct of the school must translate these general goals into goals appropriate to the specific curriculum. These goals must be stated in terms readily understood by the persons responsible for the program of instruction. Agreement among instructors on the objectives of the particular curriculum is necessary. Considerable attention was given to the development of statements of objectives of the curriculum in a previous chapter. Here we need only to emphasize that all persons associated with the educational program who will be involved in the evaluation process must know, understand, and agree with the goals of the curriculum at the outset. This does not mean that goals are static. On the contrary, the goals of any program of education should be periodically reviewed and revised to accommodate the changing needs of society and its constituents. Once the statement of goals is agreed upon, it then becomes the basis for the evaluation of learning outcomes.

Issues arise in the instructional process when the role expectations of the doers, or learners, are perceived differently by those making formal or informal evaluations. This applies to persons who instruct but who do not have direct responsibility for developing the statement of objectives, such as physicians, nutritionists, nursing practitioners and administrators, and social workers, in the case of nursing students. Their evaluations of a student's performance frequently are influenced by their own professional orientation and expectations. If these persons are expected to contribute in any way to the evaluation process, they must be informed of the specific goals and expectations of the students in a particular phase of the curriculum or of the overall goals of the specific curriculum.

DETERMINING NORMS

The statement of goals provides the participants in the evaluation process the fundamental directions for evaluation of the learner. In addition to goals or objectives, standards of performance must be developed against which the learner is evaluated. Determining the standard or norm is perhaps one of the most difficult tasks in the evaluation process. Frequently the same observed behavior relating to the same objective is judged differently depending upon the particular standard or norm of adequacy used in making the judgment. Several types of norms that may be useful in the evaluation process are described.

It is possible to identify some tasks that are sufficiently unitary to be completed on an *all-or-none basis*. The essential task to be accomplished or certain aspects of the task are described to include a general statement of adequacy of performance. The student did or did not contaminate the sterile equipment during the process of changing a dressing on the patient's wound. The evaluation problem is to observe the behavior in the situation and to judge whether adequate performance was or was not demonstrated.

A second type of norm is drawn from the *experience of a selected group*. In educational activities norms of behavior and achievement frequently are based on a relative measure, such as central tendency, or most common performance level. For example, if raw scores on a paper-and-pencil test were arranged in a frequency distribution, the most frequently attained score might be used as a norm or standard to judge the performance of other groups.

Another standard that may be used to evaluate performance is the *individual student's capacity* to perform the designed task. These measures compare present with past accomplishments. Present academic performance of the student may be evaluated in relation to previous performance in an effort to appraise what is being done now in comparison with what the student has been able to do in the past.

A fourth norm or standard is *socially or educationally desirable behavior*. The teacher or other person making the evaluation develops model patterns or descriptive behavior characteristics which they apply to the student, another teacher, or practitioner and then makes value judgments about these individuals on the basis of this conception of desirable behavior. The model or descriptive behavior characteristics should be developed so that the social and educational expectations are as explicit as possible in operational or behavioral terms. These statements can be formulated by listing and organizing the behavior believed to be normative for a given professional, student, or personal role at a particular point in time and in relation to a specific curriculum objective. In an effort to validate this conceptual analysis of normative behavior, comparisons should be made among the various appropriate conceptions of actual and perceived normative behavior. Frequently this normative basis for making value statements about the behavior of students, teachers, or practitioners is hidden and remains personal with the evaluator. Evaluation procedures should make it possible for social and educational expectations to be recognized for the important role they play in educational evaluation.

The theory and methodology of evaluation may be understood better if the distinction between the *roles* of evaluation and *goals* of evaluation is reemphasized here. The goal of evaluation is always the same: to determine the worth of something. The roles of evaluation depend on what that something is and on whose standards of value will apply. The something may be a single student's performance, the performance of a group of students, textbooks, or learning environment, or any other variable that influences curriculum and instruction. By this definition it is inappropriate to claim that all evaluation should focus on student performance, that all educational evaluation should focus on goals specified by the curriculum designer. There are other important roles for evaluation than to determine the extent to which teaching objectives have been attained. As people have different uses for evaluation information, the roles of evaluation will differ.

The various roles of evaluation and the types of norms to be utilized will suggest the kinds of information that will be needed for decision-making. To obtain the information, appropriate observations must be made, recorded, analyzed, and summarized. Procedures and instruments must be developed and utilized to facilitate data collection relevant to the behavior or entity to be evaluated.

EVALUATION OF INSTRUCTION

Evaluation of curriculum and instruction may use a variety of procedures and instruments to obtain data. Instruments should be appropriately related to the criteria that define the model. Instruments may be selected for any of the following purposes:

1. Determining the progress of students in development of appropriate cognitive, affective, and perceptual-motor behavior
2. Determining the teacher's effectiveness
3. Determining the influence of the learning environment
4. Determining the contributions of allied professional personnel (nutritionists, social workers, physicians, occupational, and physical therapists)
5. Determining community involvement

The general procedures and instruments appropriate for each purpose are described. It is suggested that the reader review the authoritative literature to learn more about the construction of the various instruments.

STUDENT PROGRESS

The process of evaluation of instruction begins with the objectives of the educational program. Since the purpose is to see how well these objectives are being realized, it is necessary to have procedures that will give evidence about the kinds of behaviors implied by each of the major educational objectives. Unless there is some clear conception of the sort of behavior implied by the

TABLE 11. Situations Which Provide for Expression of Terminal Behaviors

Description of Educational Objectives	Situations Which Provide for Expression of Behavior

1. Knowledge
 	
  a. Items of specified information, including definitions of terms in the field
  b. Sequences or patterns of items of information, including sets of rules, procedures, or classifications for handling information
  c. Comprehension or understanding of internal relationships in the field and the way in which terminology applies within the field
  d. Understanding of relations between the knowledge of this field and that of other fields
  e. Application of the rules, procedures, and concepts of the field to appropriate examples
	1. Information (a, b) shown in performance of:
	    Recital tasks
	    Discrimination tasks
	    Completion tasks
	    Labeling tasks
	  Comprehension or understanding (c, d, e) manifested in:
	    Analyzing
	    Synthesizing
	    Evaluation
	    Problem-solving
	    Applying concepts, rules, principles to selected situations

2. Motivation (attitude and values)
  a. Attitudes toward course
  b. Attitudes toward subject matter
  c. Attitude toward learning, reading
  d. Attitude toward nursing
  e. Attitude toward teacher
  f. Attitude toward classmates, school, and society
  g. Attitude toward self
	2. Attitude manifestations:
	    Usually demonstrated simultaneously with display of knowledge
	    Responses to questionnaires, projective tests, Q sort techniques, etc.
	    Characteristically have a passive-active dimension

3. Performance skills (nonmental)
  a. Perceptual-motor
  b. Psychomotor
  c. Motor
  d. Social
	3. Performance skills shown in:
	    Natural situations
	    Laboratory
	    Simulated situations

4. Clinical knowledge and skills
  a. Application of knowledge from various sources to clinical problems
  b. Utilization of perceptual-motor and psychomotor skills in clinical situation
  c. Establishing priorities for action based on knowledge, motivation, and values
	4. Application of knowledge and skills in clinical situations:
	    Problem-solving
	    Establishing priorities
	    Expression of concern for values, feelings, attitudes, and interpersonal dynamics
	    Use of appropriate methods, skills, equipment

objectives, one has no way of telling what kind of student behavior to look for to see to what degree these objectives are being realized.

The next step in the evaluation procedure is to identify the situations that will give the student the chance to express the behavior implied by the educational objectives, the terminal behavior. The only way that one can tell whether students have acquired a given type of behavior is to give them an opportunity to demonstrate this behavior. This means that situations must be found that not only permit the expression of the behavior but actually encourage or evoke this behavior. Table 11 lists situations that may give the student an opportunity to express the terminal behavior.

After the objectives have been clearly defined and situations listed which give opportunity for the expression of the terminal behavior, available evaluation instruments are examined to determine their usefulness in the evaluation process. In reviewing the instruments already available (tests, guides, checklists, etc.), it is necessary to check each proposed evaluation device against the objectives to determine whether it utilizes situations likely to evoke the kind of behavior desired as educational objectives. It is likely that the instructor will find available instruments quite satisfactory for certain educational objectives and other available instruments that can be modified somewhat and made appropriate for other educational objectives. There may be, however, some objectives for which no available evaluation instruments can be used. For these objectives, it will be necessary to construct or devise procedures or instruments for getting evidence about the student's attainment of these objectives.

In constructing an evaluation instrument, it is necessary to decide upon the terms or units of observation that will be used to summarize the behavior observed. The terms or units indicate the degree or quality of the behavior that has been expressed by the student in relation to the expected behavior described in the norm. All evaluation involves decisions about the characteristics to be appraised in the behavior and the units of observation to be used in the measurement or summarization of these characteristics. Any summary of human performance should not only include the terms indicating the quality of the performance but should also record the particular strengths and weaknesses.

An important part of developing evaluation instruments requires taking steps to insure the validity and reliability of these devices. The reader is encouraged to seek out available information about these from appropriate literature.

The time schedule for collecting data on student behavior is determined in part by the purpose of the evaluation. In general, one of the following three procedures can be used:

1. Data collected at one point in time. This schedule allows for a comparison of the student's behavior with the model or norm expectation of behavior at a specific point in time, such as the end of a course, end of a semester, or at a specific level of instruction.

2. Data collected at two points in time, as exemplified by use of pretests and posttests. This schedule allows for an analysis of change and a comparison of the observed change and the expected change, as defined by the norm or model.

3. Longitudinal evaluation, or collection of data about student behavior over a longer period of time (that is, over a major portion of the curriculum). The critical times are specified by a model. This schedule allows for an analysis of behavior change as in the description of data collection at two points in time, but with a greater degree of specificity. The major effort in the longitudinal type of evaluation is to assess the student's behavior in relation to a specific concept or problem which is identified as a curriculum theme. As the theme is developed throughout the curriculum, the concept characteristics change and the variables affecting problem-solving increase. The student's behavior is compared with the models that describe the expected behavior of the student at various points in the curriculum. Evaluation of a student in relation to her development of communication skills might follow the pattern shown in Diagram 9.

The selection of a specific time schedule for evaluation is determined by the particular role that the evaluation has in the total evaluation design.

Some of the techniques and instruments that may be used for collecting and evaluating data about student behavior are described below:*

Observations: (1) The act or process of observing (usually complex) conditions or activities as a means of gathering descriptive or quantitative data. (2) A verbal, numerical, or coded datum recorded as representing a condition or aspect of behavior, especially a value expressed in relation to a scale, such as a measurement or test value; the value derived for a given time, place, object, or event through calculation of statistical index or index number. (3) The ability to see analytically, in details; directed preception, which is almost entirely an acquired skill; its uses arise from the individuals desire to record her sense impressions, to clarify her conceptual knowledge, and to build up her memory.

* From A *Dictionary of Education* by C. V. Good. Copyright 1959 by McGraw-Hill Book Company and used with their permission.

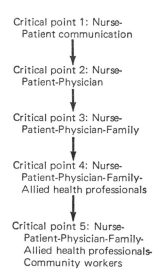

Critical point 1: Nurse-
Patient communication

Critical point 2: Nurse-
Patient-Physician

Critical point 3: Nurse-
Patient-Physician-Family

Critical point 4: Nurse-
Patient-Physician-Family-
Allied health professionals

Critical point 5: Nurse-
Patient-Physician-Family-
Allied health professionals-
Community workers

DIAGRAM 9. Critical stages in evaluation of student development of communication skills.

Standardized test: A test for which content has been selected and checked empirically, for which norms have been established, for which uniform methods of administering and scoring have been developed, and which may be scored with a high degree of objectivity.

Teacher-made test: A teacher-made or locally constructed test, of either objective or essay type, for local classroom use.

Essay test: The traditional type of examination in which the examinee is asked to discuss, enumerate, compare, state, evaluate, analyze, summarize, or criticize.

Objective test: A test so constructed that different scorers working independently will arrive at the same or essentially the same score for a given performance; usually has alternate-response, multiple-choice, matching, or completion type of questions; scored by means of a key of correct answers, any answer disagreeing with the key being regarded as wrong.

Achievement test: A test designed to measure a person's knowledge, skills, and understandings in a given field taught in the school, for example, a mathematics test, biology test, or nursing test.

Aptitude test: A device or test designed to indicate a person's potential ability for performance of a certain type of activity, as a musical aptitude test or a mathematics aptitude test.

Diagnostic test: (1) An examination intended to measure achievement in a narrow subject field or in related subfields, particularly to determine specific weaknesses of students as a basis for remedial measures. (2) An examination the results of which permit a broad, general diagnosis of student weaknesses and strengths; a standardized instrument for the identification of a specific characteristic or set of characteristics of the individual.

Performance test: (1) Commonly a test in which the person responds by overt action rather than by making a verbal or written response. (2) Broadly, any test intended to measure actual accomplishment rather than potential ability or aptitude, regardless of how the subject is instructed to respond.

Inventory: In the field of evaluation, a test or check test used to determine the examinee's ability, achievement, aptitude, interest, or likes, generally in a limited area.

Questionnaire: A list of planned, written questions related to a particular topic, with space provided for indicating the response to each question, intended for submission to a number of persons for reply, commonly used in normative survey studies and in the measurement of attitudes and opinions.

Rating scale: A device used in evaluating products, attitudes, or other characteristics of instructors or learners.

Case method: (1) In research, the use of detailed studies of single individuals as a basis for induction of principles. (2) A diagnostic and remedial procedure based on thorough investigation of a person to acquire knowledge of his history, his home conditions, and all the other influences that may cause his maladjustment or behavior difficulties.

Teacher-student conference: The face-to-face communication of the teacher with the individual student or with a small group of students, designed to help direct learning efforts through conference activities in such areas as planning, evaluation, expectations, responsibilities, behavior, cultivation of new interests, goal-setting, and discussion of pertinent material in the student's personal record.

Anecdotal record: A series of notes containing exactly what a student said or did in concrete situations; as observations are accumulated, a variety and continuity of information yielding a picture of the student's behavior patterns, development in various directions, interests, attitudes, strengths, and problems can be seen.

Self-appraisal: Methods, techniques, materials, and tools made available to and used by students to gain evaluative data about their growth and development [5].

These instruments may be used singly or in combination, depending upon the kinds of information about the student that is being sought. It is obvious that the more information we obtain about the student, the more valid our evaluation will be.

Since every educational program involves several objectives, and since for almost every objective there will be several scores or descriptive terms to summarize the behavior of students in relation to this objective, it follows that the results obtained from a set of evaluation instruments will not be a single score or descriptive term but an analyzed profile or a comprehensive set of descriptive terms indicating the student's present achievement. These scores or descriptive terms should be comparable to those used at an earlier date, so that it is possible to indicate whether educational progress is taking place. It is, therefore, essential to compare the results obtained from the several evaluation instruments before and after given periods in order to estimate the amount of change taking place.

Analysis of the results of student evaluations may suggest strengths and weaknesses in the curriculum. Therefore it is also desirable to examine the data for possible explanations or hypotheses for particular patterns of performance. If such hypotheses seem to be consistent with all the data available, the curriculum may be modified in the suggested direction. A second evaluation like the first should show whether there is any improvement in student achievement attributable to the modifications made.

Implied in all of this is that curriculum planning is a continuous process. As material and procedures are developed, they are tried out, their results appraised, their inadequacies identified, and suggested improvements indicated; there is replanning, redevelopment, and then reappraisal.

TEACHER EFFECTIVENESS

Teacher evaluation of students is only one dimension of the total evaluation program. The other equally important aspect of this twofold process is the evaluation of teacher competence or teacher effectiveness. Teaching is an extremely complex process, with numerous variables affecting teaching and learning. It is not surprising that after all these years of teaching experiences and research educators still know very little about the qualities and characteristics that are needed for effective teaching. Evaluation of the effectiveness of teaching is one of the most important functions of an educational leader. If the best teachers are to be selected or appropriately recognized, it is essential that a sound basis be established for identifying the best teachers.

Teacher effectiveness has been described as the extent to which teachers help students to attain the objectives of the curriculum. Some factors that make it difficult to determine the effectiveness of teaching are (1) ability level of the students, (2) previous attainment of students, (3) previously learned work habits of students, (4) differences in cultural learning opportunities outside of school and (5) available teaching facilities and resources. Growth and development result from many experiences encountered by the student. Thus, it is difficult to distinguish the effects of the teacher from those of other persons, agencies, and institutions in the student's environment.

Teachers frequently object to traditional plans of evaluation because of the general unreliability and secrecy associated with such plans. Many of the criticisms of devices and procedures used in rating teachers are subjective. There is sufficient evidence to indicate that different people observing the same teacher or studying data about her may arrive at quite different evaluations. Many rating procedures call for a record of opinion only, and not an actual observation of teaching. Whether evaluation of teaching is to be used for teacher evaluation by authorities or for self-improvement by the teacher, it is necessary for teachers to know the objectives they are expected to achieve.

Ideally, teaching success should be judged primarily in terms of changed behavior in students. One method of judging teacher effectiveness, often referred to as student gain, attempts to measure the learning that students experience under the guidance of a given teacher over a period of time. The method attempts to measure the knowledge, skill, or other behaviors before and after teaching. The exact division between teaching and learning remains unsettled. It is not known exactly how or to what extent teaching contributes to or causes learning. Educators are aware that certain teaching situations may activate desirable behavior changes that do not become obvious until some later time. One issue that influences teacher effectiveness is the needs of students in the various stages of their development. Some research findings indicate that students in the beginning phase of the curriculum (freshmen) make different demands on teachers than those near the end of the educational program. Freshmen frequently rate teachers in relation to their ability to give them emotional and personal support, whereas seniors judge teachers for their competency in their subject matter.

Many people are in a position to evaluate the teacher either formally or informally and should be involved in the evaluation process. Several types of ratings are practiced, such as (1) self-ratings, (2) peer ratings, (3) student ratings, (4) supervisor ratings, and (5) expert ratings. Extensive research has been undertaken in an effort to formulate teacher qualities and characteristics in terms of (1) intelligence, (2) knowledge of subject matter, (3) experience, (4) cultural background, (5) socioeconomic status, and (6) other aspects such as attitude, aptitude, job interest, and voice or diction. Although all of these factors may be important in the teaching-learning process, research has failed to show a significant correlation between these qualities or characteristics and teacher competence or effectiveness.

Numerous rating scales and evaluation instruments are available for those interested in evaluating teachers. The data provided by these instruments assist the teacher or prospective teacher in gaining insight into her strengths and weaknesses. It should be kept in mind that the use of such scales is based on the assumption that the qualities and characteristics reflected in the instruments are appropriate criteria for evaluating teacher competence and effectiveness.

The involvement of students in the evaluation of teaching and learning has become more widespread in recent years. The acceptance of this practice may be attributed to a greater understanding of the nature of the learning process. It seems logical to assume that one of the most valid sources of data in evaluating the teaching-learning situation and determining teacher effectiveness is students. The gathering of evaluative data from students is a complex problem involving both formal and informal techniques and direct and indirect procedures. Numerous devices are being used by teachers in an effort to understand better the student's perception of the teaching-learning climate.

The efforts of the faculty of The Catholic University of America School of Nursing to develop criteria for the evaluation of teaching effectiveness may be useful. In this university a charge was given to all schools and colleges to recognize an outstanding teacher periodically by making an appropriate award to her. The faculty realized that in order to make such an award, some standard or model must be constructed that would suggest criteria of effective teaching. Although literature in this area appeared plentiful, the nursing faculty developed a plan whereby their model of effective teaching could be made available for the purposes of evaluation. While the project was not yet completed at the time of this writing, the progress to date is noted here.

The initial step was identifying teaching behaviors. Undergraduates, master's and doctoral students, and faculty members who agreed to participate were asked to respond to the following directive: Think of the teacher you have known whose teaching was outstanding. Describe the characteristics that made this person an outstanding teacher.

Approximately 70 percent of the total group responded, and their responses were reviewed. The characteristics recorded could be grouped into three major areas: (1) teaching style, (2) knowledge of subject matter, and (3) personal and interpersonal behavior.

The specific characteristics that were identified under each of these headings including the following:

1. *Teaching Style*

   Engages the learner in determining the goals for learning

   Interprets the goals of learning to the learners

   Makes clear what is expected of the learners and of the teacher in attaining the goals

   Makes assignments that are meaningful and possible (in terms of time and ability of the learners)

   Sequences instruction according to some rational plan that is visible to the learners

   Engages in instructional activities appropriate to the status of the learners and the personality and skill of the teacher

   Inspires student to independent effort

   Creates desire to investigate problems of interest to learners

   Provides opportunity for learners to select materials to be studied

   Provides appropriate reinforcement but does not make learner dependent upon it

   Provides sufficient guides or cues to give direction to learning

   Selects and utilizes materials that stimulate the learners

   Utilizes materials that provide for depth, breadth, and diversity of learning

   Draws upon personal and professional experiences appropriately (for illustrative purposes), including clinical practice demonstrations

   Conveys interest and sincerity when talking with learners

   Provides ample time and privacy when discussing learner's progress

   Utilizes evaluation devices that are appropriate to the subject and goals

   Holds in confidence information pertaining to learner's progress

   Provides opportunity for self-evaluation

   Provides opportunity for course evaluation

   Provides opportunity for teacher evaluation

2. *Knowledge of Subject Matter*

   Displays knowledge of authoritative literature in the field

   Demonstrates knowledge of past and current research efforts specific to the subject

Demonstrates a commitment to the subject area based on an amalgamation of knowledge from a variety of sources

Displays rich and extensive perceptions about subject field

Provides knowledge from other areas that adds new dimensions to the subject area

Examines, evaluates, and incorporates materials relevant to the subject offered by students and others

Deletes outmoded and outdated content from presentations

Evaluates content in light of current conditions, and is adaptable to new content

3. *Personal and Interpersonal Behavior*

Reads and studies current data

Pursues significant research

Attends professional meetings

Seeks ways to share acquired knowledge

Makes known information about available resources

Distributes materials to appropriate persons

Uses voice inflection effectively

Adjusts voice volume and tone appropriately

Uses precise qualitative vocabulary

Stimulates development of productive ideas

Displays positive, supportive orientation

Has strong sense of integrity, morals, and values

Is loyal in speech and in manner

Is courteous and polite; expects others to be the same

Shows an interest in others as individuals

Has confidence in others

Shows trust in others

Respects the opinions of others

Has a sense of humility

Evidences personal convictions

Is flexible and adaptable

Wears appropriate attire

Behaves in a mature, secure manner

Is receptive to constructive suggestions; tries to modify practices accordingly

Has an honest, just, straightforward manner

Is sincere, kind, and compassionate

Uses data judiciously
Keeps confidences in trust

In a second phase of the study, each of these characteristics was rated by all the participants on a 3- or 5-point numerical or verbal rating scale. The four forms used were: (10–30–50), (10–20–30–40–50), (minimum-average-maximum), (low-medium-high). The following directions were given:

1. Select a teacher you have had in a recent course (within the past five years). Rate this teacher in relation to her/his overall teaching performance. The identification of this teacher by name is not necessary.
2. Keeping this same teacher in mind, rate the teacher according to the specific characteristics on the accompanying scale.
   You will note that there are presented several types of scales.
   You may select any point on the various scales that reveals the characteristics of "your" teacher.
3. Record general reactions and comments concerning the overall structure and format of guide in relation to its purposes.
4. Indicate the type of scale that you found easiest to use in making your assessment.
5. Record the approximate amount of time required to complete the questionnaire.

The respondents were also requested to provide information pertaining to their personal, educational, and professional characteristics.

The purpose of the second review by students and faculty is the validation of the characteristics initially identified. Efforts will be directed to determining those characteristics that appear to be most important for effective teaching in contrast to those describing the performance of poor versus good teachers. Finally, it may be demonstrated that respondents perceive effective teaching according to their personal, educational, and professional characteristics.

The Committee on Improved Teaching of The Catholic University of America School of Nursing, which is responsible for this endeavor, believes that this project will contribute to the improvement of teaching through the identification of the criteria for effective teaching.

ALLIED PROFESSIONAL PERSONNEL

Teachers of nursing frequently utilize allied professional personnel in their instructional programs. These have included physicians, nutritionists, social workers, physical therapists, rehabilitation counselors, and members of the clergy. All of them may be considered to be resource persons in the instructional process. A resource person in this instance is an individual who possesses special knowledge or skills that may supplement certain educational objectives. This person may be drawn from within the educational institution or from the community. Depending upon the qualification and activities of the resource person, he may provide opportunities for students to broaden their base of knowledge and gain insights into the use of this knowledge in practical situations.

In an effort to assess the quantity and quality of the allied professional personnel used, some general purposes for utilizing resource persons are identified:

1. The use of resource persons enriches the instructional program by providing for greater depth and breadth of certain curricular activities.

2. The utilization of different types of learning activities provides variety to the educational program. Just meeting people of varied intellectual and professional interests tends to stimulate and motivate learning.

3. The utilization of allied professional persons as resource persons may facilitate the interpretation of the roles of these persons in the health care of the patient and family.

4. When resource persons represent certain community activities and agencies, their contacts with students brings the community and school into closer relationships.

Criteria for effective use of allied professional persons should be formulated and agreed upon by the faculty. These may be used for the evaluation of the quantity and quality of their contributions to the instructional program. Criteria that were utilized by one nursing faculty included the following:

1. Continuity of learning is assured through preplanning by the instructor and resource person.
2. The resource person is made aware of the level of knowledge and other characteristics of students and the overall goals of the instructional activity.
3. Adequate time is alloted to the resource person.
4. Discussion periods are made available in an effort to utilize the contributions of resource persons in specific learning activities of the students.
5. Resource persons are selected on the basis of their unique knowledge

and/or skills, which offer vital and enriching experiences to the students in certain curricular activities.

While these criteria provide a means for the evaluating of the use of allied professional persons in teaching-learning situations, some precautions should be noted. Use of too many resource persons may fragment learning. If these persons are not available at the appropriate time, the sequence of learning activities may be disrupted. It is possible that the use of resource persons may overemphasize one aspect of learning to the neglect of another. Careful selection of the resource person is necessary to prevent the presentation of a biased view of an issue. Finally, not all specialists are good teachers. They may need some assistance in planning activities so that the experience will be meaningful and enjoyable to students. Instruments that may be developed and used to determine the quantity and quality of allied professional involvement include interview and observation schedules and questionnaires.

COMMUNITY INVOLVEMENT

The involvement of the community in curriculum and instruction may be either direct or indirect. Every school of nursing utilizes one or more community agencies for the purpose of providing appropriate learning opportunities for students. Community agencies that participate in the health and welfare of citizens are brought into focus so that a clear definition of their purposes can be interpreted to students.

When instructors identify the learning opportunities that will probably assist the student to attain the objectives of instruction, they also must identify where these learning opportunities may be obtained. Certain criteria are established which assist teachers to select those institutions and agencies that will most likely serve the purposes of the educational programs. Such criteria may include the following:

1. Availability of the types and variety of nursing problems of patients and families
2. Availability of nursing care to patients and families
3. Availability of allied health services, such as medical, social service, nutrition, rehabilitation counseling, dental, and others
4. Interest of agency personnel in cooperating with school of nursing
5. Location of agency in reasonable geographical proximity

6. Acceptable financial arrangements, including utilization of human and
    material resources of agency

The kinds of arrangements between the agency and the school may be informal, perhaps with only a verbal agreement between the cooperating groups
concerning the use of the agency facilities and resources by the school. Periodically the faculty assesses the quantity and quality of this community involvement against the stated criteria.

An arrangement between the community agency and the school may be
formalized in contractual agreements. The statement of agreement indicates
the responsibilities of the cooperating groups in an effort to provide appropriate learning opportunities for students. Usually the provisions contained in
the documents are reviewed annually; these may be revised or renewed for another period of time.

An indirect involvement of the community in curriculum and instruction
may be viewed from the standpoint of consumers of nursing. In this instance
those who have the responsibility to deliver nursing service to the public are
expected to evaluate the product or graduate of the school. Instructors usually
initiate this process whereby the staff of the community agency are asked to
assess how well the graduate is able to assume and carry out the functions for
which she was employed. This information may be obtained by means of interviews and questionnaires. The kind of relationships the school has developed with the community agencies will influence the objectivity and usefulness
of the data obtained.

As a member of a faculty who had the responsibility to provide some leadership in curriculum development, the author interviewed several directors of
nursing service concerning the major strengths and weaknesses of beginning
professional practitioners and supervisors. These questions did not focus upon
the graduates of a particular school but upon all those prepared for professional practice and supervisory activities. The responses of the directors were
unanimous in several areas and were invaluable for the purposes of curriculum
review and revisions. The directors indicated that the graduates of baccalaureate curriculum demonstrated outstanding proficiency in giving nursing
care to one or two patients and families. When more patients were assigned,
the practitioners were overwhelmed. One could infer that these practitioners
were deficient in some measure in skills of priority-setting and utilization of
other nursing personnel in the plan of nursing care. The director of nursing
service of the Baltimore City Health Department stated: "These nurses give

efficient and effective care to five families, but I have to assign one hundred families to each of them." The evaluative comments made by these directors concerning the supervisory personnel had direct curriculum implications. The directors indicated that the supervisor was the key person in the nursing service who determines the quality of nursing care. In many instances those persons holding the position of supervisor were in that position because of years of service rather than increased competency in nursing. Since the educational and practice orientation of these supervisors was primarily that of agency management rather than nursing management, they frequently did not appreciate the extensive nursing knowledge of baccalaureate graduates and did not allow them freedom and initiative in planning and giving nursing care. When the beginning practitioner needed assistance in analyzing a nursing problem, the supervisors frequently were unable to provide the necessary nursing knowledge to be helpful to them. Inferences that could be made from these evaluations might suggest that curriculums for the preparation of supervisors should be well anchored in in-depth studies of phases of nursing practice.

Other types of community involvement in curriculum and instruction include the participation of community representatives in direct teaching activities. These were discussed in a preceding section. Whether the community is a well-defined geographic area or one that is more sprawling, participation of the community in the curriculum activities provides opportunities for the development of a more dynamic and relevant curriculum. The school is a product of its community and frequently reflects the kind of community in which it is situated. Public information and public participation are two of the most powerful tools for improving schools.

STRUCTURE OF EVALUATION DESIGN

Evaluation design is the preparation of a set of decision situations for implementing specified evaluation objectives. The definition indicates:

1. One must identify the evaluation objectives to be achieved
2. One should identify and define the decision situations in the procedure for achieving the evaluation objective
3. For each identified decision situation the evaluator needs to make a choice among available alternatives. The completed evaluation design would contain a set of decisions as to how the evaluation is to be conducted and what instruments will be used

The structure of the evaluation design is the same for any kind of evaluation. The structure includes six major parts: (1) focus of evaluation, (2) collection of information, (3) organization of information, (4) analysis of information, (5) reporting of information, and (6) administration of evaluation.

Focusing of evaluation. The purpose of this part of the evaluation design is to spell out the objectives of the evaluation and to define the policies within which the evaluation must be conducted. To achieve this purpose the following steps are suggested:

1. Identify the major levels of decision-making for which evaluation information must be provided (national, regional, state, school, course)
2. Identify and define the decisions to be served at each level, and describe each in terms of its focus, locus, criticality, timing, and composition of alternatives
3. Define criteria for each decision by specifying variables for measurement and standards for use in the judgment of alternatives
4. Define policies within which the evaluation must operate, that is, self-evaluation or outside evaluation needed; define limits of access to data for evaluation team (accrediting teams—professional, regional, state board)

Collection of information. Planning for the collection of information will include the following steps to achieve this purpose:
1. Identify the sources of the information to be collected as well as the present state of information (recorded or unrecorded)
2. Specify instruments for collecting the needed information: tests, interview, and observation schedules
3. Specify the sampling procedure to be employed. Where possible, administering too many instruments to the same person should be avoided.
4. Develop a master schedule for the collection of information

Organization of information. This part of the evaluation design provides the format of the information to be collected and also designates a means for coding, organizing, storing, and retrieving information.

Analysis of information. The analysis of information requires the selection of the appropriate procedures for performing the analysis.

Reporting of information. Reporting includes the following several steps:

1. Define the audiences for the evaluation reports
2. Specify means for providing information to the audiences
3. Specify the formats for evaluation reports or reporting sessions
4. Schedule the reporting of information

Administration of evaluation. This final part of the design includes the plan for executing the evaluation. The following steps achieve this purpose:

1. Summarize the evaluation schedule
2. Define staff and staff requirements and plans for meeting these require-ments
3. Specify means for meeting policy requirements in the conduct of the evaluation
4. Evaluate the potential of the evaluation design for providing informa-tion that is valid, reliable, credible, timely, and pervasive
5. Specify and schedule means for periodic updating of the evaluation design
6. Provide a budget for the total evaluation program

The methodology of evaluation includes four major functions: collection, organization, analysis, and reporting. Criteria for assessing the adequacy of evaluation include validity (is the information what the decision-maker needs?), reliability (is the information reproducible?), timeliness (is the in-formation available when the decision-maker needs it?), pervasiveness (does the information reach all decision-makers who need it?), and credibility (is the information trusted by the decision-maker and those he must serve?).

ISSUES AND PROBLEMS IN EVALUATION

Education has unprecedented opportunities to improve and expand curricu-lums and programs. Society is annually providing billions of dollars through federal, state, and foundation sources to education agencies at all levels. These opportunities have carried the requirement that educators evaluate their plans and programs. In some instances the law explicitly states that fund recipients will make at least annual evaluation reports. As a consequence, many educa-tors are having to cope with requirements for formal evaluation. Funding agencies and the public have the right to know whether their huge expendi-tures for education are producing the desired effects. Even more important than this, educators need evaluative information to make rational choices among alternative plans and procedures.

While educators have been busy doing evaluations, the fruits of their efforts have not always provided the information needed to support decision-making related to the program being evaluated. Though such information may be pertinent to the concerns of decision-makers, it usually lacks the credibility required by decision-makers to defend their decisions, and seldom can such information be of material use in making important decisions.

The lack of adequate evaluation information persists because of several fundamental problems that must be solved before educators can improve their evaluations. These problems include a lack of trained evaluators, a lack of appropriate evaluation instruments and procedures, and a lack of an adequate evaluation theory or conceptualizations of the nature of evaluation, which are needed to accommodate educational programs. Other problems in educational evaluation are identified for further exploration.

DEFINING REQUIREMENTS FOR EVALUATION

To evaluate, one must know what is to be evaluated. Gaining knowledge of what is to be evaluated is currently a difficult task. Programs to improve education depend upon a variety of decisions, and a variety of information is needed to make and support those decisions. Evaluators charged with providing this information must have adequate knowledge about the relevant decision processes and associated information requirements before they can design adequate evaluations. At present adequate knowledge of decision processes and associated information requirements relative to educational programs does not exist.

The decision-making process is usually considered to be a rational process whereby the decision-maker begins with some awareness of a problem that she must resolve and assembles alternative ways of responding to that problem; she chooses from among the alternative responses the one that appears to have the highest success probability, and then she implements the choice. Frequently, the range of possible responses is not great, and the choice among alternatives is not usually made on the basis of explicit, well-understood criteria.

DEFINING EDUCATIONAL EVALUATION

Usually educators have defined evaluation as the science of determining the extent to which objectives have been achieved. The first step in making this definition operational is to state program objectives in behavioral terms. Then one must define and make operational criteria for use in relating outcomes to the objectives. Making such criteria operational includes the specification of instruments for measuring outcomes and standards for use in assigning values to the measured outcomes. Standards may be either absolute or relative; however, regardless of the type of evaluation standard used, the data from such studies are analyzed only after a complete cycle of the program to determine the extent to which the objectives were achieved.

Evaluation based on the above definition of evaluation yields data about gross program effects, and then only in retrospect. Such data are useful for making judgments about a project after it has run full cycle, but they certainly are not adequate to assist educators in initial planning and in the actual carrying through of programs. The major concern seems to be that reports yielded by current evaluation programs are not sufficiently specific or timely to influence educational programs. Evaluation has come to have a utility for judging not only a product (student achievement) but also a process (the means of instruction). Some disadvantages accrue from this definition, namely, (1) heavy emphasis is placed on objectives so that they are difficult to use in identifying and to defining behaviors, (2) the evaluation in relation to student behaviors tells little about related aspects of program activities, and (3) evaluation becomes a terminal technique—the data become available only at the end of a long instructional period.

LACK OF CRITERIA AND INSTRUMENTS

Most evaluators agree that the mere collection of data does not constitute evaluation; there is always the concern of making judgments about the data in terms of some implicit or explicit value structure. It is unusual to speak about whether objectives are achieved, rather one speaks of how well they are achieved. At present, no adequate methodology exists for the determination of values, even though such determination may be the most critical professional task that the evaluator performs. Another question that arises in this domain is how to achieve consensus about the values that are to be invoked on evaluations. In a pluralistic society in which multiple values necessarily exist side by side, which values will be served? When such multiple values are applied, will it not be almost inevitable that the same data when interpreted in terms of different value standards will give rise to antithetical evaluations?

The problem of describing precisely what is to be taught and what is to be measured as an outcome of instruction is a problem of educational planning and evaluation. Contributions to the question of behavioral specification of instructional outcomes stem largely from the work of Ralph Tyler. Focusing on criteria of demonstrated effectiveness suggests the appropriateness of providing program-assessment data in the form of stated performance characteristics that indicate what contribution a particular program is actually making toward the attainment of the specified instructional objectives.

When criteria have been determined, they have been primarily concerned with the effects of specific teaching-learning situations. The evaluator's most usual focus has been microscopic, that is, the individual student, or group of students, rather than macroscopic, that is, the curriculum or program. This microscopic focus serves the evaluator badly when he is confronted with evaluation problems at superordinate levels. The instruments and techniques that have been developed for use at the microscopic level are not appropriate to obtain data for the macroscopic evaluation. The data obtained at the microscopic level may not always have meaning for overall curriculum or program evaluation. The introduction of various levels of evaluation introduces problems that are by no means resolvable through the application of techniques, methods, criteria, and perspectives developed at the microscopic level.

Most contemporary evaluations of instruction begin and end with achievement testing. Many of these tests, both standardized and teacher-made, have been developed to discriminate among individual students. Discrimination among students is important for instruction and guidance, but for development and selection of curriculums, tests are needed that discriminate among curriculums. Different rules for test administration are possible, and different criteria of test development are appropriate when tests are to be used to discriminate among curriculums. Since the items of a standardized achievement test are meant to be fair to students of all curriculums, they are aimed at what is common to all. By intent, the standardized achievement test is unlikely to encompass the scope or penetrate the depth of a particular curriculum being evaluated.

Concepts such as success, progress, achievement of students, and the procedures and instruments for evaluation need reexamination because of the current emphasis upon innovation at all levels of education. Educators can no longer depend so heavily upon the assumption that success in schools or colleges as they are now operating is an acceptable criterion for validating a measuring instrument. The current trend is to seek innovation to get the institution active in learning how to serve its new clients. Evaluation instruments for this purpose must avoid using criteria based on the current judgments of schools and colleges because these criteria perpetuate the conviction that these institutions are, at present, satisfactory for the tasks to be done. Different approaches are required to attack the problems of curriculum evaluation on the various levels.

CURRICULUM EVALUATION AND RESEARCH

The means for evaluation have been developed to serve the ends of evaluation as these have been conceived traditionally. The inadequacy of available methodology is revealed when one examines the designs educators use to evaluate their programs. If they use a design at all, it typically is an experimental design.

The application of experimental design to evaluation problems conflicts with the principle that evaluation should facilitate the continual improvement of a program. Experimental design prevents rather than promotes changes in the treatment being considered because treatments cannot be altered in process if the data about differences among several treatments are to be unequivocal. The experimental design type of evaluation is useful for making decisions after a project has run full cycle but is almost useless as a device for making decisions during the planning and implementation of a project. Experimental design evaluation reflects back on whether a project did whatever it was supposed to do. At that time it is too late to make decisions about plans and procedures that have already determined the success or failure of the project.

Experimental design type of evaluation is well suited to the "antiseptic" conditions of the laboratory but not the "septic" conditions of the classroom or clinical environment. Although internal validity may be gained through the control of extraneous variables, such an achievement is accomplished at the expense of external validity. If the extraneous variables are tightly controlled, one can have much confidence in the findings pertaining to how an innovation operates in a controlled environment. However, such findings may not be at all generalizable to the real world, where the so-called extraneous variables operate freely. It is important to know how educational innovations operate under real-world conditions. Evaluations are designed not to establish universal laws but to make possible judgments about some phenomenon. In this situation, one not only does not want to establish highly controlled conditions in which possible extraneous influences are filtered out, but one wishes to set up conditions to invite interference from all factors that might influence a learning transaction. The use of laboratory-research designs and techniques poses conditions that are simply inappropriate for the purposes for which one does an evaluation.

Stake describes four kinds of studies that can be called applied research [6]. Each of these types of studies deals with the practical, everyday components of education. They differ, however, in regard to generalizability. The findings from *instructional research* are more generalizable than the findings from other types. Studies of problem-solving, content-sequencing, reinforcement, modeling behavior, and achievement need are usually considered to be instructional research studies. These studies are expected to generalize over subject matters, curriculums, school settings, student and teacher types, and time.

Formative evaluation yields findings that can be generalized to a lesser degree than does instructional research. This type of evaluation seeks information for the development of a curriculum or instructional device. The developer wants to find out what arrangements or what amount of something to use. The results of formative evaluation are generalized over school setting, teacher and student types, and within the various versions of the particular instructional device, but they are not generalized across subject matters and curriculums.

Summative evaluation is concerned with providing the educator with information about the merits and weaknesses of a particular curriculum or a specific set of instructional materials. The findings from this type of evaluation are expected to be generalized across large numbers of schools, teachers, and students. A large responsibility for the local educator is to determine how similar her uses, teachers, and students are to those described in the evaluation report.

Institutional evaluation is directed at a specific curriculum or instructional device, but it is also oriented to a specific setting, with its unique goals, classrooms, teaching staff, and student body. In any institutional evaluation, the curriculum, setting, staff, and students are specified. External norms are not of highest importance. The reader of the institutional evaluation report has relatively little need to know how her educational setting and personnel compare to others. She is little concerned about generalization to other settings or to other curriculums. She is concerned, however, about the congruences and contingencies for inputs and outcomes for a specific teaching situation.

A first concern in organizing and designing an evaluation study is deciding

TABLE 12.   Generalizability of Evaluation Results According to Type of Evaluation and Curriculum and Instruction Variables

Curriculum and Instruction Variables	Evaluation Results According to Type of Evaluation			
	Instructional	Formative	Summative	Institutional
Subject matter	+	−	−	−
Curriculum	+	−	−	−
School setting	+	+	+	−
Student type	+	+	+	−
Teacher type	+	+	+	−
Time	+	+	−	−

+ means results can be generalized beyond the locus of the evaluation project.
− means results cannot be generalized beyond the locus of the evaluation project.

on the degree to which the findings should be generalizable across subject matter, curriculums, school settings, teachers, and students. Different restrictions placed upon these variables call for different data-gathering plans.

COMPARATIVE EVALUATION

The results of the efforts to evaluate new curriculums have been remarkably uniform. Comparing students taking the old curriculum with students taking the new one, it usually appears that students taking the new curriculum do better on the examinations designed for that curriculum and worse on those designed for the old curriculum, while students taught by the old curriculum perform in the opposite way.

A legitimate reaction is to look into the question of whether one should not weight the judged merit of content and goals by subject matter experts a great deal more heavily than small differences in level of performance on assessed criteria. If we do this, the relatively minor improvements in performance on the right goals become valuable, and in these terms, the new curriculum looks considerably better. Another reaction is to ponder whether the examinations are really doing a good job testing the depth of understanding of the people trained with the new curriculum.

One might try to rate a curriculum on certain variables without also simultaneously looking at the performance of other curriculums on these variables. When the curriculum is evaluated, as opposed to merely describing its performance, then the question of its superiority or inferiority arises. In cases of comparisons among significantly different teaching instruments, no real under-standing of the reason for a difference in performance is gained from the dis-covery that one of them is notably superior to the others. No one knows which of the ingredients is responsible for the advantages. Educators are in-terested, however, in questions of support, encouragement, adoption, reward, and refinement. These are extremely important questions that can be given useful, though in some cases incomplete answers by the mere discovery of su-periority. Noncomparative evaluations will probably give the data needed for future improvement in that more variables are examined in greater detail.

CONTROL-GROUP EVALUATION

These experiments are designed to examine one treatment (curriculum component or instructional device) against a control group. The control-group experiments are rarely definitive enough to justify their cost. The lack of definitive results is itself a useful kind of knowledge. "No difference" is not "no knowledge." Educators cannot conclude from a null result that all the techniques involved in a new curriculum are worthless improvements. They must go on to make other studies that will enable them to see whether any one of them is worthwhile. Control-group study is inadequate as a total approach to curriculum research.

In an educational experiment it is difficult to keep subjects unaware that they are in an experimental group. It may be impossible to neutralize the biases of the teacher. One is never certain whether any observed advantage is attributable to the educational innovation as such or to the greater energy that teachers and students put forth when a method is fresh and experimen-tal. If one control group is used, it is impossible to tell whether it is the en-thusiasm or the experimental technique that explains a difference. If several experimental groups are used, the size of the enthusiasm effect can be estimated.

RESEARCH AND EVALUATION METHODS

Some fundamental similarities and differences in research and evaluation methods are noted. Research scientists and evaluators are observers. They each obtain their data by means of observations. Both the researcher and the evaluator endeavor to make generalizations from their observation data. The majority of researchers and developers of educational devices are manipulators, evaluators are not. Evaluators are only free to manipulate themselves into better positions for observation.

Scientists, particularly in basic research, are not governed by the demands of social utility; their responsibility is revelation of knowledge. The evaluator must assume the responsibility of utility. She must anticipate the uses of the evaluation. The educational evaluator's obligation is not to discover the essence of human learning but to discover the diversity of viewpoints and explanations of what is going on in the school. The inquiry methods of both the researcher and the evaluator are orderly, constrained, deliberate, and based on reason.

SUMMARY

The concern of educational evaluation focuses on questions such as, how well does the course or learning opportunity achieve its goals? rather than, how good is the course, or learning experience? It is obvious that if the goals are not worth achieving then it is useless to determine how well they are achieved. The success of this kind of relativism in the field of evaluation rests entirely upon the premise that judgments of goals are subjective value judgments. A nursing curriculum that requires simply the memorization of facts and procedures would be absurd; it could not possibly be said to be a good curriculum no matter how well it attained its goals. Nor could a curriculum that does not enable the student to develop certain perceptual-motor skills be considered adequate no matter what else it conveyed. This kind of value judgment about goals is not beyond debate, but good arguments to the contrary have not been forthcoming.

Evaluation must include, as an equal partner with the measuring of performance against goals, procedures for the evaluation of the goals. The key to any evaluation program is the quality of the observations being made. One major tool for knowing whether you are looking at behavior that would enable you to draw worthwhile conclusions about goal achievement is to have these behaviors validated by carefully defined objectives.

Judgments concerning the adequacy of the behavior observed are determined by what norm is used. Different norms ask different questions about the adequacy of the same behavior. Any one or all of these norms might be important and necessary to any adequate planning for future learning behavior. The roles of individuals in the various phases of the evaluation process clarify what self-evaluation means and define the kinds of communication among individuals in the evaluation process. If the evaluation is to be essentially educative for the learner, the various kinds of communication are necessary.

It is possible to distinguish between the observations of an individual in a dynamic clinical situation and those in a structured test situation. In the test situation the behavioral responses are limited and are usually categorized and scaled as a series of discrete responses. In the clinical situation with broad limits for the actual response, the behavior is usually ongoing, complex, and interactive. This latter kind of evaluation situation forms the common fabric of the teacher's day and may be more important to teaching and learning than the more formal test appraisal. A great deal more is known about test construction and use than about clinical observations and evaluation.

The real concern in learning and teaching is whether changes are taking place in the behavior of the learner. Any single set of observations can say very little about change. Multiple observations are required to make an adequate assessment of behavior change. Questions for educators related to the assessment of change in student behavior that have bearing on curriculum and instruction include the following:

1. Is initial data on learners—their achievement, their motivation, their personalities available?
2. Is initial data on teachers—their strategies, their motivations, their knowledge, their personalities available?
3. Do objectives for curriculum and learning clearly specify the type of behavior change expected?
4. Has the appropriate norm against which the behavior change will be evaluated been agreed upon?
5. Are the instruments for obtaining and recording information about the behavior change accessible?
6. Have method of summarizing and using the information obtained through the evaluation process been determined?

Educators evaluate in order to tell someone about an individual student, a group of students, or an instructional program. The quality of the evaluation will not exceed the quality of its communication. One of the greatest constraints upon evaluation today is the low quality of the language of evaluation. Our capacity to share meaning with others needs to be enlarged. All language is an approximation of the thought process. Most words and descriptions are simpler than the phenomena they represent.

REFERENCES

1. Stake, R. E.   The countenance of educational evaluation. *Teachers Coll. Rec.* 68:529, 1967.
2. Stufflebeam, D. L.   Toward a science of educational evaluation. *Educ. Techn.* 8:5, 1968.
3. Scriven, M.   The Methodology of Evaluation. In A. B. Smith [Ed.], *Perspectives of Curriculum Evaluation.* Chicago: Rand McNally, 1967. P. 41.
4. Macdonald, J. B., Anderson, D. W., and May, F. B.   *Strategies of Curriculum Development.* Columbus: Merrill, 1965. P. 119.
5. Good, C. V.   *A Dictionary of Education.* New York: McGraw Hill, 1959. Pp. 75, 121, 299, 372, 435, 440, 449, 494, 556–565.
6. Stake, R. E.   Language, Rationality and Assessment. In W. H. Beatty [Ed.], *Improving Educational Assessment and An Inventory of Affective Behaviors.* Washington, D.C.: Association for Supervision and Curriculum Development, National Education Association, 1969. P. 23.

SUPPLEMENTARY READINGS

Dressel, P. L., and Mayhew, L. B.   *General Education Exploration in Evaluation.* Washington, D.C.: American Council on Education, 1954.

Finn, J. D.   Institutionalization of evaluation. *Educ. Techn.* 9:14, 1969.

Hastings, J. T.   Curriculum evaluation: The whip of the outcomes. *J. Educ. Measurement* 3:27, 1966.

Leeper, R. R. [Ed.].   *Assessing and Using Curriculum Content.* Washington, D.C.: Association for Supervision and Curriculum Development, National Education Association, 1965.

Lumsdaine, A. A.   Assessing the Effectiveness of Instructional Programs. In R. Glaser [Ed.], *Teaching Machines and Programed Learning, II, Data and Directions.* Washington, D.C.: National Education Association, 1965.

Macdonald, J. B., Anderson, D. W., and May, F. B.   *Strategies of Curriculum Development.* Columbus: Merrill, 1965.

Metfessel, N. S., and Michael, W. B.   A paradigm involving multiple criterion measures for the evaluation of the effectiveness of school programs. *Educ. Psychol. Measurement* 27:931, 1967.

Stufflebeam, D. L.   A depth study of the evaluation requirement. *Theory into Practice* 5:121, 1966.

Stufflebeam, D. L.   Toward a science of educational evaluation. *Educ. Techn.* 8:5, 1968.

Tyler, R. W.   *Basic Principles of Curriculum and Instruction.* Chicago: University of Chicago Press, 1950.

Tyler, R. W.   Assessing the progress of education. *Phi Delta Kappan* 47:13, 1965.

Tyler, R., Gagné, R., and Scriven, M. *Perspectives of Curriculum Evaluation.* Chicago: Rand McNally, 1967.

Walbesser, H., and Carter, H. Some methodological considerations of curriculum. Evaluation research. *Educ. Leadership* 26:53, 1968.

Wilhelms, F. T. *Evaluation as Feedback and Guide.* Washington, D.C.: Association for Supervision and Curriculum Development, National Education Association, 1967.

IV THE INSTRUCTIONAL PROCESS

13 THE NATURE OF INSTRUCTION

THE instructional process involves both instruction and teaching. Although these terms are frequently used interchangeably, some difference in meaning is noted and described. *Instruction* refers to the broad range of activities that take place in the classroom, laboratory, and clinical setting. The term includes both material and human resources and variables. Instruction is differentiated from teaching in that instruction encompasses more of the situational elements. *Teaching* refers primarily to the human interaction between teacher and student. Further exploration of instruction and teaching, the relation of these processes to learning, the nature and development of theories of instruction and teaching, and efforts to study these phenomena are included in this chapter.

INSTRUCTION AND TEACHING

The process of instruction involves arranging the conditions of learning that are external to the learner so that the most efficient and effective learning can take place. These conditions need to be constructed in such a manner that each stage in the instructional process takes into account the previous acquired capabilities of the learner, the requirements for the retention of these capabilities, and the specific situational events needed for the next stage of learning. Instruction is an intricate, complex, and demanding activity. Instruction includes communicating verbally with the student for the purposes of informing her of what she is striving to achieve, noting what she already knows, directing her attention and activities, and guiding her thinking in certain directions. These events are planned and instituted for the purpose of establishing the appropriate external conditions for learning. Instruction involves the network of activities that are the heart of the educational process. Instruction is relatively easy to accomplish under those conditions in which a single teacher interacts with a single student. Instruction becomes increasingly more difficult when the teacher communicates with a group of students.

The purpose of instruction can be stated in terms of either the terminal behaviors it should generate or inferences about the kind of organismic development it should encourage. What should the student be like after her involvement in certain instructional activities? Siegel describes the instructional process as teaching, learning, and miscellaneous interpersonal processes occurring among persons other than teachers and learners [1]. Similarly, although the classroom, laboratory, and clinical units are environments for instruction, more remote environments that may affect instructional outcomes are the home, residence hall, and other extraclass settings. The participants in instruction include students, teachers, and ancillary participants—persons other than teacher and student.

The analysis of the instructional process is a part of the analysis of the learning process. Both processes involve much of the same kind of interaction between the organism (learner) and her environment. For learning of any kind to occur, certain conditions must be satisfied. Although there is not unanimous agreement as to what these conditions are, there is some evidence that certain behaviors can be acquired simply through the learner's observation of the environment. Other learned behaviors appear to require that the learner observe her environment, respond to it overtly, and then observe the effects of the response upon the environment.

The kind of learning commonly said to involve instruction appears traditionally to be defined in terms of two major characteristics: (1) the learner is presented with a formal subject matter to be mastered, and (2) learning is mediated by a specially qualified instructor.

The instructional process encompasses all situations involving the acquisition of the behavior viewed as the desired outcome of instruction. This process may sometimes be spontaneous or accidental and may involve unintentional learning. There is an intended subject matter or content of instruction, and there may be also an unintentional content accompanying the intentional content. A nursing student can come to appreciate a certain area of nursing because of her instructor's enthusiasm for her subject.

Sometimes the instructional process is carefully rehearsed or proceeds according to some predetermined plan, such as a demonstration of a specific nursing procedure or technique. Sometimes the instructional process involves only the learner and her environment, as in the case of the student providing nursing care to a specific patient. More frequently the process is mediated by another person (an instructor) or by the instructor's surrogate (textbook, programmed text). Sometimes the process involves a single person, sometimes a group. Sometimes the process prepares the learner for immediate practical interaction with the environment, such as learning to manage a patient with a particular physical disability. At other times the process prepares the learner for contingencies remote in time, space, and probability, such as learning to manage a group of people in a community during a disaster in an effort to prevent the occurrence and spread of a communicable disease.

Learning and instruction deal with the interaction of the individual with her environment. To the extent that instruction, even when presented to a group, prepares the individual to observe her environment and the consequences of alternative responses to the environment, it would be expected to be successful. Two kinds of instruction are identified by Jahnke, formal and informal [2]. *Formal instruction* refers to that which occurs in the typical American classroom. Its primary objective is usually to communicate a particular formalized content. The content is usually verbal and is mediated by an instructor or her surrogate. While these characteristics apply to the usual classroom as it is known today, they may not apply to the classroom of the future. Some of the techniques are in need of critical examination with respect to their effectiveness in facilitating instruction. Skinner has observed that there is a lack of skillful programs for presenting the content of formal instruction [3]. He indicates that some features of classroom conduct are inconsistent with some of the best known principles of the behavioral sciences. Skinner has noted that the reinforcers used in the classrooms, such as grades, diplomas, and social approval, are weak and unnatural [4]. He has maintained that reinforcers are not used often enough or promptly enough and that classroom behavior is too frequently controlled by essentially aversive techniques.

The content of *informal instruction* is idiosyncratic in the sense that what the learner carries away from her observation of the environment cannot be predicted and frequently is not communicated verbally. Informal instruction does not require the participation of a specially qualified instructor; it frequently involves an interaction only between the learner and her environment. Self-instruction, in the sense of learning from one's own experience, is an example of informal instruction. Many basic perceptual, motor, and social skills learned informally during infancy and early childhood are the foundations upon which formal classroom instruction builds at a later period in time.

Teaching implies action or behavior. Because teaching depends on one or more human beings functioning in an interaction process, it requires the continuous adjustment of behavior. When teaching is viewed as an interactive process, the context, methods, materials, media, and evaluation of teaching gain a new vitality. They become means by which a teacher creates conditions that help students to learn. Teaching becomes the translation of knowledge—knowledge about the subject, about students, about learning and teaching—into action through a personal teaching style.

A fundamental premise of education is that behavior can be changed and improved. One of the essentials for the improvement of teaching behavior is to have an opportunity for the kind of analysis of teaching that will help prospective teachers learn behaviors which will in turn produce effective learning experiences for students. Teaching, as a dimension of instruction, has been studied and analyzed by authorities in the field from different frames of reference.

TEACHING—A SYSTEM OF ACTIONS

Teaching is defined by Smith as a system of actions intended to induce learning [5]. The comprehensiveness of this definition suggests that teaching is everywhere the same, irrespective of the cultural content in which it occurs. Teaching actions may be performed differently from culture to culture or from one individual to another within the same culture, depending upon the state of knowledge about teaching and the teacher's knowledge and skill. Teaching actions are varied in form and content; however, they are related to the behavior of students whose actions in turn are related to those of the teacher. Learning occurs as a result of the execution of these actions and the interactions of teacher and student. A theoretical conception of teaching includes all the actions of teachers necessary to explain and predict the behavior of students, but the occurrence of learning through such explaining and predicting cannot be made from these actions alone. These actions which constitute teaching take place in an environment of social factors (mores, organizational structures, cultural resources) and physical objects and persons. A pedagogical model adapted from Smith's concept of teaching presents all the

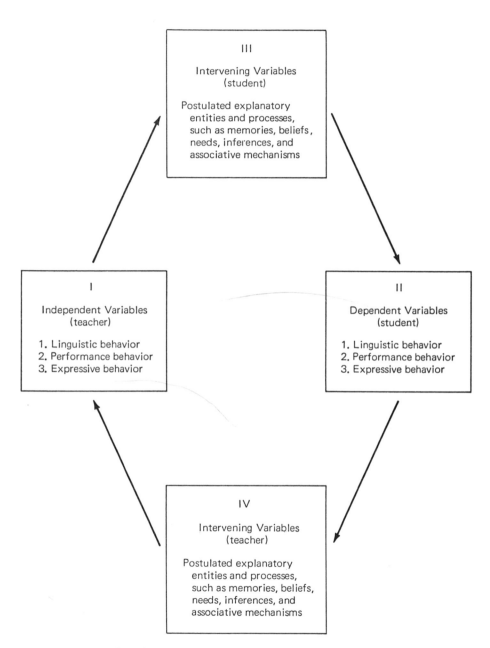

DIAGRAM 10.   A pedagogical model of teaching. (Adapted from B. O. Smith, A Concept of Teaching. In B. Bandman and R. S. Guttchen [Eds.], *Philosophical Essays on Teaching*. Philadelphia: Lippincott, 1969, p. 11.)

variables involved in and related to the actions that make up teaching (Diagram 10). These can be classified into four categories, but the teaching actions belong to only one of these. The categories include the (1) independent variables, (2) dependent variables, (3) intervening variables pertaining to students, and (4) intervening variables pertaining to the teacher. The actions of teaching belong to the first of these.

Learning, as achievement, is an intervening variable. The index of its presence is student behavior, and this behavior is a dependent variable. The teacher can see the student's behavior, but she cannot observe interests, motives, needs, and beliefs. These psychological entities and processes are inferred from student behavior. The teacher may infer from the reactions of the student that the student is interested and motivated to learn. The model also shows that the student's action brings into operation intervening variables in the teacher. These variables in turn lead to teacher actions, and at this point the cycle begins again. In this way, the process of teaching is continued until the teacher believes that the student has achieved what the teacher intended or that it is not profitable to continue teaching at the moment.

Teaching, according to this scheme, implies someone to give instruction as well as someone to take it. If the student is working on an out-of-class project, she is no doubt learning, but no teaching is going on. Teaching acts can occur, however, without the physical presence of students. A teacher giving a lecture or a demonstration over a television network is not in the physical presence of students. In this instance the teacher is probably directing her teaching behavior to a generalized student group. Classroom teaching usually involves more than one student, and the teacher's perception of student behavior is likely to be some sort of generalized picture of the general state of the class as a whole. Her actions are more likely to be shaped by those general considerations and by her habits than by the psychological requirements of any one student.

Teaching acts consist largely of verbal behavior in what is done with and to the student. The fact that language is the primary medium of teaching is not as important as the things done with language. If educators are to understand teaching, they must know what the actions are that are performed linguistically. It may be assumed that changes in the effectiveness of teaching will follow upon changes in the execution of such verbal actions. Smith describes the verbal and nonverbal actions that the teacher takes and the corresponding student actions in relation to the independent and dependent variables in teaching.

I. Independent variables—teacher actions
  A. Actions that the teacher performs with language
    1. Logically relevant actions
      a. Defining—rules for using words
      b. Classifying—putting something in a category
      c. Explaining—accounting for a state of affairs or an event
      d. Conditional inferring—the consequence, effect, or outcome of a set of actions
      e. Valuating—rating some object, expression, event, or action
      f. Designating—identifying something by name, word, or symbol
    2. Directive actions
      a. Tells student what to do in the performance of an operation or skill
      b. Gives direction in which student will move
    3. Admonitory acts
      a. Praises, commends
      b. Blames, reprimands
  B. Nonverbal actions
    1. Performance actions—may be accompanied by verbal behavior
      a. Serve to show, rather than to tell something to students
      b. Facilitates the learning of something else
    2. Expressive behavior—posture, facial expression, tone of voice, expression of eyes
      a. Are not usually purposeful nor addressed to anyone in particular
      b. Taken by students as signs of the psychological state of the teacher
II. Dependent variables—student actions
  A. Parallel the independent variables, but the purpose is different—student's purpose is not to teach but to bear witness that she is taking instruction
  B. Directive verbal behavior of student occurs on occasion when she plays the role of teacher, as chairman of class discussion
  C. Admonishing behavior—classroom conventions do not usually permit the student to praise, blame, or advise the teacher with respect to her work
  D. Performance behavior—student practices actions herself rather than to instruct anyone, that is, student practices a nursing procedure

E. Expressive behavior—smile, frown, or slump is not intended to communicate, but it functions as a sign to the teacher about feelings, ideas, and intentions [6]

Teaching is described by Smith in terms of functions of teacher behavior, verbal and nonverbal. Teacher behavior may be directed to an individual, group, or large class. The verbal and nonverbal behavior of teachers is the language of responsible actions designed to influence the behavior of students.

TEACHING—AS DECISION-MAKING

It is clear that there is a difference between seeing effective teaching in terms of the qualities and behaviors of the person *per se* and considering effectiveness in teaching as the result of dynamic interactions between a number of vital aspects of the teaching-learning situation and a teacher. If teaching may be described as decision-making in interaction, then the product of the teacher's decision is the response she makes to the individual with whom she is interacting. Herrick identifies the decision-making aspects of the teaching situation:

1. Objects found in the teaching situation
   a. Dynamic, purposeful human beings who have personalities, goal perceptions, and self-concepts. These human beings can be further divided into four levels: (1) teachers and learners, (2) supervisors and administrators, (3) parents and other adults with primary relation to the student, and (4) other adults (nurses, physicians, social workers)
   b. Objects devised to contain and develop educational programs, such as textbooks, films, and teaching machines
   c. Objects not specifically designated to convey educational programs—classroom furniture and equipment
2. Geographic space and structure—Teaching always takes place somewhere and demands space and some arrangement of objects in this space.
3. Social structure—power structure and related authority or prestige roles played by teacher and student. Structure relates to other social systems that make up the school relationship of one class to another, the relationship of a course to the curriculum, and the relationship of the curriculum to other school activities (social and recreational activities).
4. A communication system—the methods and procedures for communi-

cating ideas, needs, interests, and aspirations of the various human beings in the system

5. Educational structure—the educational plans that include the objectives, curriculum areas, teaching plans, and instructional strategies [7]

Teaching is seen as a complex act. It is concerned primarily with efficient achievement of educational objectives and involves the responsible decision-making and action of a teacher. It takes place in different kinds of social-physical settings and can be motivated by different educational rationales.

The model of teaching as decision-making suggests some characteristics and requirements of teaching behavior. Teaching requires appropriate responsiveness to the data the individual and group are contributing to the situation. The searching and exploring activities of individuals or groups can be rewarded in this way. Teaching requires a progressive reduction in the controlling functions exercised by the teacher. Growth in the student obtains when the teacher allows her to pursue pathways that are not structured by the teacher. Teaching requires that the classroom be well managed so that the activity of learning may receive full attention. Teaching requires that the environment be accepting of and supportive to each individual. Rapport is built through empathy and support from one who is a significant person in another's life. When people have a chance to talk and listen to one another, common problems, concerns, and agreements evolve. The concept of teaching as decision-making emphasizes the roles of teachers and students in relating action to the objectives toward which they are working.

RELATIONSHIP BETWEEN TEACHING AND LEARNING

There is some question whether learning must result if the teacher's actions are to be called *teaching*. Most definitions of teaching keep teaching and learning apart, that is, teaching is seen as an attempt to bring about learning. Some definitions make teaching dependent on the successful outcome called *learning*, that is, if there is no learning, there is no teaching. Most educators accept the former notion. Nevertheless, the research and writings of some teachers reflect the latter. Indeed, the relation between teaching and learning remains unsettled. It is not known exactly how teaching contributes to or causes learning. Part of the problem is that there is confusion as to which learning is being talked about and just what constitutes learning.

Learning as a subject of scientific study embraces more than what goes on in schools. It is the process by which an activity originates or is changed through reacting to an encountered situation, provided the change cannot be explained on the basis of growth and development or temporary states of the organism (for example, fatigue or reactions to drugs) [8]. Learning is considered to occur in all areas of life, not merely in the formal educational setting. The effects of propaganda, psychotherapy, child-rearing, social groups, and teachers are seen as forms of learning. One readily concedes that advertisers, psychotherapists, parents, and discussion group leaders may be viewed as teachers. Ordinary discourse restricts the term *teaching* to school situations.

A position that some psychologists take implies that if the teacher has an adequate theory of learning, then she must act upon that theory. The teacher, if she is to produce learning, must do what the theory of learning stipulates as necessary for learning to occur, or as Gage says, teaching must be a kind of "mirror image" of learning [9]. It is a recognized fact that teaching does not always produce learning, and that learning occurs in situations where there is no teaching.

Gowen, utilizing the framework provided by Gilbert Ryle in his book *The Concept of Mind,* relates the terms teaching and learning to the language used to describe tasks and achievements [10]. The language of doing is different from the language of achievement, which is the outcome of a process. Achievements are recognition that certain episodic performances have come to a close and are judged endings in experience. Some judgment is made denoting achievement, which takes into account factors over and above the doing. It appears that there are words implying process and words implying outcomes. The criterion by which achievements, or outcomes, are distinguished from something directly given, or process, is to be found in the judgment of the relation between means and end. The end of the process may not be the aim of the process. Therefore, it is necessary to analyze achievements in terms of means-end relations.

"Teach" is seen as a task word, and "learn" is the parallel achievement word. Achievement words signify occurrences or episodes, and some achievement verbs express a continued process. Task verbs always signify some sort of activity or extended proceedings. It is acceptable to state that the task teach is performed skillfully, carefully, successfully, or ineffectively. One may speak of teaching successfully but not of learning successfully. The verb teach signifies proceedings between two or more individuals, involving some sort of deliberation with adjustment of mutual claims and interests in expectation that some result will ensue. Without interaction there can be neither teacher nor student. Teaching is the process for which the true ending has to be a judgment about another process—learning.

Another notion presented by Gowen indicates that teaching is the task for which learning is the outcome. Teaching would have "learn" as an outcome, but the student apparently would not be an active participant in the learning process. "Learn" is not an activity in this analysis, but rather it is the judged ending to a process. It seems that if one tries to specify the relation between teaching and learning using this analysis, he becomes aware that teaching is independent of the student's effort and activity in learning.

In an effort to clarify the relation of teaching to learning, Gowen offers the notion "thirdness." He describes thirdness as "the triadic relation existing between a sign, its object and the interpreting thought" [11]. In this instance the teacher puts forth an idea, diagram, or proposition, and the student responds to the idea, diagram, or proposition. From the teacher's standpoint, there is a conception about the thing (idea, diagram, etc.) not only in its relationship to the teacher but also as a thing capable of being grasped by the student. Similarly the student responds to the idea or diagram in a way that is a function of the teacher's relationship to the thing. Meaning is the distinctive quality of behavior in relation to things, so that a response to another's act involves a response to the thing as entering into the other's behavior. It is in this sense that thirdness accounts for meaning. To teach is to deliberately change the meaning of experience. Teaching need not result in immediate behavior change. If meaning is changed, then the student would act as if her experience had changed. Dimensions of changes are as broad as the dimensions of meaning.

Gagné describes the relation of teaching to learning in a concise manner by stating that there are two broad classes of variables that influence learning, those within the learner and those in the learning situation [12]. These sets of variables undoubtedly have interactive effect upon learning. The external variables cannot exert their effect without the presence in the learner of certain states of motivation, prior learning, and development. Nor can the internal capabilities themselves generate learning without the stimulation provided by external events. The learning problem is that of finding the necessary relationship that must obtain among the internal and external variables in order for change in capability to take place. Teaching as one of the external variables affects and is effected by the internal variables or the characteristics of the learner. From Gagné's point of view learning and teaching are constantly interacting and interdependent.

THEORIES OF TEACHING AND INSTRUCTION

Theories of learning have been formulated and have been subjected to some experimental verification. Most frequently these experiments have been conducted in controlled laboratory settings utilizing animal subjects. Teachers have experienced difficulty in making direct application of learning theories to the practical problems of teaching and instruction. The conditions of learning in the laboratory bear little resemblance to conditions in the typical classroom environment. Theories of learning do not appear to provide useful theoretical guidelines for teaching and instruction.

If adequate theories of learning were available, theories of teaching would not be needed. Teachers need to know how students learn and how they depend on motivation, readiness, and reinforcement. Teachers also need to know how to teach and motivate students, assess their readiness, act on assessment, present the subject, maintain discipline, and shape a cognitive structure. Theories of teaching would make explicit how teachers behave, why they behave as they do, and with what effects. While theories of learning deal with the ways in which a person influences an organism, theories of teaching deal with the ways in which a person influences an organism to learn. Although theories of learning are necessary to the understanding of prediction and control of the learning process, they cannot suffice in education. The goal of education—to produce learning in the most desirable and efficient way possible—would seem to require an additional theory of teaching.

Gage identifies some reasons for the lack of theories of teaching:

1. The attempt to develop theories of teaching is seen by some persons as implying the development of a science or technology of teaching. This notion is rejected by some writers who indicate that one should not attempt to eliminate the phenomenal, idiosyncratic, and artistic aspects from teaching. Gage reacts to this concern by stating that although teaching requires artistry, it can be subjected to scientific scrutiny. The power to explain, predict, and control that may result from such scrutiny will not dehumanize teaching.

2. Learning theories have been presumed to be adequate for teaching. Theories of learning deal with what the learner does. Changes in education must depend upon what the teacher does. Changes occur in how learners go about the business of learning in response to the behavior of their teachers or others in the educational establishment [13].

Much of our knowledge about learning can be put into practice only by teachers. The ways in which these teachers put this knowledge into effect constitute part of the subject of theories of teaching. The implications drawn from learning theory must be translated into hunches about the behavior of teachers. Teachers will act on these hunches in ways to improve learning. Theories of teaching and the scientific study of teaching may enable teachers to make better use of their knowledge about teaching. Theories of teaching should be concerned with explaining, predicting, and controlling the ways in which teacher behavior affects the learning of students.

THE NATURE OF THEORY

Pursuant to further exploration of theories of teaching and instruction, some attention will be given to the nature and characteristics of theories.

A theory is a deductively connected set of laws. It is dependent upon having a series of broad generalizations about the phenomenon in question. These generalizations must be related to each other in a coherent pattern or system. Generalizations may also be called general facts, laws, or hypotheses. A theory, then, is comprised of general facts, laws, or hypotheses related to each other in a systematic, noncontradictory way. Therefore, the theory describes and explains the phenomenon to which it is addressed. The theory also serves as a means of predicting certain consequences in the phenomenon in view of certain given antecedents.

The necessary characteristics of a theory include the following:

1. Formal coherence, or systematic relationships, of the statements that comprise the theory
2. Observational verification—correspondence of the statements within the theory to that which can be experienced
3. Observational predictiveness—derivation of statements from the theory about what will happen in experience.

In any science the aim is to understand the phenomena studied. A phenomenon is understood when it can be accounted for by means of a set of principles that are sufficiently general to apply in various combinations to other phenomena. The principles are checked through testing the accuracy of predictions made from the principles. Finally, control may be achieved over the phenomena by appropriately using the principles. Theory becomes a summary of existing knowledge that provides an explanation for observed events and relationships and predicts the occurrence of as yet unobserved events on the basis of explanatory principles embodied in the theory. A theory is always held with some tentativeness, no matter how great the accumulation of findings consistent with theory. The theoretical explanations reduce a number of different phenomena to underlying general principles. The more diverse observations a theory can explain, the greater our confidence in using the general principles it embodies for the purposes of prediction. Theory increases the fruitfulness of research by providing significant leads for inquiry, by relating seemingly discrete findings, and by providing an explanation of observed relationships. The more research is directed by systematic theory, the more likely are its results to contribute directly to the development and further organization of knowledge.

The term *theory* has been misused in a variety of ways. Theory has been used to imply a nonpractical orientation, as in the statement, "She is a theoretical nurse." Also the term theory may convey the notion that a specific course was not useful because it was "too theoretical." A common use of the concept theory is as a synonym for speculation or supposition; for example, "It is my theory that students do better with limited controls placed upon them." Finally, the term theory is used to express a series of "oughts," that is, a set of rules that tells us how to perform certain functions.

Merton, in referring to sociological theory, has identified the several distinct activities carried on by sociologists [14]. Although he describes these activities in relation to the subject matter of sociology, the approach and process of theory development are applicable to other scientific endeavors.

METHODOLOGY

Sociologists and others engaged in scientific work must be methodologically oriented. They must be aware of the design of investigations, the nature of inference, and the requirements of a theoretical system. Theoretical and empirical inquiries should be guided by a concern for the logic of procedures. Merton observes that as a discipline matures, less direct attention typically is paid to the details of procedures and their justifications. All too frequently the methods of a mature science are taken as methodological prototypes by a fledgeling discipline, with little attention to the difference in research experiences of the disciplines. The implication here is that education, and more specifically teaching, may need to develop its own methodologies for investigation different from those of the natural sciences.

GENERAL ORIENTATION

The chief function of the orientation is to provide a general context for inquiry and to facilitate the process of forming hypotheses that are congruent with the general orientation. The general orientation indicates the relevance of some structural variables. The orientation of inquiry into teaching suggests variables for consideration that are different from the variables presented by other types of human phenomena.

ANALYSES OF CONCEPTS

The specific concepts identified by a discipline do not constitute theory, but they do enter into a theoretical system. When these concepts are related in an orderly scheme, theory begins to emerge. Concepts constitute the definitions of what is to be observed. They are the variables between which empirical relationships are to be sought. The selection of concepts used to guide the collection and analysis of data is crucial to empirical inquiry. A function of conceptual clarification is to make explicit the character of data subsumed under a concept. The concept "reinforcement," which is frequently found in educational literature, requires defining and description to determine which instances of reinforcement are to be included and which are not. The concept defines the situation, and the research worker responds accordingly.

EMPIRICAL GENERALIZATIONS

Empirical generalizations are isolated propositions summarizing uniformities of relationship between two or more variables. Generalizations of this nature may be of greater or lesser precision, but this does not affect their place in the structure of inquiry. The theoretical task and the orientation of empirical research toward theory begin when the bearing of such uniformities on a set of interrelated propositions is tentatively established. Empirical inquiry is so organized that if empirical uniformities are discovered, they have direct consequences for a theoretical system. Nursing education is full of generalizations that have not been assimilated into educational theory. An example of a generalization might be that among nursing students who have difficulty in conceptualizing, the larger number comes from culturally deprived environments. The two variables entering into a relationship are inability to conceptualize and culturally deprived environments. The relationship between these variables must be sought in relation to many types of conceptual learning tasks before it can become a part of the theoretical system.

INTERPRETATIONS AFTER THE FACT

There are instances in which data are collected and then subjected to interpretive analysis. The observations may be recorded in nursing-care studies in which the interpretations are made after the observations have been noted rather than through the empirical testing of a predesignated hypothesis. The implicit assumption underlying this activity indicates that a body of generalized propositions has been established that can be applied to the data at hand. Explanations of the data are consistent with the set of observations, since only those hypotheses that do accord with the observations are selected. Explanations after the fact remain at the level of plausibility rather than being "compelling evidence" on which to base a decision to use one of the methods studied. The absence of a high degree of confirmation stems from the failure to provide distinctive tests of the interpretations apart from their consistency with the initial observations.

Observation of performance is the primary technique for obtaining information about the student's competency in the practice of nursing. Although this method of securing relevant information is obviously necessary, it may not produce all the information needed to make inferences. The student may execute certain nursing activities in an appropriate manner, and we infer that her practice is based on scientific principles or concepts. In some instances when the student carries out activities in a way that is considered acceptable, she may not be able to describe the scientific rationale for her actions. Then another procedure must be used to obtain this information to assist educators in making more accurate inferences. The most useful one is the clinical conference, which provides opportunity for teachers to confirm their interpretations about the student's performance.

SCIENTIFIC THEORY

Another type of generalization is the so-called scientific law. The place of these generalizations in theory illustrates the function of theory. It indicates that theoretical relevance is not inherent in empirical generalizations but appears when the generalization is conceptualized in higher-order abstractions. An isolated uniformity might be illustrated by the generalization that teaching microbiology prior to teaching basic clinical nursing facilitates the learning of nursing practice. An abstraction of a higher order might be stated as the sequence of instruction influencing the effectiveness of learning.

After establishing the theoretical relevance of a uniformity, effort is directed to accumulating both theory and research findings. Reformulation of the empirical uniformity gives rise to various consequences in fields of conduct remote from the initial focus. Inquiries into motivation, reading ability, and previous background experiences of students may be related to the problems of learning. The successive exploration of implications increases the usefulness of research.

If theory is to be fruitful, it must be precise, in other words, it must be testable. Verified predictions derived from a theory do not prove or demonstrate that theory. They do, however, supply a measure of confirmation. It is always possible that alternative hypotheses drawn from different theoretical systems (such as in the example given, motivation theory) can account for the observed phenomena. Theories that permit precise predictions and are confirmed by observation take on strategic importance, since they provide an initial basis for choice among competing hypotheses.

The activities that comprise theory development seem to be applicable to the development of theories of instruction and teaching.

THEORIES OF INSTRUCTION

Theories of instruction must be related to scientific data rather than only to data from personal experience. Such theories will consist of propositions relating conditions of learning to the extent to which objectives are achieved. The statements will have to refer to variables demonstrably related to the achievement of various objectives excluding student characteristics, tasks (learning), and teacher characteristics.

A useful theory of instruction is a statement of empirically established ways of achieving a great range of different goals. The user of such a theory will decide what goals she wishes to achieve and refer to the theory to determine the best ways to achieve her goals. The theory of instruction itself would not specify what goals should be achieved and hence could be used by those who subscribe to fundamentally different educational philosophies.

Scientific theories are empirically based. For each statement in the theory, there must be data from which it is derived, and the data must be reproducible. The data are linked to the propositions of the theory through a set of protocols that precisely summarize the data. Protocols must have a precision which places them largely above dispute before they can be used as the foundation for deriving theoretical statements. In order to be of value as protocols, there must be no doubt about what is meant by the terms used. In the statement "positive motivation facilitates the learning of a specific nursing task," there must be precise definition of what is meant by positive motivation. If there is any ambiguity in the term, there is no basis for comparing the results of one study with those of others. Lack of comparability between the definitions used in different studies is a common problem in classroom and clinical studies. It is much less of a problem in experimental research in the laboratory, where the apparatus available defines the situation with considerable precision. Attempts to provide operational definition by alluding to educational situations do not always provide completely unambiguous statements. Completely unambiguous operational definitions of basic terms are rarely found outside the experimental sciences. The definition of terms used in communicating educational research lack the precision of definitions achieved in experimental sciences, but the level of precision could still be vastly better than it has been in the past. A theory of instruction can be no more clear and unambiguous than the protocols on which it is based.

FUNCTIONS OF INSTRUCTIONAL THEORY

The value of an instructional theory can be determined by the amount of theory-based research carried on in both laboratory and classroom that elucidates and quantifies the relationships among the variables presented in the definition. Other functions of instructional theory include the following:

1. Theory construction forces the theory builder to bring together in a concise form the knowledge that is currently available—to review carefully what is known and to separate that knowledge from both tenuous speculation and the body of ambiguous findings.

2. Theory replaces the large number of protocols found in supporting studies with a relatively few generalizations that are inductive inferences from them, and it leads to better predictions and control.

3. In this way the development of theory simplifies the communication of knowledge that has been acquired.

4. Scientific theory based on the known is a guide for the exploration of the unknown.

The immediate approaches of the teacher in a classroom tend to be primarily intuitive. There is no reason, however, why that intuition cannot be grounded in instructional theory learned by the teacher. An instructional theory stands outside the teacher and specifies the teacher as one of the inter-acting set of variables. As such, the teacher cannot invoke this or that theory of instruction at a given moment because she is a variable in the situation. However, she can be sensitized to the total instructional situation, including goal, student, and the characteristics of the instructional setting.

In instructional process there is the stage of planning where instructional theory can be injected. This is the time when the teacher is planning her in-structional strategies. A theory of instruction can specify a set of relationships between student behavior and aspects of the instructional setting other than teacher behavior. Under these conditions the teacher might be able to use the theory consciously in a preoperational planning stage to manipulate the nonteacher variables such as those related to media, sequence, level of ab-straction, length of time, class size, and organization.

CRITERIA FOR ASSESSING INSTRUCTIONAL THEORIES

The Commission on Instructional Theory has developed criteria for as-sessing the formal properties of theories of instruction [15]. These criteria in-clude the following:

1. A statement of an instructional theory should include a set of postulates and definitions of terms involved in these postulates.
   A. Student characteristics must be specified together with their relation-ship to goals. The characteristics must be demonstrably related to learn-ing. These characteristics include biosocial variables such as age, sex, social class, and level of physical maturity; and psychological variables such as, level of intellectual development, academic achievement, cog-nitive style, self-concept, and achievement motivation.
   B. The characteristics of the instructional situation must be specified to-gether with the relationship they have to goals. The situational charac-teristics include:
      1. Organizational variables, such as time, space, class size, and class composition
      2. Content variables, such as tasks, media, and sequence
      3. Teacher personality, such as warmth, openness, and control style
      4. Teacher behavior variables, including the acts the teacher is directed to perform and management techniques
   The characteristics of the instructional situation must be specified to-gether with their relationship to student characteristics.

    C. Goal characteristics should be dimensionalized.

        Objectives should be described in terms of change with respect to specific dimensions. The outcomes should be specified along a scale. These outcomes are describable as performances on a task. A task specifies the kinds of actions that have to be undertaken to reach a goal. These objectives must take into account the student variables.

    D. A change in student characteristics leads to change in instructional situation characteristics. This change must be observable and be described.

    2. The statement of instructional theory should make explicit the boundaries of its concern and the limitations under which it is proposed. Theories that are stated generally lose their relevance by trying to incorporate the universe. What is proposed must be encompassed by a description of bounds or the theory begins to leak, either because too many factors are uncontrolled or because the theory has to be stretched beyond reason to embrace the growing examples of deviant phenomena.

    3. A theoretical construction must have internal consistency—a logical set of interrelationships.

    4. An instructional theory should be congruent with empirical data, that is, the propositions of the theory should be properly derived from the data on which they are based. The statement of the theory should be properly documented so that the reader can go back and examine the protocols and the data on which protocols are based.

    5. An instructional theory must be capable of generating testable hypotheses. The postulates have to be stated in such a way that hypotheses are clearly suggested.

    6. An instructional theory must contain generalizations that go beyond the data. Unless links can be made between the findings of a particular investigation and those of other investigations, the work does not lend itself to prediction. The accumulated bits and pieces of empirical studies have utility only when they can be woven into a set of generalizations at a higher level of abstraction than the conclusions themselves.

    7. An instructional theory must be verifiable.

    8. An instructional theory must not only explain past events but also must be capable of predicting future events.

    9. At the present time, instructional theories may be expected to represent qualitative synthesis. Ultimately, a theory should be expressed in terms of quantitative relationships among variables.

CURRENT STATUS OF INSTRUCTIONAL THEORY

This review of the requirements of instructional theory and of the general approaches to the development of theory gives some indication of the current status of instructional theory. The characteristics of theory help to clarify the nature of present descriptive studies of instruction. Attempting to develop descriptive classifications rather than correlational or casual data, the researcher may identify a series of behaviors exhibiting common characteristics; group such behaviors into one category because of their common characteristics; and designate the category by some term with appropriate connotations, such as "opining," "integrative," or "controlling." The researcher may have as many of these categories as he deems necessary to handle his data. Such categories and their labels are the concepts invented by the researcher.

It is concepts that generally distinguish one field of knowledge from another. Concepts are said to be meaningful if they are sufficiently defined in terms of the observable characteristics or descriptive features they designate. Concepts are significant only when they are connected with other concepts, that is, when they enter into generalization or laws. For example, the connection between the concept "reinforcement" and the concept "retention of learning" may be stated as a generalization: reinforcement facilitates the retention of learning. The discovery of connections between concepts is not the intent of descriptive studies. The significance of concepts resulting from such studies is dependent upon subsequent investigations.

The time is overdue for investigators to stop arguing whether one mode of presentation is as good as another and to undertake instead investigations of those conditions thought to optimize the realization of educational objectives. Such investigations require precision in conceptualizing the purposes of education and the settings or learning environments that may be provided to accomplish these purposes. From a practical standpoint, the relative importance of objectives within the cognitive, affective, and psychomotor domains have significant implications for structuring the learning environments. The view of the classroom as an environment for transmitting knowledge is in contrast to the view that cognitive accomplishments depend upon affective involvement for behavior modification. The former position suggests that the learner is a manipulatable object to whom something is done by the teacher and her resources. The latter stresses the importance of "independent discovery" and leads to a view of teaching and learning in which teacher and learner roles are reversed.

Lectures or televised courses may tend to dispense more information; seminar courses may tend to encourage more student involvement and participation. But some students may become vitally involved in lecture courses, while certain students remain personally uninvolved even in seminar classes. The observation that students respond differently even when exposed to an apparently uniform instructional environment calls attention to the heterogeneity inherent in such gross categories as lecture, seminar, televised class, or conventional class. These designations are predicated primarily upon aspects of the physical environment in which the course is conducted, neglecting variations within each condition. Gross comparisons between conditions so designated tend to neglect factors other than classroom environment that also bear upon teaching and learning.

Siegel and Siegel have described the instructional gestalt as a paradigm of instructional variables conceptualizing the formal educational process in a broad framework [16]. Appropriate attention is given to the variety of instructional settings, teaching procedures, simultaneously exposed learners, and multiple criteria of effectiveness, without sacrificing either the essential flavor of the instructional process or the specificity of its conditions.

Instruction may be thought of as the institution and arrangement of external conditions of learning in ways that will bring out the internal capabilities of the learners. Instruction thus deals with manipulation of the conditions of learning situations by commanding attention, by presenting essential stimuli, and by giving verbal directions to the learner. Theories of instruction will explain how conditions may be controlled in relation to the specific learners involved in the instructional process.

THEORIES OF TEACHING

Descriptive studies of teaching are essential prerequisites to subsequent investigation; no studies as yet yield the broad predictive generalizations that are the long-range goals of inquiry into teaching. Descriptive studies do not provide principles and generalizations, which are useful in the control and resolution of teaching problems. They can only help the teacher classify elements of teaching and thereby better understand the teaching process.

There is need for continued study of teaching, with the goal of producing theories of teaching that will allow teacher education to assume the characteristics of a discipline—a discipline inextricably tied to the improvement of practice in its enterprise. Koerner indicated that "education as an academic discipline has poor credentials. Relying on other fields, especially psychology, for its principle substance, it has not yet developed a corpus of knowledge and technique of sufficient scope and power to warrant the field's being given full academic status" [17].

There have been varied attempts to study teaching. A substantial proportion of past studies has been directed at appraising qualities or some aspect of teaching performance. Such studies fall short of contributing broad, predictive generalizations about teaching. Biddle and Ellena state that "few, if any, facts are now deemed established about teacher effectiveness, and many former 'findings' have been repudiated. It is not an exaggeration to say that we do not today know how to select, train for, encourage or evaluate teacher effectiveness" [18].

Researchers have differed in the kinds of inquiry they believe could be legitimately designated as research on teaching. Because teachers engage in a variety of activities other than the direct contact with students, such as faculty committee work and administrative functions, questions are raised as to whether these activities should be the forms of inquiry. The *Handbook of Research on Teaching* gave attention to three categories of variables: (1) teaching methods, (2) instruments and media of teaching, and (3) teacher's personality and characteristics [19]. Research on teaching, as described by the contributing authors, is aimed at (1) identifying and measuring variables in the behavior and characteristics of teachers, (2) discovering the antecedents or determiners of these central variables, and (3) discovering the consequences or effects of these variables. Other variables that relate to antecedents, consequences, or concomitants of the central variables were referred to as relevant variables. Two clusters of relevant variables include social interaction in the classroom and social background of teaching, both of which affect teacher behavior. Site variables are those that are held constant and characterize the situation in which other variables are studied. The site variables considered in these studies are grade level and subject matter [20].

For purposes of these endeavors, the authors propose definitions of teaching and research. Teaching is defined as any interpersonal influence aimed at changing the ways in which other persons can or will behave. The influence has to impinge on the other person through his perceptual and cognitive processes, through his ways of getting meaning out of objects and events of which his senses make him aware. How the other person can or will behave refers to his capabilities for maximum performance, such as habits or attitudes, that constitute the objectives of instruction. The behaviors and intervening variables mediating them may be classified in many ways, such as the cognitive, affective, and psychomotor domains of behavior [21].

Research is defined as an activity aimed at increasing our power to understand, predict, and control events of a given kind. All of these goals involve relationships between events or variables, and research must seek out the relationship between variables. Research on teaching is defined as research in which at least one variable consists of a behavior or characteristic of teachers and leads to the development of teaching theory [22].

From this point of view, it is suggested that theory of teaching will consist of (1) a statement of the variables comprising teaching behavior, (2) formulation of the possible relations among the variables, and (3) hypotheses about the relations between the variables comprising teaching behavior and the variables descriptive of the psychological and social conditions within which teaching behavior occurs.

Teaching is also described as a system of actions that involve an agent, a situation, and an end in view. Within the situation there are certain variables over which the teacher has no control, such as the size of the classroom and the physical characteristics of students. Over other variables in the situation the teacher has direct control, and these become the means of teaching actions. These variables include the procedural and material means by which the teacher manipulates the subject matter and the instructional paraphernalia (material). The procedural means include large-scale maneuvers or strategies and small movements or episodes. The episodes are considered to be the tactile elements of strategies and are concerned with psychological and logical movements. The verbal exchange between two or more persons directed toward filling in the gaps with information make up the psychological episodes. These may be further described as reciprocating episodes, such as questions and answers, a unit of discourse, as in the monologue or lecture, and coordinating episodes or discussions among several persons. The logical episodes are described as rule-guided behavior and include such actions as defining, designating, classifying, and reporting [23]. Diagram 11 presents a model of the analysis of teaching.

Whatever approach to teaching is taken, the formulation of the possible relations among the variables identified and the statement of hypotheses about the relations between the variables become the subject and process of theory development in teaching. There appears to be some agreement that a single theory of teaching will not suffice to explain the variables concerned with the actions of teaching. Multiple theories of teaching will probably result

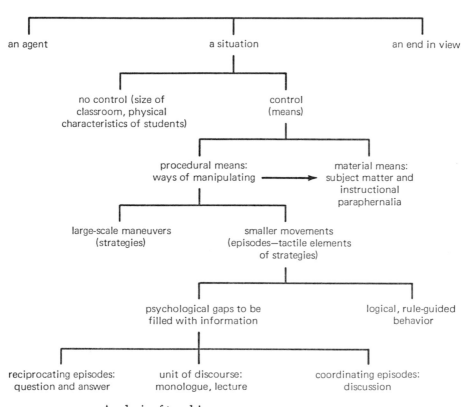

Teaching—A System of Actions Involving

DIAGRAM 11.   Analysis of teaching.

from the efforts of the researcher and theorists in education as they turn more of their attention to the examination of teaching itself. Each single theory of teaching will offer an explanation for limited aspects of teaching. The hypothesis for each theory will designate the independent and dependent variables and the relationship that exists between them. A statement of hypothesis might evolve according to the model suggested in Diagram 12.

The development of multiple theories of teaching will have significant impact upon teacher education and the enterprise of education in general. Such theories will result from cumulative, systematic inquiry into the nature of teaching. These theories will be comprised of related generalizations of a pre-

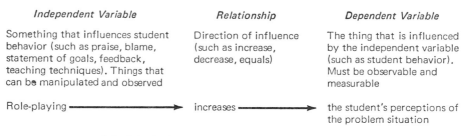

Independent Variable	Relationship	Dependent Variable
Something that influences student behavior (such as praise, blame, statement of goals, feedback, teaching techniques). Things that can be manipulated and observed	Direction of influence (such as increase, decrease, equals)	The thing that is influenced by the independent variable (such as student behavior). Must be observable and measurable
Role-playing ⟶	increases ⟶	the student's perceptions of the problem situation

DIAGRAM 12.   Model of a hypothesis.

dictive nature. The concepts, generalizations, and theories will constitute a body of knowledge with demonstrable power to describe, explain, and control various dimensions of teaching. Such knowledge ultimately will become the principal substantive content of the professional aspect of teacher education.

Research on the climate and activities of teaching makes a fundamental contribution to a theory of instruction. These contributions consist of identifying general patterns of teacher influence that produce predictable student responses and thus establish cause-and-effect principles.

RELATIONSHIP BETWEEN THEORY AND RESEARCH

Theory building and research are related activities, although they are not the same. Research follows and precedes theory. Research provides the means through which theories are tested, so in this sense it follows theoretical development. At the same time, research provides the information on which theories are based and by which they are modified and improved. In this sense, research precedes theories.

Research cannot exist at any advanced level without theory. There is no doubt, however, that a theory can exist without research and without any kind of direct evidence as to its validity. The value of such a theory is highly questionable. Unless a theory is subjected to empirical test through the research process, there is no way to judge its validity. The first requirement for a scientifically sound theory is that it be amenable to test and that such testing be performed. It must be possible to devise a situation in which the theory could be disproved, and the research process should be applied. Research, then, cannot exist without theory, and useful theory cannot exist without research. They are interdependent.

THE STUDY AND ANALYSIS OF TEACHING

In the absence of theories of teaching that have been subjected to test and validation, teachers and psychologists have endeavored to study and analyze teaching from several points of view. Some approaches to the study of teaching have been made, giving consideration to (1) the dynamics of the instructional group, (2) the classification of teacher statements, (3) interaction analysis of verbal and nonverbal behavior of students and teachers, and (4) the behavior of effective teachers. These approaches are identified and described because they appear to be representative of the current activities in this endeavor.

DYNAMICS OF INSTRUCTIONAL GROUPS

All groups, including the classroom group, have some characteristics in common. All groups have a common goal to achieve, they have participants who come together for the purpose of achieving the goal, the activities of the group are founded in some type of control or leadership, and the group has either implicit or explicit relationships with other groups. Although all groups have common characteristics, each group has certain unique characteristics. Getzels and Thelan have identified the unique characteristics of the classroom group [24]. The classroom group comes together for the purpose of learning. It becomes a planned situation where learning is held the primary concern for the group's being together. Not only is learning the prescribed objective of the classroom group, but also that which is to be learned and the means by which learning is to be accomplished are given. There is an implicit or explicit curriculum of instruction that specifies the desired outcomes and kinds of procedures to which both teachers and students must adhere.

The second unique feature of the classroom group is its membership. Participation in the classroom group is considered to some extent to be compulsory or mandatory. Membership in the group is determined by factors over which the student has little control. The composition of the group may be considered to be casual and haphazard. To the extent that the nature of the learning process is affected by the nature of social interaction, the compulsory and random selection of students will have an effect on what is learned, and the compulsory and random nature of the classroom group can be considered a distinctive feature of the classroom as a working group.

The third characteristic described by Getzels and Thelan is the nature of the control or leadership. This control and leadership is invested in the teacher. The authority is sanctioned by law and/or custom and is supported by the fact that the teacher is an expert, trained professionally to exercise authority. Most frequently the teacher is older, more mature, and presumably wiser than her students. Authority can be delegated for certain functions to the students, but such delegation does not occur without the teacher's permission. Students have little or no control over the selection of their leader; they normally have no recourse from her leadership, no influence on her method of leadership beyond that granted by her, and no power over the tenure of her leadership.

The classroom group is distinctive in the nature of its relationships to other groups and institutions. Any class is one link in a sequence, and what it may or may not do or what it must and must not do is defined as much by what other groups have done or can do as by what any particular class wants to do. In nursing the class in prevention of infections and communicable diseases is integrally related to the class in microbiology, and the class in social problems is very much a part of the class in prenatal care. On a single day the individual student is a member not solely of one classroom group but of several overlapping groups: a sociology group, a nursing group, a philosophy group, a literature group. She must accommodate herself to each group, and each group must be in tune with all other groups. Over and above the interacting participants in the classroom group, there are numerous other groups whose pressures and influences are felt but not seen directly. These include the peer group, the dormitory, sorority, and family group.

The multiple pressures that are exerted upon students are also felt by teachers. The teacher's situation may be even more complex, since conflicting expectations for her in the school, community, family, and profession are perhaps less clearly defined than they are for the students. The teacher seldom knows with certainty how to assess her work in relation to the expectation of the school, the profession, and the community.

The nature of the interaction between the school and other institutions in the community determines the extent to which the school will be an instrument for changing other institutions as distinguished from supporting them as they are. In certain kinds of interactions, the school can exist only to hand down that which is traditional, while under other conditions it can be at the forefront of change. There is nothing that goes on in the classroom that is not of ultimate consequence for the social order, and there is not much that is of immediate consequence for the social order that is not reflected in some way in the classroom. This places the teacher in a prime position for determining the classroom climate, the quality of leadership, the relationships among classroom participants, and the content of instruction. Also, the teacher provides the channel of communication between the social system of the classroom and other systems operating within the school and the larger society.

Getzels and Thelan describe the social system as involving two classes of phenomena that are conceptually independent but phenomenally interactive:

1. Institutions (classrooms, schools) with certain roles and expectations that will fulfill the goals of the system
2. Individuals with certain personalities and need dispositions inhabiting the system, whose observed interactions comprise what is called social or group behavior.

This behavior can be understood as a function of these major elements: institution, role, and expectation—which constitute the *normative* dimension of activity in a social system—and *individual*, personality, and need disposition, which together constitute the personal dimension of activity in a social system. To understand the behavior and interaction of specific role incumbents (teacher-student) in an institution, both the role expectations and need dispositions must be known. Needs and expectations may be thought of as motives for behavior, one deriving from personalistic sets and propensities, the other from institutional obligations and requirements.

Two other dimensions are relevant to this representation of a social system. One is the *biological* dimension, in which the individual is thought of as having certain constitutional potentialities and abilities. The second dimension is the *anthropological* dimension, which is related to the values and mores of the institution.

Utilizing this model for the analysis of teaching within a classroom group, issues and problems may be discovered that may interfere with the teaching-learning process. It may be noted that there are conflicts between the cultural values outside the classroom and the institutional expectations within the classroom. There appears to be some conflict between the values that nursing instructors place on the role of the nurse as an agent of change and the values of this role in the practice setting. There may be conflicts between role expectations and personality dispositions. Some studies of the personality characteristics of nursing students indicate that they are not overly aggressive. They tend to be more submissive than dominant on the scales that were used.

Our role expectations of the professional nurse as a leader among her own group and among other professionals may be in conflict, a fact which may lead to frustration and dissatisfaction. Finally, conflict may occur when a role incumbent is required to conform simultaneously to a number of expectations that are mutually exclusive, contradictory, or inconsistent. Examples of these problems are described in nursing literature, which indicates that the role of the nurse is perceived in a variety of ways by the various workers in the health system. Finally, personality conflicts arise when there is a discrepancy between the needs and potentialities of the role incumbent. The student who aspires to become a professional nurse but has questionable intellectual or personality equipment for that occupation is an example of personality conflict.

The application of this model to the classroom group as a social system emphasizes the problem of changing behavior in the teaching-learning situation. In terms of the model, changing behavior may involve adaptation of personality dispositions to role expectations. Or, changing behavior may involve the adaptation of the role expectations to personality dispositions. In attempting to achieve change, the teacher as the group leader works within these extremes, emphasizing the one or the other, or attempting to reach an appropriate balance between the two.

Three types of teaching style may be identified in this process:

1. Teaching is oriented to the normative dimensions of behavior and therefore places stress on the requirements of the institution, the role, and the expectations rather than on the requirements of the individual, the personality, and the need disposition. The assumption here is that if roles are clearly defined and everyone is held equally responsible for doing what she is supposed to do, the required outcomes will ensue regardless of who the particular role incumbent might be, provided she has the necessary technical competence.

2. Teaching is oriented to the personalistic dimension of behavior and places stress on the requirements of the individual, the personality, and the need disposition rather than on the requirements of the institution, the role, and the expectation. The assumption underlying this approach is that the greatest accomplishment will occur, not from enforcing adherence to rigorously defined roles, but from making it possible for each person to seek what is most relevant and meaningful to her. The teacher draws from the students the focus and direction of teaching rather than developing in advance detailed prescriptive lesson plans.

3. Teaching is oriented to a combination of or intermediate to the two preceeding styles. The notion here is that since the goals of the social system must be carried out, it is necessary to make explicit the roles and expectations

required to achieve the goals. Also since the roles and expectations will be implemented by the efforts of people with needs to be met, the personalities and dispositions of these people must be taken into account. The aim is to acquire a thorough awareness of the limits and resources of both individual and institution within which the teaching-learning process may occur.

In developing a balance between the institution and the individual, the group develops a culture or a climate which may be analyzed into the constituent intentions of the group, and the group climate represents another general dimension of the classroom as a social system.

The flexibility of the group in moving between the normative and personal dimensions depends upon the belongingness that the individual feels within the group. The greater the sense of belongingness, the greater the ease of communication between teacher and student and among students. The group becomes more of a planned and voluntary group, which offers greater autonomy and heteronomy for the individual student.

The ideal model of the classroom as a social system is offered by Getzel and Thelan in Diagram 13. In this social system each individual identifies with the goals of the system so that they become part of her own needs; each individual must believe that the expectations held for her are rational if the goals are to be achieved, and each individual feels that she belong to a group with similar identifications and rational beliefs. The nature of the group is determined by the way the teacher responds to the specific behavior of the students. The judgment of the teacher on how to respond depends not merely on her ability to perceive the behavior to which she is responding as an immediate act but to look behind the act and to comprehend the behavior as a transaction within the social system as a whole [25].

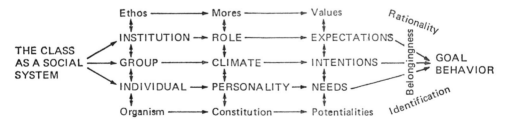

DIAGRAM 13.   Model of the classroom as a social system. (Reprinted from J. W. Getzels and H. Thelan, The Classroom as a Unique Social System. In *The Dynamics of Instructional Groups.* Fifty-ninth Yearbook of the National Society for the Study of Education. Chicago: The University of Chicago Press, 1960, p. 53.)

CLASSIFICATION OF TEACHER STATEMENTS

Another approach to the study and analysis of teaching is the classification of teacher statements. Data for classification has been obtained by means of typescripts of class activities. Recent efforts to arrive at a conceptual system by categorizing these statements have revealed the major teaching categories as procedural statements, substantial statements, and rating statements [26]. The functions of the statement categories are described as follows:

1. Procedural statements serve the function of making or keeping student purposes similar to those of the teacher.
2. Substantive statements serve the function of helping students learn subject matter.
3. Rating statements serve the function of providing students with feedback about the adequacy of their substantive responses.

Teacher statements are further divided into initiatory or reflexive moves. Initiatory moves are determined solely by the teacher's goals. Reflexive moves are determined largely by student responses to initiatory moves of the teacher. Within the category of procedural statements, the initiatory move is called activating; the reflexive move is called maintaining. Under substantive statements, the initiatory moves are informing and cuing; the reflexive moves are reacting, informing, and reactive cuing. Rating statements are all reflexive and are positive, negative, or neutral. The classification system developed by Waimon includes descriptive subcategories within each major type of teacher statement [27].

Classification System

1. *Procedural:* The teacher develops and maintains a predisposition for learning.
    1.1. Activating: The teacher makes student goals similar to his own.
        1.11. Teacher gains attention.
        1.12. Teacher gives instructions.
        1.13. Teacher states goals.
        1.14. Teacher poses problems.
        1.15. Teacher points out importance of goals.
        1.16. Teacher invites student to react to goals.
    1.2. Maintaining: The teacher keeps student goals similar to his own.

1.21. Teacher prevents student from moving class in a new direction.

1.22. Teacher reminds students to continue to pay attention.

1.23. Teacher comments on the cause of unsatisfactory progress.

1.24. Teacher offers encouragement.

1.25. Teacher points out progress being made.

1.26. Teacher invites questions or acknowledges student with a question.

2. *Substantive:* The teacher helps student acquire, comprehend, or use subject matter.

   2.1. Informing: The teacher tells student subject matter to be remembered.

      2.11. Teacher defines terms.

      2.12. Teacher states facts or generalizations.

      2.13. Teacher explains facts or generalizations.

      2.14. Teacher evaluates a subject.

   2.2. Cuing: The teacher asks student questions requiring a substantive response.

      2.21. Teacher helps student recall subject matter.

      2.22. Teacher helps student demonstrate comprehension of subject matter.

      2.23. Teacher helps student discover new subject matter.

      2.24. Teacher helps student apply subject matter to problem solving.

   2.3. Reacting Informing: The teacher improves a student's substantive response.

      2.31. Teacher rephrases or restates student response.

      2.32. Teacher adds new information to student response.

      2.33. Teacher relates various student responses.

   2.4. Reacting Cuing: The teacher helps a student improve a substantive response.

      2.41. Teacher helps student to rephrase or restate a response.

      2.42. Teacher helps student add new information to a response.

      2.43. Teacher solicits additions to a response from other students.

3. *Rating:* The teacher gives an evaluative reaction to a substantive response.

   3.1. Positive: The teacher lets student know a substantive response is correct.

3.11. Teacher gives an explicitly positive rating.

3.12. Teacher gives a mild or equivocally positive rating.

3.2. Negative: The teacher lets student know a substantive response is incorrect.

3.21. Teacher gives an explicitly negative rating.

3.22. Teacher indicates a reservation.

3.23. Teacher disagrees with a response.

3.3. Neutral: The teacher acknowledges a student response but does not let student know it is correct or incorrect.

3.31. Teacher gives a positive reaction to part of a response, a negative reaction to another part.

3.32. Teacher acknowledges having heard the response without evaluating it.

3.33. Teacher gives an ambiguous evaluation to a response.

The classification system provides a means of looking at the basic elements of teachers' verbal contacts with student. In contrast with the previous approach in which teacher actions were viewed in relation to a system of actions, the classification of teacher statements analyzes teaching at the microscopic level. Although the system is meant to be descriptive of what actually transpires in the classroom, evaluation of teacher behavior is possible. In an effort to develop a teaching style that is compatible with her philosophy, personality characteristics, and teaching skill, the teacher may use the results of the classification of teacher statements to modify her own behavior. The teacher may modify her behavior to gain a more appropriate distribution of emphasis upon the three types of teacher statements.

INTERACTION ANALYSIS OF VERBAL AND NONVERBAL BEHAVIOR OF TEACHERS AND STUDENTS

A third approach to the study and analysis of teaching utilizes the system of interaction analysis devised by Flanders. The basic assumption underlying this procedure is that language is both the instrument and the vehicle of teacher-student interaction. Observation bears out the fact that classroom instruction is inescapably involved in the use of language, written and, above all, spoken. Because language and instruction are so intimately related, a study of teaching involves the study of how teachers and students use language in their classroom activities.

VERBAL BEHAVIOR

Verbal behavior has a dimension of meaning that cannot be found merely in spoken words: it is the act of speaking and the occasion of its performance. There is a sense in which we shall want to speak of using words. When we consider what is being said as well as who is saying it, we want to know what action the speaker performs. How is he using the words to do it? Words are instrumental in the execution of various kinds of actions. A given kind of language activity has acquired certain meanings through generations of repeated use, and habits, conventions, or ground rules are built into its performance. The performance varies, even though the same words and statements may be used from one activity to another. What is said on a given occasion is partly determined by the conventions or ground rules governing the kind of language activity in which one is engaged.

Verbal acts have meaning and purpose that are best understood when they are viewed in the context of their performance. Only the context can tell us the difference between two actions performable with identical sets of words. Ascher defines a verbal act as one performed by an individual in making an utterance [28]. The utterance may take the form of speech, gesture, signal code, or writing. Ascher further describes the many wordless elements in verbal behavior. These include such things as punctuation, capitalization, and paragraphing. These do in writing what is effected in speech by means of tonal stress and pitch, pauses, and voice inflection. Since these wordless acts are as effective as words in verbal exchange, they count as verbal behavior [29].

We seek to discover which kinds of verbal actions on the part of the teacher can more effectively induce learnings of various kinds on the part of the student, first by tracing relationships between what teachers and students do and say in the context of instruction, and second by comparing the measured learning increments of a given population with data describing the classroom situations and verbal interactions of the same teachers and students. Studies in progress are attempting to trace relationships between the amount and kinds of productive thinking that certain types of teacher questions may be found to promote in the student.

One aspect of the educational problem is that of determining the most appropriate situations and the most effective ways the teacher can put various kinds of questions to the student to use her potential capacity for productive thinking to the fullest. The analysis of verbal behavior as it is carried on in class sessions can provide the investigator with an indispensable means of determining what the current teaching practices may be. The educator can hope eventually to discover the effects of various instructional practices and classroom experiences upon specific learning outcomes.

The Flanders' system of interaction analysis is an observational procedure that can be used to classify the verbal behavior of teachers and students [30].

TABLE 13. Flanders' Interaction Analysis Categories (FIAC)*

Teacher Talk	Response	1. *Accepts feeling.* Accepts and clarifies an attitude or the feeling tone of a pupil in a nonthreatening manner. Feelings may be positive or negative. Predicting and recalling feelings are included. 2. *Praises or encourages.* Praises or encourages pupil action or behavior. Jokes that release tension, but not at the expense of another individual; nodding head, or saying "Um hm?" or "go on" are included. 3. *Accepts or uses ideas of pupils.* Clarifying, building, or developing ideas suggested by a pupil. Teacher extensions of pupil ideas are included but as the teacher brings more of his own ideas into play, shift to category 5.
		4 *Asks questions.* Asking a question about content or procedure, based on teacher ideas, with the intent that a pupil will answer.
	Initiation	5. *Lecturing.* Giving facts or opinions about content or procedures; expressing *his own* ideas, giving *his own* explanation, or citing an authority other than a pupil. 6. *Giving directions.* Directions, commands, or orders to which a pupil is expected to comply. 7. *Criticizing or justifying authority.* Statements intended to change pupil behavior from nonacceptable to acceptable pattern; bawling someone out; stating why the teacher is doing what he is doing; extreme self-reference.
Pupil Talk	Response	8. *Pupil-talk–response.* Talk by pupils in response to teacher. Teacher initiates the contact or solicits pupil statement or structures the situation. Freedom to express own ideas is limited.
	Initiation	9. *Pupil-talk–initiation.* Talk by pupils which they initiate. Expressing own ideas; initiating a new topic; freedom to develop opinions and a line of thought, like asking thoughtful questions; going beyond the existing structure.
Silence		10. *Silence or confusion.* Pauses, short periods of silence and periods of confusion in which communication cannot be understood by the observer.

* Taken from N. A. Flanders, *Analyzing Teaching Behavior.* Reading: Addison-Wesley, 1970, p. 34.

Using this system, verbal behavior in the classroom is classified into ten categories. Of the seven categories for teacher behavior, four are classified as indirect influences: (1) accepting pupil feelings, (2) praising or encouraging, (3) accepting pupil ideas, and (4) asking questions. The three categories of direct teacher influences are (5) giving information or opinion, (6) giving directions, and (7) criticizing.

Two categories of student talk used in the system are (8) student response to the teacher, and (9) student-initiated talk. Category (10) is used to indicate silence or confusion. Each number in the classification designates a particular kind of communication. During observation of student-teacher interaction, numbers corresponding to the type of communication are recorded. This involves a classification of each response, not a judgment or an evaluation of the communication.

Flanders indicates that the major feature of this category system lies in the analysis of initiative and response, which are characteristics of interaction between two or more individuals. To initiate means to make the first move, to introduce an idea or concept for the first time, to express one's own will. To respond means to take action after initiation, to amplify or react to ideas that have already been expressed, or to conform to or comply with the will expressed by others. Utilizing this system, an estimate of the balance between initiative and response can be inferred from the percent of time taken by teacher talk, pupil talk, and silence or confusion. A more accurate estimate of the initiative-response balance of the classroom interaction can be made by comparing the teacher talk in Categories 1, 2, and 3 with those in 5, 6, and 7 [31]. Table 13 lists the ten categories with descriptive elements of the Flanders' Interaction Analysis Categories.

The completed matrix gives the observer a picture not only of the percentage of interactions falling in each category but also of the general sequence of responses. Although an exact representation of the sequence of the entire lesson is not shown, recording the numbers in an overlapping fashion preserves the sequence of adjacent numbers. Diagram 14 presents an example of an interaction analysis matrix.

Interaction analysis provides an objective technique for analyzing teacher-student interaction and offers a procedure for a systematic inquiry into one's own teaching behavior. Opportunity for self-study may provide answers to such questions as: What kind of student-teacher interaction is taking place? Should some change in this interaction be considered? What kind of change in interaction would result in an improvement?

Time Sequence

Categories:	1	2	3	4	5	6	7	8	9	10	Total
1											
2											
3											
4											
5											
6					1				1		2
7						1	1				2
8							1				1
9											
10											
Total					1	1	2		1		5

DIAGRAM 14.   Interaction analysis matrix. Taken from N. A. Flanders, *Analyzing Teaching Behavior*. Reading: Addison-Wesley, 1970, p. 81.

NONVERBAL BEHAVIOR

Efforts have been directed to the study of the nature and effects of non-verbal behavior of teachers. Nonverbal behaviors are those typically thought of as expressive but which have neither address nor direction. When a person speaks or gestures, he is not merely showing his mood or expressing his feelings but also acting. People regularly guide their actions toward others by observing facial expressions and other indications of feelings and reactions. Undirected expressive behavior may evoke response, verbal or otherwise. Smiles and frowns and many other expressive behaviors are more often taken as signs than signals. Verbal behavior and unaddressed expressive behaviors tend to blend and shade into one another. Either type of behavior can produce either type of response. Instances of either type are observable in the routine context of classroom interaction.

BEHAVIOR OF EFFECTIVE TEACHERS

Another approach to the study of teaching is concerned with the characteristics of effective teachers. Medley and Metzel sought to discover what patterns of classroom behavior were characteristic of those graduates who were considered to be effective teachers [32]. The investigators made the following assumptions:

1. The most promising approach is a quantitative one. No general theory of classroom behavior can be formulated until ways of quantifying classroom behaviors have been developed and a large body of measurements of behaviors using these methods has been assembled.

2. It is necessary to study behavior in the classroom. It is not necessary to assume the existence of laws of learning that are uniform across subjects, learning tasks, learning environments, and species.

3. Any effect that the teacher has on the student is mediated by some overt behavior on the teacher's part. Each behavior that a teacher exhibits has a purpose (conscious or unconscious) and may be effective in achieving that purpose to a greater or lesser degree. The competence of a particular teacher cannot be assessed unless the effects she is seeking to achieve are known. It is possible to measure certain effects of her behavior and see which of her behaviors are followed by effects in which investigators are interested. The competent teacher is able to select those modes of behavior which will produce the effects she intends to produce.

4. What the teacher does is an important factor in determining what the student learns. The student's capacity, maturation, school, and community environment are not ruled out.

5. Once effective patterns of teacher behavior have been identified, it will be possible to teach students of education how to exhibit them. Investigators choose to assume that teachers could learn to behave more effectively without undergoing basic personality change, if only enough were known about effective behavior to teach them how.

Very few of the things that teachers do in classrooms today are done because they have been demonstrated to be effective ways of behaving. Scientifically based knowledge of effective teacher behavior must be sought in studies that attempt to relate teacher behavior to teacher effectiveness. If the quantitative scientific method is to be used, each study must incorporate objective measurement of both types of variables. Few studies have been reported that attempted to measure teacher effectiveness and that also incorporate objective measures of behavior.

Problems inherent in measuring teacher effectiveness are concerned with philosophical or definitional issues and relate to the selection of the behavior changes to be measured. Also, some difficulties have to do with the removal of influences on student growth other than the teacher's behavior. Effectiveness of a behavior is judged in terms of outcomes that are chosen for study. What the teacher needs to know to achieve competence is the probable effect of each behavior, so that she can exhibit those behaviors that will achieve her purposes most efficiently.

Two or more teacher behaviors are seldom identical in all observable respects. What would seem to be the same behavior can have quite different impact according to who exhibits it. The setting or situation in which a behavior occurs also alters its effect. Moreover, when a particular teacher does a particular thing at a particular time, it does not necessarily have the same effect on all of her students. Medley and Metzel summarize these points under the heading, problems of heterogeneity of effect of behavior [33]. Behaviors may be categorized as follows:

1. Those behaviors that tend to have the same effect on most students when exhibited by most teachers in most situations. These are the most useful behaviors to know and are the ones that should be taught in general methods courses.

2. Those behaviors that have some effect on most students in most situations; which are useful to certain teachers but worthless to others. If these behaviors are teachable, they must be the result of individualization of instruction in teacher education programs.

3. Those behaviors that are effective with certain types of students only. Courses on methods for handling exceptional children should feature this kind of behavior.

4. Those behaviors that are contingent upon the classroom situation. Among the many factors that are relevant would be socioeconomic factors in the students' backgrounds, the particular subject being taught, and the type of school organization.

5. Those behaviors that are probably not worth trying to teach. It is impossible to train teachers to a point where every teacher knows exactly how to behave in every situation with every student.

In this frame of reference, effectiveness of a behavior is a function of the total number of teachers, students, and situations in which the behavior has a particular effect. Few behaviors have been identified that are effective in a majority of situations in which they occur. A skillful teacher's repertoire may include many different behaviors likely to produce a certain effect, and she selects one or another of them according to her perception of the situation that prevails at a given time.

The study of effective teacher behavior reported by Medley and Metzel proposes an operational definition of effectiveness which suggests the following method. The observer counts the number of times each teacher exhibits the behavior during a certain time and measures the effectiveness of the behavior over the same period. Effort is made to determine whether teachers who exhibit the behavior most frequently are the ones who are most effective in terms of their average effect on all the students in the class. These authors state that if behavior is to be measured objectively through observation, the task of the observer should be to record behavior only. Their approach indicates that observations should be made of a large number of teachers, recording all the behaviors of each one. Measure the effectiveness of each teacher, and use item analysis to discover which behaviors characterize highly effective teachers. Within sampling limits these behaviors may be taken as defining the domain of effective behaviors. The effectiveness of any individual behavior may not be very high; therefore, groups of behaviors that show some psychological consistency are used to determine the correlation with the criterion (the average student effect) [34].

The four approaches to the study and analysis of teaching are not the only or the best ones in use today. They do appear to be representative in both focus and methodology. The dynamics of instructional groups look at teaching in terms of the social climate and the factors that influence teaching within that climate. The classification of teacher statements analyzes and categorizes verbal behavior of teachers from which the nature and process of teaching may be inferred. Verbal interaction introduces student and teacher behavior and provides opportunity to classify the types of behaviors of each. The results of the analysis of student-teacher interaction offer useful information for the teacher to examine, reinforce, or modify her behavior in relation to her purposes and objectives of teaching. The study of effective teacher behavior presents a method for quantifying teacher behaviors for the purpose of determining effective teacher behavior. Each of these approaches provides different kinds of data that may be useful in exploring the nature and process of teaching.

SUMMARY

The instructional process is concerned with both instruction and teaching. Although these terms have been used interchangeably, some differences are noted and described. For the purposes of this publication, instruction is concerned with the various conditions of learning that are external to the learner. They may include such elements as physical and social environments, teaching strategies and procedures, and the subject matter arrangement. These conditions are manipulated by the teacher for the purposes of efficient and effective learning. Teaching is viewed as the interaction between teacher and student for the purpose of students' acquiring specific behaviors. Teaching implies continuous action on the part of the teacher. Since teaching is interaction with students, continuous adjustment in behavior on the part of the teacher is necessary. Teaching is described as a system of action intended to induce learning. The concept of teaching developed by Smith presents the variables involved in and related to the actions that make up teaching. These variables can be classified into four categories, (1) independent variables, (2) dependent variables, (3) intervening variables pertaining to students, and (4) intervening variables pertaining to the teacher. The actions of teaching belong to the first of these.

While teaching is a system of actions, these actions are the responses of the teacher in making decisions about the students with whom she is interacting. Teaching is seen as a complex act concerned primarily with efficient achievement of educational objectives. It involves responsible decision-making and actions of a teacher.

The relation of teaching to learning remains unsettled. Learning embraces more than what goes on in schools and occurs in all areas of life, not merely in the formal educational setting. Although teaching is seen as intending to bring about learning, some definitions make teaching dependent upon learning. Analysis of the concepts of teaching and learning describe teaching as a task and learning as an achievement or outcome. Other viewpoints suggest that learning is a process that cannot be assessed or judged. The notion of "thirdness" is presented, which describes learning as the development of a shared meaning of a concept or idea by teacher and student. To teach is to deliberately change the meaning of experience, which may or may not result in an immediate change in behavior.

Learning has long been the subject of scientific study. Theories of learning have been formulated and subjected to experimental verification. Since most of these endeavors have taken place in controlled laboratory settings using animal subjects, teachers have experienced difficulty in making direct applications to the practical problems of teaching. Teachers need to know how students learn and how they depend on readiness, motivation, and reinforcement. They also need to know how to teach, to motivate students, to present the subject, and to shape a cognitive structure. While theories of learning deal with the ways in which a person influences an organism, theories of teaching deal with the ways in which a person influences an organism to learn. Theories of teaching should be concerned with explaining, predicting, and controlling the ways in which teacher behavior affects the learning of students. Theories of teaching will consist of (1) a statement of variables comprising teaching behavior, (2) formulation of the possible relations among the variables, and (3) hypotheses about the relations between the teaching behavior variables and the variables descriptive of the psychological and social conditions within which teaching behavior occurs. There appears to be some agreement that a single theory of teaching will not suffice to explain the variables concerned with the action of teaching.

In the absence of theories of teaching that have been subjected to test and validation, teachers and psychologists have endeavored to study and analyze teaching. The approaches that have been made focus on different variables within a specified conceptual framework. One approach views the classroom as a social group and identifies the factors affecting the dynamics of the instructional group. These factors have a direct bearing on the teaching-learning situation and the behavior of the teacher. A second approach classifies the statements of teachers, and from these statements verbal behaviors are identified. A third approach analyzes the interaction of student and teacher. The verbal interaction is classified according to the Flanders' system, and teacher behavior is described. The last approach endeavors to quantify teacher behavior in an effort to determine its effectiveness. Although these approaches are not the only ones being used in current explorations, they are representative of the types of studies of teaching and the analysis of teaching behaviors.

REFERENCES

1. Siegel, L. [Ed.]. Integration and Reactions. In *Instruction: Some Contemporary Viewpoints*. San Francisco: Chandler, 1967. P. 317.
2. Jahnke, J. C. A Behavioristic Analysis of Instruction. In L. Siegel [Ed.], *Instruction: Some Contemporary Viewpoints*. San Francisco: Chandler, 1967. P. 181.
3. Skinner, B. F. The science of learning and the art of teaching. *Harvard Educ. Rev.* 24:86, 1954.
4. Skinner, B. F. *Science and Human Behavior*. New York: Macmillan, 1953. P. 80.

5. Smith, B. O.   A Concept of Teaching. In B. Bandman and R. S. Guttchen [Eds.], *Philosophical Essays on Teaching*. Philadelphia: Lippincott, 1969. P. 5.
6. Ibid., p. 14.
7. Herrick, V. E.   Teaching as Curriculum Decision-Making. In J. Rath, J. R. Pancella, and J. S. Van Ness [Eds.], *Studying Teaching*. Englewood Cliffs: Prentice-Hall, 1967. P. 116.
8. Hilgard, E. R.   *Theories of Learning*. New York: Appleton-Century-Crofts, 1956. P. 3.
9. Gage, N. L.   Theories of Teaching. In *Theories of Learning and Instruction*. Sixty-third Yearbook of the National Society for the Study of Education. Chicago: University of Chicago Press, 1964. P. 275.
10. Gowen, D. R.   Teaching, Learning and Thirdness. In B. Bandman and R. S. Guttchen [Eds.], *Philosophical Essays on Teaching*. Philadelphia: Lippincott, 1969. P. 86.
11. Ibid., p. 98.
12. Gagné, R. M.   *The Conditions of Learning*. New York: Holt, Rinehart & Winston, 1965. P. 26.
13. Gage, op. cit., p. 268.
14. Merton, R. K.   *Social Theory and Social Structure*. London: Free Press of Glencoe, 1957. P. 86.
15. Commission on Instructional Theory.   *Criteria for Theories of Instruction*. Washington, D.C.: Association for Supervision and Curriculum Development, National Education Association, 1968. P. 16.
16. Siegel, L., and Siegel, L. C.   The Instructional Gestalt. In L. Siegel [Ed.], *Instruction: Some Contemporary Viewpoints*. San Francisco: Chandler, 1967. P. 261.
17. Koerner, J. D.   *The Miseducation of American Teachers*. Boston: Houghton Mifflin, 1963. P. 4.
18. Biddle, B. J., and Ellena, W. J. [Eds.].   *Contemporary Research on Teacher Effectiveness*. New York: Holt, Rinehart & Winston, 1964. P. vi.
19. Gage, N. L. [Ed.].   *Handbook of Research on Teaching*. Chicago: Rand McNally, 1963.
20. Ibid., p. vi.
21. Ibid., p. 96.
22. Ibid., p. 97.
23. Smith, B. O.   Toward a Theory of Teaching. In A. A. Bellack [Ed.], *Theory and Research in Teaching*. New York: Teachers College Bureau of Publications (Columbia University), 1963. P. 1.
24. Getzels, J. W., and Thelan, H.   The Classroom as a Unique Social System. In *The Dynamics of Instructional Groups*. Fifty-ninth Yearbook of the National Society for the Study of Education. Chicago: University of Chicago Press, 1960. P. 53.
25. Ibid., p. 80.
26. Waimon, M. D.   Classifying Teacher Statements. In E. Amidon et al. [Eds.], *The Study of Teaching*. Washington, D.C.: Commission on the Implications of Recent Research in Teaching, The Association for Student Teaching, 1967. P. 56.
27. Ibid.

28. Ascher, M. J.   The Language of Teaching. In B. Bandman and R. S. Gutt-chen [Eds.], *Philosophical Essays on Teaching*. Philadelphia: Lippincott, 1969. P. 25.
29. Ibid.
30. Flanders, N. A.   *Analyzing Teaching Behavior*. Reading: Addison-Wesley, 1970. P. 35.
31. Ibid., p. 35.
32. Medley, D. M., and Metzel, H. E.   The Scientific Study of Teacher Behavior. In A. A. Bellack [Ed.], *Theory and Research in Teaching*. New York: Teachers College Bureau of Publications (Columbia University), 1963. P. 79.
33. Ibid., p. 86.
34. Ibid., p. 89.

SUPPLEMENTARY READINGS

Commission on the Implications of Recent Research in Teaching.   *The Study of Teaching*. Washington, D.C.: The Association for Student Teaching, 1967.
Haugh, J. B., and Duncan, J. K.   *Teaching: Description and Analysis*. Reading: Addison-Wesley, 1970.
Hyman, R. T.   *Teaching: Vantage Points for Study*. Philadelphia: Lippincott, 1968.
Kneller, G. F.   *Logic and Language of Education*. New York: Wiley, 1966.
Raths, J., Pancella, J. R., and Van Ness, J. S.   *Studying Teaching*. Englewood Cliffs: Prentice-Hall, 1967.
Report of the Seminar on Teaching.   *The Way Teaching Is*. Washington, D.C.: Association for Supervision and Curriculum Development and the Center for the Study of Instruction of the National Education Association, 1966.
Scheffler, I.   *The Language of Education*. Springfield: Thomas, 1960.
Siegel, L. [Ed.].   *Instruction: Some Contemporary Viewpoints*. San Francisco: Chandler, 1967.
Smith, B. O., et al.   *A Study of the Logic of Teaching*. Urbana: Bureau of Educational Research, College of Education, University of Illinois, 1963.
Tolman, E. C.   A Psychological Model. In T. Parsons and E. A. Shils [Eds.], *Toward a General Theory of Social Action*. Cambridge: Harvard University Press, 1952.

14 VARIABLES IN THE INSTRUCTIONAL PROCESS

ALTHOUGH the classroom is a site of teaching, it does not constitute the entire context for learning. Students arrive with a history, their activities there are but a small fragment of their ongoing daily regimen, and their concerns during each fragmented learning session reflect the interaction of this history with other aspects of the immediate world both in and out of the classroom.

Variables in the instructional process are those persons, events, and environmental characteristics that can be expected to have some bearing upon instructional effectiveness. Variables considered are those that are measurable or amenable to categorization and classifications. These variables can be manipulated along some unidimensional continuum. There is reason to believe that each variable is fundamental to the teaching-learning situation. Four classes of independent variables are identified and described. These include learner characteristics, teacher characteristics, the learning environment, and teaching strategies.

LEARNER CHARACTERISTICS

A constellation of characteristics of the learner may be considered to be variable in the instructional process. These may include certain personal characteristics such as age, sex, physical and mental health as well as intelligence, academic ability, scholastic aptitude, and others. Considerable attention was given to the nature of the student population in a previous chapter. For the purpose of describing additional variables that have profound effect upon learning, the concerns of motivation and previously learned capabilities are presented.

MOTIVATION

The motivation of human behavior is a large and complex subject. Many investigations of motivation have been and are being made, and there are many publications on the topic. Many students of the educational process believe that the problem of controlling and developing motivation is the most serious issue faced by schools. The broad conceptualization of the motivational problems includes a consideration of the motives that make the student want to seek knowledge, to utilize her talents, to desire fulfillment as a human being, to relate to other people in a satisfying manner, and to become an effective member of society.

In all theories of learning there is some aspect of the learning process that can be called motivation. Motivation is that which impels one to move, whether such impulsion is conscious or unconscious. It is not clear whether specific motivation is more fundamental to the process of learning or to the demonstration of behavior that is the outcome of learning. In other words, does one *learn* better under particular conditions of motivation, or does one simply *perform* learned acts better?

Motivation as a process may be thought of as both the internal or personal condition and the external situation to which one responds. The first aspect may be designated as motive, and the second as incentive. Some phase of need theory must be invoked as the basic personal condition for motivation. Incentives that satisfy needs or are perceived as satisfying needs will be most potent in directing learning and behavior. *Intrinsic* motivation, in which needs are directly satisfied by the learning itself, is most efficient and probably produces the most effective, pervasive, and permanent learning. *Extrinsic* motivation, in which secondary or intermediate incentives are used to carry the learning, is frequently necessary but not as effective as the primary type.

Most of the empirical investigations have dealt with various extrinsic motivations. A great majority of these have been concerned with aspects of reward and punishment. Findings are consistent in indicating that the incentives defined as reward are more facilitative of learning than are punishments. Whether one sees the reward as acting directly upon learning or as a mediating cue to the learning, it has become clear that rewarding a correct response (or a desired response) permits sufficient satisfaction for the student to adhere to that response and makes the response more likely to occur again under similar conditions. Few of the investigations have been able to demonstrate 100 percent efficacy for the defined reward or zero effect for the defined punishment. This is to be expected if reward and punishment are defined subjectively according to the learner's own motivational system. What the investigator plans as reward may not be so to the learner.

Several types of motivation are inherent in the instructional process and have direct impact upon learning.

Motivation to Attend School

It is evident that students must want to place themselves in the environment where instruction occurs in order to be affected by it. Although young children may have a rather weak motivation to attend school, it is assumed that college students are in the school environment because they want to be there. Even though this is true in most instances, it must be recognized that many young people are in school for external reasons. The desire to please the family or former teachers is frequently the motive that sends students to college. The director of the counseling center of a large state university indicated to the author that one of their most perplexing problems is the large number of students of high academic ability who flunk out of college. Upon investigation it is found that many of these students are in college because of parental pressures. It is not unreasonable to assume that many decisions are influenced by people and events and that these motivations are usually weaker and less enduring than those that are internalized within the student. Ensuring positive motivation toward school is something that must be dealt with by family and community. If the student's family accepts and values the school, the chances are she will also. This does not mean that the family urges or pressures the student against her will.

Motivation to Achieve

In addition to the motive to attend school there is motivation to achieve. This implies that the student not only desires "to learn something," she also has the motivation to learn something specific, that is, to be able to do something as a result of learning. The nursing student is motivated to learn, but she also possesses the motivation to be someone quite different from what she is.

From infancy onward there is motivation to achieve, to be able to do something. The individual conceptualizes her goals in terms of action. The action itself may be more or less socially useful. Much use is made of specific motivation as a basis for learning in the school. Teachers know the powerful effect of telling a student what she will be able to do when a particular learning session or topic is completed. The nursing student is told that the learning of certain principles of physiology will enable her to give nursing care to patients with specific types of illnesses. The key to achievement motivation is the conception of action on the part of the student. She must want to be able to do something.

One of the most important functions of the teacher is to provide adult guidance for the student. By assuming such a role, she is able to teach the principles that make it possible for the student to associate the specific achievement goals of a particular type of instruction with larger, more general goals.

There are available in the literature numerous studies dealing with the need to achieve and the need to avoid failure. Cronbach identifies two categories of motivation, constructive and defensive [1]. The student who is high on achievement motivation and low on anxiety is designated as constructively motivated; the one with the opposite pattern, as defensively motivated. The constructively motivated show their best persistence when led to think they are dealing with problems where there is moderate risk. The defensively motivated are most persistent when led to think the chance of success is very low. Given simple instructions to get to work and to do a task, constructives achieve well; adding pressure lowers their score. The same pressure, pacing, and stern supervision improves the work of the defensives. Telling the low-anxiety student that she has done poorly improves her work, while favorable comment improves the work of the defensives.

Defensives will learn most if the teacher spells out short-term goals, gives a maximum of explanation and guidance, and arranges feedback at short intervals to keep the student from getting off the track—in general, if the teacher maximizes opportunity for dependence. Constructives should face moderately difficult tasks where intermediate goals are not too explicit; feedback should be provided at intervals for the purpose of teaching them to judge themselves. Some learning psychologists proclaim that learning cannot be sufficiently motivated without anxiety and that the teacher's job is not to remove anxiety from the learning situation but rather to regulate its level so that there is neither too much nor too little.

Waterhouse and Child endeavored to determine the effect of frustration upon quality of performance [2]. The theory underlying these investigations indicated that the effect of frustration upon quality of performance would vary with the extent to which the individual has general habits of responding to frustration with internal responses of a potentially disruptive sort. Attempts to verify this prediction were made by using a personality questionnaire in which the subject reported her habits of response to frustrations. Scores resulting from the questionnaire permitted the subjects to be grouped according to overall interfering tendencies, and the groups were referred to as the High Interference Group and the Low Interference Group.

The effect upon the quality of performance did turn out to vary with this measure of personality in the predicted manner. In the High Interference Group frustration produced a slight decrement in performance; in the Low Interference Group frustration produced a large increment in performance. The presence of frustration increases the drive to do well. In the Low Interference Group this increase in drive leads to more effective performance, but in the High Interference Group the increase in drive is balanced by an increase in interfering responses, so that the net effect is that of performance similar to what would be found in the absence of frustration.

It appears that people who, according to self-ratings, tend to react to frustration with interfering responses tend, in test situations without frustration, to produce internal responses that motivate them to do well. Those who have a low tendency to react to frustration with interfering responses, and hence are able to work at peak efficiency when motivated by frustration, appear to be relatively lacking in motivation under nonfrustrating conditions.

Motivation to Engage in Learning

What makes an individual want to undertake learning? How can one establish the kind of motivation required for the student to be selectively attentive to the stimulus events that will bring about changes in behavior? If a student is to respond to stimulation, she must have a state of alertness that corresponds to the term *attention*. Alertness appears to be a function of certain physical and mental states, such as sleepy, fatigued, or under the influence of drugs. Alertness is also affected by the learning environment. For purposes of conducting instruction, alertness must be present in the student. Little learning is likely to occur without it.

Curiosity is almost a prototype of the intrinsic motive. Attention is attracted to something that is unclear, unfinished, or uncertain. Attention is sustained until that matter becomes clear, finished, or certain. Merely the search to clarify it is what satisfies.

The drive to achieve competence is another intrinsic motive for learning.

A person becomes interested in that which she can do well. It is difficult to sustain interest in an activity unless one achieves some degree of competence in it. To achieve the sense of accomplishment requires a task that has an obvious beginning and end. If the tasks are "silly," meaningless, arbitrary, or without visible means for checking progress, the drive to completion is not stimulated by interruption. Unless there is some meaningful unity in what is being done and some way of telling how well it is being done, the person is not very likely to strive to excel.

There is a strong human tendency to model oneself and her aspirations after some other person—a competence model. The teacher, especially if she is an effective competence model, is likely to become a part of the student's internal dialogue, a person whose respect she wants and whose standards she wishes to make her own.

Bruner has identified another intrinsic motive, which he calls reciprocity [3]. This involves a deep human need to respond to others and to work jointly with them toward an objective. When joint action is required, the process of reciprocation carries the individual into the learning situation. Bruner further states that a group cannot have both reciprocity and demand that everybody learn the same thing or be "completely" well-rounded in the same way all the time. If groups operate in a reciprocal manner, each member stimulates and gives support to learning in relation to individual contributions. The interlocking of participant roles encourages the operation of reciprocity in a group.

If teachers seek to produce some particular kind of behavior in a person, they should see to it that the person wants to behave in that way. The difficulty with this statement is that it is too general; it tells nothing about how to proceed in any given instance. It is necessary to abandon the general rule and seek in any given situation those particular conditions that maximize performance: the question of how to regulate motivational variables in a training situation so as to maximize performance in that situation. The classical finding is that performance improves as motivation increases. Motivation should be in some sense relevant to the task. The task itself often provides intrinsic motivation. People desire to complete tasks they have started, particularly if the task is one in which the trainee has some ego involvement. Success in the task serves as a goal if the trainee is motivated to excel her fellows or to compete with them.

Related to motivation to succeed is the concept of "level of aspiration." The performance an individual thinks she can do is as important as what she actually accomplishes. If the person's goal is set too high, she may experience too much failure. If her goal is set too low she has no experience of success to spur her on.

MOTIVATION TO CONTINUE LEARNING TASKS

The learning of an entire topic or subject requires the learner to persevere toward the goal she has set for herself during a period of time in which she may be engaging in quite a variety of activities. A way must be found of keeping up her motivation to continue the learning task until it is finished. In this case the learner must undertake to achieve subtasks along the route. If the accomplishment of subtasks are to become sources of motivation, it is evident that they must be systematically communicated to the student. One cannot expect her to infer the goal of the next subtask before she has even begun it. In order to use this achievement as a source of motivation, it must be communicated to her prior to the occurrence of learning. Obviously, to do this for every subtask to be learned requires very careful planning of the whole instructional sequence.

To develop a so-called love of learning, the student must be progressively weaned from dependence on the teacher or another agent external to herself. This means that she must develop her own standards against which she can compare her achievements as they develop stage by stage during the learning of a topic or a subject. A second kind of motivational development, extending over a period of years, is an increased dependence on self-generated "instructions" in the prosecution of a learning assignment. It should be possible for college-level students to provide their own guidance and to acquire a variety of learning strategies that will enable them to take control of the learning situation.

Learning proceeds best when the student is motivated to learn, wants to learn, and puts forth effort to learn. Achievement of these conditions is aided when the learner considers course goals and learning tasks as having intrinsic worth for immediate or eventual use. Goals need not be vocational to be so valued. But the learner must be helped to recognize how her achievement will contribute to her development. Instructors who recognize and accept the importance of this condition of learning will find opportunities to point out real-life applications of course principles, values, or skills. They may demonstrate by their own obvious commitment to the discipline that it merits serious study and attention.

Grades can be an integral part of the learning experience. The grades themselves can be important sources of motivation for the student and result in significant changes in behavior. The potential effect of grades as a reinforcing contingency was examined among university students. Essays were written by students defending positions on attitude-related issues contrary to their previously assessed positions. Good and poor grades were randomly assigned to the essays and reported to the student. The effects of these procedures on attitude change were evaluated, and good grades were demonstrated to serve a reinforcing role in contrast to the effects of a poor grade or no grade.

Grades motivate most students but not in the same ways nor to the same extent. Students sometimes hesitate to achieve the level of academic performance of which they are capable for fear of incurring peer-group displeasure or fear of being labeled "brains." The highly secure, highly able, low-achieving student may be satisfied with attaining a C grade without challenging herself to do either the quality or quantity of work of which she is capable. The high-drive, middle-ability student, on the other hand, may work inordinately hard to achieve a B grade, which is her symbol of success.

School policies on testing and recognition of students also are involved in any efforts made to prize human differences. Examinations, like school marking systems, usually involve standards for substantive subjects rather than for individual students. Honors and awards commonly bring satisfaction to only a few students, and they often are the ones who least need the glow of satisfaction provided by distinguished achievement. Means of helping to motivate the average and below-average students remain a part of the challenge of developing the individual learner.

PREVIOUSLY LEARNED CAPABILITIES

Research and experience show quite clearly that there are differences in students' ability to profit from learning opportunities presented at any point in time. Some students appear able to grasp ideas, concepts, or notions and assimilate them in their learning experiences, while others have difficulty in comprehending new and abstract ideas. A part of this difference may be traced to their previous experience and practice.

Differences of several kinds can be observed in the experience background of any group of college students. In the same class, for example, there may be both freshmen and seniors, whose acquaintance with college traditions, study techniques, or college knowhow will vary considerably. And unless prerequisites are enforced, students who are well grounded in the discipline may be enrolled in a course along with some making their first contact with it.

Differences in experience also stem from the varieties and amounts of work in which students have engaged, of travels they have completed, or of significant cultural experiences to which they have been exposed. Still other differences relate to their advantaged or disadvantaged cultural or economic backgrounds, as discussed in Chapter 7.

The occurrence of learning is inferred from the difference in the performance exhibited before and after being placed in a learning situation. The presence of the performance does not make it possible to conclude that learning has occurred: it is necessary to show that there has been a change in performance. The inability to exhibit the performance before learning must be present as well as the ability to perform after learning.

The existence of prior capabilities is slighted or even ignored by most of the traditional learning prototypes. The initial capabilities, or previously learned capabilities, of the learner play an important part in determining subsequent learnings. One important implication of the identification of learning activities is that these activities must be carefully planned before the learning situation is entered into by the student. In particular, there needs to be planning in terms of the student's capabilities before and after any learning enterprise. The acquisition of knowledge is a process in which every new capability builds upon a foundation established by previously learned capabilities.

RECOGNITION OF INDIVIDUAL DIFFERENCES

Teachers-in-preparation should learn about a wide variety of differences among and within individuals. In addition to the differences that originate in heredity and environment, they should have called to their attention the physical, intellectual, perceptual, emotional, social, and economic differences. Teachers need to know that differences can be very wide yet usual; they need to expect variation among individuals as one of the facts of professional or nonprofessional life.

Learning to expect wide individual differences among and within learners is a first step toward understanding the implications of those differences; but professional education must include careful examination of just what those facts mean in terms of student and teacher behavior. If students vary in ability and present achievement, what does this mean to the teacher who is planning and structuring the learning environment?

One area in which the implications of individual differences are particularly important is that of learner's goals. So central are goals within the learning process that teachers cannot afford to ignore them. Not only do individual learners vary widely in their levels of aspiration in and out of school, they also vary just as widely in their choice of particular goals to which to aspire. Knowing about differences as facts is not the same as accepting variation as normal, challenging, and in some ways desirable. Success in introducing the flexibility of instruction required to meet the needs of students possessing different goals, abilities, and backgrounds is dependent to a great extent on the security of the teacher. The teacher's security in the content to be taught is based on a complex of her knowledge and understanding of ideas in a given field of study, her competence in selecting and using sources in that field, her skill in identifying significant study techniques appropriate to the field, and her overall feeling that she knows how to be an effective guide to others.

INFLUENCE OF ACADEMIC ACHIEVEMENT

Constancy of academic attainment is partly attributable to constancy of academic aptitude and motivation. But when these factors are controlled, it is reasonable to attribute some of the obtained relationships between earlier and later educational levels to the cumulative effects of variables in the cognitive structure induced by previously learned capabilities.

An introductory course in a given field might normally be expected to establish the type of cognitive structure that would facilitate later assimilation of more advanced and highly differentiated material in the same field. Where new learning is substantially relatable to existing knowledge, the facilitating effect of increased knowledge can be attributed to the higher degree of discrimination the learner is able to attain. Where the new learning material is not substantially relatable to previously learned principles, general background knowledge probably facilitates learning and retention by increasing the familiarity of the new material and hence the learner's confidence in coping with it.

NATURE OF READINESS

There is little disagreement about the fact that readiness always influences the efficiency of the learning process and often determines whether a given intellectual skill or type of school material is learnable at a particular stage of development. Postponement of learning experience beyond this stage of readiness wastes valuable and often unsuspected learning opportunities, thereby reducing the amount of subject matter content that can be mastered in a designated period of schooling. On the other hand, when a student is prematurely exposed to a learning task before she is ready for it, she not only fails to learn the task in question but also learns from the experience of failure to fear, dislike, and avoid it.

The concept of readiness refers to the adequacy of existing capacity in relation to the demands of a given learning task. Maturation encompasses those increments in capacity that take place in the absence of specific practice experiences such as those attributable to genic influences and/or incidental experience. Maturation is not the same as readiness but is merely one of the two principal factors (the other is learning) that determines the organism's readiness to deal with new experiences. Whether readiness exists does not depend on maturation alone but in many instances is solely a function of prior learning experience and most typically depends on varying proportions of both maturation and learning.

It is important to appreciate that the current readiness of students determines the school's current choice of instructional method and materials; it is also important to bear in mind that this readiness itself is partly determined by the appropriateness and efficiency of the previous instructional practices to which they have been subjected.

LEARNED CAPABILITIES—A CONDITION FOR BEHAVIOR CHANGE

The viewpoints of several authorities in the field of learning have direct relation to the concern of previously learned capabilities. Ausubel describes the use of expository organizers to facilitate the learning and the relation of meaningful verbal materials [4]. His notion of advance organizers is based on the premise that if the organizational principle of progressive differentiation of an internalized sphere of knowledge does prevail, then new meaningful material becomes incorporated into cognitive structure insofar as it is subsumable under relevant existing concepts. When undergraduate nursing students are exposed to organizers presenting relevant and appropriately inclusive subsuming concepts of microbiology, they are better able to learn and retain unfamiliar ideational material dealing with pathogenic microorganisms, their effect upon body defenses, and the beneficial and necessary action of microorganisms on body physiology.

Advance organizers, according to Ausubel, probably facilitate the incorporability and longevity of meaningful verbal material in two different ways. First, they explicitly draw upon and mobilize whatever relevant subsuming concepts are already established in the learner's cognitive structure and make them part of the subsuming entity. Second, advance organizers at an appropriate level of inclusiveness provide optimal anchorage. Thus, the use of advance organizers renders unnecessary much of the rote memorization to which students resort because they are required to learn the details of a discipline before having available a sufficient number of key subsuming concepts.

For maximally effective learning, a separate organizer should be provided for each unit of material. Sequential organization of subject matter can be very effective, since each new increment of knowledge serves as an anchoring post for subsequent learning. Most complex learning tasks, particularly those that are sequential in nature, can be analyzed into a hierarchy of component sets or units. Serious breakdown in learning can often be attributed to inadvertent omission of a logically essential component unit from the total task or to its inadequate integration with other components.

A viewpoint expressed by Gagné indicates that behavioral changes acquired by learning involve different categories of behavior [5]. Human activities are not all the same, and the inferences one makes about underlying processes are different for different performers. Gagné defines knowledge as that inferred capability that makes possible the successful performance of a class of tasks that could not be performed before learning was undertaken. Beginning with the final task, Gagné asks the question, What kind of capability would an individual have to possess if he were to perform this task successfully with only instructions? The answer to this question identifies a new class of tasks having several important characteristics. By this procedure an entity of "subordinate knowledge" has been defined, which is essential to the performance of the more specific final task. Gagné proposes the hypothesis that learning sets, or subknowledges, mediate positive transfer to higher-level tasks. The measurement of transfer of training implies that a second task is learned more rapidly when preceded by the learning of an initial task than when not so preceded.

The notion of the structure of knowledge is also explored by Bruner [6]. Characteristics of structure indicate that organization provides the means by which new material and information are related to that which is already known. Bruner identifies four specific advantages of teaching the structure of a discipline. Comprehension is increased because knowledge of structure provides a framework to which otherwise isolated, unrelated facts and information can be assimilated. Structure promotes memory by placing details into a simplified organization of principles, which fact greatly increases the chances of recall in that the memory of one aspect of the pattern may quickly lead to recall of other related elements. Knowledge of structure appears to enhance the possibility of transfer of training. Finally, the advantage of learning the structure of subject matter is that the material will be kept up to date.

Several factors that influence changes in behavior have been found by psychology. One is individual differences. A curriculum that sets out to change behavior must take account of the fact that change occurs differently in different individuals. Another is motivation. This becomes a problem of identifying what kind of motivation will bring about the particular kinds of changes in behavior that may be contemplated by curriculum builders and how these motivations may be established in the human being.

TEACHER CHARACTERISTICS

The characteristics of teachers, their roles and activities in the teaching-learning environment, present another cluster of variables in the instructional process. The manner in which the teacher utilizes her talents, personal traits, and teaching skill to bring about changes in the behavior of students relates to the concept of teacher effectiveness. The way in which the teacher behaves both in and outside the classroom has a direct influence upon student learning. Considerable attention is being given to the nature and assessment of teacher effectiveness at all levels of education.

TEACHER ROLES

The roles that the teacher assumes in most educational settings are many and varied. A Commission on Teacher Education has identified six roles, which may be organized into three categories [7]. The first category includes the role of the teacher as a director of learning. In this role the teacher has the responsibility of selecting and organizing the learning opportunities that are appropriate for the specific behavior changes desired. Also this role implies that the teacher structures the environment of the learners (physical, social, and psychological) to facilitate the attainment of the learning outcomes. One of the most basic roles of the teacher as a director of learning is that of being a model to her students and to all who think of her as a teacher. This role properly held need not be a burden nor appear to be presumptuous. Accepted and used with skill and humility, this role greatly enriches the teaching. The teacher is a mediator of the varied experiences that are the means of learning for the student. The words, thoughts, and skills that flow through the teacher's personality are given special life and meaning. Every experience in the classroom and often those out of it are seen by the student in relation to the teacher.

The quality and power of the teacher's example vary in terms of the nature of effectiveness of the teacher. This variation is complex. In a sense the more effective the teacher the more powerful she is as an example. The traits and qualities that make her skillful in the teaching-learning situation, those that give imagination, life, meaning, are the ones that make her a powerful example. They tend to establish the open, emotion-toned relation that makes possible and even promotes the flow of feeling and thought between persons, especially the younger and the older, that is basic to influence.

It may be equally true that the very poor teacher also has an especially powerful influence as a person in setting an example essentially for the same reasons that hold for the excellent teacher. Her sarcasm, pettiness, meanness, arbitrariness, favoritism, cruelty, defensiveness, or lack of sympathy are sufficiently alive to have great power, though often negative.

Pullias and Young enumerate the ways in which example expresses its power:

1. Basic attitudes: the psychological posture taken toward important problems, such as, human relations, religion, work, play, the self.
2. Speech and diction: the use of language as the chief vehicle of thought.
3. Work habits: the style with which one does the work which comprises a large portion of every person's life.
4. Attitude toward experience and mistake: an understanding of the relation between breadth of expression and the inevitableness and value of mistakes.
5. Dress: the material extension of the self that is a vital part of that self and is a continuous and revealing expression of the whole personality.
6. Human relations, especially under stress: the quality given to all human intercourse—social, intellectual, moral, and aesthetic.
7. Thought processes: the way the mind works when it is faced with problems.
8. Neurotic behavior: defenses which are habitually used to protect the personality and often used to hurt others.
9. Taste: the system of preferences (likes and dislikes) which persistently and subtly reflect a person's values.
10. Judgment: the rational and intuitive skills used in evaluating all kinds of situations.
11. Health: the quality and tone of body, mind, and spirit, which reflect

themselves in energy level, perspective, poise, enthusiasm, and a genuine zest for life.

12. General style of life: what one believes about every aspect of life and the way in which those beliefs are translated into large and small actions [8].

Modeling, or learning by imitation, helps the individual to learn how to behave in most unfamiliar situations. Mager reports the work of Bandura concerning the nature and dynamics of modeling [9]. It appears that students learn more by imitation if the model has prestige for the student. If the student sees the model being reinforced for her performance, the student will perform more of the imitated behavior. On the other hand, when a student sees a model being punished, the student will tend not to engage in the kind of behavior that was punished. Finally, when a student sees a model doing things she should not do and sees that there is no aversive consequence to the model, there is an increase in the probability that the student will do those undesirable things. This last condition is the source of great frustration to teachers in clinical practice situations, where staff nurses and others appear to be practicing nursing in a manner that is unacceptable to the clinical instructor. Recent research has confirmed the fact that when a teacher teaches one thing and models something else, the teaching is less effective than if the teacher practices what she teaches. If educators would like to increase the frequency with which their students think critically or openmindedly, they have a better chance of succeeding if they demonstrate these qualities themselves.

The role of the teacher as the director of learning may be considered to be that of *promoting student growth*. The second category of roles, the *liaison* roles of the teacher, include the third role, the teacher as mediator of the culture, and the fourth role, the teacher as a link with the community. The school has been identified as the social institution that is established to serve the purposes of society. Some of these purposes include the school as the preserver and transmitter of the cultural heritage, the school as an instrument for transforming the culture, and the school as an instrument for individual development. The school's purposes are largely derived from the pressures of the society on the local, state, and national level. The teacher as an agent of the school has the responsibility of translating the school's purposes into action. This means that the teacher must be knowledgeable about the larger culture, which has impact upon the school, and the specific component of that culture, the profession of nursing. The teacher must be able to transmit to the student the aspects of culture that are undergoing rapid change (technologies) and the influence that these changes have upon other aspects of nonmaterial cultures (values, attitudes). Changing cultural characteristics must be viewed from the framework of their impact upon people's lives, styles of living, health, work, and recreation. The teacher brings to the classroom and clinical setting varied experiences that help students to understand, interpret, and live with some degree of comfort in the dynamic cultural environments. In her role as mediator of the culture, it is necessary for the teacher to provide learning opportunities to attain the curriculum objective. To achieve this end, the teacher must keep in close touch with the community. This means that the teacher must be familiar with and maintain beneficial relations with the various institutions, organizations, and agencies that can provide useful experiences for the students.

Finally, the *program-building* roles include the teacher's fifth role, that of member of the school staff, and her sixth role, that of member of the profession. Planning for curriculum and instruction is a group process. It implies that teachers and students come together in a cooperative relationship to plan appropriate curricular activities and instructional procedures. Working together as a group implies that each member brings to the group some knowledge and skills unique to the individual. Respect for individual talents, values, and attitudes is inherent in any successful group enterprise. The more effective the teacher is in working with the staff of the school, the more successful she will be as a teacher. The teacher in nursing has two professions to which to relate, that of nursing and that of teaching. It is incumbent upon every teacher in nursing to maintain active affiliation with these professional groups. The nursing profession provides the teacher with the necessary information about the ongoing developments in nursing, which become the content of the curriculum. The profession of teaching gives the teacher the current information pertaining to the field of curriculum and instruction. An appropriate balance of knowledge and skills in these areas offers the necessary professional equipment for the teacher in nursing.

TEACHER ACTIVITIES

In any teaching-learning situation, a dynamic process of teacher-student interaction takes place. This interaction has specific purposes that are contained in the objectives of the specific learning situation. In order for the interaction to culminate in the predetermined outcomes, teachers must engage in certain well-defined activities. Eight types of activities in which teachers engage in an effort to assist the student to achieve the objectives of the learning situation are identified.

IDENTIFIES THE EXPECTED OUTCOMES OF THE PROCESS

Considerable attention has been given to the need for identifying the specific behavioral changes that are desired in a particular phase of learning. These changes include those concerned with the attainment of information, the development and use of concepts, the application of principles and the recall of ideas, and facts that are pertinent to the subject matter under consideration. The cognitive outcomes will vary in depth and complexity from simple recall to the application of concepts and principles in some creative fashion. It is one thing to be able to name the factors that have contributed to increased life span of our citizens. It is quite another thing to design a nursing-care plan for an elderly man of low income living alone in a rooming house. The latter objective requires marshalling concepts and principles from a variety of disciplines and utilizing considerable creativity in the application of this information in a plan of nursing care. This type of learning requires recall of information but goes beyond the relatively simple type of learning to a much advanced level of thinking and reasoning.

The affective behaviors have to do with the way students feel, their emotional reactions, and motivational trends in specific nursing situations. What kinds of emotional responses do teachers wish students to develop? What are students' attitudes about certain kinds of patients? How can these attitudes be modified so that nursing care will be truly therapeutic? Because we believe that the emotional reactions of students (and all nurses) have considerable impact upon the quality of nursing care, it is necessary to explore the mechanisms of behavior change in this area in some systematic manner.

The psychomotor behaviors or outcomes rely heavily upon the affective and cognitive learning in the performance of some activity of nursing care. Even though psychomotor skills add a third dimension in the process of learning nursing, any disregard for the implications of knowledge of scientific facts and concepts or the impact of feeling tones could hardly be considered professional behavior. Although the three types of outcomes contribute to each other, they are delineated separately only for the purpose of instructional planning. When the teacher looks at each of these behavioral outcomes, she must ask herself what activities are implied or desired in the instructional process and might be the anticipated results of these activities for the future behavior of the learner.

MAKES ANALYSES OF THE STUDENT

After the teacher has formulated some ideas about the behavior changes that are desired as the result of a learning episode, the teacher must attain some knowledge of the characteristics of the students involved in the learning situation. The teacher must acquire some information about the students' present state of knowledge, their academic and clinical skills, their aspirations, and their reactions to previous study and learning. Time and energy of both students and teachers can be put to efficient use if the teacher has knowledge of the present status of the students before trying to improve or change it. It is wasteful and boring to repeat information that the student has already acquired. On the other hand, it is unfair to students and it may be disastrous for them to assume that they have acquired a certain body of knowledge and skills when in fact they have not. To plan for the articulation of learning sequences, the teacher must assess the characteristics of the students.

SPECIFIES THE OBJECTIVES OF TEACHING TO THE LEARNERS

After decisions have been made about the outcomes of instruction and assessment has been made regarding the characteristics of the students, the teacher is in a position to state the specific objectives of the learning situations. The specification of the objectives of teaching provides the teacher with the necessary information for continued planning for instruction. The teacher must share these objectives with the student so that they will have information about the changes in behavior they will undergo. Knowledge of the objectives of the teaching-learning situation enables the students to visualize the various steps that must be taken to achieve their final goals. Without this information the students may feel that they are groping in the dark with insufficient direction and confusion as to the purposes of their activities.

SELECTS INFORMATION AND MATERIALS

The formulation of specific objectives give an indication of the desired behavior changes in students. The teacher is in a position now to select the appropriate materials that may facilitate the changes which should occur within the student. This implies the selection of subject matter to be dealt with and the various clinical situations to be encountered. These activities require that the teacher have extensive knowledge of her field and be fully aware of the availability of authoritative literature, teaching materials, and technological aids, and the necessary clinical resources and facilities. The teacher must decide what materials should be used and how these are to be organized to bring about the desired results in the students. This requires that the teacher make decisions as to how she will use herself, others, and the materials she has selected in the learning process, that is, what methodological approaches she will use. Whether she will use a lecture, group discussion, self-instruction, or clinical observation and activities will depend upon several factors: (1) behavior change desired, (2) available resources, (3) available time, and (4) size and composition of class. Fortunately there are at hand a vast array of teaching approaches at the disposal of the teacher for her to select from, taking into consideration her personality characteristics and the factors mentioned above.

INVOLVES THE STUDENTS IN THE LEARNING ACTIVITIES

After the preliminary planning has been accomplished, the teacher involves the student in the designated activities, which should result in the students' progressing toward the specified outcomes. The teacher creates and manipulates learning situations that will stimulate students to think critically, solve problems, discuss pertinent issues, ask meaningful questions, engage in activities in clinical nursing appropriate to expected learnings, and make evaluations of herself, the learning situations, and the teacher's effectiveness.

DIRECTS AND GUIDES THE LEARNING ACTIVITIES

Although involvement of the student in various learning activities is necessary for learning to occur, the teacher must assume the responsibility for directing and guiding the learning activities of students. This implies that the teacher selects the appropriate procedures and events for the specific occasion for the particular student to assist her in achieving her goals. No two students are alike, and no two teaching-learning episodes are the same. Decisions must be made on the spot as to what teaching strategies might be useful for the particular students involved.

Teachers do not have the same degree of skill in involving and directing students and their activities. Although teachers all hope that they will make the correct decisions at the right time, they know that they will on occasion fall short of this goal. Probably no one knows better than the sensitive teacher that she has made an inappropriate decision. The effective teacher can, however, use these experiences to improve her teaching skills and competencies.

PROVIDES SITUATIONS FOR USING THE LEARNINGS INVOLVED

Any learning that the student may acquire is made more effective and meaningful if it has some long-range value. If the student has the opportunity to use the new concept, principle, attitude, or skill in situations beyond those in which they were learned, the learning takes on broader usefulness. The teacher can facilitate this extension of learning by providing learning opportunities that incorporate previous learning materials in a variety of different situations which have reality to the students. Repetition of previously learned information and skills in the same situation is boring and wasteful of time. If the knowledge and skills are repeated in new and varied situations, the usefulness of the knowledge and skills becomes apparent.

EVALUATES THE OUTCOMES OF THE PROCESS

Evaluation of the teaching-learning process is continuous throughout any instructional endeavor. The teacher is sensitive to the effect of each learning episode, each teaching procedure, and each interpersonal event upon the development of the student. These are viewed in relation to their effectiveness in assisting students to obtain the desired outcomes. Evaluation may be informal or formal in nature; however, every teacher must obtain necessary information at one stage of learning to give direction to the next stage of learning. Evaluation of student attainment is necessary for the student as well as the teacher. Students must have accurate information about their status, strengths, and weaknesses. The program of evaluation includes a variety of techniques and procedures that focus on the various aspects of behavior change, namely, verbal, affective, and psychomotor. Appropriate tools must be developed and utilized to assess each category of behavior. The data obtained by means of the evaluation program provide information that assists students and teachers to make wise decisions.

Activities of teachers usually are not this systematic and orderly, and certainly not this sequential. A number of these activities may go on concurrently, and some degree of evaluation goes on throughout the total process. All of the activities are equally important if the teaching-learning process is to effect optimal changes in student behavior.

CONCEPT OF TEACHER EFFECTIVENESS

The analysis of teacher roles and activities implies that teaching is a rational and logical process. Although this may be true, there is considerable variation in teacher behavior and style. Teaching is a highly individualized process in which the teacher's personality in interaction with students is a variable. Two teachers dealing with the same material and having very similar objectives will present very different pictures to the classroom observer.

There is considerable evidence that the particular personality characteristics of the teacher have a discernible influence on the behavior, learning, and adjustment of students. There is little evidence that certain personality characteristics are more desirable than others for teaching in general. Increasingly, it is being accepted that effective teaching depends upon appropriate matching of a particular personality with a particular teaching situation.

Ryan defines teacher behavior as the behavior or activities of persons as they go about doing whatever is required of teachers, particularly those activities that are concerned with the direction or guidance of the learning of others [10].

An implication of this definition is that teacher behavior is social behavior. In addition to the teacher, there must be students who are in communication with the teacher and with each other and who are presumably influenced by the behavior of the teacher. Not only do teachers influence student behavior, but students influence teacher behavior as well. What the teacher does is a product of social conditioning and is relative to the cultural setting in which she teaches. Teacher behavior is good or bad, right or wrong, effective or ineffective, only to the extent that such behavior conforms or fails to conform to a particular culture's value system or set of objectives relating to (1) the activities expected of the teacher, and (2) the kinds of student learning desired and the methods of teaching to be employed to bring about this learning [11].

Certain environmental influences and the learned and unlearned characteristics of the individual teacher determine the nature of teacher behavior. Some postulates that evolve from this assumption may include the following:

1. Teacher behavior is characterized by some degree of consistency and therefore is predictable.

2. Teacher behavior is characterized by a limited number of types of responses. This includes the number of responses the individual teacher is capable of making and the number of stimulus situations and organismic variables that may affect a teacher's behavior.

3. Teacher behavior is always probable rather than certain. All human behavior must be considered in light of probability instead of from the standpoint of invariable cause-effect relationships.

4. Teacher behavior is a function of personal characteristics of the individual teacher. Teacher behavior is determined in part by the teacher's personal and social characteristics (such as intellectual, emotional, temperamental, attitudinal, and interest characteristics), which have their sources in both the genetic and the experiential background of the teacher.

5. Teacher behavior is a function of the general features of the situation in which it takes place.

6. Teacher behavior is a function of the specific situation in which it takes place. Teacher behavior is determined, in part, by unique features of its setting at a particular time [12].

DETERMINING TEACHER EFFECTIVENESS

For the purpose of describing, analyzing, and interpreting any teaching situation or episode, information about various characteristics must be obtained. The data that is obtained will provide some clues to better understanding the process and consequences of the teaching act.

In order to make judgments or predictions about teacher behavior, criteria must be employed. The criteria become a standard that provides a frame of reference for judging whether some phenomena occurs and the degree to which it occurs. The complexity of a criterion is in direct proportion to the breadth of the behavior with which the investigator is concerned. Research in the area of teacher effectiveness has been slow to evolve, largely because of difficulties inherent in defining criteria adequately and obtaining criterion measures of teacher competence.

In studies directed by Barr, efforts were made to measure and predict teacher effectiveness [13]. Difficulties that arose in this endeavor stemmed from the facts that teaching means many different things and that the teaching act varies from person to person and from situation to situation. Teachers teach different subjects and at different grade levels; some may not teach a subject but direct activities of a clinical nature. Besides classroom instruction teachers are presumed to be friends and counselors of students, members of a school community, and members of various local, state, and national associations of professional workers.

Another difficulty arose in these studies out of the fact that the concept of efficiency is not well defined. Opinions are varied among teacher educators, administrators, and teachers in relation to the nature of efficiency. It has been noted that the judgments of a group of supervisors, administrators, and teacher educators, all observing the same teacher at the same time under identical conditions, may vary from "among the best" they have observed to "among the very worst."

The criteria of teacher effectiveness employed in these investigations were of two sorts, namely, efficiency ratings and pupil gains, as measured by tests administered to the pupils before and after instruction. More specifically, the criteria included the following:

1. In-service rating
   a. By the superintendent
   b. By the principal
   c. By other supervisory officials
   d. By teacher educators
   e. By departmental personnel
   f. By state department personnel
   g. By self-rating
2. Peer rating
3. Pupil gain score
4. Pupil rating
5. Composite of test scores from tests thought to measure teaching effectiveness
6. Practice teaching grades
7. Combination or composite of some or all of the above criteria [14]

CHARACTERISTICS OF SUPERIOR TEACHERS

The instructor's personality and manner of dealing with students are potential influences upon student performances. Katz identifies some personality characteristics and their effects upon student behavior [15]. The authoritarian, caustic, or impatient instructor may seriously inhibit or otherwise adversely affect the quality of student contributions in her class, cause students to avoid needed interviews, or build lasting negative attitudes toward the course. The permissive, relatively undemanding, understanding instructor, on the other hand, may encourage high-level performance and good attitudes toward learning. But in the case of either instructor, there may be students who will react quite the opposite. The critical authoritarian instructor may be regarded by some as "tough" but a stimulus to perfection. The permissive instructor may be labeled a "pushover for an A" or "too easy to please."

Knapp reports the findings of surveys and studies which endeavored to identify the characteristics of superior teachers [16]. One early study (1930) lists in descending order of importance some eighteen qualities that are attributed by students to the ideal professor. Of these, the four most frequently mentioned—"interest in students," "fairness," "pleasing personality," and "humor" —refer to social and moral qualities. "Mastery of subject" is placed fifth, and such qualities as "keenness of intellect" and "wide range of information" rank far down the list.

Another study (1940) concerned with the image of the ideal professor revealed that the order of attributes appeared to have shifted in that "mastery of subject" was placed second, with "organization of material" in fourth place and "a clear exposition" in fifth place. "Fairness" occupies the highest position, and "interestingness of delivery" is in third place.

A third study (1950) attempts to summarize the attitudes of a group of presidents of liberal arts colleges concerning the ideal qualifications of faculty for instructing in the first and second years of college. "Encouragement of individual thought," "emotional stability," "friendliness," "tolerance," and "sympathy with problems of college students" are ranked in top position. Among the fifteen desirable attributes listed, there was no allusion to high scholarly attainment.

Knapp reported several studies of great teachers that were concerned with the attributes of teachers of known or acknowledged distinction [17]. Teachers who were rated as great were primarily characterized by interest in students; "sympathy," "helpfulness," "sincerity," and "enthusiasm" were the characteristics mentioned most frequently.

Ratings of college teachers by former students were the focus of other studies of teacher characteristics. Among those qualities correlating with high effectiveness of the teacher in motivating her own students to pursue their professional fields were three general constellations. "Masterfulness," "warmth," and "intellectual distinction" appeared to characterize highly effective science teachers.

An extensive survey of student and faculty ratings of the effectiveness of college teachers indicated a substantial agreement in the ratings assigned by the two groups. The faculty, however, tended to rate scholarly attainments as more important, and the students accentuated specific personal and teaching qualities. Size of class and field of specialization of teachers were not significant factors in the ratings.

A study of ratings of former teachers made by graduate students and alumni indicated that the most esteemed qualities were "thoroughness of knowledge in the subject matter taught," "familiarity with recent developments in the field," "logical and forthright presentation," and "stimulation of discussion."

Finally, a study was conducted that involved the rating of college instructors at a large metropolitan college by both faculty and students. The teachers were rated for "effectiveness as a teacher," "as a personality," and for "creativeness." The ratings on the three variables all showed high positive correlations for both rating groups. The estimate of teaching effectiveness is influenced in college ranking by "creativeness," although students tend to rate teaching more as a function of "good personality."

The teacher's behavior both in and out of class constitutes the strategies and tactics of teaching. Whereas learning environments describe the physical setting and structure provided for the course, the instructor variables describe the unique contributions to a given learning environment made by the teacher. The intellectual climate developed by the instructor and the involvement of students in the learning process are important variables in defining the structure of the learning environment. Finally, the personal characteristics of the teacher, her philosophy of life, and her relationships with students and others have tremendous impact upon the teaching-learning process.

THE LEARNING ENVIRONMENT

No matter what man's philosophy of behavior may be, he is not likely to deny that the world about him is important. Behavior must be appropriate to the occasion within a particular environmental setting. In studying the important independent variables that lie in the immediate environment, one may begin with a physical description. What is the structure of the world that one sees, touches, and smells? The learning environment, however, includes other events and phenomena that influence learning: the relationships of student to teacher, of students to students, of teachers to teachers, all of which give an indication of the social structure of the learning environment. Lastly, the complex of stimuli that press upon the individual and to which his behavior is a response is known as the psychological environment of the learning situation. Educators are interested in all these conditions or events because they have an effect upon behavior.

PHYSICAL ENVIRONMENT

When John Dewey was organizing his experimental school in Chicago in the 1890's, he searched for appropriate equipment and furniture to supply the kind of environment he desired for an active, working class. It was reported that a perceptive salesman told him that he was seeking equipment that encourages working, whereas all conventional school furniture was designed to encourage listening.

Today's schools have available a variety of facilities and furniture with both specialized and multipurpose uses. The typical classroom today does not have "listening" seats fixed in permanent rows but is flexible enough to lend itself to instant rearrangement for various purposes. The imaginative teacher can reorganize classroom furniture and space for a variety of activities.

In our affluent society within a wide range of differences, it is highly probable that the schools of a community will be consistent with the homes of a community in architecture, space, and equipment. The culture tends to perpetuate itself by providing school buildings that influence teachers and students in the direction of the community norm. Consciously or unconsciously, the typical teacher uses the physical environment of the school to instruct the students in attitudes toward the protection and care of property and the importance of their physical environment. More subtle learnings in the use of color and harmony in decoration, and values concerning interaction between people and things, are also transmitted.

Nursing schools have not always been favored in the allocation of appropriate physical facilities. All too often in the past, faculties and students were relegated to outmoded and out-of-the-way classrooms and offices that had been discarded by others. It was not always easy to convince administrative officials that a school of nursing needed equipment and facilities beyond a nurses' residence and a hospital. More recently, and with the advent of federal legislation for school construction, nursing school facilities have shown marked improvement. Modern, attractive classrooms and offices have been made available to faculties and students in schools of nursing. In addition to the very basic equipment, many schools display an elaborate array of teaching aides and devices. In many instances newer buildings are being equipped with multimedia instructional equipment, including closed-circuit television. This is, indeed, a far cry from the basement facilities where many nurse educators began teaching. It seems rather obvious that new and different variables have been introduced into the instructional process. The variables in the learning environment may be defined by the physical setting and characteristics of the classroom or other instructional site and by certain events transpiring in the physical environment. Other kinds of physical environments include the library carrel, the language or autoinstructional laboratory, and the room at home where an off-campus telecourse is taken.

Some of the specific variables entering into the composition of the environment include the following:

1. Class size
2. Physical characteristics of the classroom
3. The physical presence or absence of an "authority figure" in the classroom

4. The methods by and extent to which audiovisual devices of various kinds are used

5. The availability of accessory facilities, such as study rooms, lounges, lavatories, eating facilities, coatrooms, and lockers.

The control of the external events in the learning situation is what Gagné refers to as "instruction" [18]. These are the events that are manipulated by the teacher, the textbook writer, the designer of films or television lessons, and the developer of self-instructional programs. A major part of the instructional complex that may be controlled or manipulated is the stimulus situation. By this is meant the objects or events that are the focus of learning interest. In reading, the stimuli are printed words on a page; in science the stimuli may be plants or tissues or chemical solutions; in mathematics, they may be symbols of drawings of geometrical figures; and in nursing the stimuli may be patients, nurse practitioners, and allied health workers as well as considerable physical equipment. The objects and events that make up the stimulus situation for learning vary according to what is being learned. The desired content of instruction will determine whether the stimulus situation is primarily composed of contacts with specific patients, community groups, or nurse practitioners or the manipulation of clinical equipment and materials.

SOCIAL ENVIRONMENT

The teacher deals not with isolated individuals but with a group of people who are organized in a social structure. The interaction of students in a class is characterized by various patterns of friendship, enmity, cooperation, competition, acceptance, rejection, and role expectation. For various activities, the roles enacted by individuals will shift. There are many ways for the teacher to utilize the social structure of the class to enhance or interfere with the teaching-learning process. The way in which classes are organized according to grade level, ability, achievement, or other criteria will affect the conditions under which teaching occurs.

Social interaction is concerned with the behavioral transactions among human beings in the school learning situation. Realization of the very great influence of the classroom group upon individual learning follows from a consideration of the implications of research in social psychology. These studies capitalized on the view of the classroom as a social milieu in which learning and instruction occurred. They identified four functional interrelationships between the individual and the group in which the classroom group helps the individual to learn, to progress toward self-realization, to test social concepts, and to adapt to her culture. The studies emphasized the need to understand the individual learner's frame of reference within the context of the group values and pressures in the classroom situation. This understanding requires the development by the teacher of the ability to conceptualize the internal frame of reference of each learner and to ascertain how she can use group forces and group problem-solving mechanisms to bring about learning [19].

A three-dimensional investigation is required, which includes (1) the teacher's actual behavior in the classroom and her comprehension of the learner's self and social perceptions, (2) the learner's perception of the instructional activities, and (3) the group-life context in which the teacher and learner interact. The teacher can best fulfill her function in the classroom group as a skilled practitioner of evocative leadership. The teacher, in this role, helps learners to identify common goals, common values, and roles of members. The studies identified the specified needs of class members as individuals and as group members. The close interdependence of personal needs and group needs were emphasized. The fulfillment of personal needs appears to depend upon the fulfillment of the individual as a group member. Individuals in the learning situation have to help insure the satisfaction and resolution of group needs if their private personal needs are to be met optimally.

It was observed that productivity of a class, the achievement of its members as individuals, and the members' satisfactions with the class are a function of the relationships among the following dimensions: problem-solving, authority-leadership, power, friendship, personal prestige, sex, and privilege. A group is characterized by the interaction of its members; each person is changed by the group and changes as the group changes. A collection of individuals becomes a group as members accept a common purpose, become interdependent in implementing this purpose, and interact with one another to promote its accomplishments.

Referring to the classroom as a social system, Getzels and Thelan have this to say:

It is not the image of a social system in equilibrium. It is rather the image of a system in motion or, if you will, in dynamic disequilibrium. It is the image of a group continually facing emergent complexity and conflict (if not confusion) and dealing with these realities, not in terms of sentiment but in terms of what the complexity and conflict suggest about the modifications that have to be made in the goals, expectations, needs and selective perceptions of the teachers and learners. It is through this experience of recognizing and dealing with complexity, conflict and change in the classroom situation that we can educate children to take their places as creative and autonomous participants in the other social systems that constitute the larger social order [20].

These observations seem to imply that the social environment presents a purpose to education as well as variables in the learning environment. The analysis of group endeavors enables the teacher to determine and assess the effect the individual has upon the group and the effect the group has upon the individual student and the teacher.

PSYCHOLOGICAL ENVIRONMENT

The psychological environment has been defined as the complex of stimuli that press upon the individual and to which his behavior constitutes a response. H. A. Murray (1938) introduced a taxonomy for classifying both the environmental pressures and the characteristic ways in which an individual strives to structure the environment for himself. He called the external pressures *press* and their internal counterparts *needs*. Murray proposed a system for classifying the organizational tendencies that appear to give unity and direction to personality. Although he called these tendencies needs, the terms *drive* and *motive* have also been used to refer to the objectives that a person characteristically strives to achieve for himself. Whatever they be called, they stand for something inferred from a person's actions. The actions themselves may be quite diversified and lend themselves individually to many different explanations in other contexts, but they are given a unified theme in the interpretation placed on them. The simplest indirect source of this information about students is the responses they give when asked to indicate preferences among verbal descriptions of various possible activities. The Activities Index (Stern, Stein, and Bloom) provides for the measurement of these needs [21].

The external counterpart of the personality need is called an environmental press. It has been used to describe the private world of the individual, the unique view each person has of the events around him. There is a level at which the person's private world merges with that of others like him, with people who share a common ideology. Both the private and the mutually shared press are of interest in their own right, but in the final analysis it is the inferences made by observers that provide us with useful classifications of situational differences.

The source of indirect information about press comes from a participant's acknowledgment of characteristic events occurring in the environment. The College Characteristic Index (Pace and Stern) is a measure of thirty kinds of press, analogous to the needs scales of the Activities Index but restricted to the description of activities, policies, procedures, attitudes, and impressions that may characterize various types of undergraduate settings [22]. Both needs and press are inferred from characteristic activities and events, the former from things that the individual typically does, the latter from things that are typically done to him in some particular setting.

Utilizing these questionnaires, Stern investigated the characteristics of the intellectual climate in college environments [23]. It was evident from the relationship demonstrated that the intellectual climate of an institution is closely related to the quality of its student body and to their academic achievements after graduation. Some of the characteristics of these college environments that were considered to be "high intellectual" included the following:

Alma Mater seemed to be less important than the subject matter.
Faculty put a lot of energy and enthusiasm into their teaching.
School has good reputation for academic freedom.
Main emphasis in learning is on breadth of understanding, perspectives, and critical judgment.
There is respect for nonconformity; students are encouraged to be independent and individualistic.

Among the characteristics of students in college with high intellectual climate are the following:

Students enjoy engaging in mental activities requiring intense concentration.
They would like to understand themselves and others better.
They are interested in learning the causes of our social and political problems.
They dislike working for someone who always tells them exactly what to do and how to do it.

McFee endeavored to determine the relationship of students' needs to their perception of a college environment [24]. Using the same questionnaires, he failed to find any significant correlation between scale scores of individuals on the College Characteristics Index and their parallel scores on the Activities

Index, nor was there strong relation found between personality need and the students' perceptions of environment press.

It has been found that the faculties at institutions whose graduates attain doctoral degrees in greater numbers than would be expected on the basis of aptitudes of their entering classes are perceived differently from the faculties at less productive institutions. Some students making the decision to seek graduate or professional training during the college years attribute their decision to the influence of college teachers. An interpretation of these observations is that some colleges are more successful than others in creating learning environments that motivate students to seek advanced training and that these differences are in part traceable to faculty behaviors and activities.

Thistlewaite sought to identify the characteristics of the environment that appeared to motivate students to seek advanced learning in specialized fields [25]. The students included in the study were exceptionally talented students who had received scholarship or honorary recognition awards. The most important result of the study is the finding that students exposed to some educational treatments can be shown to have raised their degree aspirations more than comparable students exposed to other educational treatments. Teachers who exert press for independence tend to be more effective in stimulating students in social sciences or humanities. Students who were influenced to raise their aspirations more frequently reported that "there are many facilities for individual creative activity," "the faculty is not too busy to invent ways of encouraging initiative among students," "there is opportunity for pursuing independent study," and "the main emphasis is on critical judgment."

Teachers who are supportive appear to have the greatest influence upon student aspirations. Such teachers are distinguished by the following attributes: willingness to discuss student goals, to help students discover their special talents, to give special tutoring or counseling to students having difficulty, and to help students obtain redress of grievances.

Thistlewaite in another study endeavored to obtain information relative to the holding power and attractiveness of different fields of study, the characteristics of students and faculty in these fields, the effects of the intellectual and social atmosphere upon motivation to seek advanced training, and the traits of instructors that had the greatest influence upon talented students. The study turned up the following information:

1. After three years of college, one third of the students are planning to do graduate study required for the doctoral degree, while one in seven expect to get a professional degree in law or medicine.

2. Sixty-five percent of those majoring in the biological sciences have raised their goals, while somewhat less than 50 percent of the students in other fields report such changes.

3. The natural sciences and the arts and humanities are most dissimilar in faculty and student press. The natural science faculty exhibited pragmatism, achievement, and compliance, and relatively little enthusiasm, affiliation, and supportiveness. They also demonstrated a weak press for humanism and independence. The student subcultures show strong press for reflectiveness and aggressiveness and a weak press for humanism.

4. The arts and humanities faculty tend to be enthusiastic, affiliative, and supportive and demonstrate a strong press for humanism and independence. They exhibit a weak press for pragmatism and achievement. The social science faculty resemble those in the arts and humanities. They exhibit a weak press for compliance. The student subcultures emphasize reflectiveness, breadth of interest, and competition [26].

It appears that college environments characterized by faculty affiliation or enthusiasm or faculty emphasis upon achievement, humanism, or independence are associated with increased motivation to seek advanced degrees in the arts, humanities, and social sciences; college environments characterized by a lack of faculty emphasis upon student compliance are associated with increased motivation to seek advanced degrees in the natural and biological sciences.

These studies show that certain aspects of the learning environment are conducive to the realization of their potentials. The student reports provide abundant evidence that college press differ considerably. The most striking feature of these results is that one type of college environment is associated with achievement in the natural sciences while a different kind of environment is related to accomplishment in the arts, humanities, and social sciences. There is not yet available comparable information about the press of environments in nursing. Nurse educators have reason to believe that some nursing programs place heavy emphasis upon the natural sciences while others stress the behavioral sciences. It would be interesting to discover the nature of the student cultures that are associated with these environments in relation to the characteristics of the different college environments.

There are many other critical areas that influence the teaching process. The nature of the community, the experiences provided by mass media, and the administrative arrangements in the school are among the external conditions with which the effective teacher must deal in planning instruction and creating a learning environment. The prospective teacher must somehow acquire a wide array of understandings concerning knowledge of purposes, materials, techniques, and appropriate attitudes toward learners and the social milieu in addition to a mastery of skills in weaving these together in the complex process of teaching.

TEACHING STRATEGIES

A strategy is a plan for purposeful action. A strategy of teaching is a plan of specific activities that will assist the student to modify or change her behavior in specific, predetermined ways. The strategy incorporates several activities that are designed in a certain fashion because of the specific requirements of the learner and the conditions of the learning environment. The particular activities that are selected and the way in which they are arranged will depend upon the objectives of the defined teaching episode. Although larger strategies may encompass all of the various activities, smaller strategies may utilize as few as two or three activities. The activities that may be included in strategies of teaching include the following:

Setting behavioral goals
Informing learners of objectives
Presenting the stimulus
Providing cues for learning
Controlling attention
Stimulating recall of previously learned capabilities
Arranging for reinforcement
Encouraging generalization
Measuring and assessing behavior

SETTING BEHAVIORAL GOALS

A first and foremost component of teaching strategy is the identification of the goals to be attained during the student-teacher-environment interaction. These goals may involve an almost infinite number of behaviors, including a wide range of verbal behaviors, specific motor and manipulatory behaviors, and those concerned with feelings and emotions. It is important to specify as precisely as possible those behaviors that should evolve as the result of the teaching-learning process. In doing so, it is necessary to give consideration to the initial behaviors of the student, or the repertoire of learning that the student brings to the learning situation. This requires that some assessment be made of the initial behaviors to provide the teacher with a starting point from which change may be initiated and measured.

It is equally important to define the desired change precisely so that it will be possible to determine the steps to the goal and the point at which the goal is achieved. It is surprising how many nursing goals for students are so ill-defined that nurse educators really do not know when they have been achieved or to what degree they have been attained. Goals should include precisely the defined steps for their achievement, with each step an important link in the learning process. Although it is a temptation to design objectives that designate a wide array of behaviors, teachers must be realistic about the specific purpose of the unit of instruction and include only those objectives that are directly pertinent to the goals.

Perhaps the greatest difficulty with teacher-set goals is their lack of precision. It is likely that every nursing curriculum, as well as those in other fields, includes an objective concerned with "good citizenship" as a desirable outcome. If one considers all the possible behaviors that could be included or excluded, depending upon who is defining the term, then one realizes how vague and general this objective is. It is only when these goals are broken down into their particulars that sufficient specificity to guarantee understanding is achieved.

It is relatively easy to determine the criteria for the goal if the objective is some simple behavior. Most nursing behaviors are not simple but very complex and involving many subbehaviors. The analysis of these behaviors reveals many varied behaviors pertaining to verbal and psychomotor skills. Each of the particular behaviors must be analyzed and assessed in terms of the degree of attainment expected of the student. It has been observed that when certain specific behaviors are neglected in assessment and teaching, the process of behavior modification is hindered. Assessment involves developing appropriate measures for the specific behaviors. The result of such testing procedures gives the teacher firsthand information about the behavior repertoire of each student, which facilitates individualizing instruction. Testing in this sense utilizes any legitimate way in which the teacher can get at the desired behavior, be it verbal, affective, or psychomotor.

Teacher-set goals should be expressed in such a way that they can be readily understood by the student. Such statements as "advanced knowledge of pathophysiology" or "increased skill in communication," while implying certain behaviors, do not specify them precisely. The qualifying words "advanced" and "increased" may be perceived differently by student and teacher to the point that there may be lack of congruence in the goals set by teacher and student. Both teacher and student may end up being frustrated because there is lack of communication as to the goals. Terminal behaviors, therefore, must be precise and stated in such a way as to enable students to follow a clear procedure to the final goal.

Specific terminal behaviors are those determined by the teacher to meet the objectives that she has set for the student. They may involve the learner in some verbal activity or in some physical activity or both. Whatever they are, they must be stated so that teacher and student can determine the point at which they have been achieved. The subbehaviors or components of the terminal behavior are considered to be steps toward the attainment of the terminal behavior. The emphasis or degree of attention given to each of the subbehaviors is dependent upon the initial assessment of the student and the diagnosis of her strengths and weaknesses.

INFORMING THE LEARNER OF THE OBJECTIVES

A requirement of teaching that may transcend other conditions of learning is that the learner be informed of what is expected of her. It make little difference in what is done, or said, or what kinds of environment for learning are created if the learner does not know about the nature of the performance expected of her when learning is finished. The procedure of informing the learner of the objectives of learning establishes a continuing set that facilitates learning by making possible reinforcement at several points in a rather lengthy sequence of activities. If the learner is aware of the various components or subbehaviors of the terminal behavior, reinforcement is likely to occur as the learner accomplishes each of the steps toward the achievement of the terminal behavior.

The statement of objectives provides the learner with knowledge of the specific types of behavior (verbal, affective, psychomotor) modification in which she will engage. With this knowledge, she can make some self-assessment of her initial behavior to determine where she is and where she needs to go. This information also reveals to the learner something of the nature of the learning situations and the conditions of learning necessary for modification of her behavior. It is likely that this knowledge produces a set for learning and facilitates the movement of the student toward optimal behavior change.

Set induction or preinstructional orientation helps the teacher prepare students for the class so that maximum learning may take place. Set is more than introductory remarks. Its purpose is to clarify the objectives of instruction, utilizing the initial behaviors of the student to get them involved in the learning process. The presentation of an overview of the unit including the behavioral expectations is related to Ausubel's concept of advance organizers and provides a link between previous learnings and those to come.

PRESENTING THE STIMULUS

A stimulus is any condition, event, or change in environment of an individual that produces a change in behavior. A major task in any learning situation is the careful selection and arrangement of the stimuli to which the student will respond. A stimulus usually refers to a specific event that calls for specific behavior. It is that aspect of the environment which is responsible for producing the behavior. In an instructional situation one may assume that the learner attends to those parts of the stimulus situation that are necessary for her to produce a correct response. It may be necessary to present the stimulus in a variety of ways so that the student's answer indicates that she is responding to a particular stimulus.

Selecting the proper stimulus requires decisions. If objectives of the unit of learning indicate the desired behavior changes, the selection of stimuli must be directly related to this behavior change. If any behavior change is to occur, the student must be given an opportunity to deal with the behaviors. If objects must be learned, the object itself must be presented. It may be represented initially by a word, but eventually the object itself or a simulated version of the object must be presented as a stimulus to which the student may respond. If the behavior change implies the manipulation of objects, then opportunity must be provided for the student to practice the manipulatory skills. The learning of verbal behavior necessitates the presentation of verbal stimuli.

When an individual responds in a certain way to a given stimulus, that stimulus can be considered to control behavior. The number of stimuli that control or influence behavior increases with maturity. The behavior of a very young child is determined by relatively few, primarily internal stimulus conditions, such as hunger, pain, or thirst. As he matures, the child learns to respond to more and more external stimuli. The development of complex forms of behavior is possible because of an individual's increasing responsiveness to new sources of stimulation in his environment. Since instruction is concerned with the manipulation of subject matter stimuli in the environment of the learner, the process requires first the identification of those stimuli that currently control the behavior of the learner and then the placement of these stimuli under the management of the teacher. The teacher can then use the present behavior of the student to guide her to new forms of behavior. This process is greatly helped by the detailed specification of the behavior that the teacher wants the student to perform. For each stage of learning, the subject matter stimuli (words, symbols, formulas, patients) to which the leaner can respond and the kind of response that each of these requires (writing, problem-solving, developing a nursing-care plan) should be specified in terms of observable behavior.

At the beginning of any instructional program, the student is asked to make responses that are already familiar to her. As the learner proceeds to perform subsequent subject matter activities that build upon these, she transfers her original responses to new subject matter content and also attaches newly learned responses to the new subject matter. An evident characteristic of learning that leads to subject mastery is the increasing precision of the student's responses. In learning complex behavior, the student's initial performance is variable and often quite crude; it rarely meets the criteria of competence. Effective instructional procedure tolerates the student's initially crude responses and gradually takes her toward mastery. To accomplish this, the instructional process must involve the establishment of successively more rigorous standards or criteria for the learners' performance and must present the appropriate stimuli to evoke the desired responses.

PROVIDING CUES FOR LEARNING

Providing cues for learning requires that a part of the response is shown before there is an opportunity for an overt response. The purpose of providing cues is to assure that the correct response will be made, which reduces the possibility of errors. A cue is that aspect of the environment that provides an individual with information about what she is to do if she is to receive reinforcement. Varieties of cuing that have been or could be employed include (1) denotative prompts and (2) connotative cues. The former includes the use of physical controls, such as underscoring or italic type. The latter includes the use of sentence structure, relational words, opposites, and rhyming. Pictures and diagrams can also be used as connotative cues. A prompt is a highly specific cue intended to promote a rapid emission of an already learned response. The prompt helps the student by greatly increasing the chance that she will make a correct response. Prompts may be verbal, or nonverbal, as when the teacher presents an object or a picture.

The teacher is concerned with providing a classroom environment in which new and increasingly difficult stimuli (materials, activities) are presented with a considerable number of clear cues and prompts. As material is presented and correct responses made, cues and prompts are gradually eliminated until minimal cues are sufficient to elicit correct responses.

The teacher, acting as a model for the student, is actually providing very precise cues to the student as to what she is expected to do, cues so precise that the probability of incorrect responding is quite low. Modeling is a valuable tool in teaching. By demonstrating exactly what she wants her students to do and by reinforcing their successful efforts at imitation, the teacher can overcome problems that would otherwise consume much time and effort. The technique is particularly useful when the subject being taught requires highly specific kinds of motor behavior. Although modeling can serve as a shortcut to learning, the teacher serving as a model must be careful that her performance is free of errors so that the students do not pick up incorrect behavior. Videotape recordings are extremely useful in this regard, in that a teacher can view her performance and can correct responses before presentation to her students. Visual techniques, such as movies and videotape, can themselves be used, with the teacher filming or taping a performance to enable students to imitate the model's recorded behavior.

Certain students may themselves appear to be modeled by other students. If a student learns behavior that is particularly successful in obtaining reinforcement in the classroom, others may emulate the behavior and emit similar responses to obtain reinforcement.

The use of human models in instruction is hardly new. Apprenticeship programs from the time of the early guilds up to the present have based much of their training on the use of models. The teacher demonstration of a procedure and the return demonstration by the student is inherent in all nursing instruction. Some of the problems that may be encountered include (1) oversimplification of activity or skill, (2) adoption of personal characteristics of others, (3) lack of opportunities for immediate practice, and (4) requirement of a clear definition of the skill the teacher is trying to demonstrate.

The optimal amount of cuing has not been determined, presumably because students differ in the amount they need. However, unless cuing is adequate, the student can easily get lost and is likely to lose motivation. It is therefore believed that control of excessive errors through cuing procedures is important, despite the fact that no optimal level of control can yet be named. If the student cannot respond, why should she not be given maximal help? The teacher helps the student respond on a given occasion so that she will respond on similar occasions in the future. In traditional face-to-face teaching, this problem is solved by using only as much of a prompt or cue as is needed to evoke a response. It is inefficient to continue to prompt behavior when learning has taken place, but if prompting is stopped too quickly, the student may have to guess, and wrong responses may not contribute to further learning. Students who have learned how to study know how to limit the help they receive from prompts and cues.

CONTROLLING ATTENTION

Attention may be considered a first step in learning, and unless a student attends to relevant features of a problem, she will not be able to learn it. Controlling attention of the student is integrally related to presenting stimuli and providing cues for learning. It has been noted that extraneous stimuli may distract students and that students have a difficult time learning to make important discriminations among stimuli in such an environment. Skinner indicates that the student can be induced to act selectively to special features of the environment by arranging contingencies of reinforcement [27]. The student can be taught that some features of the environment are worth responding to. To attend to something as a form of self-management is to respond to it in such a way that subsequent behavior is more likely to be reinforced.

Problem-solving begins with essentially chance or random responding. As the student progresses, she no longer attends to those aspects of the problem that do not contribute to finding a correct solution. The sooner the learner abandons irrelevant cues and attends to those that are relevant, the faster her rate of problem-solving will improve. Teachers should systematically select those cues that are critical to the solution of the problem and accentuate them while simultaneously avoiding cues that are irrelevant and distracting. By planning for the systematic presentation of relevant cues that are both numerous and accentuated, and by eliminating distracting materials, the teacher can expect to increase the rate of learning by controlling the attention of the student.

Although verbal statements are the most commonly used means of directing attention, there are other ways. Gestures made by the teacher can be equally effective. The movement of objects is another kind of event that is likely to direct attention to it, such as the movement of a piece of equipment to the bedside of a patient for explanation and demonstration. When illustrations are used as a part of instruction, a variety of means of directing attention are available, including contrasting colors, arrows, underlining, italicizing, and bold type.

Directions that guide the student's discovery of concepts or principles are often in the form of questions. The question of how much guidance is necessary to maintain the attention of the student is individual. Too little guidance or questions that may be too difficult may discourage the learner, and her attention to the instruction may diminish. Too much guidance and questions that are relatively simple will reduce the challenge of the problem and diminish attention.

Some techniques of getting and maintaining attention involve physical constraints. Earphones reassure the teacher that only what is to be heard is going into the student's ears. Less coercive practice is to make what is to be seen or heard attractive and attention compelling. The teacher induces the student to look at an object by isolating it from other things or by showing it suddenly or moving it about. She induces the student to listen to what she is saying by speaking loudly or varying her speech or intonation. So-called audio-visual materials, brightly colored books, and animated films are made attractive by the same principle.

STIMULATING RECALL OF PREVIOUSLY LEARNED CAPABILITIES

Verbal directions may tell the learner to recall something she has learned previously. Verbal directions may include a question about previously learned responses or a direct statement. Such a statement as, "You remember what emphysema is and its effect upon respiratory action," directs the student to recall previously learned information. When more complex principles are being acquired, it may be desirable for the directions to require a restatement, as, for example, "Explain the mechanisms of gas exchange in respiratory activity."

The necessity for recall of previously learned responses immediately prior to the new act of learning is probably an indication of the importance of contiguity of learning. The attempt to learn something when some "piece of content" cannot be recalled results in delays and frustration to the learner. The use of verbal instructions in inducing recall is a highly important feature of the total instructional process.

Bruner's concept of the spiral curriculum requires the learner to continually look back upon ideas, notions, or activities that were previously learned, so that they can be further explored, expanded, and examined at higher levels of development in the various stages of learning [28].

Other techniques and procedures that may assist the student to recall previously learned capabilities include (1) the presentation of an overview of new learning incorporating important issues of previous learnings, (2) the assignments that require a recall of important ideas previously learned, (3) the constant calling of the learner's attention to the ideas or notions that have become the organizing themes or centers of the curriculum, and (4) the use of questions that stimulate the learner to remind herself of pertinent aspects of knowledge.

ARRANGING FOR REINFORCEMENT

A reinforcement is an environmental event that increases the rate of a response that it follows. The consequences of an individual's actions are critical in the modification and maintenance of behavior. Behavior is acquired or modified under conditions in which a response produces a consequent stimulus event, such as a reward, that strengthens or maintains that response. The stimulus event that the response produces is referred to as a "reinforcer" or "reinforcing stimulus." The occurrence of a reinforcer as a consequence of behavior is called reinforcement. The arrangement of an environment that will yield reinforcing stimuli only when specified behaviors occur is the process of providing reinforcement.

Reinforcement may be positive or negative. Praising the student for a good paper involves the use of positive reinforcement because a stimulus (praise) is presented following the desired behavior (good paper). Negative reinforcement consists of removing something that could be punishing so that the student avoids or escapes the punishing event by doing whatever is required: "If you don't hand your paper in on time, you will get a failing grade." Presumably the student will hand in the paper on time to avoid getting the failing grade. Negative reinforcers require the presentation of a threat, usually through some verbal means, and then the removal of the threat following compliance. Punishment is an environmental event that decreases the rate of the response that it follows.

It is not always easy to ascertain just what is reinforcing and what is punishing for an individual student. It requires alertness to administer reinforcement in a consistent manner. Some principles pertaining to the use of reinforcers are suggested:

1. Positive and negative reinforcers are defined only in terms of how they affect the learner, not how the teacher thinks they might affect the learner.

2. The effects of positive and negative reinforcers are automatic.

3. Reinforcers should be very closely related to the desired terminal behavior. The teacher must be aware of exactly what she is trying to reinforce and then make certain that the reinforcement is contingent only on that behavior.

4. The teacher must be consistent in how she responds to a student if she wishes to achieve specific educational objectives in a predictable manner.

5. Reinforcers should closely follow the behavior on which they are contingent. In trying to gain, maintain, or eliminate specific behavior in the classroom, the teacher will have greater effect on the behavior of the student by using immediate reinforcers than by using delayed outcomes.

6. Generally it is desirable to reinforce more frequently and with more potent reinforcers on tasks involving new learnings.

7. The student's work should be programmed so that there are many steps to be reinforced.

The various kinds of reinforcers that are available include:

1. Consumables—food pellets that are used in experimental studies and that do not lend themselves to the ordinary classroom
2. Manipulatables—toys, trinkets, hobby items
3. Visual and auditory stimuli—signals from the teacher, confirmation of results of learning
4. Social stimuli—peer approval or disapproval
5. Tokens—grades, honor certificates, money (such as scholarship awards)

The teacher in the college setting has two categories of reinforcers available to her: visual and auditory stimuli, and tokens. The teacher can select reinforcers from these stimulus events that are appropriate to the learning situation.

ENCOURAGING GENERALIZATION

The more general objectives of instruction usually include the aim of generalization or transfer of learning. It is to be expected that there will be sub-

written nursing-care plan. Although these are useful demonstrations of student's learned capabilities, the teacher must have clearly defined and prepared in written form the criteria by which the student will be assessed. These criteria should be made available to the student at the beginning of instruction so that she will have full knowledge of the kind of behavior change expected of her.

Some behaviors that are essential to the practice of nursing can be assessed only by observation of practice. This means observing the behavior of the student as it is taking place. Observation and recording of human behavior is plagued with all the problems of changing environmental conditions: distractions, subjectivity, and forgetting. In an effort to overcome these problems, the teacher should formulate clearly the kind of practice behavior that is expected of the student at the various stages of her development. This takes into consideration the various types of learnings expected to occur, such as technical competence, skills in communication and interpersonal relationships, and the application of scientific concepts and principles. Since there will be differences in the behaviors among a group of students, these definitions of practice behaviors should include descriptions of the behavior that might be termed minimally acceptable, average, and outstanding. Again, the student should have full knowledge of these behavior characteristics so that she can engage in self-evaluation of her own behavior.

Accurate knowledge of the results of learning provides the student and teacher with the necessary information for decision-making. If the student has achieved what is considered to be satisfactory, she is then ready to move on to other, perhaps more difficult, learnings. If she has not achieved satisfactorily, some diagnosis of learning difficulties is required to prescribe appropriate remedial activities. Immediate knowledge of results of learning provides the student with the opportunity to correct wrong responses and reinforces correct answers or behavior. Knowledge of results through measuring and assessing behavior also tends to have a positive motivational value in guiding ongoing learning activities.

SUMMARY

Variables in the instructional process are those persons, events, and environmental characteristics that can be expected to have bearing upon instructional effectiveness. The variables are those that are measurable or amenable to categorization. They also can be manipulated along some unidimensional continuum, and the effects of the manipulation can be observed. Four classes of independent variables are identified: (1) learner characteristics, (2) teacher characteristics, (3) the learning environment, and (4) teaching strategies.

The characteristics of learners that have a profound effect upon learning are described as motivation and previously learned capabilities of the learner. Motivation of the student is a challenge to the learning psychologist and the classroom teacher. Almost all theories of learning include in some way the effects of motivation upon the learning process. Many studies pertaining to motivation of the learner have been published; however, there is no conclusive evidence as to exactly what motivates students. It is known that for students to learn, they must be motivated. Beyond this, it is the concern of the teacher to discover the individual factors that relate to the motivation of the learner. Some of these may include (1) the motivation to achieve, (2) the motivation to engage in learning, and (3) the motivation to continue learning tasks.

Differences in the learning outcomes of a group of students may be attributed to differences in previously learned capabilities. Differences of several kinds can be noted in the experience backgrounds of any group of college students. These may stem from the arrangement of courses within various curriculums, the length of time the student has been in school, and the other kinds of out-of-school experiences the student has had. The bearing of individual differences upon the instructional process must be recognized and used in structuring the learning environment. This includes a clear conception of the learner's goals as she sees them, not as the teacher conceives them. In addition, assessment of the existing academic background of the learner in relation to goal attainment is a prerequisite for future planning. The concept of readiness implies that the student has the necessary knowledge and skills to move forward. Readiness often determines whether a given intellectual skill or type of school material is learnable at a particular stage of development and always influences the efficiency of the learning process. Authorities in the field of learning have noted the issues and concerns in providing for sequence in learning materials.

Another cluster of variables in the instructional process includes those pertaining to the teacher. The manner in which the teacher utilizes her talents, traits, and skills to bring out changes in the behavior of students relates to the notion of teacher effectiveness. The roles that teachers assume in the educational setting include (1) director of learning, (2) mediator of the culture, (3) member of the school staff, (4) link with the community, and (5) member of the profession. In each of these roles the teacher exercises her influence, the effect of which may be seen in the behavior change of students.

In any learning situation, teacher-student interaction is ongoi..g and dynamic. In order for this interaction to facilitate the attainment of the objectives, the teacher engages in several related and interdependent activities: (1) identifies the expected outcomes of the process, (2) makes analyses of the student, (3) specifies the objectives of teaching to the learner, (4) selects information and materials, (5) involves the students in the learning activities, (6) directs the learning activities, (7) provides situations for practice of the learning involved, and (8) evaluates the outcomes of the process. It is obvious that some of these activities should precede others, and several activities may be going on at the same time.

The concept of teacher effectiveness is prominent in the literature today, but it is a concept that is difficult to define and describe. Teaching is a highly individualistic process in which many teacher characteristics are involved. Even though there is evidence that certain characteristics have a discernible influence on the behavior of students, there is little confirmation that certain traits have greater influence than others. Numerous investigations have been reported that endeavor to measure and predict teacher effectiveness and to describe the characteristics of superior teachers.

A third cluster of variables in the instructional process relates to the learning environment. The environment can be further designated as the physical, social, and psychological environment. The physical environment includes the school facilities such as classrooms, offices, library, lounges, instructional equipment, and materials. Not only is the availability of the facilities important for learning, but also the ease and attractiveness of these aspects of the physical environment for use by students and teachers become influential conditions for learning. The social environment includes the aggregate of relationships promoted in the classroom setting. These include teacher-student, student-student, and teacher-student-other relationships. The manner in which the teacher utilizes the social structure and relationships within the classroom has direct impact upon the behavior of students. It has been observed that the productivity of a class, the achievement of its members as individuals, and member satisfaction with the class is a function of the relationship between various group dimensions, such as leadership, power, friendship, and authority. The psychological environment refers to those stimuli that press upon the individual and cause her to respond in a specified way. Murray's concepts of personality needs of students and college press have stimulated much thought and research on the effect of the psychological environment on student behavior. Studies have identified the characteristics of the college environment that are influential in directing the behavior of students with certain personality structures.

The last set of variables in the instructional process are those that may be called teaching strategies. A strategy of teaching pertains to planning and directing specific activities that assist the student to modify or change her behavior in specific, predetermined ways. The strategy includes a number of activities organized to meet the requirement of a specific learning situation: (1) setting behavioral goals, (2) informing learners of objectives, (3) presenting the stimulus, (4) providing cues for learning, (5) controlling attention, (6) stimulating recall of previously learned capabilities, (7) arranging for reinforcement, (8) encouraging generalization, and (9) measuring and assessing behavior. The selection and organization of one or more of these activities becomes a strategy of teaching for a specific instance. While smaller teaching episodes may call for few of the activities, the larger movements in teaching will require that all activities be considered.

REFERENCES

1. Cronbach, L. J.   How Can Instruction be Adopted to Individual Differences? In R. M. Gagné [Ed.], *Learning and Individual Differences*. Columbus: Merrill, 1967. P. 34.
2. Waterhouse, I. K., and Child, I. L.   Frustration and the Quality of Performance. In J. P. DeCecco [Ed.], *Human Learning in the School*. New York: Holt, Rinehart & Winston, 1963. P. 117.
3. Bruner, J. S.   *Toward a Theory of Instruction*. Cambridge: Belknap Books, Harvard University Press, 1966. P. 125.
4. Ausubel, D. P.   *The Psychology of Meaningful Verbal Learning*. New York: Grune and Stratton, 1963. P. 214.
5. Gagné, R. M.   The acquisition of knowledge. *Psychol. Rev.* 69:355, 1962.
6. Bruner, J. S.   *The Process of Education*. New York: Vintage, 1960. P. 17.
7. Commission on Teacher Education.   *Teacher Competence, Its Nature and Scope*. Burlingame: California Teachers Association, 1961.
8. Pullias, E. V., and Young, J. D.   *A Teacher is Many Things*. Bloomington: Indiana University Press, 1968. P. 72.
9. Mager, R. F.   *Developing Attitude Toward Learning*. Palo Alto: Fearon, 1968. P. 61.
10. Ryan, D. G.   *Characteristics of Teachers*. Washington, D.C.: American Council on Education, 1960. P. 15.
11. Ibid.
12. Ibid.

13. Barr, A. S., et al. *Wisconsin Studies of the Measurement and Prediction of Teacher Effectiveness.* Madison: Dembar, 1961.
14. Ibid.
15. Katz, J. Personality and Interpersonal Relations in the Classroom. In N. Sanford [Ed.], *The American College.* New York: Wiley, 1962. P. 365.
16. Knapp, R. H. Changing Functions of the College Professor. In N. Sanford [Ed.], *The American College.* New York: Wiley, 1962. P. 303.
17. Ibid.
18. Gagné, R. M. *The Conditions of Learning.* New York: Holt, Rinehart & Winston, 1965. P. 216.
19. Stern, G. G. Environments for Learning. In N. Sanford [Ed.], *The American College.* New York: Wiley, 1962. P. 690.
20. Getzels, J. W., and Thelan, H. A. The Classroom Group as a Unique Social System. In N. B. Henry [Ed.], *The Dynamics of Instructional Groups.* Fifty-ninth Yearbook of the National Society for the Study of Education, Part II. Chicago: University of Chicago Press, 1960. P. 82.
21. Stern, G., Stein, M., and Bloom, B. *Methods in Personality Assessment.* Glencoe, Ill.: The Free Press, 1956. P. 123.
22. Pace, C. R., and Stern, G. G. Approach to the measurement of psychological characteristics of college environment. *J. Educ. Psychol.* 49:269, 1958.
23. Stern, G. G. Characteristics of the intellectual climate in college environments. *Harvard Educ. Rev.* 33:5, 1963.
24. McFee, A. The relation of students' needs to their perception of a college environment. *J. Educ. Psychol.* 52:25, 1961.
25. Thistlewaite, D. L. Fields of study and development of motivation to seek advanced training. *J. Educ. Psychol.* 53:53, 1962.
26. Thistlewaite, D. L. College press and changes in study plans for talented students. *J. Educ. Psychol.* 51:222, 1960.
27. Skinner, B. F. *The Technology of Teaching.* New York: Meredith, 1968. P. 121.
28. Bruner, J. S. *The Process of Education.* Cambridge: The Belknap Books, Harvard University Press, 1960. P. 52.

SUPPLEMENTARY READINGS

Allen, D., and Ryan, K. *Microteaching.* Reading: Addison-Wesley, 1969.
Anderson, H. A study of certain criteria of teaching effectiveness. *J. Exp. Educ.* 23:41, 1964.
Atkinson, J. W. *The Psychology of Motivation.* Princeton: Van Nostrand, 1964.
Atkinson, J. W., and Reitman, W. Performance as a function of motive strength and expectancy of goal attainment. *J. Abnorm. Soc. Psychol.* 53:361, 1956.
Ausubel, D. P. The use of advance organizers in the learning and retention of meaningful verbal materials. *J. Educ. Psychol.* 51:267, 1960.
Bandura, A., and Walters, R. H. *Social Learning and Personality Development.* New York: Holt, Rinehart & Winston, 1963.
Biddle, B., and Ellena, W. [Eds.]. *Contemporary Research on Teacher Effectiveness.* New York: Holt, Rinehart & Winston, 1964.
Bowers, N. D., and Soan, R. The influence of teacher personality on classroom interaction. *J. Exp. Educ.* 30:309, 1962.

Brown, J. S.   *The Motivation of Behavior.* New York: McGraw-Hill, 1961.

Bruner, J. S.   The act of discovery. *Harvard Educ. Rev.* 31:21, 1961.

Carpenter, F., and Haddon, E. E.   *Systematic Application of Psychology to Education.* New York: Macmillan, 1964.

DeCesso, J. P.   *Human Learning in the School.* New York: Holt, Rinehart & Winston, 1963.

Dewey, J.   *The School and Society.* Chicago: University of Chicago Press, 1909.

Gage, N. L.   A method of improving teacher behavior. *J. Teacher Educ.* 14:261, 1963.

Gagné, R. M., and Bolles, R. C.   A Review of Factors in Learning Efficiency. In E. H. Galanter [Ed.], *Automatic Teaching: The State of the Art.* New York: Wiley, 1959. P. 13.

Hall, J. F.   *Psychology of Motivation.* Philadelphia: Lippincott, 1961.

Henderson, K.   Theoretical models for teaching. *School Rev.* 72:384, 1965.

Jersild, A. T.   *When Teachers Face Themselves.* New York: Teachers College Press (Columbia University), 1955.

Mandler, G. and Sarason, S. B.   A study of anxiety and learning. *J. Abnorm. Soc. Psychol.* 47:166, 1952.

McClelland, D. C., Atkinson, J. W., Clark, R. A., and Lowell, E. L.   *The Achievement Motive.* New York: Appleton-Century-Crofts, 1953.

Meacham, M. L., and Wiesen, A. E.   *Changing Classroom Behavior.* Scranton: International Textbook, 1969.

Medley, D., and Metzel, H.   A technique for measuring classroom behavior. *J. Educ. Psychol.* 50:86, 1958.

Metzel, H. E.   Teacher Effectiveness. In C. W. Harris [Ed.], *Encyclopedia of Educational Research.* New York: Macmillan, 1960. P. 1481.

Murray, H. A.   *Explorations in Personality.* New York: Oxford University Press, 1938.

Pullias, E. V., and Young, J. D.   *A Teacher is Many Things.* Bloomington: Indiana University Press, 1968.

Rath, L.   What is teaching? *Educ. Leadership* 13:412, 1956.

Ryans, D. G.   Predictions of Teacher Effectiveness. In C. W. Harris [Ed.], *Encyclopedia of Educational Research.* New York: Macmillan, 1960. P. 1486.

Ryans, D. G.   Assessment of teacher behavior and instructions. *Rev. Educ. Res.* 33:415, 1963.

Sears, P., and Hilgard, E. R.   The Teacher's Role in the Motivation of the Learner. In E. R. Hilgard [Ed.], *Theories of Learning and Instruction.* Sixty-Third Yearbook of the National Society for the Study of Education. Chicago: University of Chicago Press, 1964. P. 192.

Smith, B. O.   A conceptual analysis of instructional behavior. *J. Teacher Educ.* 14:294, 1963.

Taba, H., and Elzey, F. F.   Teaching strategies and thought processes. *Teachers Coll. Rec.* 65:524, 1964.

Taber, J. I., Glaser, R., and Schaeffer, H. H.   *Learning and Programmed Instruction.* Reading: Addison-Wesley, 1965.

White, R. W.   Motivation reconsidered: The concept of competence. *Psychol. Rev.* 66:297, 1959.

Withall, J.   The development of a technique for the measurement of social-emotional climate in classrooms. *J. Exp. Educ.* 17:347, 1949.

15 INSTRUCTIONAL MODES AND MEDIA

THE phrase "instructional modes and media" is used to refer to the various kinds of components of the learning environment that are used to stimulate the learner. Although the teacher is usually a major source of such stimulation, there are various objects and devices ranging from books and pictures to television sets and computers. Inanimate systems can perform their function effectively only when they provide stimuli designed by people who also have in mind the purpose of instruction. Instructional modes and media are viewed from the standpoint of their importance in the educational process and the rationale for their use, with descriptions of several modes and media currently in use in nursing. Some attention is given to the concept and processes of educational technology.

NATURE AND IMPORTANCE OF INSTRUCTIONAL MODES AND MEDIA

The importance of instructional modes and media in the teaching-learning process is being recognized. Educators no longer assume that the essential ingredients in the process are simply the teacher and the curriculum guide. Guidance in the selection of media has been minimal, frequently only a list of reference books, films, activities, or methods of teaching. Selections have included very limited consideration of concepts to be taught, behavioral objectives sought, strengths and weaknesses of students, instructional environment, or effectiveness of the teacher. An improvement in the selection of modes and media is needed. The determination of the influences of these on the teaching-learning process cannot be made in isolation; it is a complex process.

The term *modes* is used here to designate the types of conversation between teacher and student and between students for the purpose of attaining specific instructional objectives. Examples of instructional modes include lecture, discussion, seminar, demonstration, and laboratory. The term *media* is designated to refer to those devices that are utilized in instruction to extend the learning situation beyond that provided by the teachers alone. These devices may employ various components of the human and material environment, either singly or in combination. Instructional media include such devices as programmed instruction, television, films, computer-assisted instruction, and simulation. This chapter provides some information pertaining to the nature of modes and media and their use in nursing education.

RATIONALE FOR USE OF INSTRUCTIONAL MODES AND MEDIA

There is obvious need for many different kinds of modes and media to facilitate the conduct of the various activities of teaching and learning that were identified in Chapter 14. The more or less traditional library materials, such as textbooks, supplementary books, reference books, periodicals, charts, graphs, microfilms, and documents are important segments of instructional resources. But of equal importance in today's teaching programs are the newer nonbook materials, such as films, filmstrips, slides, transparencies, television programs, tape and disk recordings, and computerized materials for teaching. All of these materials and the various services for providing them are sufficiently complex and interrelated to merit some examination of the rationale for their use in teaching.

A first point in such a rationale is that the modes and media of instruction should follow, not dictate, teaching aims. The most essential question is, What should be taught or achieved? Then follows the question, What instructional resources are needed? There is some danger of the instructor's losing sight of this fact when she is faced with the vast array of electronic and mechanical aids to learning that are now appearing on the market. This is not to discourage their use but to warn against allowing gadgetry to usurp more than its share of educational decision-making resources.

Another point in the rationale is that time and effort are required to effect changes in the utilization of various forms of teaching resources, but the results are often worth it. In higher education particularly, it frequently seems easier to continue doing things as they have always been done and to leave experimentation to others. The instructor may not wish to abandon practices that have proved useful, particularly not for alternative practices in which she is unskilled or with which students are unfamiliar. Neither does the instructor look with favor upon surrendering some of her freedom of operation to other individuals or organizations. Some newer teaching media do require electronic equipment, and frequently the service of another person is required. If teaching is to be improved, it must be studied continuously; creative, experimental approaches to teaching must be tried, evaluated, and improved. The everyday management of classroom activities provides many opportunities for testing one's ideas about teaching and for evaluating the efficacy of varied presentations.

A third point in the rationale is that media of instruction do not replace teachers; they supplement and enlarge their capabilities. Experience demonstrates that some teaching media (teaching machines, for example) relieve instructors of the need to make certain class explanations or demonstrations, thus freeing them for other, more important in-class or out-of-class activities. It is difficult to conceive of the major responsibility for instruction being taken over by mechanical or electronic devices without continued full and direct instructor participation. It seems more realistic to regard teaching resources of all kinds more as a means of improving the instructor's performance than of replacing her. Television, teaching machines, books, slides, and recordings are media through which functionally varied learning experiences are presented. They extend the instructor's powers and help to free her from the monotonous role of the lecturer.

A fourth point in the rationale is that no one instructional resource is superior to others. Each type of instructional material has some special (but not necessarily unique) advantages and potentialities for teaching. Its worth depends on the adaptation of the resource to the educational purpose for which it is used.

A fifth point in the rationale is that there are many acceptable ways of using teaching resources. Numerous research studies concerned with instructional resources have been undertaken to determine whether one pattern of use is better than another. Patterns investigated have included the use of film alone (without instructor participation), the multimedia approach, the extent and roles of instructor participation in the uses of materials, and student participation in activity as materials are presented versus absence of such participation. The results of these studies show that some patterns of use are superior to others for certain purposes and under certain circumstances. No single method seems to be universally superior.

A sixth point in the rationale is that no instructor should expect to use all the instructional resources described. She should analyze her own teaching aptitudes and requirements and give highest priority to improving her skills in using those that promise to contribute most toward the achievement of the objectives.

A final point in the rationale is that individually tailored instructional materials sometimes make especially effective contributions to college teaching. Many of the instructional resources used in today's institutions of higher education have been developed from plans of professors working cooperatively with campus specialists in graphic communication. Instructors are often led to improved ways of teaching when they are given opportunities to think through their own classroom problems and are given expert assistance in developing materials tailored to their particular requirements.

AREAS OF RESEARCH NEEDED

Problems concerning the various instructional resources and their effects on instruction that should receive the attention of research include the following:

1. What are the effects of instructional strategy on the value of media?
2. What are the effects of media on instructional strategy?
3. What are the effects of various combinations of media?
4. What is the interaction of media with different types of students, teachers, organizational settings, and instructional climates?
5. How are media produced in accordance with the emphasis on learning specifications?

DESCRIPTION OF INSTRUCTIONAL MODES

The need for preparing for instruction is acknowledged by any self-respecting teacher. The effective teacher will not meet a class without having given considerable attention to the substance of the lesson, checked on the details of fact, and assembled accessory materials. In addition, the teacher will make some decision about the specific mode or modes of presentation suggested by the objectives of instruction and the appropriate activities of the student. Each mode requires the teacher to engage in preliminary activities, giving consideration to the characteristics of the learners, the size of the class, and the specific instructional situation. Planning instructional method is a requisite for effective teaching. This involves deliberate selection among the possible teaching approaches of those most appropriate to the particular class or lesson.

Planning the instructional method to be used does not require plotting every detail. A detailed, predetermined plan might result in a rigid, inflexible environment that would not promote effective learning. Planning does, however, require the teacher to ask herself, which of the possible ways of teaching this topic are most promising and feasible, what instructional media would be most useful, and what kinds of learning opportunities would be beneficial to students? In planning for a particular lesson it must be viewed as part of the whole, that is, each lesson should contribute to the attainment of the objectives of the unit of the course; it follows one lesson and precedes another. The teacher will find it desirable to plan individual lessons as she sees the sequential development of the whole unit. To plan the unit as a whole provides opportunity to select the desired methods or modes for the various lessons in relation to their appropriateness for the specific subject matter topics. The teacher can better determine when to use the lecture, group discussion, laboratory, demonstration, and other instructional modes.

LECTURE

The lecture is the most common mode of teaching at the college and adult levels of learning. Despite the many criticisms that befall the lecture, it is appropriate at this stage of education. It is economical of time at a period in learning when time is of the essence. The lecture makes available to large groups of students the knowledge and skills of an outstanding teacher or scholar. It not only enables the students to obtain pertinent information, but it also provides the stimulation of a competent personality.

The lecture is at times the only appropriate method to use. The lecturer, who has spent years of her career pursuing in depth the vital elements of a particular field of study, can present the essence of the subject matter in a way in which no other instructional mode can accomplish. Informing students of recent research in a specific aspect of the subject is best attained by means of a lecture. For students to gain this information on their own would require an undue amount of time and effort. To listen to a lecture that is well organized and carefully presented can be an exciting experience. The delicate combination of an individual teacher's personality and intellectual competence can stimulate students' thinking to a greater degree than can other forms of instruction.

The oral communication by the teacher can provide all of the required instructional activities. Not every lecture situation calls for all these activities, and in some instances another mode may be more effective than the lecture. Nevertheless, the lecture can provide means for implementing these instructional activities:

1. Selecting behavioral goals
2. Informing learners of objectives
3. Presenting the stimulus (limited)
4. Providing cues for learning
5. Controlling attention
6. Stimulating recall
7. Arranging for reinforcement
8. Encouraging generalization
9. Measuring and assessing behavior (limited)

To be effective as a lecturer, one must remain in continuous contact with the audience. In a lecture, opportunity for student participation is not as frequent. To compensate for the restriction of students' verbal expression, the lecturer must utilize other forms of feedback from students to sense how students are responding. As with other modes of instruction, the lecture should provide opportunity for clarification of thought, assimilation of ideas, and reflection. A criticism of the lecture is that students are so completely occupied in note-taking that they cannot reflect on the content of the lecture. Providing students with an outline of the lecture may eliminate the need to take copious notes. Allowing time for discussion at the end of the lecture will provide opportunity for recall and reinforcement of ideas presented. The use of study questions pertaining to the content of the lecture stimulate students to pursue related issues and problems in accord with their individual interests and talents. The postlecture assignment enables the student to apply principles presented in the lecture to problem-solving situations. The content of the lecture may be enhanced by the use of certain instructional media, such as pictures. These may implement those instructional activities that the lecture does less effectively.

Planning the lecture requires the teacher to note carefully the objectives to be attained. The lecture outline defines the scope of the content. Prior to the lecture the teacher develops and distributes study questions, guides, and assignments. If instructional media will be used, these are prepared and made ready for use. The plan also includes opportunity for discussion of topics presented and a summary of ideas and further issues to be explored.

GROUP DISCUSSION

A mode of instruction frequently employed in college and adult education is the discussion. It is an effort to have students learn by thinking and talking together as a group, developing through the group process a shared appreciation of subject matter. This mode of instruction seems to be appropriate in instances when the outcomes of a course are attainable from deliberation and exchange of thought following from some prior attention to the specific ideas, issues, or problems.

The group discussion provides opportunities for learning certain behaviors that are not realizable through other means. It enables a student to organize and present her thoughts and to broaden her understanding of a particular subject as a result of questions posed by group members. Group discussion provides opportunities for mutual exchange of ideas and feelings, through which may come a deeper respect for individuals engaged in a collaborative effort.

Instruction by means of the group discussion presents learning opportunities in the group roles of leader and member. Under the supervision of the teacher or another observer, the students can gain skills in effective group processes. This implies that the goals of group activity must be clearly identified and made known to all participants. Periodic assessment of progress toward the goals indicates the effectiveness of the group enterprise. The role of the teacher in group discussions may vary with her philosophy of teaching and the requirements of the particular learning situation. With students who are relatively inexperienced in the group process, the teacher may feel the need to become involved in the group discussion. The objectives of the discussion must be realized to some degree, or valuable instructional time is lost. With a more sophisticated group, the teacher's role fosters students' initiative and freedom to express ideas without relinquishing her responsibility for keeping the discussion within the bounds of relevance. Students should carry the burden of the discussions, and should feel free to differ with one another and the teacher. The discussions of the group presuppose that the individual members have given thought to the issues and that their remarks are based on substantial information as opposed to opinion.

The group discussion, like other forms of instruction, requires planning. It means delineating those objectives that can be readily attained by this mode of instruction. Review of the subject matter of the discussion must be planned. This may be accomplished in several ways, such as assigned reading, outline of a previous lecture, study questions, or film presentation. A specific problem is identified, which becomes the focus of the group discussion. Following a relatively exhaustive treatment of the problem, the discussion should summarize the major points or ideas expressed and the unresolved issues. A post-discussion conference might examine the group process in relation to the various roles enacted by the students.

PANEL DISCUSSION

Similar to the group discussion, the panel discussion is primarily a dialogue among individuals concerning topics of interest to the panel members. The panel usually consists of persons who have expertise in the subject matter of discussion. The process involves an interplay back and forth among the panel members with agreement, disagreement, qualification, and elaboration of pertinent points. The panel chairman participates to keep discussion to the point, to invite nonparticipants to talk, and to give an occasional summary. The major focus in panel discussions is upon trying to solve problems through group thinking. After the panel has made its presentation, other members of the class may be invited to ask questions and to make comments or observations. The chairman usually presents a summary of the discussions at the end.

SEMINAR

The seminar offers another form of conversation between students and faculty members. It is usually reserved for graduate students or those who have acquired considerable background information about the subject of the seminar. The discussion is focused upon a problem or issue that is of interest to the group and provides for an interchange of ideas relating to the problem. The discussions should enable the students to gain additional information, insights, and approaches to problem-solving. The success of the seminar depends upon careful preparation, reading, or laboratory work prior to the session.

Also the mode of presentation of the various points of view by individual members will enhance the effectiveness of the seminar. The role the teacher assumes will influence the active participation of the seminar members. The major role of the teacher is to bring out the ideas of the students and say as little as possible herself except at those points where her comment may be needed.

DEMONSTRATION

The demonstration as a mode of instruction provides opportunities for manipulation of objects so as to display an event or a set of events. The demonstration helps students to focus attention on steps and procedures involved in certain manual operations and performances of physical and social phenomena. Whether a student or a teacher is presenting the demonstration, some basic requirements must be met if the demonstration is to be useful to the observers.

1. The specific objectives and content of the demonstration must be identified. The present level of understanding or skills possessed by the student must be taken into consideration. The key terms, ideas, principles, or problems which will be introduced must be specified.

2. The purposes of the demonstration and the expected outcomes must be made known.

3. It is usually helpful to make a trial run of the demonstration to insure that all necessary materials, equipment, and facilities are on hand.

4. The conversation of the demonstrator with the students during the demonstration will hold their attention and focus on pertinent points.

5. The demonstration should be paced to enable most of the students to follow it. Periodic check should be made to determine whether points need to be repeated.

6. The demonstrator should encourage students to participate in the demonstration by engaging in some of the operations.

7. At the end of the demonstration the students should be given an opportunity to ask questions and to evaluate what has been learned.

LABORATORY INSTRUCTION

The major purpose of laboratory instruction is to give students real opportunities to discover things for themselves whether or not those things have been discovered by others. The laboratory enables students to carry out the steps in problem-solving and helps students to develop skill in making accurate observations and arriving at their own conclusions.

Laboratory experience is possible as a learning activity for all kinds of courses. It gives the student opportunities to deal with the raw data of which the particular subject is concerned. The raw data of the natural sciences are chemical or biological elements and their interactions. The data of the social sciences include the various interrelationships of individuals and groups in a social context. The raw data of nursing are the human responses of individuals, families, and the community to nursing intervention. The laboratory provides the student with opportunities to make observations of the data, to manipulate aspects of the environment, and to observe the resulting effect.

The value of laboratory instruction lies in the opportunities for the student to experience learning in a natural setting, to utilize theory in practical problem-solving, to develop, test, and apply principles, and to learn methods of procedure. The student can use her initiative and creativity in designing an approach to the problem and can use her own insights in the interpretation of the outcome of the problem-solving activity. The teacher can observe how the student approaches the problem, organizes her materials, initiates problem-solving activities, and draws conclusions from the laboratory experience. The teacher may find it necessary to intervene to correct mistakes and guide the student's actions.

Other instructional modes and media may be used in conjunction with laboratory instruction. The teacher may precede the laboratory activity with a lecture concerning the problems under study. A manual is frequently used to guide the student in using the appropriate steps to study the problem, including questions and assigned readings to assist the student to extend her knowledge beyond that of the immediate situation. Tapes that present clues to observing and making inferences may also be used to provide explanatory information about the specific study problem.

The important role of the teacher in laboratory instruction is guiding the student. Whether it be a science or a clinical laboratory, the teacher must be able to analyze the teaching situation and to know when she should offer help and when she should withhold it. Preparation for laboratory instruction requires the teacher to reflect upon what the students will be doing, the verbal instructions they will require and the problems they will encounter, and to determine the kinds of questions through which their work can be appraised and their learning experience can be improved.

TEAM TEACHING

Team teaching is a method of organizing teaching personnel to improve the content and process of instruction. The method involves two or more instructors who are assigned to work together in teaching the same group of students. The teachers are selected primarily on the basis of their expertise in the subject matter to be taught. The usual procedure entails identifying the specialized aspects of the content and giving each teacher specialized responsibility for certain portions or activities of the course. Planning instruction for the phase of nursing dealing with aging persons, the psychiatric, medical-surgical, and community health nurse instructors all might share in developing and imparting the content of nursing in this area.

Team teaching, from the opinions of its advocates, offers these distinct advantages: (1) Instructors are given the opportunity to specialize in the aspects of the course for which they are best qualified, (2) instructors are stimulated to do better teaching because of their close association with their peers, and (3) students are stimulated by the various points of view and the different personalities to which they are exposed.

Although the advantages are important in efforts to improve teaching, some further considerations should be made. Instructors must have sufficient time to prepare for the presentation. This means that the teachers must meet together to plan the content, teaching approaches, and instructional media. Personalities of individuals may determine the success or failure of team teaching. Team teachers must be able to share, to relinquish some vested interests, and to become part of a team. Economics are affected in that several teachers, rather than one, must invest time to plan for the class, develop tests and other evaluation devices, and make the final evaluation of students in the class.

CONTRACT TEACHING

Contract teaching had its origin in elementary school in the 1930's under the name of the Dalton Plan. It was initiated in an effort to individualize instruction. With the advent of other teaching approaches, such as ability grouping, contract teaching lost its popularity. There has been little application of this plan to teaching at the college level. More recently some schools of nursing are attempting to use contract teaching in baccalaureate programs.

With the contract plan the student is given individual assignments known as contracts. Details of each assignment are clearly outlined so that the student may work on it independently at her own speed. The outcomes of learning are defined to give the student directions for study. A specific course may include a definite number of contracts to be completed by a set date. When the student completes one contract, she requests the next one to work on. It is possible that a student might complete all contracts before the end of the course. In some contract teaching plans the student may also select the level of work she feels she can attain. In this instance she may select a contract that describes the work to be done to acquire an A, B, or C grade. Contract teaching places considerable emphasis on individualized, self-directed instruction.

DESCRIPTION OF INSTRUCTIONAL MEDIA

The characteristics of various types of instructional media are presented. The use of specific media in nursing education is described and attention is given to research findings where appropriate. In some instances the experimental endeavors made use of a single medium, while in others a combination of media are used. In evaluating the findings, the reader should always take into consideration the purpose and conditions of the teaching endeavor.

PROGRAMMED INSTRUCTION

Teaching machines and programmed books of various sorts promise to play increasingly significant roles in higher education. These are self-study devices designed to provide immediate and regular feedback. Both devices can elicit student response and participation throughout the exercise. The branching programs or "scrambled textbook" presents information, invites immediate response or reaction to the presentation, and directs the reader to different pages (in scrambled, not sequential, order within the textbook), depending upon her particular response. If the response is correct, the reader will have her choice confirmed and will receive directions for proceeding to the next step. If, on the other hand, a wrong answer is chosen, the reader will be informed and asked to retrace her steps to make another response.

Some programmed books or manuals arrange subject matter into a series of sequential steps in a supposed order of familiar to unfamiliar. The student reads and reacts as she goes from one page to the next. Programs are also presented in sheet or roll form to be inserted in various autoinstructional machines. Teaching machines themselves range from the simple to the very complex, including push-button devices, flashing lights, score recorders, and branching facilities which lead from printed problem statements to slides and motion pictures.

The use of teaching machines or programmed book materials in instruction present special problems that merit consideration by the instructor:

1. If programmed materials are to be used, programs will need to be found or developed that meet one's expectations and specifications.

2. Programs requiring nonportable machines will require special rooms; someone must be responsible for loading machines, keeping them functioning, and reclaiming and analyzing residual answer sheets.

3. Instructors who use programmed materials sometimes find that it is possible to devote more time to class discussion and explanation of misunderstandings arising from out-of-class study of programmed materials and less to lecturing or other instructor presentation techniques.

4. Instruction must be given to students in how to use programmed materials and equipment.

Seedor introduced the concepts and methods of programmed instruction to nursing education. In her initial study she indicated that "the method has not been used in the field of nursing," and her project was concerned with the possibility of applying the method to nursing education [1]. A unit on asepsis was developed, and experimentation took place in two junior colleges. The experimental group consisted of students using the programmed instruction materials by means of the Auto-Tutor, and the control group consisted of students receiving instruction in the same curriculum materials by conventional methods. The results of the study indicate that nursing curriculum content, such as asepsis, can be programmed successfully. The majority of the students using teaching machines learned the material in roughly half the usual time. The majority of students who learned the subject matter on the Auto-Tutor were satisfied with the new teaching method. Also, the instructors who were involved in the study indicated satisfaction with programmed instruction as a method of teaching. Following the same pattern of programming, Seedor developed another unit concerned with aids to diagnosis to be used in the course in fundamentals of nursing.

Krueger undertook an investigation for the primary purpose of constructing a model visual-verbal program for teaching a manipulative nursing skill, and determining whether nursing students in a generic baccalaureate nursing program could learn the scientific knowledge and motor skills needed to perform the nursing procedure using the program as the sole instructional material

[2]. A model visual-verbal program using both linear and branching styles of programming was constructed to teach the scientific knowledge and motor skills needed to administer a hypodermic injection. The program was subjected to experimental test to determine whether students using only the program could achieve the learning outcomes intended by the program. Achievement was measured by analyzing each student's performance on discrete items on two specially constructed evaluation instruments: a paper-and-pencil test measured comprehension of scientific knowledge; a performance test measured achievement of motor skill learning. The results showed that the nursing students using the program acquired most of the scientific facts and principles and most of the motor skills intended by the program. Most of this learning could be transferred to the clinical setting or to an actual nursing practice setting. The program enabled each student to determine the amount of self-directed learning activity required to learn the program content.

Another study, by Hinsvark, had the following purposes: (1) to explore the feasibility of applying procedures of instructional programming developed in other fields to nursing knowledge and skills, (2) to determine appropriate learning tasks in nursing for programming, (3) to develop illustrative programs for such tasks, revising them on the basis of student data, (4) to study the use of programmed materials in a nursing course, and (5) to determine whether the use of programmed materials could save faculty time and student time [3]. One field of study, nursing in the operating room, was selected because it was the field with the lowest number of students per teacher. Twenty-eight collegiate nursing students were given a four-day period of planned instruction that included programmed materials. This was followed by clinical practice. The students were tested prior to and directly following the clinical practice to determine the amount of content learned and retained, adeptness of procedural skills, and effects of different kinds of programs for the different types of learning tasks. The results indicated that programmed instruction could be used successfully in nursing education if the learning tasks and necessary knowledge and skills were clearly identified. A saving of teacher time was effected, and there was no increase in student time when programmed materials were used.

Craytor and Lysaught developed and tested a programmed unit called An Introduction to Radiation Therapy for Nursing Students [4]. The unit was used with a class of college juniors and a class of second-year students in a diploma program in nursing. The purpose of the investigation was to determine whether the unit could be taught as effectively as a traditional lecture presentation of materials. Students in each type of nursing program were divided into control and experimental groups by class sections. Evaluation was based on pre- and posttesting. All students showed an increase in knowledge about the subject matter. If the control groups in each program were combined and the experimental groups were likewise combined, no statistically significant differences between the groups on the posttesting was found. Students did learn at least as well by means of the self-instructional unit as they did by a conventional lecture presentation. The programmed unit reduced the spread of individual achievement scores, but this reduction was not statistically significant.

Another study of programmed instruction was made by Hart, who endeavored to determine the effectiveness of programmed instruction in teaching metrology to nursing students [5]. The investigator developed a course in programmed instruction concerned with the science of weights and measures as these relate to the arithmetic of dosage and solutions. The programmed instruction presented this content using the Skinner single-step method to lead the student through a series of very simple steps to the acquisition of the knowledge. A comparison was made of the achievement of two groups of nursing students; one group of sophomore students took the metrology course by means of programmed instruction, and the other group of sophomore students took the traditional didactic course. The results on the metrology achievement test taken by the two groups demonstrated that the experimental group's achievement level was markedly higher than that of the control. It was evident, in this instance, that the use of programmed instruction reduced the amount of time spent in student-instructor contact and increased the amount of student time needed to master the content of metrology.

The rapid development of programmed materials led Noth to develop a guide for nurse educators to use in the selection of programmed materials [6]. The author indicated that current selection techniques used to evaluate textbooks and educational tests were found to be inadequate for programmed materials. Through a survey of the literature the essential characteristics of efficient, effective programs were determined. Based on these criteria, questions were developed and submitted to raters for evaluation of pertinence and importance. Two rating forms were developed, and six reviewers were asked to evaluate available programmed instruction materials in nursing by means of these forms. The results of the study indicated that the rating form helped nurse instructors to know what to look for in a program.

Early efforts in the development of programmed materials in nursing focused on learning of specific manipulative skills. More recently, however, attention has been directed to the use of programmed instruction in other aspects of nursing. Currey, Swisher, and Kruse utilized the Management Improvement Program (M.I.P.) of the Human Development Institute to teach skills in human relations [7]. This programmed text required interactions between partners as well as a group program in which all met together to work through the general discussions. Three instruments were used to determine the effectiveness of the program: (1) Group Perception Inventory, a part of the M.I.P., (2) the Barrett-Lennard Relationship Inventory, and (3) the Clinical Awareness Scale. The results indicated that the Management Improvement Program had a significant impact on the human relations skills of the nurses participating in the project. Furthermore, the Management Improvement Program assisted these nurses in their roles as team members and team leaders.

Programmed instruction has been developed and tested in other curriculum areas, including nutrition, legal aspects of nursing, nurse-patient relationships, medical-surgical nursing, and maternal-child nursing. Programmed instruction has also been developed and utilized for inservice education in hospitals and for refresher courses for nurses who have had to interrupt their professional careers.

Programmed instruction is a system of teaching and learning in which pre-established subject matter is broken down into small discrete steps and carefully organized in a logical sequence in which it can be learned readily by the students. Each step builds deliberately upon the preceding one.

There are two general types of programs: linear or single-step and extrinsic or branching. The linear type of program is based upon Skinner's theory of small-step progression of material in a logical sequence. Reinforcement is central to his theory. Reinforcement may be built into the program, as in the sequencing of the items, which increases the likelihood that the student will get the correct answer to the problem. The material itself may serve as a reinforcer. Extrinsic reinforcement may take the form of ringing bells or flashing lights when the subject selects the correct response to the stimulus. Skinner believes that a major shortcoming of the present education system is the lack of reinforcement of the student's behavior. When reinforcement of the desired behavior is given by the teacher, it often is not properly timed, and its effectiveness is thus destroyed. Much of the student's behavior may be governed by aversive stimulation (unpleasant situations to be avoided). The student's behavior is governed by such things as the desire to avoid criticism or the teacher's displeasure; getting the correct answer to the problems is less significant.

The second type of program is the extrinsic or branching program. In this type the student may progress to the next problem in the program if the correct response to the question is given. However, if an incorrect response is given, the student may be referred to another part of the program for additional information. This type of program also allows the student to select her own method of organization of materials.

Programmed instruction may be offered by means of machine, programmed textbook, slides, television, or videotapes. The program may be presented to groups or to individuals.

TELEVISION

Motion pictures and television are generally considered more efficient than printed matter in adding realism to vicarious experience, and the use of these media is recommended for the demonstration of perceptual motor skills in which realism is important to instruction.

Some studies in which the relative effectiveness of television and conventional instructional methods have been evaluated involved university extension and on-campus courses and teaching in the United States armed forces. Generally speaking, these studies have tended to show that television is more often than not as effective in teaching as is the teacher in the classroom. Schramm's summary of this literature at all levels from elementary school through graduate study counts a number of studies in which no significant differences were found between televised and conventional courses in effectiveness as measured by student achievement [8].

Nursing literature reports several exploratory studies in the use of instructional television. There is also evidence that closed-circuit television is being used more extensively than formerly by personnel in nursing-service administration and nursing education. Okamoto reports a study that tested the effectiveness of television in teaching students about the establishment of meaningful relationships with patients [9]. The problem was to determine whether such relationships could be demonstrated through television. Weddige and Kinsella have reported the use of instructional television with New York City's Office of Nursing Education and Nursing Service of the Department of Hospitals [10, 11]. Televised lessons included a series on the legal aspects of nursing, the evaluation of nursing service personnel, and a training program for nursing aides in nursing homes.

At the Ohio State University, Dilley used television to demonstrate how to change an occupied bed [12]. Instructors found that return demonstrations by the students were as good as or superior to the performance of students taught by other methods in previous years. Closed-circuit television has been used to instruct classes of seventy to eighty students in such procedures as making beds, bathing patients, administering injections, and making physical examinations.

Instructors in nursing have a dual concern in the instructional process: meeting the educational needs of students, and protecting the safety and well-being of patients. With increasing numbers of students in schools of nursing, both concerns are vital in planning learning opportunities for students. These issues became the focus of a study conducted by Griffin, Kinsinger and Pitman [13]. The major question of the study was, How can an instructor satisfy the safety factors involved in working with hospitalized patients and at the same time meet the needs for individualized instruction of an increased number of nursing students? Seven questions evolved from the central problem of study:

1. Is it possible for an instructor to satisfy safety factors involving work with hospital patients while at the same time meeting the needs for individualized instruction of an increased number of nursing students?
2. Are there differences in nursing students' skills that result when the instructor uses closed-circuit television to teach and to evaluate student performance?
3. Will patients accept what they might consider an invasion of privacy involved in this type of teaching?
4. Do faculty and students resist teaching and learning by closed-circuit television?
5. Is there resistance to this system of instruction from hospital personnel?
6. Will normal hospital operations be affected by using television in this way?
7. Can nursing instructors readily adapt their clinical teaching skills to the use of closed-circuit television?

The data of the study revealed positive answers to these questions and identified some specific characteristics of this form of instruction. Observation of the student is more frequent and is free of distraction and completely centered on the activity of the student and patient. Communication is instantaneous and individualized. Gross details are easily observed; however, fine details may be missed. The instructor cannot herself demonstrate a point or a procedure. Since she is observing more students, she must develop an awareness of the need to be specific in her attention to student performance. Finally, she must learn to use words to replace actual demonstration, a process which requires a thorough knowledge of the various components of a procedure.

The approach of this study was not merely to add new devices to make it easier to do things in the old way. It was hypothesized that with this system the teacher could manage the learning environment in a different, more effective manner, and the student would be able to learn in ways not previously possible. The general conclusion of the study indicated that under optimum conditions the number of students that existing nursing facilities can teach might be more than doubled if closed-circuit television were generally employed in hospitals for clinical instruction. This increase could be accomplished without loss of instructional quality.

The increase in enrollments in schools of nursing is causing faculties to explore means by which the quality of instruction can be maintained or improved using the available qualified teachers. The purpose of a study conducted by Westley and Hornback at the University of Wisconsin was designed to determine whether procedures taught in the course Fundamentals of Nursing were learned by students as effectively through videotaped television demonstrations as through conventional (face-to-face) demonstrations [14]. Selected nursing procedures were prerecorded on videotapes, to be played back according to a prearranged schedule. Four television lessons were chosen for testing from among the fifteen that were presented on television during the course, (1) making the unoccupied bed, (2) taking the vital signs, (3) bandaging, and (4) insertion of the nasal catheter. Since the focus of the study was on teaching certain manipulative techniques, criteria of effectiveness of performance were developed to be used when observing student's performance. No significant differences in performance were found between television and conventional classroom groups for the four lessons combined. It would appear that basic skills in nursing may be taught by means of videotape recordings. Thus, a course that usually had to be taught to small groups because close observation is necessary could now be taught to a larger group of students. Although extra effort is required of the teacher initially to make the recordings, a considerable net saving of her time and effort would be possible, since the videotapes can be reused until procedures must be revised.

Another study attempted to evaluate the effect of weekly discussion classes (follow-up sessions) as a means of supplementing television instruction. Follow-up sessions consisted of review, movies, question-answer sessions, and tests. Dearden and Anderson utilized television instruction in anatomy and physiology with and without follow-up sessions [15]. Freshmen students at five diploma schools were subjects, and they were divided into three experimental groups. Group 1 had television lessons and one class hour of follow-up discussion per week conducted by the person serving as the television teacher. Group 2 students had television lessons without follow-up discussions. Group 3 had television lessons and one class hour of follow-up discussion per week by a nursing instructor from the school faculty.

A comparison was made of the averages on the mid-quarter and final examinations; the final examination was used as a retention test four months later. Statistical analysis of test scores indicated no statistical differences in the achievement of groups when compared on the mid-quarter and final examinations. Students having follow-up sessions achieved higher average test scores than those who did not have follow-up sessions. Students not having follow-up discussion periods exhibited a noticeable decrease in interest in the courses in anatomy and physiology.

Claims, substantiated by experience and research, are made for the use of televised instruction techniques in general and professional education. Television instruction permits the especially well-qualified instructor to reach more students than could normally be accommodated in an ordinary classroom. Televised instruction reduces unit costs and keeps tuition fees within the reach of more students than would otherwise be possible. Television instruction makes feasible the concentration of considerable effort upon one fairly brief presentation. The activities involved in this effort include determining objectives, planning approaches, developing visual or audio materials to illustrate points, and practicing delivery.

The behavior of the teacher will be affected by her participation in television instruction. The teacher must learn to function effectively as a member of a production team. A second effect of television teaching is that it changes the teacher's ways of interacting with students and colleagues. The teacher who teaches several hundred students at a time on a closed-circuit network appears on numerous screens and loudspeakers over the campus. Much of her success will depend on her ability to project her personality in a forceful, interesting manner and upon her capacity to use the sometimes slim feedback to improve future presentations.

MOTION PICTURES

Motion picture films are capable of enlarging, slowing down, or speeding up action, portraying the unobservable, bringing to life the distant past, heightening interest, and juxtaposing experiences for emphasis and clarification. Films have been found useful in teaching facts; what might not have been expected is that on some occasions they have been found to be almost as effective by themselves in teaching these facts as were instructors with their usual methods of teaching. Studies of film use have suggested their utility in teaching concepts as opposed to strictly factual learning. They have also been shown to be helpful in modifying motivations, interests, activities, and opinions.

The relation between motion pictures and still pictures is analogous to that between demonstrations and objects. Demonstrations can present events as stimulus situations rather than simply the objects that participate in these events. The advantage of motion pictures is that they enormously extend the range of stimulus situations that can be brought into the classroom. Basically what motion pictures do in a highly effective way is to present the stimulus situation to the learner. Motion pictures are an excellent medium for presenting problem situations whose solutions are not known but are to be the subject of later class discussions.

Motion pictures can provide the external prompting needed for a student to learn procedures. They are often effective in communicating to the learner the kind of terminal performance expected. Motion pictures are seldom used by themselves to perform instructional functions. Sound track is usually added. When this is done, the range of functions that can be performed is greatly increased, since all the advantages of oral communication supplement the stimulus-presentation function. The oral communication directs students' activities, describes the performance to be learned, guides the thinking process, raises questions for assessment purposes, and provides feedback.

Certain assumptions underlie the use of motion pictures in teaching. They include the following:

1. The audiovisual presentation can serve as stimulus material to evoke discussions among students fostering a broader awareness of behaviors or aspects of themselves, work, family, education, and community.

2. The audiovisual presentation can communicate important elements of behavior that can be referred to only indirectly in a lecture or print, such as nonverbal behavior.

3. The level of comprehension for each individual in a group will not vary as widely with an audiovisual presentation as with written or printed material.

4. The dynamics of group discussion will reinforce the audiovisual stimulus elements.

5. Audiovisual presentations can be designed to establish for a group the conditions for principle-learning and problem-solving, which otherwise may take hours of individual instruction and guidance.

Some recommended instructional activities of the teacher in using film presentations suggest that the teacher should be familiar with the film to be used. The film should be previewed in advance, paying attention to the emphasis of the film's key words and terms. Suitable questions should be developed, which may later be used to focus student attention during viewing. The teacher should endeavor to develop a favorable motivational set for seeing or studying the film. The film should be introduced to the students, indicating what they are expected to learn from it, discussing the meaning of key terms to provide better communication, and explaining the follow-up activities to be conducted after the film showing. The teacher should stimulate appropriate student participation during film showing. Special attention should be directed to the original points identified prior to film showing. Finally, the teacher should conduct suitable follow-up activities. This calls for discussion of original points called to the viewing attention of students, with some analysis of each point. Tests may be given to check student comprehension. The use of related assignments and study guides appears to increase depth and breadth of learning. Finally, reshowing all or portions of films facilitates clarification of points and correction of misinformation. The usefulness of this medium of instruction has been substantiated by numerous research projects. It is a superior form in promoting retention of learned materials and in imparting knowledge dealing with performance.

TAPE AND DISK RECORDINGS

In recent years, offerings of prerecorded tapes and disks have become so numerous, so varied, and of such high quality that they must now be regarded as one of the most important of the many teaching resources. Tape recordings can be altered easily and effectively in a number of different ways for a number of different purposes. They can be edited to remove unwanted or unnecessary material, or to reduce playing time, and the sequence of events on tapes can be rearranged to fit some special teaching situation. The tapes or disks can be played back more slowly than they were recorded to permit studies of sound details.

Nursing literature provides information about the varied uses of tape recordings in nursing education. The tape recorder provides a means through which the instructor can obtain accurate information about the clinical performance of the student without disturbing the student-patient relationship.

It is frequently difficult to arrange opportunities for the nursing student to do patient teaching under direct guidance of the clinical instructor. The reasons for this include the numbers of students in the clinical field in relation to the available instructors and the spontaneous nature of the setting. An alternate method to develop skills in patient teaching would be to provide the student an opportunity to practice teaching-centered patient conversations outside the clinical area. Monteiro designed a study to investigate the use of tape-recorded patient conversations to which the students could listen and respond, as a method to develop the nursing student's ability to teach patients [16].

Eleven teaching-centered conversations of a nurse with different hypothetical medical-surgical patients were written as scripts, reviewed by a panel of experts, and recorded on tape. The sequence of each script was such that the participant heard the patient's remark, was given time to respond (into a tape recorder), and then heard a nurse's response, which was patient teaching in nature. It was assumed that during the course of the series of eleven recorded conversations, the learner's response would become more similar to the taped response and that the amount of factual information in the response would increase.

Collegiate students in two New England nursing programs participated in the study. A similarity scale was developed to measure the closeness of the student's response to the taped response. The findings of the study indicated that there was a tendency for the student's response to become similar to the taped response. Also, the factual teaching content of the subject's responses showed a definite increase.

Tape recordings were used in another project to ascertain the needs of certain types of patients [17]. The area of study was the preoperative nursing care of patients undergoing open heart surgery. This selection was prompted by the desire to ascertain the needs of such patients, particularly during the immediate preoperative period. It was assumed that patients about to undergo such an operation would have certain psychosocial and intellectual needs and that they could make valuable contribution to nurses' assessments of these needs.

Five collegiate nursing students participated in the study. These students interviewed the patients on three occasions: (1) two days before surgery, (2) the morning of the day before surgery, and (3) the evening before surgery. A guide was developed to assist the students to cover the same areas in the interview. The first interview was to include (1) finding out how much the patient knew about his condition, surgery, and hospitalization, (2) giving him a review of preoperative instruction, and (3) determining the probable impact of the operation on the patient's family and his economic status. The second interview focused on the patient's feelings concerning his condition and his decision to have surgery, and the third, on the immediate pre- and postoperative period and the patient's anxieties about impending surgery.

Each interview was recorded on tape. The investigators listened to the tapes as a group. Consensus concerning the significance of each statement was determined, and the statements were categorized according to patient's preoperative needs. The tape recorder did not prove to be a hindrance to meaningful nurse-patient interaction. The investigators found the tape recorder to be an important tool for evaluating and improving communication skills. They also found that the taping method had one limitation, namely, the meaning of many of the statements could not be fully comprehended because the nonverbal communications that had accompanied them were not available.

The problems of evaluating clinical performance were the focus of another study in which tape recordings were used. In community health nursing, when each student is in a different part of the community at the same time, direct observation by an instructor is impossible. Also, an instructor's presence as a third person on a home visit may change the course of the conversation and distort the situation.

Stevens designed a project in which the student taped her interview with the patient in the home setting [18]. The student listened to her tape and made her own evaluation of the visit. The instructor listened to the tape and reviewed the notes taken by the student pertaining to the nonverbal communication. The student and teacher shared each other's evaluations. The instructors believed that the taped interviews were an effective way to help a student to evaluate her verbal communication skills. The students frequently heard on the tape bits of conversation they had not heard during the interview. The tape recordings enabled the students to hear the silences, to hear who broke them, and to note the length of the silences. Tape recordings appeared to be useful in evaluating how well students used some of the principles of interviewing. Lastly, the tapes revealed how well students teach patients. Do they overwhelm the patient with too much material? Do they utilize feedback from the patient? Do they have sufficient knowledge about a subject? The tapes were also used for group discussions of students having similar clinical experiences.

The combination of television and tape recordings extend these media to include both sight and sound. The use of videotape eliminates some of the shortcomings experienced in each media when used singly. Videotapes provide opportunities for repeated playblack for differential analysis. Both verbal and nonverbal behavior of participants in the situation are made accessible. Griffin and his colleagues designed a research study to test the hypothesis that regular analyses of patient care by means of immediate videotape playback would affect student learning [19]. It was believed that viewing videotapes of the nursing student's performance could change the behavior of nursing students who would be seeing themselves with other students in nursing situations with which they could identify. The students could see the situations as correct or incorrect, as appropriate or inappropriate, or as something they themselves had done or might be required to do in the future. The students could make changes in their behavior if they felt that change was indicated. It was the purpose of the study to evaluate whether the behavior of nursing students did change as a result of viewing videotape recordings of students performing in the clinical area.

Four groups of students were assigned to a unit where they were instructed by closed-circuit television and videotape, and four groups of students were assigned to a unit where they were taught in a more conventional manner, two groups by closed-circuit television only, and two without closed-circuit television. The experimental groups viewed videotapes during postclinical conferences. The videotapes of actual nursing practice were made during the students' clinical sessions using students in the two groups. The content of the videotape was dependent upon the relationship of clinical practice to the weekly clinical nursing objectives that were developed by the nursing faculty participating in the project. At the beginning of each postclinical conference, the instructor reviewed the objectives with the students. The review was followed by the playback of the videotape and the group discussion. The discussions focused on the tape content with emphasis on the relation of the content to the clinical objectives and then moved into a broader discussion of other individual experiences and problems. The use of videotape gave structure to the postclinical conference.

For the purpose of the research project, the instructors developed several instruments: (1) clinical performance scale, (2) clinical analysis record, (3) participation scale, and (4) a questionnaire. The findings of the study revealed no significant differences in total performance as measured by the clinical performance scale. There was a significant interaction between videotape recording variables and the closed-circuit television variables. Students who saw videotape recordings and were taught by the conventional method (with closed-circuit television) scored significantly higher in total performance than any other group. These results seem to indicate that the use of videotape recordings with the television method of clinical teaching may be less satisfactory than the use of videotape recording with the conventional method of teaching. The levels of learning as measured by the scores of the clinical analysis record and the final examination showed no significant differences between the videotape recording and nonvideotape recording groups. The quality of responses in the postclinical conferences was significantly greater for the nonvideotape recording groups than for the videotape recording groups. The quality of response did show significant differences in some areas. The closed-circuit television groups had a significantly higher percentage of factual and probing responses. Also the level of clinical performance of the closed-circuit television and the non–closed-circuit television groups was not significantly different. Responses to questionnaires concerning the use of videotape recordings were favorable.

Observations made by the faculty indicated that the greatest asset in using videotape recordings was probably the feeling of immediacy or of being right in the room with the patient and the student. The greatest drawback in the use of tapes was the quality of the sound, which made it difficult or impossible at times to follow the spoken word.

The combination of television, films, and tapes introduces the concept of audiotutorial instruction. This approach to teaching utilizes visual and auditory aids that can be duplicated and used by students as needed. The assumptions underlying this process indicate that greater opportunity is provided to the student for self-directed learning, which presumably increases learning efficiency. Also instructors have more student contact in individualized learning events of a less routine nature. The audiotutorial method permits students to progress at their own speed and places on them the responsibility for learning. The use of this approach to teaching and learning is described by Deegan, Dieter and Voelker, in which an integrated science program was offered, using a combination of lectures, conferences, and the audiotutorial laboratory [20].

The traditional type of lecture was given, which preceded the laboratory experiments. All laboratory work was accomplished by the audiotutorial method, which permitted students to progress at their own speed. The student's booth in the learning laboratory was equipped with a tape recorder, an 8-millimeter film loop projector, a slide viewer, a microscope, and all routine laboratory supplies. In addition, each student had her own dissecting and culture material, her own fetal pig, petri dishes, and materials for experimental work. Each student conducted her own experiments at the direction of taped message and under the tutelage of an instructor. A script for the master tape had to be prepared in advance, with attention to the fact that the student would be hearing the material for the first time.

The taped message directed the entire laboratory period. On occasion the student was told to select a film loop that gave visual support to a directional message. There were instances in which the student saw the instructor on film carrying out her own recorded instructions during the dissection. The student could run and rerun the tape and film until she felt prepared to begin the laboratory work. If she felt unsure of herself, she could always seek assistance from the instructor. When the laboratory work was completed, the tape suggested to the student that she complete the exercises in the manual. Weekly student conferences in groups served as quiz sessions to review and reinforce major principles involved in the laboratory work of the week. It appeared that the course was completed faster and more thoroughly than on previous occasions utilizing the traditional laboratory experiences. Students and instructors had an opportunity to work closer together.

The availability of many prerecorded tapes and disks suggests that instructors should utilize criteria for the selection, such as the following:

1. The content of the tape should be that which can be best presented by this medium.

2. The topics presented should encompass the essential content.

3. The teacher should audition the material to become familiar with it. Attention should be given to the organization of the recording, its main points of emphasis, its unusual vocabulary, and the questions that might grow out of its use.

4. The teacher should prepare for class listening by providing an overview of the recording contents and showing how it relates to the work under way in the class. The use of handouts to guide students' thinking about the topic under discussion facilitates listening and learning. Explanation of key vocabulary and the use of assignments related to the topic aid in comprehension of materials.

5. The presentation should be relatively short and should help the student to organize and challenge her thinking. Variety in presentation will foster continuing interest.

6. The student should listen to the recording without interruption.

7. The notion of individual and self-directed study should be stressed. The student should be encouraged to use the recording as she sees fit, which may involve slowing down or replaying the tape.

8. The teacher should involve students in group discussion and other follow-up activities. The completion of study questions, assignments, and check tests are means of evaluating the comprehension of the materials contained on the tape.

COMPUTER-ASSISTED INSTRUCTION

Specialists in the field of instructional media estimate that the major new educational developments of the late 1950's and early 1960's were the teaching machine and programmed instruction. The major development of the late 1960's and early 1970's will probably be the computer-assisted instruction movement.

The underlying premise of computer-assisted instruction is to investigate ways of maintaining stable interactions between men and machines. The study of man-machine interaction cannot be maintained for very long unless man gets some sense of satisfaction and achievement from the activity. The machine must hold the man's interest. It must provide him with things to do and to think about; otherwise, his attention wanders, and the machine cannot be guaranteed to achieve anything at all. A stable interaction between a man and a machine is an interaction in which man must of necessity be learning something of interest to him. The machine must have some of the characteristics of a teacher.

Teaching, regarded as the control of learning, is concerned with providing opportunities to a student to learn about something relevant to the subject matter. An optimal system of teaching will maximize the student's rate of learning. The instructional situation is defined in terms of problems that have a solution within the field of attention. Performance of the skill is conceived as the act of solving these problems. Provision must be made for comprehending the student's problem-solving process and the mechanisms that underlie these processes.

The major types of computer-assisted instruction at the moment include (1) didactic instruction in which linear or branching program techniques are used, (2) tutored dialogues in which the student is relatively free to query the computer, (3) inquiry approaches in which the student attempts to explain a phenomenon by using the computer as a resource tool to seek necessary information, and (4) gaming or problem-solving in which the student is led into a simulation of a real-life problem and in which the computer controls the sequence and nature of simulated events.

One of the major advantages of computer-assisted instruction is that of individualization of instruction through specifically designed, highly adaptive programs. Students are allowed to progress at their own rate. These teaching methods can be extended to the case of controlling the learning of a group of persons. Group learning is usually discussed in terms of computerized classrooms. With the aid of a centralized computer that is time-shared among a group of students, detailed records can be compiled of each student's progress. Insofar as the computer performs these operations in place of the teacher, the classroom is necessarily run according to a predetermined scheme.

If some teachers are threatened by the advances of computer technology and fear that they will be replaced by machines, they may be assured that there is little likelihood of computers becoming surrogate teachers in widespread use. Computers are presently performing some low-level teaching tasks in schools that can afford them, such as record-keeping, scheduling, and in a few cases storing occupational and educational information. Computer-assisted instruction may in the future cast the teacher in a new role of instructional designer and strategist. This new role requires a high degree of professionalism. It is not the existing computer technology that stands in the way of developing computer-assisted systems which will free the teacher to do more of the kind of productive work that is beyond the capability of a machine. Present-day hardware is adequate. The problem is one of money. The man-hours of thinking and effort by experts from engineering and other specialty areas needed to develop the kinds of systems that are seen as possible realities cost more than anyone can afford.

Molnar identifies the critical obstacles in the development and use of computer-assisted instruction:

1. Availability of individuals with appropriate competent skills
2. Sufficient funds for implementation
3. Sufficient funds for research and development
4. Attitudes of faculty
5. Lack of sufficient incentives to stimulate preparation of educational software

6. Poor documentation of educational software
7. Existence of a communication gap between educators and representatives of industry [21]

SIMULATION

Simulation has been defined as the creation of realistic games to be played by participants in order to provide them with lifelike problem-solving experiences related to their present or future work. Simulation experience is a natural activity among children in all cultures. While many traditional childhood games provide little more than social experience, modern educational games are designed for specific practice in communications, problem-solving, scientific inquiry, information management, and decision-making. Simulation is usually employed in any of three ways: (1) to evaluate or analyze an existing system (operations analysis), (2) to develop and evaluate a model or plan for a new system (experimentation, prediction), and (3) to provide a learning environment that represents a life situation (training, transfer).

In each instance relevant conditions are presented, and assumptions, hypotheses, or courses of action are observable. Consequences often shape conditions or sequential patterns. Simulation designs range from abstraction to reality. Beck and Monroe have identified the characteristics of simulation as a tool in training [22].

1. It starts with an analogous situation. The analogous circumstances provide a setting in which the learner can function. It is assumed to have enough of the characteristics of the real environment to provide practice in meeting contingencies that would occur in the learner's life.

2. It provides for low-risk input. The learner can make a response without irrevocable commitment and without destroying the original circumstances.

3. It feeds back consequences symbolically. The simulation system tells the learner the consequences of her responses. It delivers a message without modifying the physical or psychological learning climate.

4. It is replicable. Simulation provides opportunities for iterative procedures in arriving at best solutions.

Common uses of simulation techniques in education include role-playing, simulation games, and logic games. Almost all of these uses of simulation involve the use of prestructured situations with relatively complex rules. The designers attempt to anticipate logically the possible contingencies in the playing of the simulation setting. Many of these simulations depend for various reasons on win-or-lose motivations to maintain participant interest. Using traditional teaching methods such as lectures, discussions, or seminars, it is very difficult for students to learn with feedback any very complex or personal set of behaviors appropriate to particular situations. Even demonstrations of these behaviors have limited value for most students. Simulation strategies of one sort or another remain the most likely strategies for learning and practicing new behaviors. The use of simulation is particularly appropriate in teaching problem analysis, decision-making, strategy change, goal-setting, planning and executing action, and evaluation of change. Many of these objectives involve learning or sharpening the behavior of students in leading or managing group processes.

Simulation has been employed in programs for the preparation of students for teaching [23]. In one project specific teaching problems were identified. Videotaped incidents, role-playing, written incidents, and various combinations of techniques were employed in simulating problems. These situations were utilized in a research project that was designed to (1) examine the methodology of simulation in order to judge its effectiveness in presenting teaching problems and (2) determine whether exposure to simulated teaching problems and subsequent decision-making would have any observable effect on a subject's student-teaching behavior. The results of the study indicated that the first purpose was "accomplished very successfully as evidenced by the developed materials, the two simulators and student's reaction to simulation training" [24]. The second purpose did not receive clear-cut support. Although it was evident that students utilizing simulation appeared to have fewer problems, significant effects of simulation on other aspects of teaching behavior were not noticed.

ROLE-PLAYING

In role-playing, hypothetical but representative circumstances involving interpersonal relationships are established verbally, and trainees are assigned to roles in which they talk and act extemporaneously according to their notions of the role incumbent's motives and behavior. At the conclusion, the group discusses and assesses what happened in the role-playing. Role assignments may be exchanged and the situation reenacted. Such sessions demonstrate consequences of interactive behavior and provide a basis for testing behavior strategies to achieve particular objectives.

While role-playing seems to fulfill the requirements set for simulation, the question may be raised as to whether it is truly replicable. It may be that the simulation model is changed in light of intervening experience of the participants.

GAMES

Games vary widely in their concepts and processes; some may be classified as simulation and some not. Learning via games that are valid simulation for educational purposes is transferable, so that the learner after experiencing simulation is better prepared to cope with real events. One such game that may be useful in relating concepts applicable to nursing is The Disaster Game. This game simulates citizens' roles under disaster conditions and encourages players to cooperate, organize, and plan.

COMPUTER-BASED SIMULATION GAMES

Although games and role-playing offer attractive opportunities for personal interaction among learners and teachers, simulation using computer facilities may be more effective in reaching certain instructional objectives. With computer-based simulation, it is possible to design complex programs for teaching problem-solving or decision-making. In the problem-solving design, the process required to arrive at a specified answer is learned. In the decision-making pattern, a learner acts upon a series of contingencies supplied by the computer, which evaluates and describes consequences of learner's responses.

The decision-making type of program would not have just one correct answer but would teach the learner how to apply and evaluate alternative courses of action at the choice points. The computer could print out successive status reports, and the learner could decide whether she was satisfied with the state of affairs; if not, she could go back to the beginning and again work through the problem, making alternate choices.

A computer-mediated learning program combining simulation and role-playing is also possible. In this a whole system involving a number of people playing various roles could be the basis of testing the efficacy of the decisions of the individuals in the roles and the effect of the individual's decisions on group objectives. To teach a group of students some of the responsibilities involved in providing nursing service to patients, three roles can be programmed: the director of nursing service, the clinical supervisor, and the nurse-clinician. The data base contains a description of the objectives of nursing service, the location of a specific unit and the number of people who staff it, and the time dimensions of the activity. From this common data base, a program developed for students in each of the three various roles requires decisions as part of the advance planning for the activity. As the students make their responses, the computer processes them and feeds back a scenario of the developing plans for evaluation by the team. This is followed by a computer programmed "field test" of the plans, with intervening events introduced. Decisions based on these events and outcomes can be assessed by the students at the conclusion of the simulation program.

Bitzer designed a project to determine the feasibility of adapting the subject matter of nursing to an automatic teaching system [25]. A two-hour class section of medical-surgical nursing was chosen for the experiment. In the regular class this theoretical material is usually presented by lecture, discussion, assigned readings, and study of case histories and nursing-care plans of patients whose clinical picture is typical of the conditions being studied. The lesson material, covered in the regular class in two hours, was programmed into a ninety-minute lesson on the PLATO system. Conferences were held with the regular instructors to assure that the same material would be covered in both groups. In order to help convey an image of a real patient, a three-minute film was incorporated into the programmed lesson. The objectives of the film were to acquaint the student with the patient's socioeconomic background, his present family situation, and his outlook on life. The patient's past medical history and treatments along with information concerning factors precipitating his condition were also presented.

A special set of rules was programmed into a high-speed digital computer to accommodate this method of teaching. The students could experiment with the patient by giving drugs and nursing care and then obtain the effects on the patient by checking his condition in the condition mode. Upon completion of the lesson for the PLATO group and of the regular classroom instruction for the control group, both groups were tested on the lesson material covered. The results of the study seem to indicate that the lesson material was appropriate for this type of presentation. Most of the students found the answers by experimenting. The difference between the means on the posttest was significant. A comparison of the posttest scores indicated that the students who inquired instead of guessed were able to answer more questions correctly on the posttest. All of the students except one stated that they felt this was an effective way of presenting lesson material. A simulated clinical situation could prove a useful inbetween step where stress would be at a minimum. Also the simulated laboratory of the automatic teaching system provides opportunities for immediate application and immediate feedback.

The use of computer-based simulation in medical education is occurring with greater frequency and sophistication. The development of a computer-controlled manikin is being used to teach skills required in anesthesiology and surgery. It is speculated that if these skills could be taught through simulation, the achievement of the skills could be accomplished in less time than is now needed. It is also important to note that patients would be spared potential discomfort and harm.

Simulation techniques are presently being used in various types of training programs. The major advantages of simulation include the following:

1. Simulation can provide experience in a wider range of educational objectives: affective as well as cognitive, process as well as content, evaluation by self and system criteria as well as by the instructor.

2. With simulation there may be greater transfer from the training situation to the life situation.

3. Simulation provides a responsive environment, which may give learners a sense of immediacy and involvement.

4. Simulation can provide experiences in a low-cost model of a high-cost environment. Students can practice aspects of nursing care without the risks of harmful effects on patients or others.

5. Simulation can provide short-time experiences and feedback in long-time processes.

6. Simulation can provide a field for practice in hypothesis formulation, testing, and modification.

7. Simulation can provide systematic exercises in inquiry training.

FIELD TRIPS

Field trips help to enrich instruction by providing opportunity for the student to relate theoretical aspects of study to the practical realities of life. Field trips permit students to analyze problems in fairly unstructured ways; in the process they are expected to exercise judgment and come to conclusions about meanings or results of their study.

Successful field trips require considerable planning and effort. Assuming that the proposed trip is essential and that a suitable destination has been selected, the instructor must also do the following:

1. Make preliminary contacts with officials or others at the destination site. It is advisable that the instructor visit the location before the students make the trip.

2. Make arrangements with school or college officials as to liability coverage and absence of students from school and file appropriate records or forms.

3. Prepare a guide sheet for members of the class to be handed out well in advance of the trip. Guide sheets should contain details of the trip, location,

departure and arrival times, return time, route description, major purposes of the trip, costs, recommended clothing, names of individuals at destination, and safety rules. Time should be provided for students to discuss guide sheets.

4. Prepare a follow-up discussion and evaluation of the field trip. The follow-up should relate to the major questions and study points mentioned in the field trip guide.

As mentioned previously, field trips consume much time and effort in planning and making the trip. Teachers should make certain that they can justify the expenditure of their time as well as that of the students in relation to the outcomes of the field trip. Field trips can, however, provide an effective means for extending learning opportunities out into the community. This experience may broaden the student's perception of problem situations and the varied approaches to problem-solving.

PICTORIAL PRESENTATION

Pictorial presentations include instructional media in the form of still photographs, pictures, charts, graphs, and transparencies. The most important function of pictures and diagrams as a medium of instruction is to display the stimulus situation. Another function well performed by pictures is prompting or presenting cues for learning. Still pictures appear on the pages of books accompanying printed material and are frequently used by the teacher to accompany oral instruction.

Presenting the stimulus situation for problem-solving and thereby introducing group discussion is a specialized function that may call for a picture, graph, diagram, or chart. These may be enlarged sufficiently to be viewed by an entire class. They may also be used in developing display boards. Graphic presentations and charts may require special training in reading and interpreting them. Certain kinds of data are required when diagrams are used. Accompanying diagrams with explanatory texts or comments generally enhances understanding of the message conveyed by the diagram. The use of color in preparing the chart or diagram appears to heighten interest and facilitate communication.

Transparencies are usually developed for use with the overhead projector. Because of its wattage and optical system, this machine is capable of projecting readable images in a lighted room. Another advantage of this medium is that it permits the instructor to manipulate her projection while facing the class and maintaining eye contact with the audience. Transparencies permit the teacher to make some modification in the stimulus situation that they present. The use of overlays allows the instructor to provide additional stimuli or cues and extend the initial message conveyed by the transparencies. The use of overlays maintains the transparency in its original form. The use of transparencies as opposed to chalk-board illustrations requires less time, provides a more accurate presentation, and allows the teacher to maintain direct contact with students.

There are occasions in which pictorial presentations cannot be effectively used to inform the student of the performance to be expected as a result of learning. Media of this type cannot be used by themselves to guide the learner's thinking or to assess her performance or to provide her with feedback. Many teachers have considerable skill in developing their own charts, graphs, and diagrams. If teachers are lacking in this ability, they obviously will need to obtain assistance, lest the message becomes distorted or inaccurate.

PRINTED LANGUAGE

Books and periodicals are a traditional part of the instructional situation. Teachers and students are most dependent upon this medium of instruction in relation to other media. A college student may derive most of her instruction from the printed media of books and learned journals. Instruction by means of books and periodicals is usually a rapid and efficient process. The book can convey a great deal of information in a relatively short period of time when it is used by a student who is able to read and comprehend the subject matter. This implies that for printed media to be effective, the student must know how to read and must have acquired the necessary background knowledge.

Many books are available in nursing, which are excellent media of instruction. They provide appropriate stimulus situations, inform the learner of the nature of the performance to be learned, and facilitate learning through the use of prompts. It is the responsibility of the teacher to be certain that the books that are selected and assigned establish these conditions for learning for the particular group of students at a specific point in time.

MODELS

Three-dimensional materials may be most effective when the task to be learned is the actual manipulation of such objects, while other media are effective for teaching components of knowledge that support such manipulations.

Models are used as media of instruction at all levels of education. A series of specially constructed models may be useful in teaching certain concepts in the elementary stages of education. Simulation games often provide models of environmental objects. Problem-solving and decision-making underlie the manipulation of the models according to some theoretical formulation.

Models are frequently employed to provide visual experience with objects that are not readily available in the natural form. In nursing education, models have been constructed and used to illustrate the structure of the human body and the component parts of the body parts. Torsos of the body and models of various organs provide stimulus situations and cues to learning that are not always available in the natural form. If models are to be constructed for this use, they must replicate as nearly as possible the characteristics of the actual object. Color, size, and shape are elements of the stimulus situation that provide the learner with accurate visual input to elucidate information imparted by the printed language media.

Instructional media include the vast array of resources for instruction available to the teacher, from pictures to computers. Each type of medium, if used properly, assists in establishing the necessary conditions for learning in some different ways. Some types of media, such as books and motion pictures, are prepared by commercial groups and are readily available to the teacher. Other forms must be developed by the instructional staff to meet the specifications of the learning situation. In some instances, such as with charts and graphs, the teacher herself can prepare the materials, a preparation that requires certain technical skills that must be developed by utilizing the expertise of the teacher and the multimedia technician.

UTILIZING INSTRUCTIONAL MODES AND MEDIA

The description of various instructional modes and media indicates that these techniques and devices are used to accomplish specific purposes. They become a part of teaching strategy because they assist the student to modify or change her behavior in a predetermined way. All modes and media are not helpful in every way. One way of determining their usefulness is to view these in relation to the several activities of teaching.

Table 14, a brief summary of the use of various instructional modes and

TABLE 14.   Modes and Media in Relation to Teaching Activities

Teaching Activity	Description of Activity	Modes and Media
Setting behavioral goals	Identification of the goals to be attained during the student-teacher-environment interaction. Goals may include a wide range of verbal behaviors, specific motor and manipulatory behaviors and those behaviors concerned with feelings and emotions Identification of the initial behaviors of students Definition of steps that lead to the achievement of goals	Review of published materials, films, and videotapes to obtain information pertaining to current nursing activities in a particular phase of nursing Develop and utilize assessment devices that will indicate the initial behaviors of students prior to instruction
Informing the learner of the objectives	Make known to students the nature of the performance expected of her Provide student with behavioral description of the objectives indicating the qualitative and quantitative aspects of behavior change Present overview of unit of teaching, which provides a general summary of unit, which demonstrates a connection with previous learning experiences Provide opportunity for student assessment and possible revision of objectives	*Printed language:* written statements of objectives including terminal and subbehaviors, bibliography, other sources of information such as assignments, examinations, and required readings *Lecture:* overview of unit including explanatory information about content and learning opportunities *Motion picture:* present the kind of terminal behavior to be expected *Programmed instruction:* presenting specific areas of content for students who show the need for remedial instruction (as revealed by assessment of initial behaviors)
Presenting the stimulus	Selecting the proper stimulus requires noting the desired behavior changes described in the objectives. If any behavior change is to occur, the student must be given an opportunity to deal with the behaviors Objects, words, simulated versions of objects must be presented as a stimulus to which the student may respond	*Lecture:* description of specific behaviors to be attained *Motion picture, television, pictorial presentation, programmed instruction, tapes, simulation, laboratory,* and *field trips:* present stimuli pertaining to verbal behavior, feeling or emotional behavior, problem-solving, and manipulatory behavior

Teaching Activity	Description of Activity	Modes and Media
	Identification of the stimuli that may control the behavior of students, and presenting the stimuli so as to evoke the appropriate response in the student	
Providing cues for learning	Providing cues reduces the possibility of errors. Determination must be made of the amount of cuing that is necessary for the individual student Knowing when to withdraw cues as student learns how to go on her own	*Printed language:* utilizing underscoring or italic type *Pictorial presentations:* as pictures or diagrams *Role modeling by teacher, videotape recordings,* and *motion pictures:* provide student with information about the environment that assists her in formulating a correct response to stimuli
Controlling the attention of the student	Controlling attention is integrally related to presenting stimuli and providing cues Selecting relevant cues and eliminating distracting materials Providing reinforcement when student responds to appropriate feature of the environment Focusing on the problem to be solved	*Nonverbal behavior of teacher:* gestures, movement of objects *Physical constraints:* reduce distractions from environment *Motion pictures, pictorial presentations, simulation games, computer assisted instruction:* focus attention on specific aspects of the environment to which the student should attend
Stimulating recall of previously learned capabilities	Restatement of previously learned concepts to provide for contiguity of learning Requires teacher and student to continually look back upon ideas, notions, or activities so that they can be further explored	*Lecture, group discussion, programmed instruction, motion picture, videotape:* present ideas, problems, activities previously learned, to promote learning in greater breadth and depth
Arranging for reinforcement	Behavior is acquired, or modified under conditions in which a response produces a consequent stimulus event, such as a reward Reinforcers should be closely related to the desired behavior	Visual and auditory stimuli; signals from the teacher confirming results Peer approval or disapproval Grades, honors, awards Reinforcement by means of programmed instruction

(Table 14 continued on page 526)

Table 14 (*Continued*)

Teaching Activity	Description of Activity	Modes and Media
Encouraging generalization	Assisting students to respond to similar elements in different learning situations Providing variations of the stimulus context in which the student response facilitates the student to extend her initial knowledge and to make finer discriminations and generalizations	*Group* and *panel discussions, laboratory, team teaching, television, videotapes, computer-assisted instruction, simulation, models, printed language,* and *pictorial presentations:* present a wide range of stimulus situations which facilitate the extension of knowledge beyond the initial level of learning
Measuring and assessing behavior	Various assessing devices must be used to determine the extent to which each learner has achieved the defined objectives with which instructional planning began	*Verbal* and *nonverbal:* behavior of teacher questioning and observing *Printed language* in the form of tests *Demonstrations:* of clinical performance behavior *Tape recordings:* to assess interview skills *Television:* to observe students in clinical activities *Computer-assisted instruction:* to assess problem-solving skills

media, has some limitations. It is not intended that all modes and media that are suggested be used in relation to each teaching activity. In many instances the use of any one device may accomplish the goals of more than one teaching activity. Finally, if media are to be used, they must be available to the teacher. The specific content of the media must be compatible with the instructional process in the particular course. The teacher must take into consideration the goals of instruction and the characteristics of students involved. Many of the forms of media, such as programmed instruction and videotapes, have been developed and used with a well-defined group of students who may or may not be similar to another classroom group. The teacher will need to select those media that best meet the needs of students and the specific activities of teaching.

EDUCATIONAL TECHNOLOGY

Advances in physical science and biological science technology have implications for the tasks of education and the development of educational technology. Educational technology as a resource for education presents two distinct concepts relating to learning and behavior theory and to educational practice.

The first concept of educational technology refers to the application of physical science and engineering technology to provide mechanical or electro-mechanical tools, instruments, or hardware that can be used for educational purposes. From this frame of reference, educational technology means the use of equipment for presenting instructional materials, such as still and motion pictures, projectors, tape recorders, television, teaching machines, and computer-based teaching systems.

In the second concept, educational technology does not concern hardware as such but refers to technology in a general sense. In this sense it is the application of an underlying science to educational practice. The science of behavior, especially learning theory, has become a primary source from which applications to a technology of instruction might be anticipated. This does not exclude the contributions of other theories, such as communication and perception, to instructional activities. The interaction of both concepts of educational technology can pro. .ote the design and use of various forms of instructional modes and media to provide better control of the learning situation.

Gagné describes educational technology as the development of a set of systematic techniques and accompanying practical knowledge for designing, testing, and operating schools as educational systems [26]. Many disciplines are called upon in the development of this technology, which includes architecture for designing working space, physical sciences for the design of equipment, sociology and anthropology which design social environments, the science of human organizations which designs administrative procedures, and psychology which designs conditions for effective learning. In technology these disciplines solve practical problems through the kinds of engineering efforts known as design and development. Technology therefore forces one to consider the specific purpose and function of the lecture, the printed text, or the pictorial presentation in solving some problem in the process of learning.

Physical science technology has contributed to teaching at intervals in the past: means of supplying printed materials in quantity, which fact removes the need for dependence on the individual teacher; the invention of photography and developments in optics and illumination; sound recordings and sound-synchronized motion pictures; and most recently, the electronic audio-visual transmission apparatus of television. The development of motion picture projection equipment and of televised transmission and receiving equipment occurred in the entertainment industry almost entirely without reference to education. It was only after these media had been technically perfected that they were used as instruments of instruction. Audiovisual presentations have been used almost exclusively for presenting stimulus materials, with little attention to the response aspect of the stimulus-response paradigm of learning. Also little attention has been given to the matter of individual differences of the audiences.

The development of teaching machines by Pressy in the 1920's illustrates a change toward greater dependence on theory in the conceptualization of teaching machines and programmed learning. It is evident that Pressy and more recently Skinner incorporated principles of learning enunciated by psychologists in the development and use of programmed instruction sequences. The development of programmed instruction materials has precipitated major changes in educational practices, which were direct outgrowths of the concerns of psychologists with theory and experimentation on learning.

Educational technology means that the first step in the instructional process is the assessment of the student to determine what she already knows and what she does not know. The rationale behind the testing process is that instruction must be designed for the individual student, and it must begin where the student is. On the basis of test results the teacher prescribes learning sequences that are directly related to the objectives of instruction. The student, as she becomes involved in learning, may utilize a variety of materials that are suggested by the lesson unit and that have been made available to her. These materials may include books, tapes, motion pictures, and printed materials. These materials have been addressed to the student at a particular level of instruction in a specific phase of learning.

Periodic assessment of the student's progress is made to determine where she is, how much she has learned, and where she should go next. The teacher utilizes this information to recommend a course of further study that will best suit her individual needs. Strengths and weaknesses can be identified, and appropriate remedial activities can be initiated if necessary. Also, designs for ongoing instructional activities can be constructed. These techniques of individualized instruction are implemented by both software and hardware. They require the development of new tests, diagnostic procedures, lesson units, instructional materials such as exercises and manuals, and student performance records. All of these fall into the category of educational technology software. Hardware may also be used to implement these procedures. The student may use a tape recorder, a film projector, or a computer. In all instances, hardware offers a service to the learner. The student controls the hardware rather than the other way around. The individual student, the learner, is the focus for change. The use of hardware should always be related to the difference in individual learning it facilitates. At the present time we need to know more about these differences before we put too much stress on hardware, particularly big hardware. Small items of hardware such as the tape recorder and film projector may prove to be far more effective for the individual learner.

Programmed instruction, whether by text or machine, has its major value in teaching the student to do something. Performance objectives indicate what the capability is, and the primary purpose of instruction is the development of that capability. The orientation toward intellectual skills—toward what the student is able to perform rather than what she knows—is an important result of developing educational technology. This technology has encompassed the systematic development of procedures and techniques of instruction based on psychological theory.

SUMMARY

Instructional modes and media include the various components of the learning environment that generate stimulation to the learner. The way in which the teacher presents a particular aspect of the course, unit, or lesson is considered to be a mode of instruction. In this presentation the teacher is the major source of stimulation to the student. The teacher may use various objects and devices that provide additional inputs to the learner, ranging from printed language and pictorial presentations to complex electronic devices. These are classified as instructional media.

It is obvious that instructional modes and media are necessary to promote the teaching-learning process. In an effort to effect optimal learning, the teacher should have a clearly formulated rationale for the use of the various modes and media. A first point to be considered is that the objectives of instruction should suggest the types of modes and media that could contribute to the learning outcomes. The rationale should also give attention to the fact that time and effort are needed to effect change in the faculty's utilization of the various forms of teaching resources. It is frequently easier for teachers to continue to use familiar approaches than it is to try out new procedures. A third point is the recognition that media do not replace teachers. Teaching media supplement and enlarge the teacher's capabilities and bring to the student a vast array of stimuli. Presently, there is no evidence that any one instructional media or mode is superior to others. The worth of these resources is dependent upon the educational purpose for which they are used. Frequently, a combination of several media and modes may be more effective than one used singly. On the other hand, no instructor should expect to use all the available instructional resources within her teaching program. She should give priority to those that are compatible with her teaching aptitudes and the objectives of instruction. Lastly, instructional media developed through the cooperative endeavors of a group of teachers and technical experts offer challenging experiences for teachers as well as stimulating opportunities for students.

An extensive array of media of instruction have been developed over the past several decades. Although these are being used on all levels of education, we need to know more about the effects of these devices on the teaching-learning process. Research efforts should be directed to seeking answers to the problems of instruction that relate to the various forms of media, their characteristics, their major functions, and their effects on instructional strategy.

Instructional modes are described as the types of conversation in which students and teachers participate. In some instances the teacher may assume the major responsibility for the conversation, on other occasions the students may be the predominant speakers. The selection of a specific mode of instruction depends upon the objectives of teaching, the class size, available resources, and the total plan of instruction. The planning for an individual class should be viewed in relation to the contribution of the class to the development of the unit or course. The teacher can better determine when to use lecture, group discussion, laboratory, demonstration, and other instructional modes as she develops the total instructional plan.

The full range of instructional media are in use today in nursing education. In some instances the utilization of some types of media is primarily on the basis of intuition, while in others the specific media were selected because of some initial research findings. The research that is reported was designed and carried out in accordance with the specifications of an individual situation. The findings of these studies may not be generalized to other settings. The media that have been described include programmed instruction, television, motion pictures, tape recordings, computer-assisted instruction, simulation, field trips, pictorial presentation, printed language, and models.

The utilization of modes and media of instruction should be related to the specific teaching activities that are designed to facilitate the attainment of the objectives. All modes and media are not helpful in each of these activities, and the selection of the procedures and devices should be made in relation to the following teaching activities:

Setting behavioral goals
Informing the learner of the objectives
Presenting the stimuli
Providing cues for learning
Controlling the attention of the student
Stimulating recall of previously learned capabilities
Arranging for reinforcement
Encouraging generalization
Measuring and assessing behavior

Teachers, psychologists, and administrators are looking to the advances in physical science and biological science technology to study the problems of education. Educational technology has emerged and has become a resource for education. Two distinct concepts of educational technology have evolved. One concept relates to the use of mechanical tools or hardware for educational purposes, the other to the application of science to educational practice. The science of behavior is viewed as a primary source of theory to explain the learning process and information needed for the design and development of instructional programs. Although most of the modes and media of teaching have not been developed and utilized as an outcome of research endeavors, educational technology forces the teacher to look at the purposes and functions of the various procedures and devices in relation to behavioral science theory.

REFERENCES

1. Seedor, M. M.   *Programmed Instruction for Nursing in the Community College.* New York: Teachers College Press (Columbia University), 1963.
2. Krueger, E. A.   The Administration of a Hypodermic Injection: An Instance of Programmed Instruction. Unpublished Ed.D. Project. Teachers College (Columbia University), New York, 1964.
3. Hinsvark, I.   A Case Report of the Application of Programmed Instructional

Techniques for Nursing Education. Unpublished Ed.D. Dissertation. University of California, Los Angeles, 1965.

4. Craytor, J. K., and Lysaught, J. P.   Programmed instruction in nursing education. *Nurs. Res.* 13:323, 1964.
5. Hart, L.   Teaching metrology by programmed instruction. *Nurs. Res.* 15:20, 1966.
6. Noth, Sr. M. S.   Selecting Programmed Instructional Materials in Nursing. Unpublished Ed.D. Project. Teachers College Press (Columbia University), 1964.
7. Currey, J. W., Swisher, J. D., and Kruse, L.   Improving human relation skills through programmed instruction. *Nurs. Res.* 17:455, 1968.
8. Schramm, W.   What We Know About Learning from Instructional Television. In L. Asheim et al. [Eds.], *Educational Television: The Next Ten Years.* Stanford: Stanford University, Institute for Communicative Research, 1962.
9. Okamoto, R. H.   Nursing education and television. *Nurs. Outlook* 10:676, 1962.
10. Weddige, D.   WUHF-TV (Channel 31). *Nurs. Outlook* 11:254, 1963.
11. Kinsella, C.   Educational television for a hospital system. *Amer. J. Nurs.* 64:72, 1964.
12. Dilley, D. L.   Teaching through TV. *Amer. J. Nurs.* 61:104, 1961.
13. Griffin, G. J., Kinsinger, R. E., and Pitman, A. J.   Clinical nursing instruction and closed-circuit TV. *Nurs. Res.* 13:196, 1964.
14. Westley, B. H., and Hornback, M.   An experimental study of the use of television in teaching basic nursing skills. *Nurs. Res.* 13:205, 1964.
15. Dearden, D., and Anderson, L. D.   An evaluation of televised instruction in anatomy and physiology with and without follow-up classes. *Nurs. Res.* 18:156, 1969.
16. Monteiro, L. A.   Tape recorded conversations: A method to increase patient teaching. *Nurs. Res.* 14:335, 1965.
17. Boguslowski, M., et al.   Tape-recording patient interviews: A minimister project. *Nurs. Outlook* 17:41, 1969.
18. Stevens, D.   A tool for evaluating clinical performance. *Amer. J. Nurs.* 70:1308, 1970.
19. Griffin, G. J., et al.   New dimensions for the improvement of clinical nursing. *Nurs. Res.* 15:292, 1966.
20. Deegan, M., Dieter, C. D., and Voelker, C.   An audiotutorial approach to learning. *Nurs. Outlook* 16:46, 1968.
21. Molnar, A. R.   Critical issues in computer-based learning. *Educ. Techn.* 11:61, 1971.
22. Beck, I. H., and Monroe, B.   Some dimensions of simulation. *Educ. Techn.* 9:45, 1969.
23. Cruickshank, D. R., and Broadbent, F. W.   An investigation to determine effects of simulation training on student teaching behavior. *Educ. Techn.* 9:50, 1969.
24. Ibid., p. 54.
25. Bitzer, M.   Clinical nursing instruction via the PLATO simulated laboratory. *Nurs. Res.* 15:144, 1966.
26. Gagné, R. M.   Educational technology. *Educ. Techn.* 8:5, 1968.

SUPPLEMENTARY READINGS

American Council on Education, Committee on Television. *Teaching by Closed-Circuit Television*. Washington, D.C.: American Council on Education, 1956.

Beck, J. On Some Methods of Programming. In E. Galanter [Ed.], *Automatic Teaching: The State of the Art*. New York: Wiley, 1959.

Becker, M. E., and Mihelcie, M. R. Programming a motor skill. *J. Nurs. Educ.* 5:25, 1966.

Blyth, J. W. Teaching Machines and Human Beings. In A. A. Lumsdaine and R. Glaser [Eds.], *Teaching Machines and Programmed Learning*. Washington, D.C.: National Education Association, 1960.

Brown, J. W., and Thornton, J. W., Jr. *College Teaching: Prespectives and Guidelines*. New York: McGraw-Hill, 1963.

Bushnell, D. D., and Allen, D. W. [Eds.]. *The Computer in American Education*. New York: Wiley, 1967.

Caliandro, G. Programmed instruction and its use in nursing education. *Nurs. Res.* 17:450, 1968.

Center for Research and Evaluation in Applications of Technology in Education. *Instructional Media*. Pittsburgh: American Institutes for Research, 1967.

Cluno, B. Teaching machines and programmed learning. *J. Nurs. Educ.* 3:13, 1964.

Corey, S. M. The Nature of Instruction. In P. C. Lange [Ed.], *Programmed Instruction*. Chicago: University of Chicago Press, 1967.

Cruickshank, D. R. Simulation: new direction in teacher preparation. *Phi Delta Kappan* 47:23, 1966.

Diers, D., and Schmidt, R. L. Transcriptions and tape recordings in interaction analysis. *Nurs. Res.* 17:236, 1968.

Feldman, H. Learning transfer from programmed instruction to clinical performance. *Nurs. Res.* 18:51, 1967.

Feldhusen, J. F., and Szabo, M. A review of developments in computer assisted instructions. *Educ. Techn.* 9:32, 1969.

Gagné, R. M. *The Conditions of Learning*. New York: Holt, Rinehart & Winston, 1965.

Gilbert, T. F. On the Relevance of Laboratory Investigation to Learning of Self-Instructional Programming. In A. A. Lumsdaine and R. Glaser [Eds.], *Teaching Machines and Programmed Learning*. Washington, D.C.: National Education Association, 1960.

Glaser, R. [Ed.]. *Teaching Machines and Programed Learning, II, Data and Directions*. Washington, D.C.: Department of Audio-Visual Instruction of the National Education Association, 1965.

Green, E. J. *The Learning Process and Programmed Instruction*. New York: Holt, Rinehart & Winston, 1962.

Growel, E. C., et al. No drop-outs in this refresher course. *Amer. J. Nurs.* 70:94, 1970.

Holland, J. Teaching Machines: An Application of Principles from the Laboratory. In A. A. Lumsdaine and R. Glaser [Eds.], *Teaching Machines and Programmed Learning*. Washington, D.C.: National Education Association, 1960.

Justmas, J., and Mais, W. H. *College Teaching: Its Practice and Its Potential.* New York: Harper & Bros., 1956.

Kiang, M. H. Y. Programmed instruction in nutrition for collegiate nursing students. *J. Amer. Diet. Ass.* 57:423, 1970.

Lumsdaine, A. A. Educational Technology, Programmed Learning, and Instructional Science. In *Theories of Learning and Instruction.* Sixty-third Yearbook of the National Society for the Study of Education. Chicago: University of Chicago Press, 1964.

Maehr, M. L. Programed learning and the role of the teacher. *J. Educ. Res.* 57: 554, 1964.

Markle, S. M. Empirical Testing of Programs. In P. C. Lange [Ed.], *Programed Instruction.* Chicago: University of Chicago Press, 1967.

Meierhenry, W. C. Implications of learning theory for instructional technology. *Phi Delta Kappan* 46:345, 1965.

Merrill, I. R. Closed-circuit television in health sciences education. *J. Med. Educ.* 38:329, 1963.

Milton, A. W. The science of learning and the technology of educational methods. *Harvard Educ. Rev.* 29:96, 1959.

National Society for the Study of Education. *Programmed Instruction, the Sixty-sixth Yearbook.* Chicago: University of Chicago Press, 1967.

Pearman, E., and Suleiman, L. Test of a programmed instruction unit. *Nurs. Res.* 15:258, 1966.

Pressey, S. L. A Simple Apparatus Which Gives Tests and Scores—and Teaches. In A. A. Lumsdaine and R. Glaser [Eds.], *Teaching Machines and Programmed Learning.* Washington, D.C.: National Education Association, 1960.

Pressey, S. L. Development and Appraisal of Devices Providing Immediate Automatic Scoring of Objective Tests and Concomitant Self-Instruction. In A. A. Lumsdaine and R. Glaser [Eds.], *Teaching Machines and Programmed Learning.* Washington, D.C.: National Education Association, 1960.

Pressey, S. L. Auto-instruction Perspectives, Problems, Potentials. In *Theories of Learning and Instruction.* Sixty-third Yearbook of the National Society for the Study of Education. Chicago: Universty of Chicago Press, 1964.

Puleo, Sr. M. P. Comparison of on-the-job and at home use of programmed instruction and the lecture method in an inservice education program. *Nurs. Res.* 18:356, 1968.

Schurdak, J. J. An approach to the use of computers in the instructional process and an evaluation. *Amer. Educ. Res. J.* 4:59, 1967.

Skinner, B. F. The science of learning and the art of teaching. *Harvard Educ. Rev.* 24:86, 1954.

Skinner, B. F. Why we need teaching machines. *Harvard Educ. Rev.* 31:377, 1961.

Spence, K. W. The relation of learning theory to the technology of education. *Harvard Educ. Rev.* 29:84, 1959.

Sullivan, J., and Weber, M. Nurse's bag technique—self-taught. *Nurs. Outlook* 18:59, 1970.

Taber, J. I., Glaser, R., and Schaeffer, H. H. *Learning and Programmed Instruction.* Reading: Addison-Wesley, 1965.

Ting, T. C., and Walden, W. E. An instructional system for computer assisted instruction on a general purpose computer. *Educ. Techn.* 10:28, 1970.

Wittmeyer, A. Teaching by audiotape. *Nurs. Outlook* 19:162, 1971.

V STRATEGIES AND PROCESSES FOR CURRICULUM CHANGE

THAT changes do occur in nursing curriculums is obvious to anyone who has taught or been associated with curriculums for a period of years. To some persons, these changes come about much too slowly in view of changes taking place in society. To other persons, the changes occurring are breathtaking. Change is occurring within and among schools, but it has occurred in some schools to a much greater extent than others. It appears that nurse educators are in a period of tumultuous educational activity; however, not all of the change has reached all schools. Curriculum change is concerned with processes and strategies for change. This chapter describes the major issues and events that have initiated change in nursing curriculums.

PROCESS OF CURRICULUM CHANGE

The process of change in school curriculum presents problems that are not inherent in the change process in some other fields. In the fields of medicine, agriculture, and public health, major changes are not likely to occur until considerable research and experimentation have identified and validated a desired change. Many changes are brought about in school programs on the basis of intuition or value judgments without the benefit of research. On occasion, these changes do not bring about the hoped-for results. For a number of reasons, changes that were proved beneficial in some schools may not be satisfactory in others. Changes in school programs are made in full view of the recipients of change. This is contrary to the practice of medicine and agriculture, in which considerable laboratory testing is done before involving the recipients of the change. When a test or tryout of a curriculum innovation is made, it is often under limited or invalid test conditions.

If innovations in curriculum are to be initiated, decisions must be made about the nature of changes to be endorsed and supported. It appears that the only changes that should be tried out, tested, and diffused to other schools are those that clearly, in the eyes of skillful judges of nursing and nursing education, adhere to and enhance the basic values of American education. The changes being tested and advocated for adoption within this basic structure of fundamental values are efforts to keep curriculums in tune with changing times. Finally, innovations, experiments, and changes being tried out offer high promise of contributing to the welfare, happiness, and self-realization of the individuals who are being subjected to the practices in the school.

If prospective changes are to be judged on the basis of these criteria, some fundamental steps in developing strategies for change are essential. Nurse educators must come to some agreement about the fundamental values that should characterize nursing education programs. This will require tapping the resources of sociologists, psychologists, philosophers, political scientists, and others who have insight into social conditions in an effort to define the changing state of things under which education must be carried on now and in the future. Nurse educators must continue deep and penetrating studies of the motivations, anxieties, problems, desires and aspirations, and drives of human beings. Lastly, nurse educators should be willing to discard those practices that on the basis of evidence do not remain defensible in the face of pressure for change.

Strategy for curriculum change must involve a widespread and comprehensive effort to induce those who make decisions and who actually direct the development of learning opportunities for students to change something. *Strategy* is the means used to create curricular innovations and to facilitate their use on a continuing basis. It specifies a sequence of activities for getting an advocated innovation installed in an ongoing educational system [1]. An innovation is considered to be a deliberate, novel, specific change, which is thought to be more efficacious in accomplishing the goals of the system; innovations are willed and planned rather than occurring haphazardly. The worthwhileness of an innovation is usually justified on the basis of its anticipated consequences for the accomplishment of system goals [2].

Strategies of curriculum change may be grouped into two major categories: (1) pragmatic approach to change, and (2) directed change. The pragmatic approach to change includes attempts to resolve a major educational problem. Data upon which the innovation is designed are obtained by means of studies and surveys. The process of change is usually effected by supplying teachers with new materials (usually developed outside the school) and consultants and by providing inservice education and workshop activities. Professional organizations frequently support the suggested innovation. An individual school interprets and implements the change to the degree that it is compatible with the faculty's philosophy and resources and the interests and support of the community. Evaluation of the effects of this innovation may be made by the individual school and shared with other schools through interschool visitation, publications, and reports.

A strategy of directed change implies that certain persons outside the school make an assumption about the kind of change that is needed and formulate a plan of action. This plan calls for program design and field testing by outside forces. Usually large sums of money and expert personnel are needed for the design and testing. Whereas teachers may resist outside groups designing curriculum change, inservice education may facilitate active teacher involvement. The innovation is linked to long-term goals, a specific program plan is developed and instituted, and procedures for evaluation are utilized during the field testing. Results of the field tests are made known through publications, reports, and professional meetings.

Nursing has used the pragmatic approach to a greater extent than the directed change strategy. Descriptions of the strategies that have been utilized in the past and of some more recent strategies are provided. Although these are isolated for the purpose of description, the various strategies were not used singly. On occasion, two or more different approaches were used concurrently. The review of the process and outcomes of these strategies for change leads to the formulation of some suggested guidelines for developing future strategies.

PREVIOUS APPROACHES TO CURRICULUM CHANGE

The strategies for curriculum change that were utilized by nurse educators during the first half of the twentieth century demonstrated efforts and activity to establish nursing education in this country as a sound, respectable, and useful endeavor. The approaches that were used were pragmatic in nature. Seven strategies can be identified: strategy of reform, standard setting, organizational efforts, activity analysis, establishing new goals, group dynamics, and subject reorganization.

STRATEGY OF REFORM

The philosophy and activities of Florence Nightingale in establishing a school of nursing in London in 1860 attracted the attention of physicians in this country. The low level of nursing care was a concern of the American Medical Association, nurses, and the general public. A committee of the association was appointed to consider the question of the training of nurses. The chairman of this committee made visits to England and Germany to learn the nursing reforms in these countries.

The Nightingale School impressed the physicians; however, they suggested that the system could be improved if it were placed under the control of the medical profession. The ideas of the reformers were acceptable to nurses in this country, but the control of nursing by physicians was not. In 1873 the first three Nightingale schools were established in this country by lay groups. Communications from Miss Nightingale outlined the general principles of organization of nursing schools, which emphasized the differences between medicine and nursing. Control of the nursing staff, according to Miss Nightingale, "must be put under qualified woman heads and not under the medical or the economic staff of the hospital" [3]. Other schools of nursing that opened during the late 1800's were influenced by pioneers in this field who had visited or communicated with the Nightingale School in London. These schools provided demonstration activities in which the translation of the reform ideas into practice could be viewed and adopted by interested groups.

History shows that the social and economic conditions in this country did not nurture the growth of these schools of nursing. The lack of financial support forced education for nursing into an apprenticeship system under hospital control. The first strategy of curriculum innovation—the development of ideas of reforms—had a penetrating, though long dormant influence on nursing education.

EFFORTS TOWARD STANDARD SETTING

The years during the early 1900's saw considerable activity in the development of schools of nursing. During the period from 1873 to 1893, approximately one hundred schools of nursing were established in the United States.

The founding of these schools coincided with the appearance of colleges for women, such as Smith and Wellesley, a fact which was probably an indication of growing initiative and independence on the part of women. This new system of education proved useful and profitable to hospitals. It became evident that patients received better care by better educated women The programs were such a joy to hospitals in providing a good but cheap source of service that every hospital wanted to establish a school of nursing. In the next twenty-year period, 1893–1913, over one thousand new schools were established. This period was known to some as the "boom" period, but it proved devastating to the young profession of nursing. Standards of education varied, as did the products of these schools. During this time the curriculum was increased from two to three years; however, in most instances there was no increase in the hours of instruction offered, only an increase in the amount of nursing service given to the hospital.

Before the end of the first decade of the new century, the success of visiting nurses had created a variety of opportunities for nurses in connection with the growing public health movement. The professional organizations, the American Nurses' Association, the National League for Nursing Education, and the National Organization for Public Health Nursing, had come into being and were aware of the expanding fields of social usefulness that were opening for qualified nurses. Members of these associations were deeply conscious of the danger to society and to the profession of inadequate preparation for nursing. The influence of the hundreds of young women who had dropped out or had been dismissed from nursing schools was having a deleterious effect on nursing as a whole. The frustrations of graduate nurses, who from lack of information had entered substandard schools, were inhibiting desirable students from enrolling. Leaders in nursing education believed that institutions called schools should be expected to have definite educational standards and objectives.

The only method through which the standardization of nursing schools, so earnestly desired by the professional organizations, might be secured was the medium of legislation. Although a national standard was discussed, it was realized that the power to regulate the practice of professional and other workers is a function of state governments. When the American Nurses' Association undertook the task of securing legislation to control the practice of nursing as a protection to the public and as a means of standardizing or upgrading the preparation of nurses, it had to first promote the organization of nursing in the various states. By 1912, thirty-eight state nurses' associations had been organized, and thirty-three of them had secured nurse practice acts in the state legislatures. These laws indicated who could legally practice nursing in the states, established the minimum standards for the practicing nurse and for educational programs, and became the first means of standard setting of nursing curriculums.

The enactment of state laws regulating the conduct of educational programs was the starting point for curriculum renovation and improvement. In some instances progress was hindered by the passage of ineffective laws. Some of the laws specified curricular requirements in such detail that they soon became obstacles to progress. The absence of a definition of nursing in the nurse practice acts presented problems to upgrading schools of nursing. Considerable opposition to regulatory policies was experienced by nurses in many states. Many of the members of boards of nurse examiners were as poorly qualified for their important function as some of the nurses directing the schools of nursing. Nurses learned that legislation which controls licenses to practice must be amended at intervals to retain its usefulness [4]. The strategy of change concerned with setting standards for educational programs in nursing precipitated considerable activity in curriculum improvement.

ORGANIZATION EFFORTS TO IMPROVE CURRICULUM

Initial efforts of the nursing organizations to improve standards of nursing education led to legislation. It became apparent that other approaches would be necessary to assist schools of nursing to upgrade the quality of curriculums. The selfish and vested interest of medical and other groups and the lack of resources for nursing education delayed needed curriculum change.

The Education Committee of the National League of Nursing Education started to construct the *Standard Curriculum for Schools of Nursing* in 1914. The first edition, which appeared in 1919 stated:

The Committee on Education undertook the task of preparing a curriculum which might serve as a guide to training schools struggling to establish good standards of nursing education, and which might also represent to the public and to those who wish to study our work, a fair idea of what, under our present system, we conceive to be an acceptable training for the profession of nursing [5].

The purpose that the Committee had in mind was to arrive at some general agreement on a desirable and workable standard whose main features could be accepted by training schools of good standing throughout the country. In this way the diversity of standards that existed among schools could be overcome. The standard could also supply a basis for appraising the value of widely different systems of nursing training [6].

The *Standard Curriculum for Schools of Nursing* provided general information concerning the administration of the school of nursing, including the type and capacity of hospitals conducting schools. Specific information was given about the curriculum, including the description of courses to be offered, hours of instruction, teaching methods and materials, evaluation procedures, the placement of courses in the curriculum, and the qualifications of teaching personnel. Requirements for admission were specified, and the housing and living conditions of students were described.

This publication had considerable impact upon nursing education. The purposes of the document were realized to some degree, and many nursing schools began to reorganize their curriculums to bring them into line with the recommendations of the league's committee. The disruptions and distractions of the war and the postwar period were partially responsible for a reduction in curriculum activities. World War I brought to light several factors about nursing and nursing education. In 1918 the list of schools accredited by the state boards of nurse examiners totaled nearly 1,500, but almost 40 percent of them fell below the standards of the American Red Cross nursing service. The generally low level of nursing education was in sharp contrast to the type of service expected of nurses. The revelations of the draft alerted health workers to some fundamental problems in health care. Approximately 29 percent of the young men called had been found to be physically unfit for military service. Since many of the disabilities had been caused by preventable conditions, the findings gave tremendous impetus to the health programs of both official and nonofficial agencies. The sudden demand for an increased number of public health nurses and the indifference of young women to nursing as a career created a serious shortage of nurses in the immediate postwar period.

As the demands for public health nurses increased, questions were raised as to the scope of public health nursing practice and the educational preparation for the practice. A committee to study public health nursing education was appointed, with Dr. C. E. A. Winslow as chairman. The committee later became known as the Committee for the Study of Nursing Education. The report of the committee, with the study on which it is based, still stands as a beacon in the field of nursing education. The committee found that the objectives and structure of most nursing schools bore little resemblance to educational institutions. Certain recommendations were made regarding the (1) financing of nursing education, (2) development and strengthening of university schools, (3) special preparation for administrators and teachers in nursing, and (4) preparation and licensing of subsidiary workers. This report was made available in the publication *Nursing and Nursing Education in the United States* in 1923 [7].

The movement toward improving curriculums was strengthened by the work of the committee. A revision of the *Curriculum for Schools of Nursing* was started after the publication of the report. The revision took into consideration many of the recommendations, especially the increased emphasis on public health. This revision was completed in 1927.

Diversity in the quality of nursing programs continued to be a problem for students and nursing organizations. Participants in the postwar national recruitment program, which was sponsored by the nursing organizations and the American Red Cross, were seriously handicapped by lack of information about schools. Prospective students wanted information about schools of nursing other than the fact that a school was on the approved list of a state board of nurse examiners. Following the publication of the Goldmark report, the National League of Nursing Education set to work to secure interest and financial support of other organizations in a program for grading schools of nursing. The Committee on the Grading of Nursing Schools was organized in 1926, which included representatives from the three nursing organizations, the American Medical Association, the American College of Surgeons, the American Hospital Association, the American Public Health Association, and the field of general education. Seventy-four percent of the schools approved by the state boards of examiners (approximately 1,500) participated in the first grading, and 81 percent, in the second. Each school that participated responded to a questionnaire pertaining to various educational practices. The individual school was graded on each item of the questionnaire in relation to all other schools. The revised *Curriculum for Schools of Nursing* was the measure used by the committee in evaluating courses of instruction in the participating schools in the surveys made in 1929 and again in 1932. The schools received two reports that showed the standing of the school, item by item, in relation to all other schools. A classified list of schools, which was so greatly desired by vocational and other advisors, was not made. The committee decided that the data obtained was insufficient and that any possible list would be unjust to some schools. Some improvements in curriculum and educational practices in the schools were noted between the first and second grading [8].

After the release of the final report of the committee, which was entitled

Nursing Schools Today and Tomorrow, a committee of the National League of Nursing Education began the task of reconstructing the *Curriculum for Schools of Nursing* [9]. The philosophy and activities of the committee reflected contemporary views of education and curriculum construction. Efforts were expended in securing the participation of experts from the field of education, representatives of nursing school faculties, members of state boards of nurse examiners, and other persons interested in the project. It was estimated that during the three years of the committee's activities, between two and three hundred persons took part in the work. Study committees of state leagues were organized in many states to work with the central curriculum committee. A group of cooperating schools reviewed and tested tentative course outlines that were prepared by the production committees while the curriculum revision was in progress [10].

A *Curriculum Guide for Schools of Nursing* was published in 1937 [11]. It was intended to serve as a guide to nursing schools in building their own curriculums. It was not to be considered to be a standard to be enforced. The purpose of the guide was to encourage schools to plan ahead in their educational programs and to experiment with new methods and materials. The curriculum guide accepted the adjustment aim of education as an appropriate focus of nursing curriculum. This edition offered a definition of nursing that became the conceptual framework for curriculum objectives and activities. Standards of education, including admission and graduation requirements, were suggested. The major portion of the curriculum guide was devoted to detailed information about the required courses, indicating content, placement, hours of instruction, instructional personnel, teaching methods and materials, and suggested reference readings. The final section pertained to measurement and evaluation of educational outcomes.

The publication of the *Curriculum Guide for Schools of Nursing* evoked mixed reactions from schools of nursing. It was conceived to be most helpful to those faculties that had served on participating state committees of the curriculum revision project. Many schools could not make effective use of the guide without substantially more facilities and resources. Within some schools of nursing, the guide aroused fear and resistance to change, not an uncommon reaction to innovation in any human experience [12].

ACTIVITY ANALYSIS

One of the projects undertaken by the Committee on the Grading of Nursing Schools was an analysis of nursing activities. The rationale underlying this strategy of curriculum change indicated that before the committee could assist schools in preparing good nurses, it must discover, first, what is good nursing, and second, how can it be taught. It seemed appropriate that the committee include a project designed to show what nurses do and provide suggestions as to how they may be taught to do it.

The report of this project culminated in the publication of *An Activity Analysis of Nursing* in 1934 [13]. A major aim of the study was the definition of good nursing. To respond to this question, the study endeavored to answer these related questions: What should a professional nurse be? What should a professional nurse know and be able to do? The latter question was studied from the points of view of the patient, the physician, the hospital administrator, the community, and the nurse. Some conclusions on the functions of nurses were stated, which were based on generally accepted practice. The report defined those tasks that lie in the "middle ground of nursing practice." The tasks were those that constitute the greater part of the nursing service offered to the community and those where the welfare of many sick people is at stake [14].

The report proceeded to describe the four successive steps involved in a functional approach to revision of the nursing curriculum:

1. An analysis of the present content of nursing practice by means of checklists of duties, classified according to type, frequency, difficulty of performance, and relative importance to the patient
2. A determination of the content of professional courses that bear directly upon nursing methods and procedures and are intended to prepare nurses to perform efficiently the duties included in the checklists
3. A study of the elements of the fundamental science courses in order to select the facts and principles upon which professional methods and procedures are based
4. The organization of materials so derived into a form most appropriate for teaching [15]

A significant portion of the study was allocated to the identification of the "conditions" that require nursing care in the hospital and the community and to the rating of those conditions on the basis of frequency of occurrence. The conditions that occurred most frequently were those which were considered for curriculum content. Listing and classification of nursing activities were undertaken. These were categorized in relation to hospital bedside nursing activities, public health nursing activities, and private duty nursing activities in the home.

The study endeavored to relate the conditions and the nursing activities to the various hospital services, such as medical nursing, surgical nursing, and pediatric nursing. This became the technique for identifying and organizing the content of the nursing curriculum. The activities of nursing were then related to the specific content in science courses to determine the appropriate specifications for science instruction.

Certain disadvantages of activity analysis as a tool in curriculum development were identified. The time required to make this analysis seemed to be the major objection to the technique. It appeared, however, from the point of view of the study projects, that the advantages far outweighed the disadvantages.

ESTABLISHING NEW GOALS

During World War II the demands for national defense and military nursing required the nursing profession to focus on new goals and new content, and the means to get these into operation. The *Curriculum Guide for Schools of Nursing* outlined recommendations for quality education for nursing; however, it acknowledged that the heavy demands of the war and postwar activities upon nurses would require some adjustments in the curriculums without weakening fundamental standards. At the request of the Nursing Council on National Defense, a statement pertaining to principles and policies for guidance in the basic preparation were formulated by the Committee on Educational Policies and Resources [16]. The general thrust of the statement indicated that schools of nursing should be interested in the nursing needs of the country as a whole as well as in the needs of their own institutions and local communities. Some curriculum changes were suggested:

1. The utilization of colleges and universities for certain phases of the instructional program
2. Cooperative arrangements with several schools of nursing within a geographical area to conserve and share facilities and resources
3. The utilization of military hospitals for part of the professional preparation of the nurse
4. The use of methods of teaching that might reduce the amount of time required to complete the program

The response of schools of nursing to the statements of the Nursing Council on National Defense took several forms. Programs were streamlined as the result of a critical review of instructors in relation to the urgent needs of the times. Preclinical science courses were offered by cooperating colleges and universities. Some efforts were made to centralize schools of nursing within specific geographical areas to share resources and facilities. Advances in military medicine provided new content for the nursing curriculum. The movement of nurses to the far corners of the earth awakened the concerns of nursing beyond the immediate environs of the school to include a national and international view of health and nursing. This became a curriculum orientation that persisted beyond the war effort.

GROUP DYNAMICS

The group dynamics movement of the 1940's introduced a whole new trend of thinking and practice regarding curriculum change. Previous strategies were developed by groups outside the school setting and concerned with activities of organized groups on the national and state levels. The group dynamics movement shifted the focus of attention to the processes of changes and away from the intended change itself. The persons most directly concerned with the changes—faculties of schools—became involved in the process. New roles and titles began to appear in schools. Curriculum committees became active, and the consultants from within or outside the school were used frequently. Specialized inservice education and program development activities became useful techniques for the involvement of faculty in curriculum study. One form of this, the workshop, brought together teams of people from various schools to work together. The idea was that during the period of the workshop, the experience of working and living together would facilitate the development of common understandings, common goals, and programs that would be useful to the participants when they returned to their own schools.

The use of group dynamics in curriculum activities requires the acquisition of group process skills. Any group that does not intend to remain forever a collection of individuals must clarify its purposes, consider how it will accomplish those purposes, arrive at some conclusions upon which the group agrees, and take action upon these decisions. The history of curriculum study is marked by the number of curriculum committees that have expired because they could not cope with one or another of these steps. Reports of faculties that used group processes to bring about changes in the curriculum indicate the need for training in the basic skills of group work. Not only were faculty members instructed in the principles of group participation, but also the group leaders were instructed in leadership techniques. Nevertheless, the faculty believed that the experiences in group activities led to better committee work in the school. The group process allows for clarification of terms and concepts that facilitates communication about curriculum issues. Some reactions to this strategy suggested that the process is slow and too involved in personal problems of individual members. Many felt, however, that verbalizing ideas within a group and obtaining reactions from group members was a beneficial experience for all participants.

This strategy for curriculum change was utilized by the National League for Nursing in the initiation of curriculum conference projects. The first approach of the league in utilizing the conference technique was on the organizational level; the second approach focused on faculty participation in curriculum conferences. In 1949 the league initiated the nursing organization curriculum conference, which was a joint effort on the part of all organizations of the nursing profession. The purpose of this curriculum conference was to consider the status of curriculum activities relative to practical nursing, basic professional, and advanced programs. Committees on education and curriculum of the various organizations (American Association of Industrial Nurses, American Nurses' Association, Association of Collegiate Schools of Nursing, National Association of Colored Graduate Nurses, National Association for Practical Nurse Education, National League of Nursing Education, National Organization for Public Health Nursing, and the International Council of Nurses) were represented at the conference and presented reports of their activities. The major focus of the conference was to assess the curriculum activities of these organizations in relation to common elements and the overlapping of and gaps in content and variances of curriculum objectives. Deliberations were carried on by small group discussions, which provided opportunities for groping with and exploring various issues affecting curriculum development. It was reported that the conference was characterized by great freedom of thinking. Interest was expressed in more careful planning at the national level for curriculum activity that would avoid duplication of effort, eliminate gaps, map out a program of action, pool financial and personnel resources, and involve as many nurse educators as possible. Also stressed by the participants was the value of a conference made up of representatives of many curricular interests and from various geographic areas [17].

A second curriculum conference was held in 1950, which was concerned with three areas relating to curriculum development that evolved from the 1949 meeting. Three pivotal questions were discussed in the group meetings: (1) How can the functions of nursing be differentiated sufficiently to develop appropriate curricula, (2) how can each of us go about improving the curriculum in her own situation, and (3) how can we stimulate and share research in nursing in order to improve nursing and nursing education?

The conference utilized persons who had knowledge and expertise in curriculum work in general education. Some trends in general education were highlighted, with implications for nursing education. The trend away from the organization of the program of study in a great many narrow, specific courses and toward program organization into broader groupings was a major consideration. The interpretation of the purposes and patterns of professional nursing education within colleges and universities was explored. Attention was given to the potential contributions of community colleges to nursing education. Finally, the nature and processes of curriculum development were examined. This conference appeared to be of great value to the participants. The sharing and exchanging of ideas, the opportunity to clarify concepts and issues, and the reassurance given to individual and group efforts were stimulating experiences [18].

The National League for Nursing received funds from the National Foundation for Infantile Paralysis to conduct regional conferences in 1957. The conference technique was seen as the most effective means of involving great numbers of nurse educators, and a broad program designed to reach all faculty groups was developed. The four curriculum conferences that were held early in 1957 were designed as pilot conferences. On the basis of the experiences with the first conferences, the league planned eleven conferences for 1958. The conferences were designed primarily for instructors in basic nursing programs. The major purpose of the conferences was to provide the participants with new ideas, knowledge, and understandings that they could translate into improved curriculums in their schools. A major focus was given to mental health and rehabilitation in the curriculum.

Since curriculum development is the responsibility of the whole faculty, efforts were made to interest all of them in the conferences. Each school was invited to send two instructors to a conference. Questionnaires that were sent to the schools which accepted the invitation elicited the problems and concerns of faculty members in curriculum activities. Participants in the conferences were assigned to small groups. The groups were composed of individuals whose curriculum interests were the same or similar. As the conference proceeded, each participant became identified with his particular group, and there were many opportunities for exploring ideas and sharing one's experiences with the other members of the group [19].

The regional differences and inequalities in education have been the concern of the states within various regions of the country. The governmental arrangements that developed among the several states within a region provided a means for studying the curriculum problems specific to a region. The activities of the Southern Regional Education Board and later the Western Interstate Commission on Higher Education offered strategies for curriculum change by which faculty members within a region came together to analyze the problems in that region and to develop curriculum models, activities, and materials that would be useful to schools in that area. The state governments and state leagues for nursing, individually and as a group, provided the structure, motivation, and resources for productive group endeavors. Since the problems among schools within a region were similar, participants in the group sessions came from comparable situations with common problems. The initial endeavors of the Committee on Nursing of the Southern Regional Education Board sought to establish graduate programs in this region. The objectives, curriculum design, and clinical focus reflected the needs of this area for better qualified teachers for schools of nursing and administrators for nursing services. More recently, both the Southern Regional Education Board and the Western Interstate Commission on Higher Education Committees on Nursing have focused attention on specific projects and activities that utilize new approaches in developing and organizing the subject matter of nursing. Group process techniques have proved to be useful strategies for identifying and studying curriculum problems and designing innovations by group decision-making.

SUBJECT REORGANIZATION

Central to much of the curriculum revision activity in the 1940's and 1950's were the efforts to reorganize subjects included in the curriculum. Problem-, student-, community-, and society-centered programs were proposed in the field of general education. Variously organized, core curriculums were attempted at the secondary level, while numerous revisions of general education programs were advanced at the college level. Other curriculum notions were being explored in terms of their relevance for specific curriculums. One notion in particular related to the organization of curriculum providing larger blocks of learning subsuming many small but related courses.

Although subject organization is the usual and to some inevitable pattern for classroom studies, it has been criticized. The critics contend that it results in the splitting up of human knowledge and skills into arbitrary segments and that the student who pursues it comes out with piecemeal education. Such criticisms have led to efforts to modify subject reorganization along the lines of "broad fields." One approach to broad-fields organization is that of fusion, under which two or more subjects are brought together in such a way that they lose their separate identity and form a new pattern.

Faculties of schools of nursing found this organization of subjects useful for nursing curriculums. Considerable activity in curriculum revision took place utilizing the broad-fields approach. Some changes in subject organization revealing this influence were noted. Table 15 shows a comparison of the traditional and broad-fields organization.

TABLE 15. A Comparison of Courses in Traditional and Broad-Fields Organization

Traditional Organization	Broad-Fields Organization
Medical Nursing Surgical Nursing	Medical-Surgical Nursing
Obstetric Nursing Pediatric Nursing	Maternal-Child Nursing

Social Aspects of Nursing
Diet Therapy
Nursing Arts
Introduction to Medical
  Science (Pathology)
	Appropriate content fused
	  into all clinical courses

History of Nursing Professional Adjustments I Professional Adjustments II	History and Trends in Nursing

The traditional organization gives as separate courses the subjects that appeared in the curriculum. The courses in the broad-fields organization result from fusion of two or more subjects, some of which lose their original identity in the curriculum. This arrangement provided for fewer courses; however, the courses that evolved were broader in scope. In all of these efforts toward subject reorganization, difficulties were experienced in moving very far from the traditional courses that reflected the medical curriculum model.

RECENT STRATEGIES FOR CURRICULUM INNOVATION

By World War II America's nursing services were sorely taxed. Increased hospital construction, the expanded use of graduate nurse staffs, new fields of nursing, public health programs, and other health activities made increasingly urgent demands on the supply of nursing services. The nursing profession was looking to the future, seeking appraisal of present needs, questioning what to expect in the years ahead and what to do about it. Faculties of schools of nursing were sensitive and responsive to the demands for more and different types of nurse practitioners. The tasks that confronted nursing education required some new strategies for curriculum innovation.

IMPLEMENTATION OF STUDIES OF NURSING

In 1948 three major reports concerning nursing were published. The Committee on Nursing Problems of the American Medical Association issued a report that offered recommendations for the improvement of the quality and quantity of nursing services. Some of the recommendations were concerned with the immediate relief of shortages of nursing personnel; others pertained to future developments in nursing and nursing education. The committee recommended that professional nurses be subdivided into two groups: (1) the nurse educators who have collegiate preparation, and (2) the clinical nurses who complete a two-year training program. The committee also recommended that provisions be made for the training of practical nurses who will assist the professional nurse with routine bedside nursing [20].

The second report was the outcome of activities undertaken by the Division of Nursing Education of Teachers College, Columbia University. Since the division concentrates on preparing future teachers of nursing, it considered it desirable to secure the viewpoints of other health and social welfare professions concerning the structure of nursing and the medical needs of the community. A Committee on the Function of Nursing was formed, composed of experts in various fields of medical and social sciences who would be willing to bring their knowledge and experience to bear on the problems confronting the nursing profession and to express their views of the role of nursing in this period of rapid social change. The committee reviewed the demands for medical and health care, the economic base of nursing practice, the utilization of nursing personnel, and the existing pattern of nursing education. The major thrust in the recommendations of the committee focused on the education of the professional nurse at the collegiate level and the preparation of the practical nurse in the adult and high school vocational system. In each instance, the educational programs should be planned to meet the educational needs of the student rather than the service requirements of the hospital [21].

The third report was that prepared by Esther L. Brown for the National Nursing Council. At the request of this Council, Dr. Brown undertook to explore the organization, administration, and financing of professional schools of nursing. The study endeavored to view nursing service and nursing education in terms of what is best for society. A conceptualization of the probable nature of health services in the second half of the twentieth century and of the nursing services likely to be demanded by the evolving health services was formulated. Lastly, inquiry was made into the kinds of training and the academic and professional education requisite to prepare nurses to render the various kinds of nursing services. The Brown report recommended that efforts be directed to the establishment of basic schools of nursing in universities and colleges that would prepare the professional nurse. The hospital schools of nursing were designated to prepare the graduate bedside nurse. The report suggested that consideration be given to shortening the hospital programs by utilizing the teaching resources of junior colleges. Finally, the preparation of the practical nurse should be provided by vocational or adult education units of the public school systems. The Brown report, which was published as *Nursing for the Future,* was approved in principle by the profession [27]. The national nursing organizations formed a Committee on Implementing the Brown Report, with representatives of allied professional groups. In January, 1949, the Joint Board of Directors of the Six National Nursing Organizations was established, and the Committee on Implementing the Brown Report became a committee of the joint board. Later, its name was officially changed to the National Committee for the Improvement of Nursing Services.

The first task of the National Committee for the Improvement of Nursing Services was to consider the current status of nursing education facilities as one approach to the improvement of nursing services. A subcommittee on school data analysis was assigned the task of collecting and analyzing data submitted by schools of nursing. In addition, it was asked to present findings to individual schools and to prepare a report for publication. In the spring of 1950 the report of the school data was made available. The report was published as *Nursing Schools at the Mid-Century* and was accepted by the profession [23].

The general characteristics of nursing schools in such basic areas as organization, student health, curriculum, clinical experiences, instructional personnel, performance on state board examinations, and cost of nursing education were examined in the survey. The standards of quality against which the performance of schools in these areas was measured were those set forth in *Essentials of a Good School of Nursing*, and *A Curriculum Guide for Schools of Nursing* [24, 25]. A scoring system was developed to evaluate and to classify the schools.

The response to the survey was encouraging—as 97 percent of all schools (1,156) participated voluntarily in the questionnaire study. Schools were classified in two groups according to their educational practices. Group I included approximately 25 percent of all schools exhibiting the best practices. Group II included the middle 50 percent. About three hundred schools, including those with the lowest national standing, were not classified. This interim classification was received with shocked surprise, rebellious disbelief, and considerable misunderstanding by persons unaccustomed to thinking in comparative terms.

Funds were obtained for the development of a program of accreditation under the National Committee for the Improvement of Nursing Services. As a result of the interim classification, hospital administrators and directors of schools of nursing recommended that all schools be visited and that a list of schools be prepared as a part of the accreditation program. With foundation support, the National Nursing Accrediting Service developed a five-year plan for temporary accreditation on the assumption that with assistance many basic schools of nursing could improve their facilities and programs. Regional conferences, which were arranged by the accrediting service for faculty and other representatives of nursing schools, were stimulating sources of information and guidance. State boards of nurse examiners were encouraged to develop more flexible criteria and were becoming actively interested in the upgrading rather than standardization of schools within their jurisdictions. The first list of basic schools granted temporary accreditation was published in 1952. With the restructuring of the professional nursing organizations, the National Nursing Accrediting Service became an administrative unit of the National League for Nursing.

Temporary accreditation of professional nursing programs by the National League for Nursing ended in 1958 in recognition of the readiness of schools of nursing to apply for full accreditation. The aim of the temporary accreditation program had been to stimulate self-evaluation and self-improvement among schools that would eventuate in the termination of this type of accreditation. Nursing schools were ready to apply for full accreditation by the National League for Nursing. The nursing schools whose applications were accepted and verified by an accreditation visit were granted full accreditation; those whose applications were accepted but waited to be verified by an accreditation visit were granted provisional accreditation. The process of provisional accreditation was terminated in January, 1960.

From these beginnings the National League for Nursing has established a comprehensive program of accreditation. Criteria for self-evaluation have been prepared, and boards of review have been appointed for the various types of programs in nursing education. Accreditation by the National League for Nursing is a voluntary process and is one means by which to assist faculties of schools to improve their programs for the preparation of nurse practitioners.

Another report that contributed to a strategy for curriculum change was prepared by Dr. Margaret Bridgman. Her study, *Collegiate Education for Nursing*, endeavored to provide data upon which a philosophy of the nature and purposes of collegiate nursing education could be built [26]. Her appraisal of the status and characteristics of the hospital schools and the baccalaureate programs in view of the critical need for quantitative as well as qualitiative nursing services pointed out weaknesses and shortcomings. Attention was directed to the content of the baccalaureate curriculum that provided the major in nursing. Dr. Bridgman expressed concern that the policies of the school of nursing were consistent with the general policies and standards of the college and university of which the nursing school is a unit. Various types of curriculum patterns of baccalaureate programs were described. The report focused attention on the characteristics and quality of programs on the advanced level preparing clinical specialists, teachers, and administrators. Fundamental prerequisites were identified that the college or university must assure to initiate and conduct collegiate education for nursing. The report provided useful information to administrators of higher education, to deans and faculties, and to members of the nursing profession and health services that were concerned with the advancement of nursing.

The impetus for a more recent study of nursing and nursing education came from a recommendation in the report of the Surgeon General's Consultant Group on Nursing. The report, *Toward Quality in Nursing*, recommended a national investigation of nursing education, with specific emphasis on the responsibilities and skills for high-quality patient care [27]. After the publication of this report, the two major nursing organizations, the American Nurses' Association and the National League for Nursing, appropriated funds and established a joint committee to study the ways to conduct and finance such a national inquiry. In 1966, W. Allen Wallis, president of the University of Rochester, agreed to head such a study if adequate financing could be obtained. Approximately $450,000 was obtained from the American Nurses' Foundation, the Avalon and W. K. Kellogg Foundations, and an anonymous benefactor. Although the study commission was an outgrowth of the interests of the American Nurses' Association and the National League for Nursing, it was set up as an independent agency and functioned as a self-directing group.

Members of the commission were appointed, and at the first formal meeting of the group in 1967, Dr. Jerome P. Lysaught was appointed director of the planning and operation of the inquiry. Four key problems were identified: (1) the supply and demand for nurses, (2) nursing roles and functions, (3) nursing education, and (4) nursing careers. Two general approaches were utilized to attain the objectives of the study: the analysis of current practices and patterns, and the assessment of future needs.

The commission was funded for a three-year period, and the final report and recommendations were presented in January, 1970. Even though the group acknowledged many limitations of the study, the data that the study yielded enabled the commission to make some recommendations for change in nursing. The following are the four recommendations:

1. Funds should be appropriated from federal and private sources to increase research contracts to investigate the impact of nursing practice on the quality, effectiveness, and economy of health care.
2. Each state should create a master planning committee that will take nursing education under its purview to ensure that nursing education is positioned in the mainstream of American educational patterns.
3. A National Joint Practice Commission, with state counterpart committees, should be established between medicine and nursing to discuss and make recommendations concerning the congruent roles of the physician and nurse in providing quality health care.
4. Federal, regional, state and local governments should adopt measures for the increased support of nursing research and education. Private funds should be sought where such activities are not publicly aided [28].

The commission held a series of regional meetings to announce the findings and recommendations and to allow for comments and suggestions for implementation. Additional funds were obtained to enable the commission to begin the implementation of the recommendations of the state and local levels.

The strategy of curriculum change involving the implementation of studies of nursing brought to the attention of the profession, allied professional groups, and consumers of nursing services the need for restructuring the system of education for nursing. Groundwork was laid for the various types of curriculums and the general specifications for each. Educational standards and criteria for self-evaluation of the programs provided faculty and administration with useful guidelines for review and revision of ongoing educational programs. Perhaps the greatest impact upon the system of education and on the faculties of schools of nursing was a sense of direction that was created for future planning.

STRATEGY OF DIRECTED CHANGE

Certain assumptions underlying the strategy of directed curriculum change are advocated by some persons interested in the change process. It is assumed that persons in government, foundations, universities, and service agencies must decide on the desired goals and plan innovations to promote them. Basic research, program design, and field testing in relation to curriculum should be done by outside forces. This assumption implies that the best experts possible should be brought together to design a program based on the best available research, and it should be tested in many field situations to determine its quality and its adaptability. In addition, major instructional innovations should be introduced by the administration because they can marshall the necessary authority and bring about the decisions necessary for adoption. This prepackaged instructional system can be introduced despite original opposition or apathy on the part of teachers. The teachers will be willing to try an innovation if it is advocated by someone whose reputation they respect or if it is associated with an organization or institution that they revere. The key to successful innovation is providing assistance to teachers as they begin to implement the adopted program. Because of teacher turnover, a continuous program of in-service education in the skills necessary to implement the innovation must be available for new teachers brought into the system. The process of curriculum change contains three steps: innovation, diffusion, and integration. According to the advocates of directed change, innovation is developed on the outside, and the process described leads to diffusion and integration [29]. (See Diagram 15.)

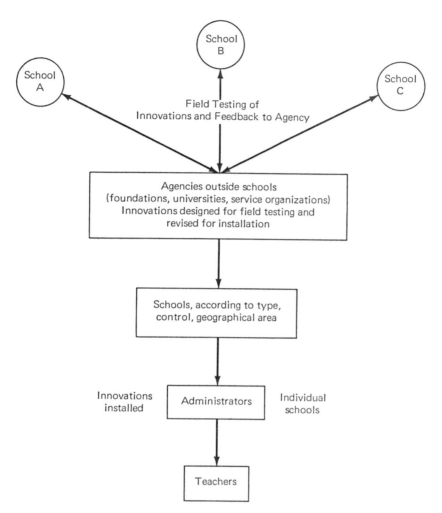

DIAGRAM 15.   Strategy for curriculum change: Directed change. (Adapted from Wiles [29]. P. 7.)

The development of junior college programs in nursing were prompted by the strategy of directed change. The participation of junior colleges in nursing education prior to 1950 was primarily concerned with the provision of general education courses to students enrolled in hospital nursing programs. In 1952 there were in all probability no more than four or five nursing programs leading to an associate degree that were conducted by institutions authorized to grant such a degree. Studies of nursing and nursing education in the late

1940's suggested the potential contribution of junior colleges in nursing education.

In 1952 the Division of Nursing Education of Teachers College, Columbia University, initiated and sponsored the Cooperative Research Project in Junior and Community College Education for Nursing under the direction of Dr. Mildred Montag. The Cooperative Research Project had as its purpose the development and testing of a new type of program preparing young men and women for those functions commonly associated with the registered nurse. The term *bedside nurse* was used to describe the type of nurse that would be prepared in this program and implies that limitations of certain activities of nursing differentiated this practitioner from the professional nurse with broader preparation.

Certain assumptions were stated, which provided the foundation of the study:*

The functions of nursing can and should be differentiated into three basic categories: the professional, the semi-professional or technical, the assisting.

The great bulk of nursing functions belong in the intermediate category, the semi-professional or technical. Therefore, the greatest number of persons should be prepared to fulfill these functions.

Education for nursing belongs within the organized educational framework.

The junior-community college, the post-high school educational institution specifically suited to semi-professional or technical education, is the logical institution for the preparation of the large group of nurses.

When preparation for nursing is education—rather than service-centered— the time required may be reduced [30].

The project was essentially a curriculum study, and it enlisted the cooperation of seven community junior-colleges and one hospital school in developing and setting up an entirely new, two-year nursing program. Questions that the study attempted to answer included the following:*

What are the objectives of this type of nursing program?

What learning experiences are best, and how may they be organized most effectively?

What kind of facilities does this program require?

How does general education and a part in college life affect the product?

Is the product of this program usable?

Will the program tap new resources of personnel for nursing?

What kind of students select this kind of program, and why?

* From *Community College Education for Nursing*. Copyright 1959 by McGraw-Hill Book Company and used with their permission.

What are the reasons for withdrawal?

How do graduates perform on the job?

Can this program become an integral part of the college in which it is established [31]?

During the five years of study activities, data were obtained through questionnaires and school reports on withdrawal and progress of students during the two-year program. The results of licensing examinations and the performance of graduates were also studied. Essential data were collected by the faculties in the cooperating schools pertaining to the activities of curriculum development and teaching.

The design of the study, the development of the curriculum plans, the field testing of the curriculum in the cooperating schools, and the evaluation of the process and the product provided an experience in directed curriculum change. The impact of this study upon nursing education is readily visible in the tremendous growth of junior college programs in nursing since the publication of the study report, *Community College Education for Nursing*.

EVALUATION OF AN INNOVATION

Although the capacity for change is an essential attribute of a socially viable school, change itself becomes meaningful only when it demonstrably leads to more effective functioning. Change is a neutral process, inherently neither good nor bad, neither progressive nor regressive. The introduction of change for the sake of change, in the absence of a clear perception of what improvements it is to effect and without evidence as to whether the expected improvement does indeed occur, becomes a dangerous experience in self-delusion.

Evaluation must be built into plans for innovation, lest the latter become nothing more than well-intentioned but aimless activity, presenting the illusion but not providing the substance of improved education. Only as the evaluation process confirms the effectiveness of a new procedure vis-á-vis some established criteria does the innovation become an educational asset.

The favorable results of a pilot program, testing nursing programs in selected junior colleges over a period of years under the auspices of the Cooperative Research Project at Teachers College, Columbia University, were called to the attention of the W. K. Kellogg Foundation. In 1958 this foundation appropriated funds to facilitate the widening of associate degree education for nursing in states selected for concentrated action. Nursing education leaders, the National League for Nursing, and the American Association of Junior Colleges suggested that certain criteria deemed essential to the successful development of the new idea in education be used by the foundation in selecting the states to be assisted. The foundation's Division of Nursing analyzed the potentialities in numerous states through responses to a series of questions pertaining to the needs, readiness, and resources for associate degree education in nursing.

On the basis of answers to the questions and additional statistical information, the states were selected for foundation assistance to community junior-college nursing programs. Funds were allocated for six major aspects of these programs:

1. Faculty preparation was necessary to assist universities through graduate education programs to prepare faculty for associate degree programs in nursing.

2. Continuing education was necessary for faculty members of community junior-colleges who were teaching in the associate degree programs.

3. Consultation was considered necessary for community colleges who had established or had indicated they wished to establish an associate degree program.

4. Demonstration centers were established to provide a pattern of effective curriculum development to be used as orientation experience for new faculty and for directors of associate degree nursing in community junior-colleges. Such centers served as laboratories for curriculum study and evaluation and for the preparation of instructional materials.

5. A preparatory planning year was instituted to enable the employment of nurse directors one year in advance of program initiation and clinical instructors at least four months in advance.

6. The evaluation of the associate degree programs and graduates provided for a systematic appraisal of the program activities as well as of the graduates in order to draw conclusions for the benefit of the profession of nursing, nursing services, and nursing education [32].

Case histories of the projects in the states were developed. These included descriptive information about the characteristics of the programs within each state and assessment of program activities and the progress being made. The activities included faculty preparation, curriculum planning and implementation, determination of characteristics of students, faculties, and resources available for programs, determination of faculty stability, evaluation of student personnel services, evaluation of student performance, admissions and graduations, employment and evaluation of associate degree graduates, and evaluation of associate degree program development.

The five-year project sponsored by the W. K. Kellogg Foundation revealed the outstanding strengths of the programs within the various states and identified some key problems that would have stood in the way of rapid development of associate degree programs. Evaluating the programs individually and as a whole highlighted the contributions such a project could make at the national and state levels. University faculties and state departments of education developed team relationships to encourage and assist in program development in the preparation of faculty for the programs. The collaboration of programs facilitated intervisitation and the sharing of materials and experiences. The junior colleges involved in the project gained a clearer understanding of their responsibilities in opening and conducting associate degree programs. Perhaps one of the major innovations in basic nursing curriculums was the concept of preparing the student for nursing in its generalized aspects. The focus of teaching was on the nursing problems of each patient in terms of the individual and in relation to his health problem.

The major problems that were identified included the high costs of the programs in relation to other types of technical programs. The content orientation of the curriculum, which was a radical departure from that suggested in the 1937 curriculum guide, puzzled state boards of nurse examiners. The variance between the educational goals and employer expectations presented employment problems. The problems of unprepared teachers appeared to be an obstacle in the ongoing development of the associate degree programs in nursing.

DEFINING THE CONTENT OF NURSING

In 1965 the American Nurses' Association published its first position paper on education, proposing a differentiation between two categories of nursing education and nursing practice using the terms *technical* and *professional* to name the categories. The position paper recommends that educational programs in nursing leading to an associate degree prepare graduates for technical nursing practice and that programs leading to a baccalaureate degree prepare graduates for professional nursing practice [33].

The concept of the team approach to nursing has legitimized the reality of the technical and professional nurse. The existence of these two types of workers is endorsed by the profession, and theoretical descriptions of their roles and activities have been formulated. The rapid development of junior college programs in nursing and the effort to utilize the professional and technical practitioners effectively have stimulated faculties to delineate more precisely the objectives and curricular requirements of professional and technical education for nursing.

The demand for nurses with highly specialized knowledge and skills has prompted the development of graduate programs in nursing preparing the clinical specialist. These curriculums provide clinical content in circumscribed areas of nursing in greater depth. The reception of the clinical specialist added a third member to the field of nursing practice.

Nursing practice has been described on a continuum along which different kinds of functions could be identified. Continuing effort is being exerted to identify the types of functions and activities of nursing that fall into the categories of technical and professional nursing. This is a major task for nursing, since the content of nursing within the various curriculums is dependent upon the delineation of the nature and scope of technical and professional practice. Some notions about technical practices have been offered that provide some guidelines for the selection of nursing content. Technical nursing is characterized by those accepted rules of action or principles of nursing practice that are common, recurring, controlled, and immediate. These nursing actions are likely to be standardized and validated through observations. Curriculums, to fulfill the goal of technical practice, must translate these general notions into more precise activities. It must deal with the questions, What are the common, recurring patient problems, and what are the well-controlled nursing actions? Nursing curriculums initially organized content around a medical diagnosis or geographical location of patients. Associate degree programs from their inception utilized a generalized concept of nursing as a frame of reference for curriculum content. One might ask, What are the elements which make up this generalized concept of nursing?

One study is reported that attempted to determine the differences in nursing practice between graduates of associate and baccalaureate degree programs. The study also endeavored to describe the actual differences in practice for the purpose of improving the utilization of nurses in service settings and of improving curriculums for both programs in nursing. Technical nurses were observed as performing routine activities of nursing, seeking supervision when in doubt, working more with the basic problems of patient care. Baccalaureate graduates dealt with problems that could be described as wider in scope, less common, and having more solutions that were often psychological in nature. The theoretical and empirical basis of technical and professional practice offered some directions for defining content in nursing [34].

Faculties of associate degree programs have used considerable initiative and creativity in attempting to resolve the problems of content orientation and selection. What is evolving frequently is a curriculum based on the concept of the continuum of health in relation to the growth and development of individuals and families. Content in nursing that is offered during the first year is defined as it pertains to the concept of health as a relative state on the health-illness continuum. Learning opportunities are oriented to maintaining normal physical and mental functions in patients of all age groups, including the newborn, young child, teen-ager, postpartum mother, middle-aged man, and elderly woman. The second year of the curriculum is focused on the relative state of illness. Skills learned are those aimed at the restoration toward wellness of those impaired functions related to the physical and mental processes, such as oxygen intake, elimination, nutrition, chemical and neural regulation, and trauma and stress. Learning opportunities are provided that include individuals of all age groups and at varying points on the health continuum.

Efforts of the organized profession, of regional groups, and of individual faculties have been directed toward identifying the major focus of nursing practice that would guide the development of the body of knowledge of nursing and the design of systematic programs of professional education. In the American Nurses' Association position paper, the profession accepted the major components of nursing practice as care, cure, and coordination. The Department of Baccalaureate and Higher Degree Programs of the National League for Nursing endorsed the position paper and further stated that the primary focus of nursing is care [35].

As these actions were being taken by the nursing organizations, nurse educators were calling for a redefinition of nursing. In a paper presented at the Conference of the Council of Member Agencies of the Department of Baccalaureate and Higher Degree Programs in 1966, Mary S. Tschudin stated:

The main difficulty that we face is the lack of agreement among our university schools as to the primary or the unique role of professional nursing, the implications or variations of this role in the nursing specialty areas, and the relationships with members of the other health professions and others within the organizational hierarchies that deliver nursing care services. The existence of such a central guiding statement delineating the professional nursing role and functions would greatly alleviate the problem that so often exists now when members of the faculty are pulled in various directions by the pressures and demands of particular specialty areas in nursing.

. . . . Were an adequate and acceptable statement defining professional nursing presently available to faculty members, the determination of subject matter content for the curriculum and the specification of the kinds of behavior to be developed through the educational program would be greatly simplified [36].

In the absence of research findings to guide decision-making, nurse practitioners and educators are faced with the problems of clarifying and differentiating the roles of technical and baccalaureate nurses and those of the clinical specialists, and defining the appropriate content in nursing for the educational programs preparing these practitioners.

The baccalaureate seminar of the Western Council on Higher Education recognized early the need for a study that would identify the nursing knowledge which should be imparted to all students in baccalaureate programs. Faculty of individual schools had attempted to identify basic concepts that constituted a core of nursing knowledge but found that it was impossible to devote the necessary time to such an undertaking while engaged in teaching. The seminar group developed a project to identify the content essential to baccalaureate preparation in nursing, which was accepted by the Western Council on Higher Education for Nursing and funded by the United States Public Health Service. The aim of the project was "to investigate the nursing content at the baccalaureate level to determine whether or not a new approach to the education of nurses at the baccalaureate level is possible through identification of a core of nursing knowledge [37]. Six schools of nursing in the West participated in the study. Throughout the project, the staff worked as a total group on most aspects of the study and in subgroups or as individuals to carry out specific assignments. The staff selected a conceptual framework that focused on the nursing needs of patients and the relationship of these needs to the patients' biophysical and psychosocial backgrounds. Data were collected on some 750 patients, which provided information on categories of nursing needs in relation to patient characteristics. The resulting statistical relationships were utilized in the development of inferences and statements of essential content. The parameters established for the study included the statement of philosophy of baccalaureate nursing education, the description of college-bound high school graduates, and the description of the graduate of a baccalaureate program in nursing. Although the study provided data for the development of guides for the identification of essential content, questions were raised in relation to the validity and reliability of the instruments used in the study.

As early as 1958 the graduate seminar of the Western Council on Higher Education for Nursing expressed the need for extensive study and research in the problems of nursing education at the graduate level. Faculty members of schools of nursing offering graduate education organized themselves into four groups for the purpose of clarifying and delineating the content in four clinical areas of nursing at the master's level. These areas were maternal-child health, psychiatric nursing, medical-surgical nursing, and public health nursing. Funds were obtained from the United States Public Health Service to initiate the project. The objectives of the study included the following: (1) to discover areas of content common to the four clinical nursing specialties, (2) to determine the basic science content of master's degree programs, (3) to identify what the nurse teacher and the nurse supervisor must know in order to improve nursing practice, and (4) to provide some uniformity of content in the master's programs in the West in order to facilitate complementary specialization [38, 39, 40, 41].

Each clinical group selected or developed a theoretical framework that seemed to be more appropriate for the study of clinical content in each area. Each of these projects enabled specialists in the area to work together to research basic science information that would provide a foundation for nursing content. The conceptual orientation of nursing selected by each group provided the structure for organizing the application of the sciences to nursing problems. The project enabled faculty members from the various schools to come to grips with the issues of defining content at the master's level and to delineate this content from that which might be included in baccalaureate nursing programs.

The Southern Regional Education Board sponsored a three-year project in teaching psychiatric nursing in baccalaureate programs. The project was funded by the National Institute of Mental Health and provided an opportunity for selected instructors from baccalaureate programs to study and describe the content of psychiatric nursing. A second aim of the project was to provide an opportunity for a group of psychiatric nursing teachers to continue their professional growth through individual and collaborated study. The major foci of the seminars were the selection and description of concepts of psychiatric nursing that would provide the framework for identifying content in nursing. The seminar work resulted in the description of selected psychiatric nursing concepts that the group members found useful in teaching baccalaureate students. These materials have been used by others in teaching psychiatric nursing and other clinical nursing courses. The group members recognized the many issues and problems involved in defining and describing concepts [42].

Faculties of many baccalaureate programs have given attention to selecting and utilizing various themes that provide structure for identifying content in nursing. Several of these activities were described in Chapter 10, Approaches to Identifying Content in Nursing. The results of any faculty or organizational endeavor facilitate the identification of nursing knowledge at a specific point in time. The dynamic nature of nursing will require a continuous search for the content of nursing as new roles and activities evolve.

INFLUENCE OF THE FEDERAL GOVERNMENT

The recognition of the vast needs for health services and the shortages of qualified health personnel awakened the interests of various groups and agencies in education for the health professions. New resources, both money and personnel, became accessible to schools from the federal government. Funds have been made available to study curriculum, to initiate new programs, to try new approaches to teaching, and to develop various forms of educational media. Many of the ideas for curriculum change came from outside the individual school and even outside the nursing profession. This strategy tended to give substantial attention and support to designing innovations and to preparing materials and equipment based on the experiences and research activities of business, industry, the military, and educational institutions.

The federal government has had a long history of giving support and direction to education, beginning at the time of the Civil War. Although education is the domain of the individual states, the federal government has intervened to make possible the creation and development of general and specialized programs that would provide the necessary resources for improved economic and social conditions.

During World War I, the federal government, through the Department of the Army, established the Army School of Nursing in several military hospitals in the United States. The purpose of this school was to provide a training program in nursing that would yield a supply of nurses who would contribute to the nursing services of the United States Army. After the critical need for nursing services of a nation at war terminated, the school was discontinued. Again during World War II, the Federal Cadet Nurse Corps provided funds to students in schools of nursing to increase the supply of nurses for civilian and military needs.

The passage of the Health Amendments Act of 1956 provided funds for graduate training of professional public health personnel. The intent of this legislation was to improve the health of the people by assisting in increasing the numbers of adequately trained professional and practical nurses and professional public health personnel. Amendments to the Public Health Service Act have extended the funding of graduate training and research in public health.

In 1961 the Vocational Education Act of 1946 was amended to provide funds for practical nurse training. Additional support for practical nurse training and for retraining of professional nurses was made available through the Manpower Development and Training Act of 1962.

The Public Health Services Act was amended again in 1969 to increase the opportunities for training professional nursing personnel. Related health legislation has provided support for programs in nursing education in the construction of facilities, purchase of equipment, faculty salaries, and traineeships for students. Special project grants have been made to schools of nursing for the improvement of nurse training. These grants have been awarded for projects designed by faculty in a variety of areas including curriculum revision, faculty development, instructional technology, program initiation, program evaluation, and remedial services to students. The special project grants authorized funds to schools of nursing, public or nonprofit private agencies, organizations, or institutions to help support the additional costs of projects for the planning, development, and establishment of programs of nursing education and to help meet the costs of improving, expanding, and strengthening the quality and effectiveness of programs of nurse training. A summary of funded projects is reported in the publication *Special Project Grants for the Improvement of Nurse Training* [43].

A demand for military support in this country and in various parts of the world increased the need for nursing services. In an effort to maintain adequate nursing service in the army hospitals, civilian nurses were recruited and employed, thus draining the supply of nurse practitioners for civilian agencies. In 1963 the Surgeon General of the United States Army proposed a cooperative arrangement with a university school of nursing to extend their baccalaureate program through the utilization of army facilities and resources. The University of Maryland accepted the invitation to participate in this arrangement and contractual agreements were negotiated. The United States Army provides the teaching and supportive personnel and the clinical facilities to the University of Maryland for the conduct of the baccalaureate program. The army pays full tuition and stipends to the students enrolled for the four-year period. The majority of the students enroll in other four-year colleges for the first two years of the program and transfer to the University of Maryland for the professional education. Students receive the bachelor of science degree from the University of Maryland and are obliged to serve in the Army Nurse Corps for three years. The Walter Reed Army Institute of Nursing was established to facilitate the ongoing activities of this cooperative enterprise.

The participation of the federal government in educational planning and change has been contingent upon the advice and direction of experts in various fields of endeavor. Periodic assessment of nursing and nursing education and future planning are the responsibility of nurses and related health workers. In the Spring of 1961, the Surgeon General of the United States Public Health Service appointed a consultant group on nursing to advise him on nursing needs and to identify the appropriate role of the federal government in assuring adequate nursing services for our nation. The consultant group studied the needs for nursing services from the standpoint of the health needs of the country and the changes in the practice of nursing. The changes in nursing education focused attention on the growth of baccalaureate and graduate programs as well as the rapid development of junior college programs. The consultant group concluded that, in spite of improvements in nursing supply and education, the profession is not keeping abreast of fast-changing health care needs [44].

Recommendations of the consultant group included allocation of financial aid from federal funds for recruitment programs, assistance to schools of nursing to expand and improve the quality of educational programs, assistance to professional nurses for advanced training, increased support for nursing research, and assistance to hospitals and health agencies to improve the utilization and training of nursing personnel. The consultant group also recommended that a study be made of the present system of nursing education in relation to the responsibilities and skill levels required for high quality patient care. Funds for such a study should be obtained from private and government sources [45]. The report of the Surgeon General's Consultant Group on Nursing furnished the profession and the federal government with a useful compilation of statistics regarding current nurse supply, preparation, and employment and established some realistic goals for the future.

The continued expansion of health services, in an effort to fulfill a commitment to the American people that health is a right rather than a privilege, has called for a review of the roles and activities of nurses in health care services. The belief that the nursing profession can and must occupy a larger and more effective place in the delivery of health services for the American people led to the appointment of the Secretary's Committee to Study the Extended

Roles for Nursing. Nurses, physicians, hospital administrators, and representatives of nursing and medical associations examined the potential for extending the contribution of nursing in the delivery of health care and the barriers that stand in the way of achieving this goal. The committee submitted to the Secretary of Health, Education, and Welfare a report that stated their recommendations. A basic problem seen by the committee was that many nurses were not practicing at their highest potential nor receiving training and experience that would enable them to extend the scope of their practice and thereby extend the availability of health service. The report delineated the elements of nursing practice in primary, acute, and long-term care and indicated those elements for which nurses now have primary responsibility, those elements for which responsibility is exercised either by physicians or nurses or by a member of the allied health professions, and those responsibilities that generally fall outside the practice of nurses who are not now utilized or prepared to practice in extended roles. The report further indicated that the delineation of the boundaries of the sphere and scope of nursing practice requires that nurses continue to examine the nature of nursing, the needs of society, and the part nurses play in the delivery of health services today and in the future. Once the profession has accepted a function as falling within the sphere of nursing, then each nurse who carries out that function must obtain the systematic instruction needed to acquire the necessary knowledge and skill to support her practice [46].

The recommendations of the secretary's committee will probably have considerable impact on curriculum activities on all levels of education as well as on continuing education for practicing nurses.

CAREER-LADDER CONCEPT

Labor organizations have made the observation that many hospital workers are employed in dead-end jobs. Most frequently these workers come from minority and economically deprived groups. Because of circumstances the hospital workers (aides, orderlies, attendants) received minimal education; however, their level of education was not always an indicator of their potential abilities. These people were often locked into a system that deprived them of advancement in their occupation. Low-paying hospital jobs prevented those who were economically depressed from obtaining the necessary education for career mobility. The enactment of federal legislation for practical nurse education and for manpower development and training offered an incentive and financial assistance to many disadvantaged workers, many of whom were already acquainted with the health fields through employment as aides, attendants, and assistants. Today more than half a million persons work in these capacities. Many administrators report that the disadvantaged, once productively employed, exhibit both the motivation and the intellectual capacity to assume far greater responsibility, responsibility that often requires additional education [47]. Although some administrators have capitalized on this discovery, many others have missed the opportunity to develop these talented individuals. With the recent move by labor organizations to adopt career ladders as a vital concept, there will be increasing pressure on health care facilities to look within their ranks to find likely candidates for professional training [48]. The executive director of one district council of the American Federation of State, County, and Municipal Employees, AFL-CIO, expressed the belief of the council in his statement:

. . . society now owes its members who have been denied entry into the system training opportunities and job opportunities so that they can put their potential to use. The difference between a black worker and the white worker in a more skilled job really boils down to the question of opportunity. We know this. When our union provides opportunity for the lower economic worker, he usually does magnificently well. This represents an entirely new trend, one in which the union wants to be a leader [49].

Nursing has endeavored to implement the concept of the career ladder through the recruitment of disadvantaged and minority groups into the profession. Frequently, talented workers who might otherwise qualify for advanced training have deficiencies in the basic skills of English, mathematics, and science. Several schools of nursing report the outcomes of specific programs that assist the students to remedy their deficiences so that they can be successful in the school of nursing [50, 51]. Whether the aide or orderly seeks entry into a vocational, technical, or professional program or the practical nurse seeks entry into a technical or professional program, the career-ladder concept implies that talented individuals be encouraged and assisted to obtain the necessary preparation for career mobility.

The development of baccalaureate programs in nursing and the demand for professional nurse services have prompted graduates of diploma programs to seek further education leading to the bachelor of science degree. Faculties of schools of nursing were initially reluctant to admit these students into the baccalaureate program because they were "different" from the other students. The registered-nurse student came with her major—nursing. Various plans were formulated to assist her to meet the requirements of the degree. In some instances the registered nurse was required to complete only the general education courses in the curriculum. In other plans the registered nurse was prepared for specialty areas of teaching or administration. Many programs for the registered nurse required little or no additional clinical training. Programs for the registered nurse varied widely, a fact which seemed to indicate that there was little agreement about the nature of professional education for the registered-nurse student at the baccalaureate level. There was considerable variation in the number of credits that were allocated for the diploma program, and the techniques for determining the credits to be allocated varied as widely as the number.

The situation seemed to indicate conflicting philosophies of baccalaureate education of the generic and registered-nurse students. At a meeting of the Department of Baccalaureate and Higher Degree Programs of the National League for Nursing, the issues and problems of registered-nurse education were discussed. It was the general consensus of the group that there should be a single program in nursing leading to the baccalaureate degree. Entry points into the program may differ for the student coming directly from high school and the registered-nurse student. The group agreed that, since nursing is the major, some upper division courses in nursing should be required of all students. Baccalaureate education in nursing prepares the general practitioner; therefore, preparation for specialized functions (teaching and administration) is not appropriate at this level [52].

Education of the registered-nurse students moved into the mainstream of baccalaureate programs, and schools of nursing applied the concepts enunciated by the National League for Nursing in different ways. Some baccalaureate programs required the registered nurse to complete all courses required in the curriculum; others attempted to assess the student's nursing background to "fit" her into the program where additional knowledge and skills were indicated. The career-ladder concept initiated by labor and the activities in general education to facilitate the student's journey through college caused faculties to take another look at the curricular requirements of the registered-nurse student. Testing programs in general education were providing students and faculties a wide range of tests that could be used to assess the student's knowledge in general education and the sciences. Satisfactory performance on these tests exempted a student from certain courses in the curriculum and enabled her to proceed at a more rapid pace. In addition, she did not become bored by repetitious instruction. Many of these tests were applicable to baccalaureate nursing education. The assessment of nursing knowledge was initially made by use of tests prepared by the National League for Nursing. More recently, however, schools of nursing have assumed the responsibility for test construction in the area of nursing. The challenge examinations and the evaluation of clinical practice have become the major tools for determining the point of entry into the baccalaureate curriculum. These procedures offer a means for determining a more rational and shorter passage for the registered nurse to fulfill the requirements of the undergraduate curriculum.

The rapid development of associate degree programs is making available an extensive resource for students in baccalaureate curriculums. Although these programs were initially viewed as terminal as opposed to a step toward professionalization, experience is demonstrating that many graduates of associate degree programs have the desire and ability to complete professional study at the baccalaureate level. College credits earned in general education in the junior college are frequently transferable to the collegiate program. In addition, the same procedures for assessing nursing knowledge of the diploma graduate are being used for the junior college graduate. Nurse educators have learned that students make career decisions for a variety of reasons. As circumstances change, so does choice of a career. Efforts should be exerted to assist practitioners to move from one type of nursing career to another as efficiently as possible and without undue expenditure of time and money.

Graduates of liberal arts colleges are being attracted to health occupations. These graduates have acquired considerable background in the liberal arts and very frequently have substantial preparation in the sciences. Liberal arts graduates offer another potential resource for baccalaureate programs in nursing, and attention must be directed to providing suitable entry for them into the curriculum. Entry should be made at a point that will enable the student to build upon her previous background and to acquire the necessary knowledge and skills for professional practice. The liberal arts graduate who completes the baccalaureate program in nursing has acquired essentially two majors. When the second major is in the natural or behavioral sciences, advancement through graduate study may be facilitated.

Several approaches for implementing the career-ladder concept in nursing curriculums are developing. The first approach is the generic baccalaureate program into which registered-nurse graduates of diploma or associate degree programs are admitted. Some of the major differences among baccalaureate programs in curriculum planning for these students include (1) the number or prerequisite courses in which the student must enroll or be exempted by examination, (2) the number of credits in nursing that may be earned by equivalency examinations, and (3) the extent to which progression through a program at the individual's own speed is encouraged, resulting in individually tailored programs. Some programs are increasing the number of both nursing and nonnursing electives and are offering the possibility of pursuing an interest in a specific clinical area. Faculties of schools of nursing who utilize this approach are committed to the belief that the structure and components of the generic baccalaureate curriculum offer the student a sound educational route to professional practice. Modification of curricular requirements can be readily made on the basis of individual needs and attainments. The goal of these programs is preparation for professional practice; the means for achieving the goal will vary in relation to the characteristics of the students enrolled.

The second approach for implementing the career-ladder concept is the program that offers several career goals and provides a curriculum that assists the student to attain these goals in a sequential manner. The curriculum provides for articulation between the associate and baccalaureate degrees. This program permits the student who satisfactorily completes the requirement of the first two years to earn an associate degree with a major in nursing. After the completion of the requirements of the first two years, the graduates are eligible to take the State Board Test Pool Examinations required for licensing as a registered nurse. Students who successfully complete the requirements of the third and fourth years receive the bachelor of science degree in nursing. Graduates from diploma and other associate degree programs may receive credit for lower-division courses in nursing and may transfer credits in general education studies. These students may continue their education on the upper-division level and may be admitted into the final two years of the program. Examinations testing cognitive nursing skills are used for placing students at the appropriate location within the curriculum.

A modification of this approach provides preparation for practical nursing during the first year. At the end of the second year, the student is granted the associate degree, and the baccalaureate degree is awarded at the completion of four years. Faculty members who subscribe to these program plans believe that there are common elements that permeate the various levels of preparation. From the point of view of teachers in the programs, the acquisition of technical knowledge and skills at the lower level of the program facilitates the attainment of professional knowledge and skills during the third and fourth years. The career-ladder models provide various points of entry and exit for students with different characteristics and goals.

There is not unanimity of opinion in relation to a particular approach to the career-ladder concept. The general idea that talented individuals be assisted to advance in the profession is probably acceptable to all; however, a specific route is not endorsed by all educators. This is probably a healthy situation because of the wide range of motivations, abilities, and goals of students entering various programs in nursing. One would not suggest that all entrants in nursing should begin the study of nursing at the technical level, that all graduates of technical programs should be encouraged and expected to enter professional programs, or that professional programs should be designed so that technical preparation is a prerequisite.

Career goals of many persons change with time. What a person sets as his goal at one stage of his life may be quite different from the one he sets at another. Cultural and economic changes, as well as varying rates of personal growth, modify the initial as well as later goals set by young people. As goals change, talented students should be encouraged to move upward on the career ladder. The system should be so ordered that what one learns at one stage has relevance and academic value at the next. Any other system is inefficient and wasteful.

SYSTEMS APPROACH TO CURRICULUM CHANGE

The application of general systems theory to the basic sciences, engineering, and the field of psychiatry has found the system model a useful conceptual framework. More recently, systems theory has been utilized to bring about changes in educational programs in a variety of settings. The failure of new programs to take root is the concern of administrators and teachers. Matthew B. Miles, in his book *Innovation in Education*, makes the observation that many experimental programs within a larger system fail because the change or innovation is perceived as creating too much disequilibrium in the system, thus preventing it from meeting its obligation in a well-ordered manner [53]. Any change in teacher-student relationship is likely to have repercussions on teacher-teacher interaction, on teacher-administration contacts, and on administration-board of trustees relationships. Any estimate of resistance that considers only the persons primarily and centrally concerned will be inadequate; repercussions elsewhere may be even more influential in the survival of the innovation. For this reason small-scale and fragmented changes may be doomed to failure before they are even launched. What is needed is a more comprehensive and coordinated approach to educational reform in which piecemeal efforts are linked together, with considerable time and attention given to the development of coordinate strategies for bringing about desired changes. Future innovations must be discussed not only in terms of what is to be changed but also in terms of how the change is to take place.

The notions underlying general systems theory originated in the biological and social sciences. The idea of society as a system of interrelated parts with a boundary, usually tending to maintain an equilibrium, was explicitly entertained by early and contemporary sociologists. There is at the base the concept of a system of elements in mutual interrelation that may be in a state of equilibrium, so that any moderate change in the elements or their interrelations away from the balanced position is counterbalanced by changes tending to restore it to its original state. The organic model of society was inspired by advances in biology. Many sociologists exploited the organismic analogy, searching out the social analogue of the heart, brain, and circulatory system. It is the general principle of "mutual dependence of parts" that makes society like an organism.

Talcott Parsons, in his functional analysis of social change, represents the social system as tending to maintain a relatively stable equilibrium by way of continuing processes that neutralize endogenous and exogenous sources of variability which would change the structure if proceeding too far [54]. Mature organisms, by the very nature of their organization, cannot change their given structure beyond very narrow limits and still remain viable. This capacity is what distinguishes sociocultural systems.

The term homeostasis was coined by Cannon for biological systems to avoid the static connotation of equilibrium and to bring out the dynamic, processing, potential-maintaining properties of basically unstable physiological systems. The constant conditions that are maintained in the body might be termed *equilibria*; however, this word has come to have a fairly exact meaning as applied to relatively simple physiochemical states and enclosed systems where known forces are balanced. The coordinated physiological processes that maintain most of the steady states in the organism are so complex and so peculiar to living beings that the term *homeostasis* is suggested as a special designation. This word does not imply something set and immobile. It means a condition that may vary but which is relatively constant [55].

In dealing with sociocultural systems, some new terminology is needed to express not only the structure-maintaining feature but also the structure-elaborating and -changing feature of the inherently unstable system. What is maintained or restored is not so much an internal state of the organism as some relation of the organism to its environment. This gives consideration to the adaptation and adjustment of the organism to the social environment and gives attention to the case in which the goal and/or norm is some state or relation that has never previously been experienced. On the sociocultural level there is no specific structure that is alone viable and normal for every society. Not only may structure change as a response to pressure on viability, but also the internal limits of structural compatibility may be great, though certainly with outer bounds [56].

The concept of system is described in relation to two models: the organismic or biological, and the mechanical or mathematical. Parsons has been deeply concerned with the concept of "order," and he and Shils use it to define the notion of "sytem":

> . . . the most general and fundamental property of a system is the interdependence of parts or variables. Interdependence consists in the existence of determinate relationships among the parts or variables as contrasted with randomness of variability. In other words, interdependence is order in the relationship among the components which enter into a system [57].

Parsons indicated further that the order must have a tendency to self-maintenance which is very generally expressed in the concept of equilibrium. There is the tendency of the social system to maintain equilibrium within certain boundaries relative to an environment, a property held to be similar to the biological concept of homeostasis. It is a fundamental assumption of Parsons that the maintenance of an established state of a social system is nonproblematic, that the tendency to maintain the interactive process is the first law of social process.

Some reactions to Parsons' functional model indicate that a social system does not have any such fixed, normal structure that if changed beyond narrow limits, leads necessarily to the system's death. In contrast to an organismic system, social systems are characterized primarily by their propensity to change their structure during their culturally continuous lifetime. Although there are limits within which the features of a social system structure may vary and still remain compatible enough for system maintenance, these limits, in comparison to an organismic system, may be relatively broad.

Other sociologists have interpreted social systems and the concept of equilibrium from a mechanical point of view. Homans rejects the biological-structure-function model [58]. For Homans the system is consistently defined in terms of the determinate, reciprocal interrelationships of all its parts, regardless of the particular structure in which these interrelationships are manifested. Deviance, stresses, and strains are integral parts of the system. A social system is a configuration of dynamic forces. Sometimes the configuration is in balance and a steady state is maintained; sometimes it is out of balance and continuing change occurs.

Homans' model of a system considers both processes of growth or elaboration of structures and processes of disorganization or disintegration of structure. He distinguishes in the total system two analytically separable systems, the external and the internal, and relates them in terms of the concept of feedback. The internal system refers to the relations among sentiments, activities, interactions, and norms viewed as responses by members to the necessity of surviving in an environment. The internal system refers to the elaboration of these elements and their relations that simultaneously arise out of the external system and feed back to it and to the system as a whole [59]. The system that Homans is describing is an open system in interaction with an environment. His recognition of this is shown in his distinction between the internal and the external system. To elucidate these notions, Homans states:

. . . Assuming that there is established between the members of a group any set of relations satisfying the condition that the group survives for a time in its particular environment, physical and social, we can show that on the foundation of these relations the group will develop new ones, that the latter will modify or even create the relations we assumed at the beginning, and that, finally, the behavior of the group, besides being determined by the environment, will itself change the environment [60].

That a system is open means not simply that it engages in interchange with the environment but that this interchange is an essential factor underlying the system's viability, its reproductive ability or continuity, and its ability to change. The response of natural, closed systems to an intrusion of environmental events is a loss of organization or a change in the direction of dissolution of the system. The typical response of open systems to environmental intrusions is elaboration or change of their structure to a higher or more complex level.

The idea of a general systems theory was first introduced by von Bertalanfly after World War II [61]. The events following the war provided a fertile climate for some of his generalizations. Some of these developments included cybernetics, information theory, game theory, decision theory, topology, and the application of the concepts of systems to concrete phenomena (general systems theory). Although systems theory in the broad sense has the character of a basic science, it has its correlate in applied science. The following fields of application can be identified:

Systems engineering, which deals with the scientific planning, design, evaluation and construction of man-machine systems.

Operations research, which is concerned with the scientific control of existing systems of men, machine, material, and money.

Human engineering, which is the scientific adaptation of systems and especially machines in order to obtain maximum efficiency with minimum costs in money and other expenses [62].

Although there is considerable overlapping, different conceptual tools are predominant in the individual fields. In systems engineering, cybernetics and information theory are used. Operations research uses tools such as linear programming and game theory. Human engineering concerned with the abilities, physiological limitations, and variabilities of human beings includes biomechanics, engineering psychology, and human factors among its tools.

Education may be considered as a special dimension of human engineering. In applying a systems approach to education, the first task involves the specific definition of what outcomes or results are desired. It is against these specifications that the system, the educational program, is to be built. The next step is to analyze the many variables that will contribute to the performance of the system. The means and strategies that can be employed to produce the desired outcomes must be identified. This involves the study of relative costs and feasibility of means and the predictability of the results.

Carter presents a series of procedures and methods that should be followed in utilizing the systems approach to curriculum change [63]. For this purpose system is defined as a bounded collection of interdependent parts devoted to accomplishment of some goal or goals and maintained in a steady state of feedback from the environment. A system is characterized as (1) organized and orderly, (2) comprised of objects, elements or components, relationships among components, and relationships between components and the whole, (3) functioning as a whole by virtue of interdependence of its parts, (4) synthesized in an environment to accomplish progress to a goal, and (5) possessed of structure, function, and development. In the application of general systems theory to curriculum, an analysis of the system involves eight steps.

1. State the need of the curriculum. The need for the curriculum is viewed

in relation to the health and nursing resources of the community. Attention is also given to whether a particular type of curriculum is needed in a specific community in light of existing programs in nursing. Description of the specific contributions of the graduates to the health and welfare of the community further elucidates the need for the particular type of curriculum.

2. Define educational objectives. The next point in systems analysis is to carefully define the objectives that will contribute to satisfying that need for which the curriculum is planned. The behaviors that the students are expected to acquire as a result of the program of instruction are specified. The goals or objectives for the program must be stated in terms of output specifications. These objectives must be directly related to and consistent with the functions and activities of the type of practitioner the program attempts to prepare.

3. Define constraints. The third major procedural point is to define the constraints within which the curriculum is developed. Constraints in this instance refers to the amount of money that can be spent, the amount of time involved in developing the program, the availability of skilled staff, and the adequacy of clinical facilities and equipment.

4. Identify and analyze alternates. The next major point calls for the identification and analysis of alternative systems that might serve the curriculum requirements. Since it is acknowledged that an objective can be attained in more than one way, several alternative procedures can be developed, subjected to evaluation, and revised. Since many curriculum patterns that have evolved give an indication of a historical perspective, decisions must be made concerning the appropriateness of utilizing this approach or of designing alternatives that present differing curriculum orientations.

5. Select the best alternative. The next point in systems analysis is to select the best of the several alternatives. The best alternative should be selected from the standpoint of which one contributes to more effective teaching and learning. The alternative selected must be realistic in terms of the constraints that have been identified. A particular approach might be deemed the best alternative, but if sufficient funding is not available, obviously this approach will not be the best at this time.

6. Implement for testing. The next step is to implement the selected alternative for testing. This calls for careful planning of the implementation of the procedures developed. This may call for the monitoring of teachers as they try to implement teaching procedures and other instructional activities. It may also require the observation of teacher-community relationships and

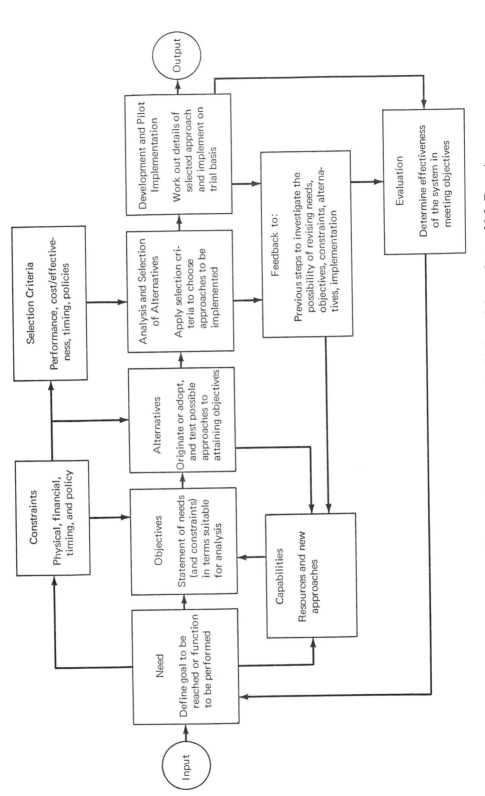

DIAGRAM 16.   Strategy for curriculum change: The systems approach. (Adapted from Carter [63]. P. 23.)

identification of administrative problems that occur during the implementation.

7. Evaluate the system. The next major step calls for the evaluation of the system developed. Careful planning for evaluation of the new procedures is implied. The evaluation activities must be planned at the very beginning of the program and are carried out as the system is installed. This may require the development of new techniques for evaluation or the modification of those already prepared.

8. Provide feedback and modification. Finally, the systems analysis procedure calls for feedback on the performance of the system and modification of the training as a result of the feedback. As the program continues, all personnel will feed back information on the program. There will be a continued modification and perfection of the system as long as it is in existence. Diagram 16 presents a schematic plan of the steps in systems analysis as it pertains to curriculum change.

Use of systems techniques means that the decision-maker will know how and when to use these techniques and will be cognizant of the factors suggesting need for change in nursing education. The forces of change that create need for change in nursing education can be summarized as (1) social and economic conditions, (2) information explosion, (3) student unrest and dissatisfaction, (4) technological change, and (5) federal aid to education. All of these forces have created changes in nursing, and the quality change is of the essence. Continued change using careful planning and evaluation is in order. Planned intervention must be implemented to optimize organization, functioning, and evaluation of nursing education programs. Knowing how and when to use system techniques can go a long way toward realizing the kind of planned intervention that is needed. Elaboration of this point can be made by (1) defining a rationale for use of systems techniques in nursing education, (2) examining concepts and principles of general systems theory as applied to nursing education programs, and (3) describing systems techniques for decision-makers concerned with programs of nursing education.

Setting up and operating nursing programs in institutions of higher education are functions of management systems. Management encompasses planning, organizing, motivating, and controlling human and material resources and relationships among resources to attain predetermined goals. Those implementing decision-making roles in programs of nursing education are concerned with optimizing outcomes. They are responsible for identifying and organizing goals and objectives, planning courses of instruction to accomplish objectives, organizing and employing resources, and evaluating results. Professionalism cannot be attained in nursing-education programs that continue to treat selection of students, design of course work, clerical practice, and use of resources as unrelated elements rather than articulated segments of a unified system. As educational systems become larger and more complex, a knowledge of the parts taken separately no longer suffices. With complex systems a knowledge of interconnections of components in the system becomes more important than knowledge of the components alone. It is incumbent upon decision-makers to achieve organized integration and orderly interrelationships in the management of these systems. General systems theory gives a framework for making such an approach, and systems techniques provide tools for implementing viable management decisions.

GUIDELINES FOR DEVELOPING STRATEGIES

Teachers and other curriculum workers who are planning curriculum change will draw upon many areas of knowledge. Not only do they deal with the knowledge and the processes of the particular disciplines underlying subject areas in the school program, but they also deal with other components of the curriculum that the learner encounters in the school, namely, the features of the school system that characterize the schools as social systems, with economic and political factors, curricular planning processes, human relations, and communication systems. Educators, psychologists, sociologists, and subject matter specialists are working together in some areas of education in an attempt to examine and to develop strategies for introducing curriculum innovations. Innovation in curriculum must be considered from the standpoint of the student in the learning environment and with reference to the school as a social system that affects the introduction of planned curriculum change. Some guidelines for developing strategies for curriculum change are suggested from these reference points.

THE STUDENT IN THE LEARNING ENVIRONMENT

Curriculum is defined as those opportunities planned for the learner within the school environment to facilitate the attainment of predetermined objectives. Teachers plan and offer these opportunities to the student. As the student takes advantage of the opportunities, she has experiences that are unique to her. Since each student brings to the classroom a different background for experiencing different opportunities, different reactions to opportunities, and different abilities, the student's experience cannot be planned. As the student deals with the opportunities that are planned for her, she encounters various events. The areas of events are essentially the components of the curriculum and include (1) content, (2) teaching strategy, (3) verbal and nonverbal behavior of the teacher, (4) the learning environment, (5) instructional materials (6) organization of time, space, and personnel, and (7) evaluation. Decisions must be made concerning each of these areas in planning and developing the curriculum by those planning strategies for introducing planned curricular innovation.

When one considers each component, it is necessary to be acquainted with current research pertaining to a particular component for the purpose of designing curriculum. Even though each component is an entity, it must also be viewed as a part of the whole. It is directly related to other parts of the curriculum.

Guideline. Teachers responsible for introducing a change in the curriculum must plan for each of the previously enumerated components. If there is to be quality in the opportunities developed with students, teachers must be knowledgeable about and have expertise in working within each area of the curriculum.

CONTENT

The information explosion, which has exerted great influence in all areas and levels of education since World War II, has brought about a rethinking of the implications of what kind of knowlege should be transmitted. Scholars of various disciplines underlying subject matter areas have expressed the need for students to understand and be able to work with the concepts of a discipline. These educators emphasize the importance of students having understandings within various disciplines in order to examine the problems of man or society, since no one can possibly cover all available knowledge or keep up with developing knowledge.

Value decisions must be made relative to sources from which the content will be derived and through which methods of a discipline will be taught. Curriculum planners in nursing must make decisions in relation to the learning opportunities that are available but which have not been traditional in nursing curriculums. Development of basic concepts of health and nursing may occur by means of learning opportunities offered by some evolving health and treatment programs in the community. Another value question involves change as a central concept in our culture. Man places high value on experimentation and invention in technology. Some areas of social change have seen notable advancement; however, other areas have been slow to change. Although the medical profession has considerable knowledge about the scientific and humane care of the aged, its programs and facilities are lagging. The health care system needs persons who have the psychological, technological, and professional freedom to change. The public needs nurses with the ability to design social and technological change within their sphere of responsibility and nurses who have the ability to create orderly processes for change. The content of opportunities encountered by learners must make provision for meeting this goal.

Attention has been given to the ordering and sequencing of content and skill development for learners. Curriculum writers frequently refer to the need for organizing the content of the curriculum. Nurse educators have learned more recently that what is logical ordering of content and skill development to the teacher often has not been a logical ordering for the student. Curriculum writers have frequently been slow to reevaluate the ordering of curriculum opportunities in relation to the changing characteristics of students. Many of the nursing students today are far more sophisticated in understanding their world than was true a few years ago. Useful information for curriculum planners is available from projects initiated by universities and secondary schools, where consideration is being given to structures and organization for teaching within individual disciplines. This question is causing schools to identify questions, problems, and themes to be explored and then to consider these matters from the structure and content of the various disciplines. Another aspect of the organization question concerns the depth and frequency of exploration of ideas. Continuous assessment of the learner's encounters in the classroom must be made in this approach to assure increasing depth and breadth rather than mere repetition of ideas.

Guideline. Teachers must deal with two basic questions of curriculum development: What shall be the ordering and sequencing of content for the learners? How shall the organization of content be placed within a framework that gives attention to current educational ideas and research?

STRATEGIES FOR TEACHING

If the content of the curriculum centers attention on the concepts or framework of the discipline by which students may develop the understandings necessary for examining problems within this framework, teaching methods or strategies are required that are different from those used when the goal of instruction is to "cover" the subject. Researchers are studying the various aspects of teaching strategies that relate to individual styles of learning, modes of inquiry, and motivation for learning.

Guideline. Teaching strategies must be designed to achieve the goals of teaching. Encounters with content of the discipline by way of concepts, ideas, or problems require new teaching strategies. Teachers planning procedures for introducing these innovations must give attention to inservice training of teachers in these strategies. Teaching materials must be developed to implement the new approaches to teaching.

VERBAL BEHAVIOR OF THE TEACHER

The teacher's use of language in the classroom seems to influence the cognitive performance of students. Some curriculum authorities believe that the most marked single influence on cognition performance is teaching strategy. Language behavior is an area within education in which much research is being done. The findings thus far are discouraging in that (1) the majority of questions raised in classrooms with learners require mere regurgitation of facts, (2) questions seeking exploration of ideas, for analysis, for generalization to be formed are infrequent, (3) many directives are given, (4) many interesting inquiries of students are turned aside, and (5) the major portion of time is spent in "teacher talk."

The student encounters in varying degrees of sophistication the vocabulary of a discipline. She may have a teacher whose understandings of a particular discipline and its language system is very limited. This situation may limit the student's opportunities to conceptualize the nature of the discipline. Conversely, a teacher who understands the language of a framework of concepts and possesses the ability to use language in developing cognitive processes will provide extensive opportunities in encounters with the student.

Guideline. The teacher's use of language in classroom and clinical settings is a crucial determinant of the quality of opportunities developed with the learner. When developing strategies for planned curriculum change, teachers must be assisted in examining and restructuring their verbal and nonverbal behaviors to achieve certain goals. The use of tape-recorded and videotaped class sessions provide opportunities for teacher self-analysis of language behavior. Ongoing inservice programs in schools may also be useful in the reeducation of the teacher in this dimension of teaching.

LEARNING ENVIRONMENT

A desirable learning environment is provided when all students know they are understood and valued by their teachers and peers and can find ways of contributing to group enterprise. Order is present in the classes, but not rigidity. The environment is characterized by an arrangement of furniture that facilitates class discussion and self-discipline in the movement of students, in the development of ideas, in the use of time and space, and in interpersonal relations.

Guideline. Teachers who are developing strategies for planned curriculum innovations must anticipate the kinds of problems they may encounter in developing a supportive environment for learning in the classroom. Attention must be given to developing strategies that will assist teachers in creating such an environment in relation to the problems of today's classrooms.

INSTRUCTIONAL MATERIAL

The increased interest in instructional materials has brought students into contact with a wide variety of materials. Individual schools are creating adaptations of instructional materials produced by others or in some instances are developing their own materials. Instructional materials can extend the horizons of the learner through a variety of stimulating experiences. Instructional materials may present a complicated new language with which the student is unfamiliar but which she is expected to comprehend and use. Media for instruction may make an exciting contribution to learning or may result in boredom, depending upon the quality and appropriateness of materials for the particular group of learners. In addition to the concern for the literacy of the viewer, the quality of presentation and the viewing environment are necessary considerations for the selection of instructional materials.

Guideline. Instructional materials must be designed for the learners in terms of the goal of the planned curriculum change. The effective use of these materials contributes to the quality of the student encounter in relation to a specific learning opportunity. Teachers may need assistance in the development and use of some of the newer instructional materials. When the purpose of the curriculum change is to stimulate independent learning, it may be necessary to aid students in selecting their own materials.

ORGANIZATION OF TIME, SPACE, AND PERSONNEL

The utilization of programmed instruction and other self-instructional procedures for individualized instruction frees some of the teacher's time, which can then be devoted to other types of teaching activities. The use of a variety of teaching techniques that engage individuals and small groups of students requires appropriate time, space, and personnel. Curriculum innovations that suggest the use of these procedures must take into consideration the need for these resources.

Guideline. Teachers planning curriculum change must give attention to the requirements for and appropriate organization of time, space, and personnel so that students may realize maximum goals for learning.

EVALUATION

As curriculum innovations are designed, a concomitant activity of teachers is the construction of appropriate evaluation procedures and devices. The changes may indicate the need for assessing short-term as well as long-range goals in relation to the growth of the student. The evaluation devices that are constructed must be designed to measure the specific student behavior that is inherent in the innovation.

Guideline. When teachers introduce planned curriculum change, they must give attention to the evaluation of the student that will assess both short-term and long-range progress of the student. Teachers should be provided with in-service opportunities to assist them in developing new evaluation procedures to measure the growth of the student in relation to the curriculum change.

THE SCHOOL AS A SOCIAL SYSTEM

The different strategies that have been employed in changing curriculums in nursing suggest some different procedures and processes. The extent to which plans are made by individual schools to utilize and implement these processes may relate to the successful outcomes of the curriculum innovation. When all aspects of school functioning are considered in terms of the change, it is likely that curriculum modifications will be expedited. A school may be viewed as a social system that has certain characteristics in common with other systems. The identification and discription of these characteristics provide guidelines for developing strategies for curriculum change.

GOAL CONGRUENCY

Curriculum changes that are introduced into a school must be compatible with the goals of the school. This requires that curriculum goals be made visible and that they be understood and accepted by members of the school staff. Continuous orientation to and discussion of the goals of the curriculum may be necessary as new members enter the school system. Innovations are possible today in relation to new learning opportunities, but these should be congruent with the statement of goals of a specific course and the curriculum as a whole. Goals must be continuously reviewed in terms of changing student characteristics, changing health and nursing needs, and changing instructional approaches and technologies.

Guideline. If effective strategies for introducing curriculum change are to be developed, the school must make provision for examining the proposed innovation in terms of the goals of the system.

RESOURCES

Designing a strategy for introducing a change in the curriculum requires those in a specific instructional area to work closely with members of related divisions in developing proposals for such items as materials, personnel, facilities, inservice training for staff, travel, and materials for evaluation. If the innovation is to become institutionalized, necessary resources must be specified and made available to the instructional staff.

Guideline. Reexamining these goals in light of changing social, economic, and professional characteristics and requirements should become a continuous process. Planning for long-term budget needs and other instructional resources must be made if the innovation is to become institutionalized.

ADEQUACY OF COMMUNICATION

If an innovation in curriculum is to be considered and effected, provisions must be made within the school system for adequate communication among all persons concerned with the innovation. Processes must be regularized so that communication of ideas may be transmitted from any position in the system. Provisions must be made for interdepartment or interschool communication. Adequacy of communication is promoted when staff are informed of intramural and extramural activities related to the innovation. This suggests the reporting and discussing of the initiation and progress of related experimental or pilot projects. Channels of communication for receiving and transmitting ideas must be open to all groups and individuals within the system. Provisions must also be made for analysis of ideas and for appropriate feedback through the same channels of communication.

Communication concerned with planning instructional activities, personnel, inservice education, facilities, and budget is necessary if curriculum changes are to be effective. When all ramifications of an innovation are explored by the various groups within the school systems, decisions on priorities can be formulated.

Guideline. The school that is considering the introduction of a curriculum change into the system must have open, regularized, and honored channels of communicating with all members of the staff.

POWER EQUALIZATION

Distribution of power within an organization is necessary if it is to operate effectively. In school situations, where power is controlled by top administration, efforts to initiate curriculum innovations are hampered. The chief administrator is reluctant to delegate power and thus becomes preoccupied by many administrative details. When lines of authority and responsibility are clearly defined in an equitable manner and made visible to everyone in the school, the system can operate more efficiently and effectively. Wide involvement in the formulation and initiation of a curriculum change contributes to the acceptance and support of the change by all members of the staff.

Guideline. The distribution of power within the hierarchy of the school and within the various subgroups is essential if action is to be taken in studying and introducing a change into the curriculum.

UTILIZATION OF RESOURCES

When curriculum changes are being planned and implemented, the talents and time of all school personnel should be used wisely. The development of curriculum innovations by teachers and others requires much individual and cooperative work of a professional nature. Teachers can become burdened with clerical and academic housekeeping chores, which consume much of their time and effort. Faculty become concerned that they can fulfill neither their expectations for themselves nor the expectations they feel administrators have for them when they are not utilizing their talents in curriculum endeavors. Faculty members who have some expertise in highly specialized areas, such as testing and evaluation, should be utilized as resource persons to faculty members who do not have comparable degrees of competence.

Guideline. If innovations in curriculum are to be initiated and installed, the school must give attention to the appropriate utilization of the staff. Determination of staff utilization must be made in relation to (1) performance of nonprofessional duties, (2) availability of sufficient supportive personnel for clerical activities, (3) utilization of the special talents of teachers, and (4) provision of adequate time for curriculum study to generate new ideas and insights.

MORALE

High-level morale of the staff of the school is necessary if curriculum changes are to be effected. It is likely that morale will be high if all of the previously mentioned aspects of system characteristics are considered to be important in the operation of the system. High morale also develops when there is mutual belief in the dignity and worth of each individual, and this belief is demonstrated in the leadership behavior.

Guideline. High morale among the staff is necessary if the school is to initiate and institutionalize a curriculum change. The composite of characteristics of a viable system should be examined when the morale of staff is being assessed. High morale among those planning curriculum change is necessary, and any situation that deters morale development should be identified and modified.

Nursing education in this country is in an era of innovation and reform. For these innovations to be studied, initiated, and institutionalized, some guidelines for developing strategies of change seem to be needed. The guidelines suggest that the school staff examine the learning environment where the student encounters the learning opportunities planned by the teacher and examine the school as a social system that will effect and be affected by the innovations in the curriculum. The development of innovations requires a competent professional staff, an environment conducive to change, and appropriate procedures and processes to insure systematic and orderly change.

SUMMARY

It appears that many schools are engaged in considerable curriculum activity in an effort to bring about innovations and reform. The changes that are occurring in nursing curriculum exhibit marked variations in the focus and rapidity of change. The processes of curriculum change require teachers to make decisions about the nature of the change to be made and the strategies to be used for insuring that the change does occur in an efficient and effective manner. Strategies for curriculum change must also give attention to the consequences of changes in curriculum and must incorporate plans and procedures for evaluating the consequences as a part of the change process.

Strategies for curriculum change may be considered from two approaches: (1) the pragmatic approach to change, which endeavors to resolve some educational problem through the implementation of ideas and suggestions of authoritative individuals and groups, and (2) the strategy of directed change in which a plan of action is designed by an expert and subjected to field testing before implementation. Nursing has relied primarily on the pragmatic approach to guide curriculum change.

The establishment and development of nursing education in this country during the first half of the twentieth century was accomplished by utilizing a number of different strategies for change that were pragmatic in nature. Seven strategies are identified that seem to reflect the status and problems of two evolving professions, nursing and education. These strategies include strategy of reform, standard setting, organizational efforts, activity analysis, establishment of new goals, group dynamics, and subject reorganization. It is noted that among these strategies for change a common characteristic is the use of forces outside the school to design and direct curriculum change.

The strategies for curriculum change which have been employed more recently suggest a trend toward greater faculty responsibility and involvement in curriculum activity. Again, most of the strategies that have been developed may be considered to be practical approaches to curriculum problems. Major studies conducted on a national level identified the problems within nursing and nursing education and made recommendations for curriculum changes. One strategy utilized research methods and procedures in the design and field testing of an entirely new nursing curriculum. While reports of surveys and commissions provide substantial data and information, major strategies for curriculum change are being designed and utilized by faculties of individual schools or of several schools within a geographical region. These strategies imply that teachers must become knowledgeable about the nature of the suggested change and the dimensions of the change process.

It is apparent that teachers in all types of nursing curriculums will be involved in designing new or redesigning established curriculums. The primary motive underlying these endeavors should be the provision of educational opportunities and an appropriate environment for learning to the student. Guidelines for the development of strategies for curriculum change should take into consideration the student in the learning environment and the school as a social system that effects the introduction of planned curriculum change. The development of guidelines in relation to the student in the learning environment should give attention to the various encounters that the student has as she utilizes the opportunities planned for her. The areas of encounter that the student experiences include (1) content of curriculum, (2) teaching strategy, (3) verbal and nonverbal behavior of the teacher, (4) the learning environment, (5) instructional material, (6) organization of time, space and personnel, and (7) evaluation. These encounters are essentially the components of the curriculum.

The guideline for developing strategies for change must also give attention to all aspects of school functioning. The general characteristics of the school as a social system identify the areas of concern for the guidelines. These characteristics include (1) goal congruency, (2) resources, (3) adequacy of communication, (4) power equalization, (5) utilization of resources, and (6) morale. The development and use of guidelines that direct attention to the characteristic of a school as a social system and to the various encounters that the student has in the learning environment by a competent, professional staff will insure systematic and orderly changes in the curriculum.

REFERENCES

1. Miles, M. B. [Ed.]. *Innovation in Education.* New York: Teachers College Press (Columbia University), 1964. P. 18.
2. Ibid., p. 14.
3. Stewart, I. M. *The Education of Nurses.* New York: Macmillan, 1949. P. 87.
4. Roberts, M. M. *American Nursing: History and Interpretation.* New York: Macmillan, 1954. P. 106. Copyright, 1954, by the Macmillan Company.
5. Committee on Education, National League of Nursing Education. *Standard Curriculum for Schools of Nursing.* New York: National League of Nursing Education, 1919. P. 5.
6. Ibid.
7. Goldmark, J. *Nursing and Nursing Education in the United States, Report of the Committee for the Study of Nursing Education.* New York: Macmillan, 1923.
8. Roberts, op. cit., p. 184.
9. Committee on the Grading of Schools of Nursing. *Nursing Schools Today and Tomorrow.* New York: Committee on the Grading of Schools of Nursing, 1934.
10. Ibid., p. 282.
11. Committee on Curriculum, National League of Nursing Education. *A Curriculum Guide for Schools of Nursing.* New York: National League of Nursing Education, 1937.
12. Roberts, op. cit., p. 283.
13. Johns, E., and Pfefferkorn, B. *An Activity Analysis of Nursing.* New York: Committee on the Grading of Nursing Schools, 1934.
14. Ibid., p. 40.

15. Ibid., p. 45.
16. Committee on Educational Policies and Resources, Nursing Council on National Defense. Nursing schools and national defense. *Amer. J. Nurs.* 42: 182, 1942.
17. Department of Services to Schools, National League of Nursing Education. *Nursing Organization Curriculum Conference, Curriculum Bulletin, No. 1.* New York: National League of Nursing Education, 1950.
18. Department of Services to Schools, National League of Nursing Education. *Joint Nursing Curriculum Conference, Bulletin, No. 2.* New York: National League of Nursing Education, 1951.
19. Elliott, F. *Viewpoints on Curriculum Development.* New York: National League for Nursing, 1957.
20. American Medical Association Committee on Nursing Problems. Report of the Committee on Nursing Problems. *J.A.M.A.* 137:878, 1948.
21. Committee on the Function of Nursing. *A Program for the Nursing Profession.* New York: Macmillan, 1948.
22. Brown, E. L. *Nursing for the Future.* New York: Russell Sage Foundation, 1948.
23. West, M., and Hawkins, C. *Nursing Schols at the Mid-Century.* New York: National Committee for the Improvement of Nursing Services, 1950.
24. Committee on Standards, National League of Nursing Education. *Essentials of a Good School of Nursing.* New York: National League of Nursing Education, 1942.
25. Committee on Curriculum, National League of Nursing Education. *A Curriculum Guide for Schools of Nursing.* New York: National League of Nursing Education, 1937.
26. Bridgman, M. *Collegiate Education for Nursing.* New York: Russell Sage Foundation, 1953.
27. Surgeon General's Consultant Group on Nursing. *Toward Quality in Nursing.* Washington, D.C.: U.S. Department of Health, Education, and Welfare, Public Health Service, 1963. P. 55.
28. National Commission for the Study of Nursing and Nursing Education. *An Abstract for Action.* New York: McGraw-Hill, 1970. P. 156.
29. Wiles, K. Contrasts in Strategies of Change. In R. R. Leeper [Ed.], *Strategy for Curriculum Change.* Washington, D.C.: Association for Supervision and Curriculum Development, National Education Association, 1965. P. 6.
30. Montag, M. L. *Community College Education for Nursing.* New York: McGraw-Hill, 1959. P. 3.
31. Ibid., p. 9.
32. Anderson, B. E. *Nursing Education in Community Junior Colleges.* Philadelphia: Lippincott, 1966. P. 16.
33. American Nurses' Association Committee on Education. *A Position Paper.* New York: The American Nurses' Association, 1965. P. 6.
34. Waters, V., et al. Differences in Nursing Practice Between Graduates of Associate Degree and Baccalaureate Degree Programs. In *Associate Degree Education—Current Issues*, 1970. New York: National League for Nursing, 1970. P. 18.
35. Department of Baccalaureate and Higher Degree Programs, National League for Nursing. Statement of Position on the Primary Focus of Nursing. In *The*

Shifting Scene—Directions for Practice. New York: National League for Nursing, 1967. P. 3.

36. Tschudin, M. S.   The Re-definition of Nursing: A Critical Need. In *The Shifting Scene—Foundations for Strength.* New York: National League for Nursing, 1967. P. 7.

37. Coe, C.   *One Approach to the Identification of Essential Content in Baccalaureate Programs in Nursing.* Boulder: Western Interstate Commission for Higher Education, 1967.

38. Lewis, L., et al.   *Defining Clinical Content, Graduate Nursing Programs—Medical-Surgical Nursing.* Boulder: Western Interstate Commission for Higher Education, 1967.

39. Fujiki, S., et al.   *Defining Clinical Content, Graduate Nursing Programs—Psychiatric Nursing.* Boulder: Western Interstate Commission for Higher Education, 1967.

40. Ford, L. C., et al.   *Defining Clinical Content, Graduate Nursing Programs—Community Health Nursing.* Boulder: Western Interstate Commission for Higher Education, 1967.

41. Highley, B. L.   *Defining Clinical Content, Graduate Nursing Programs—Maternal–Child Health Nursing.* Boulder: Western Interstate Commission for Higher Education, 1967.

42. Zderad, L. T., and Belcher, H. C.   *Developing Behavioral Concepts in Nursing.* Atlanta: Southern Regional Education Board, 1968.

43. Division of Nursing, Bureau of Health Manpower Education.   *Special Project Grants Awarded for Improvement in Nurse Training.* Washington, D.C.: U.S. Department of Health, Education and Welfare, 1971.

44. Surgeon General's Consultant Group on Nursing.   *Toward Quality in Nursing.* Washington, D.C.: U.S. Department of Health, Education, and Welfare, 1963. P. 5.

45. Ibid., p. 55.

46. Secretary's Committee to Study Extended Roles for Nurses.   *Extending the Scope of Nursing Practice.* Washington, D.C.: U.S. Department of Health, Education, and Welfare, 1971.

47. Gotbaum, V.   Influence of the labor movement in hospital affairs. *Hospitals, Journal of the American Medical Association* 44:23, 1970. With permission.

48. Ibid., p. 72.

49. Ibid., p. 74.

50. Fever, H. D.   Operation salvage. *Nurs. Outlook* 15:54, 1967.

51. Mannion, S. E.   Upgrading L.P.N.'s to R.N.'s *J Pract. Nurs.* 19:31, 1969.

52. Department of Baccalaureate and Higher Degree Programs, National League for Nursing.   *Baccalaureate Education for the Registered Nurse Student.* New York: National League for Nursing, 1966.

53. Miles, op. cit., p. 437.

54. Parsons, T.   Some considerations on the theory of social change. *Rural Sociol.* 26:219, 1961.

55. Cannon, W. B.   *The Wisdom of the Body.* Rev. Ed. New York: Norton, 1939. P. 20.

56. Buckley, W.   *Sociology and Modern Systems Theory.* Englewood Cliffs: Prentice-Hall, 1967. P. 14.

57. Parsons, T., and Shils, E. A. [Eds.].   *Toward a General Theory of Action.* Cambridge: Harvard University Press, 1951. P. 107.

58. Homans, G. C. *The Human Group*. New York: Harcourt, Brace & World, 1950.
59. Buckley, op. cit., p. 31.
60. Homans, op. cit., p. 91.
61. von Bertalanfly, L. *General Systems Theory*. New York: George Brazeller, 1968.
62. Ibid., p. 92.
63. Carter, L. F. The systems approach to education: mystique and reality. *Educ. Techn.* 9:22, 1969.

SUPPLEMENTARY READINGS

Anderson, D., et al. *Strategies of Curriculum Development*. Columbus, Merrill, 1965.

Bullough, B., and Bullough, V. A career ladder in nursing: Problems and prospects. *Amer. J. Nurs.* 71:1938, 1971.

Carnegie Commission on Higher Education. *Open Door Colleges*. New York: McGraw-Hill, 1970.

Eiss, A. F. A systems approach to developing scientific literacy. *Educ. Techn.* 10:36, 1970.

Elliott, F. Regional conferences on curriculum in 1957. *Nurs. Outlook* 6:173, 1958.

Gagné, R. M. [Ed.]. *Psychological Principles in System Development*. New York: Holt, Rinehart & Winston, 1962.

Gray, W., Duhl, F. J., and Rizzo, N. D. *General Systems Theory and Psychiatry*. Boston: Little, Brown, 1969.

Harms, M. *Development of a Conceptual Framework for a Nursing Curriculum*. Atlanta: Southern Regional Education Board, 1969.

Ingles, T. Debate—ladder concept in nursing education—pro. *Nurs. Outlook* 19: 726, 1971.

Jarrett, V. The Open Curriculum. In *Challenges to Nursing Education—Preparation of the Nurse for Future Roles*. New York: National League for Nursing, 1971.

Johnson, D. E. Competence in practice: Technical and professional. *Nurs. Outlook* 14:30, 1966.

Johnson, D. E. Professional Practice in Nursing. In *The Shifting Scene—Directions for Practice*. New York: National League for Nursing, 1967.

Lawler, M. *Strategies for Planned Curriculum Innovation*. New York: Teachers College Press (Columbia University), 1971.

Leeper, R. R. [Ed.]. *Strategy for Curriculum Change*. Washington, D.C.: Association for Supervision and Curriculum Development, National Education Association, 1965.

Leeper, R. R. [Ed.]. *Curriculum Change: Direction and Process*. Washington, D.C.: Association for Supervision and Curriculum Development, National Education Association, 1966.

Matheny, R. Technical Nursing Practice. In *The Shifting Scene—Directions for Practice*. New York: National League for Nursing, 1967.

McKean, I.   Faculty work conferences improved our curriculum. *Amer. J. Nurs.* 52:1254, 1952.

Montag, M.   *The Education of Nursing Technicians.* New York: Putnam, 1951.

Parsons, T.   *The Social System.* New York: Free Press of Glencoe, 1951.

Ramphal, M.   Needed: A career ladder. *Amer. J. Nurs.* 68:1234, 1968.

Silogyi, D. V., and Blanzy, J. J.   The systems approach in the community college. *Educ. Techn.* 12:46, 1972.

Tschudin, M. S., and Morgan, T. M.   A faculty grows through curriculum study. *Nurs. Outlook* 1:198, 1953.

Tuckman, B. W., and Edwards, K. J.   A systems model for instructional design and management. *Educ. Techn.* 11:21, 1971.

17 ROLES AND PROCESSES IN CURRICULUM CHANGE

CURRICULUM change is a complex process involving a network of human relationships. It is concerned with creating, maintaining, and improving the conditions for learning, and it requires the knowledge and expertise of teachers, students, and administrators in a variety of activities and processes. Efforts to change the curriculum mean that the direction of change has been identified and that there is some general agreement about the nature of the change to be adopted. It means that teachers, students, and administrators are ready and willing to discard certain familiar practices to try innovations. A climate favorable to change must be created at all levels at which decisions are made: classroom, school or department, college or university, and the governing board. The development of a supportive climate at the first two levels is primarily the responsibility of teachers, students, and school or departmental administrators. A school cannot change its curriculum, however, unless those occupying top positions in the hierarchy of the administrative structure of the college or university deliberately and overtly set about to build a climate for educational change. The resources for designing and implementing curriculum change are available and abundant. If, however, the goals and motivation to translate new knowledge into new professional practices, the skills to combine talents and efforts into group endeavors to realize those goals, and the insight and imagination to use the resources and opportunities creatively are lacking, the changes which are to be adopted are likely to be ineffective. Curriculum change implies the deliberate use of the organizational processes of authority, leadership, group dynamics, and decision-making. Educational change requires the identification of the roles various participants assume in the process and the development of contributory relationships among those involved in curriculum endeavors. The phenomenon of resistance to change is forever present in all aspects of curriculum development and must be dealt with, giving attention to individuals, groups, and the innovation under consideration.

ORGANIZATIONAL PROCESSES IN CURRICULUM CHANGE

The efforts of any organization to achieve its goals requires some form of structure and certain processes to insure efficient and effective operation. Whether it is big business, a small private enterprise, or a faculty organized for curriculum development, the organizational processes of authority, leadership, group dynamics, and decision-making are inherent in their structure and activities. Although these are considered to be useful in contributing to the goals of the group, conflicts may arise which produce obstacles. Brief exploration of these processes is made in relation to the concerns of curriculum change.

AUTHORITY

The nature of society gives sanction to the fact that some individuals should be in a position to exercise influence over others. It is necessary, however, that there should be a differentiation between those modes of influence that are held permissible or desirable and those that should be discouraged or even forbidden. Where such modes are institutionally legitimatized, they may be called authority. Parsons defines authority as an institutionally recognized right to influence the actions of others, regardless of their immediate personal attitudes to the direction of influence [1]. Authority is an aspect of power in a system of social interaction; it is institutionalized power over others. It is a mechanism of social control, and as such it can be said that every member of a social system has some authority.

Organizational influence upon the individual may be interpreted not as a determination by the organization of the decisions of the individual but as the determination for him of some of the premises upon which his decisions are based. Where the individual decides upon a particular course of action, some of the premises upon which this decision is based may have been imposed upon him by the exercise of the organization's authority over him. Of all of the modes of influence, authority is the one that distinguishes the behavior of individuals as participants of organizations from their behavior outside such organizations. It is authority that gives an organization its formal structure. Authority gives one person the power to make decisions that guide the actions of another. Simon describes the relationship between two individuals, one superior, the other subordinate. The superior frames and transmits decisions with the expectation that they will be accepted by the subordinate. The subordinate expects such decisions, and his conduct is determined by them. He holds in abeyance his own faculties for choosing between alternatives [2]. The willingness of the subordinate to accept a command does not imply that all or even most of his behavior choices are governed by commands. Authority refers to those situations where suggestions are accepted without any critical review or consideration. The process of authority provides that a subordinate accept a command in the absence of a choice of his own. A subordinate may also accept a command that is in opposition to a choice of his own. When there is disagreement between two persons, and when the disagreement is not resolved by discussion, persuasion, or other means of conviction, it must then be decided by the authority of one or the other participant.

The exercise of authority in a group makes possible a separation of the decision-making process from actual performance or what might be called specialization in decision-making [3]. Specialization in decision-making is possible without the use of authority. A unit of the group may be given a purely advisory status in the organization. Through its recommendations it may actually make decisions that are accepted elsewhere in the organization. If the recommendations of the unit are accepted without reexamination on their merits, the unit is really exercising authority. Such may be the case with the curriculum committee of the school of nursing. Authority functions to enforce the conformity of individuals to the norms laid down by the group or by its authority-wielding members. The core of most social institutions consists of a system of authority and a set of sanctions for enforcing it. An important function of authority is to secure decisions that are not only rational but also highly effective. To obtain expertise in decision-making, the responsibility for decisions should be allocated in such a way that decisions requiring particular knowledge or skill will rest with individuals possessing that knowledge or skill.

It may be necessary to go beyond the formal structure of authority to obtain the kinds of specialized assistance that are often needed for a single decision. Authority also functions to centralize the process of deciding so that a general plan of operation will govern the activities of all members of the organization. Procedural coordination establishes the lines of authority and outlines the sphere of activity and authority of each member of the organization.

Authority exercised in educational organizations is based on superior knowledge and technical competence in a particular element in the division of labor. The administrator has the technical training and the competence to allocate and integrate the roles, personnel, and facilities required for attaining the goals of the system. *Administrative authority* consists of certain permissions or rights: the right to act for the organization in specified areas, the right as spokesman for the organization to request that other staff members perform activities of various kinds, and the right to impose sanctions and discipline if a subordinate disregards his instructions. These rights are vested in the head of an enterprise by law and custom, and they are supported by the moral approval of society. Because of this background, employees and in fact our whole society accept the idea that the head of an enterprise has certain rights of authority and that he may reassign these rights. The rights that an administrator may transfer are more akin to authorization than they are to power. Effective delegation requires that the limits of authority be made clear to each subordinate. Written job descriptions, policies, and procedures should give some indication of the authority of each member of an organization. A subordinate gets into trouble when the limits of authority are so vague that he either goes far beyond his appropriate sphere of action or fails to exercise the initiative he should.

Legal authority is principally a matter of the relationship of outsiders to an enterprise. An organization always has a number of people who can represent it to the outside world, to other institutions and agencies. These agents can make contracts and otherwise act as legal representatives of the organization. Effecting contractual relationships with health agencies for clinical practice of students is a function of legal authority vested in representatives of the school of nursing. Although authority is an essential element in any modern enterprise, it does not confer unlimited power. In addition to inherent limitations on the authority that an administrator can delegate, virtually every organization imposes limitations of its own. An administrator is permitted to act "within company policy" and "in accordance with established procedures."

Basic to all that is occurring today within society at large is a questioning of traditional patterns of authority, a search for new methods of governance, and an insistence that all constituencies be adequately represented and that decision-making not be oblivious to their needs. The inclusion of students and faculty in the decision-making process at almost all points has become commonplace within the last few years. This represents a shift from a fundamentally hierarchical pattern of authority to one striving to be collegial and to include all parties in the affairs that regulate their lives. The debate about the best procedures of insuring order and equity is by no means resolved. For some, no valid alternative exists except participatory democracy. To others, such a procedure would result only in chaos. The central task is to create workable patterns of communal governance that vary with circumstances, that remain sufficiently fluid, that build in accountability as the prime safeguard to rights and freedom, and that enable persons from each constituent group to meet regularly to discuss alternatives. Within the realm of curriculum there exists the dilemma of being sufficiently responsive to the expressed needs and interests of students, as individuals or as a group, without being irresponsible to the experience of history and a large community of learning.

Individual autonomy cannot exist without some measure of collective support. Professors have customarily banded together within their respective disciplines to agree on curriculum matters. With few exceptions this has resulted in rigidly prescribed courses of study, with questions of methods and goals of instruction usually being ignored. Individually and collectively staff members have been successful in maintaining a high degree of control over curriculum and instruction. The staff also exercises control over its own selection and promotion practice but has measurably less influence on deciding economic rewards.

The university as an organization is unique in its decision-making process. It depends upon two types of authority or decision-making structures: the *bureaucratic* structure and the *collegial* structure. In the bureaucratic authority structure, decision-making power is based on ranking in a hierarchy, with the person at the top having the final say. It usually has as its ends efficiency and growth, defined either monetarily or in terms of members. The administration is usually associated with this authority and is concerned with decisions involving services to faculty or students, basic resource allocations, and general policy direction. The collegial authority structure is based on the logic of educational expertise, peer management, and career or discipline relevance. Since this logic is less quantifiable, measures of quality or success are more subject to ideological and personal bias and to the bias of tradition.

The concerns of this authority, usually operating in faculty units, include the processing of students through the institution, knowledge generation and dissemination, general educational, and institutional prestige.

The two types of authority structures employ different styles of decision-making. The bureaucratic authority uses delegation as well as implicit and explicit compliance with superiors. Collegial decision-making uses majority vote and consensus. Majority vote is common in departments or colleges, as in faculty senate or faculty meetings. Consensus generally operates in committee settings and in some departments. Consensus decision-making operates on the assumption that members have shared interests, values, and experiences, that open communication occurs, and that the members are essentially peers.

The extent to which either of these two models predominates within any one university is dependent on that university's history and emphasis. In the bureaucratic model, students do not have a formal position in the decision-making hierarchy. In a study by Gross, more than fifteen thousand faculty members and administrators were asked, Who makes the decisions on the major goals of the university? [4]. Students were ranked slightly above citizens of the state and slightly below alumni and large private donors in decision-making. Students are excluded from the collegial authority structures, since by definition they are neither experts nor equals of the faculty. It is assumed that they do not share the communality of interest required for consensus decision-making. The professional faculty are assumed to know what is best for the students and to act in the students' best interest. The effect of this system on student participation can be examined from the standpoints of discipline and educational expertise. Discipline expertise implies advanced knowledge in a particular field of study. To the extent that this expertise is assumed necessary for certain decisions (course content or quality of research), the current requirement of advanced preparation in the field makes student participation impossible. Educational expertise determines the educational process: what should be required, how courses should be taught, and the grading procedure. It is an assumed ability of faculty members that is due to their being on the staff of the university rather than to any special educational training they might have had. As long as educational expertise is defined in these terms, there is no way students can be equal to faculty.

The exclusion of students from both the bureaucratic and the collegial decision-making structures seems to belie the repeated exhortations to students to "work through the system." On the basis of structural considerations, students are not members of the system they are asked to work through.

LEADERSHIP

Leadership may be defined as the initiation of a new structure or procedure for accomplishing an organization's goals and objectives or for changing an organization's goals and objectives. Leadership is an influence process, the dynamics of which are a function of (1) the personal characteristics of the leader, (2) the personal characteristics of his followers, and (3) the nature of the specific situation in which the influence efforts take place. Leadership may be further defined as efforts on the part of one person (the leader) directed at influencing the behavior, attitudes, or values of another person or persons (followers) toward specified goals in a given situation. Any attempt on the part of one person to influence others is considered to be leader behavior whether or not the effort is successful. The leader's influence efforts may be directed either toward or against changing the behavior of others. This definition of leadership encompasses leader efforts directed toward influencing both the behavior of another individual and that of a group of followers.

A person does not become a leader by virtue of some combination of traits, but the pattern of the personal characteristics of the leader must bear some relationship to the characteristics, activities, and goals of the followers. The consistent failure to find a generalized personality syndrome typical of leaders in any or all leadership settings may be due to many factors. Gibbs suggests some possibilities that may account for the difficulty: inadequate measurement, lack of comparable data from different kinds of research, and the inability to describe leadership adequately [5].

Increasingly, the focus must be upon the relationship of the individual to the organization. A major source of conflict derives from discrepancies between the basic personality structure of an individual and the demands of his organizational role. Care must be exercised when one endeavors to generalize leadership characteristics from situation to situation and from one leadership role to another.

Extensive comparisons among groups designed to distinguish the major dimensions by which groups differ and thus to measure the impact of the leader have been made by Hemphill [6]. He found two dimensions, viscidity (the feeling of cohesion in the group) and hedonic tone (the degree of satisfaction of group members), to correlate more highly with leadership adequacy than did other dimensions. More recent studies reported by Hemphill identified two other dimensions of leadership: initiating structure and consideration [7]. Initiating structure relates to the behavior of the leader in establishing relationships between himself and the members of his work group and in establishing well-defined patterns of organization, channels of communication, and methods of procedure. Consideration means leader behavior that is indicative of friendship, mutual trust, and warmth in the relationship between the leader and members of his group. Some studies of leadership behavior revealed that effective leaders were those who scored high on both dimensions.

Other studies emphasize the fact that working with people in groups is a complicated undertaking and that there are many differences among groups which are of critical importance to the leader. A major source of conflict for the leader of an organization is the situation in which he frequently finds himself attempting to fulfill simultaneously the expectations of two or more reference groups that may be contradictory in nature. Persons in leadership positions are subjected to markedly different sets of leadership expectations, and the leader's behavior varies according to whether he is with superiors or subordinates. Just as conflict in expectations for the role of the leader may occur among reference groups, so conflicts may occur within a reference group.

An individual may help satisfy many different needs by assuming the role of a leader. The financial rewards given to those holding positions of considerable influence are generally greater than those realized by persons exerting relatively little influence in their work. Some individuals may also derive feelings of security simply by being in positions in which they have the power to control the behavior of others. Assumption of a position of leadership may also put the individual in a better position to satisfy both his belongingness and his esteem needs. Individuals holding positions of influence in organizations and groups usually attain higher status than those who do not, that is, the degree of prestige that an individual enjoys as a member of a group. Finally, assuming the role of a leader may provide the individual with an opportunity to help meet his self-actualization needs. Many leadership positions call on the individual to direct and coordinate the efforts of others toward the solution of complex and difficult decision problems.

The leader has certain powers to provide, withhold, or take away need satisfaction that he may utilize to ensure influence acceptance. An individual may be able to influence others because he is in a position to *reward* them if they accede to his influence efforts. The rewards that the leader has at his disposal may represent either an increase in positive need satisfaction or a reduction in need dissatisfaction. The potential ability of the individual to influence others because he is in a position to reprimand or punish them if they do not follow his wishes is a function of the *coercive* power of the leader. The professor may influence his students to attend class by virtue of his power to lower their grade if they do not do so. One accedes to the influence efforts of another person because he is attracted to him, wishes to identify with him, and wants to be like him. Such identification enables the individual to incorporate psychologically the strength of another in himself. A person may identify with groups of people as well as with an individual and that identification may provide a basis for being influenced by the values, standards, and modes of conduct considered desirable by the group. This form of leader influence is known as *referrent* power.

Expert power refers to the potential ability of one person to influence others because of his superior knowledge or understanding of a particular situation, for example, the student's acceptance of her teacher's recommendation to utilize certain references for the preparation of a term paper. The range of expert power is narrow. One tends to be influenced by another person because he is an expert within his area of expertise. The expert power of a person may be reduced if he attempts to exercise it in an area in which he is not truly knowledgeable. An individual may permit himself to be influenced by others because he believes that it is the right thing to do. A person's conscience or his own internalized value system tells him that another person has the right to influence his behavior, and that he has an obligation to accept that influence. *Legitimate* power is based on the belief that other individuals holding certain positions have the right to influence behavior. Most leaders probably derive their power from all five of the sources to varying degrees. Some leaders may rely more heavily on one source of power in some situations and on another source in others. Those in leadership positions may feel that some of their subordinates recognize their expertise and identify with them, whereas others are somewhat hostile toward them and at times can be induced to accept their influence efforts only through coercion.

Leadership process focuses attention on the degree of direction exercised by the leader in his relation with his followers. Individuals holding positions of leadership in organizations and groups differ widely as to the degree to which they attempt to direct and control the behavior of those in subordinate positions. At one end of the continuum is the pattern of leadership that is referred to as *authoritarian* leadership. The authoritarian leader makes decisions and gives directions often without consulting with his subordinates. He supervises his people closely, checks on their behavior frequently, spells out in detail how they should perform their work, and gives them little latitude in making decisions on their own. At the other end of the continuum is a type of behavior that is called *laissez-faire* leadership. The laissez-faire leader rarely sets or helps set objectives for his work group and gives his followers little or no direction. He allows them almost complete freedom to do what they wish to do. The behavior of most leaders falls somewhere in the middle of the continuum. The middle range is often referred to as *democratic* leadership. This leader sets objectives, makes decisions, gives directions, and does not give his subordinates extreme latitude in their behavior. The democratic leader does not attempt to control his subordinates closely or insist on spelling out in detail the way that they should behave. He encourages his followers to help set objectives and make decisions, gives them considerable freedom to act on their own within certain prescribed limits, and encourages their creativity and development. This leader treats his followers more as equals than does the authoritarian leader. He invites criticisms of his own ideas and welcomes the suggestions of others when they are appropriate.

Any leader, although he generally exhibits behavior that may be described as authoritarian, democratic, or laissez-faire, will vary in the degree of directiveness that he exerts from time to time. Probably the most effective leader is one who is flexible in his behavior and adjusts his influence strategies appropriately to meet the requirements of different situations. Supporters of democratic leadership have pointed out that where followers are permitted to participate in making decisions for their group or organization, they will tend to gain a greater understanding of the work in which they are involved and give greater support for the programs developed and decisions made. Some observers of modern business organizations have questioned the efficacy of the democratic pattern. Unlike the democratic and the authoritarian approaches, the laissez-faire pattern of leadership has few supporters. Most people have some needs for dependence and at times want to rely on and receive direction from a leader figure. A complete or almost complete lack of direction usually leads to a highly ambiguous and unstructured situation for the followers, tends to frustrate their dependence needs, and is likely to result in chaos and confusion and hostility toward the leader. The key question for leadership analysis is not which approach is generally most effective but rather under what specific conditions do the varying degrees of directiveness seem most appropriate.

Leadership effectiveness is a difficult process to assess. Since leadership involves a series of steps, time is required to assess the extent to which an attempted leadership act is successful or effective. The failure to attempt leadership could result in inadequate structures, ineffective procedures, and archaic goals. On the other hand, repeatedly attempting leadership would make it difficult to assess the effectiveness of any given leadership act. Frequent, continuous changes in an organization's structures, procedures, and goals can result in disorganization, disintegration, and disorientation. The assessment of leadership effectiveness entails the assessment of the objectives of the leader and the means utilized to achieve the objectives. To assess the leader's objectives, one must first appraise the values upon which they are based. Whether a particular leader's objectives are judged to be appropriate depends on one's own value system and to the extent to which one uses his values in appraising the behavior of others. One point of issue is that a leader is effective as long as his efforts are successful in inducing influence behavior that leads to the attainment of his objectives regardless of the values from which they are derived. The leader's own values are accepted as appropriate even though his subordinates may not agree with them as long as the values do not grossly conflict with the subordinate's. The question may be raised as to how congruent a leader's objectives are with those of the institution. A leader may successfully influence his subordinates to direct their efforts toward his own personal objectives; yet such influence behavior may be incongruent with the goals of the college or university. The question may also be asked, to what extent the leader's influence efforts are congruent with the needs and objectives of those he is attempting to influence. Does the leader have a moral obligation to refrain from exerting influence on teachers which, if accepted, would be detrimental to their interests? Answers to questions such as these depend upon one's own value system and the extent to which one uses his own values in appraising the behavior of others.

The assessment of the means to achieve the objectives requires the determination of the contribution of the follower's behavior in relationship to these objectives. Is the behavior of the follower going to contribute to the leader's attainment of his objectives, assuming they are appropriate? If not, the leadership must be considered ineffective, even though the leader is successful in inducing the influence to behave as he desires. For example, the leader of a curriculum committee may influence the members to adopt a course that has questionable contribution to the curriculum only because a particular faculty member has some expertise in the subject matter of the course. Finally, the evaluation of leader effectiveness reflects the extent to which the leader is actually able to gain acceptance of his influence efforts, assuming that they are appropriately directed toward the attainment of valid objectives.

GROUP DYNAMICS

The nature and characteristics of groups and group processes have been the subject of considerable study. Most of the social sciences and a number of the applied disciplines are vitally involved in small-group research at the present time. A number of social psychologists are working in the field utilizing a psychological as well as a sociological emphasis. Clinical psychology is using methods of group therapy in the treatment of the mentally ill. A number of workers among different disciplines who study the roles of family members may be considered to be students of small groups. There is lively interest among educational psychologists in studying the dynamics of classroom and instructional groups. Another interest stems from problems of administration in all sorts of settings: educational, recreational, religious, governmental, industrial, and military. The study of small groups may perform a service in clarifying how certain common concepts in social science, such as status, role, function, motivation, and culture patterns, are really only useful abstractions of the same concrete events, that is, the behavior of individuals in interaction with each other.

The small group is defined by Berelson and Steiner as:

. . . an aggregate of people, from two up to an unspecified but not too large number, who associate together in face-to-face relations over an extended period of time, who differentiate themselves in some regard from others around them, who are mutually aware of their membership in the group, and whose personal relations are taken as an end in itself. It is impossible to specify a strict upper limit on the size of the informal group, except for the limitation imposed by the requirement that all the members be able to engage in direct personal relations at one time—which means, roughly, an upper limit of around fifteen to twenty. If the aggregate gets much larger than that, it begins to lose some of the quality of a small group [8].

The various types of groups that have been studied include (1) the autonomous group, such as a circle of friends built on free choice and voluntary association, (2) the institutional group, such as the family, (3) the small group within a large organization, often called a mediating group because of its linking position between the individual and the organization, and (4) the problem-solving group, such as a committee with a task to perform [9]. Some pertinent research findings are organized and presented in relation to three areas: (1) how groups are formed, (2) how they influence their individual members, and (3) how groups operate internally.

FORMATION OF GROUPS

When people associate with one another under conditions of equality, they come to share values and norms and they come to like one another. There is a tendency for people to gravitate into groups or subgroups, which has the effect of maximizing their shared values. When an individual is caught in cross-pressures, between the norms of different groups of which he is simultaneously a member, he will probably suffer emotional strain and will move to reduce or eliminate it by resolving the conflict in the direction of the strongest of his group ties. When a great number of new members join an established group within a given period of time, the group will probably resist their assimilation. New members of a group are likely to feel inferior to established members and tend to conform to established relations. The less change there is in a group's membership, the higher the group's morale will be. When an individual is eager to become a member of a group, he will readily conform to its norms of behavior.

Related groups tend to become similar in their norms and values when there is considerable interaction between the groups. The less communication or interaction there is between them, the greater the tendency for conflict to arise between them. The less contact there is among members of different groups, the less there will be mutually recognized, proper behavior for their relations. If such contact sharply increases, there will tend to be increased tension until the proper behavior is defined and established.

INFLUENCE OF GROUPS

The small group strongly influences the behavior of its members by setting and/or enforcing standards for the proper behavior of its members, including standards for a variety of situations not directly involved in the activities of the group itself. The more stable and cohesive the group is and the more attached the members are to it, the more influential it is in setting standards for their behavior. The deviant members of the group are more likely to change their behavior to meet the standards of the model members of the group than are the model members to conform to the deviant behavior. The less certain the group is about the right standards, the less control it can exercise over its members. When the standards external to the group are not clear and definite, the group can exercise more control over itself. When neither an objective nor a group basis of judgment exists, judgments tend to be unstable, and as a consequence there is an increase in interaction within the group in order to reduce ambiguity. A single individual tends not to hold out against the weight of an otherwise unanimous group judgment, even on matters in which the group is clearly in error.

When activities are imposed upon a group from the outside, the norms that the group sets are likely to be limited in character. If the activities are determined from within the group, the norms take on the character of ideal goals to be constantly enlarged and pursued. People within a group tend to agree with the opinions of people they like, and they tend to think that the people they like agree with them and that those they dislike do not. The small group strongly influences the behavior of its members by providing them with support, reinforcement, security, encouragement, protection, and rationale for their "proper" behavior and by punishing them for deviations through the use of ridicule, dislike, shame, and threat of expulsion. The response of the group to deviation from its norms for behavior is (1) discussion and persuasion to bring the dissenting minority into line, (2) disapproval of the dissenters, (3) lowered ranking for the dissenters, and (4) their expulsion or forced resignation from the group. Small groups tend toward uniformity in attitudes and actions and in values and behavioral norms.

INTERNAL OPERATIONS OF GROUPS

In most groups, there is a rough ranking of members, implicit or explicit, depending on the extent to which the members represent or realize the norms and values of the group. The more the members realize the norms, the higher they rank. The closer an individual conforms to the accepted norms of the group, the better liked he will be; the less he conforms, the more disliked he will be. To the extent that the group's objectives are vague, undirected toward any special interest, and purely "social," the ranking of the members will be based on such personal characteristics as amiability, good nature, charm and, in general, "personality." If the group's norms are poorly defined, the ranking of the members will be less clear or definite. Conformity to the group's norms for behavior is related to prestige and security within the group in the following way: the highest ranked and most secure members feel most free to express their disagreement with the group, both privately and in public; the lowest ranked members are more likely to disagree privately but conform in public; and the average members are most likely to agree both privately and in public. The higher the rank of the member within the group, the more central he will be in the group's interaction and the more influential he will be.

The leadership of the group tends to be vested in the member who most closely conforms to the standards of the group on the matter in question or who has the most information and skill related to the activities of the group. When groups have well-established norms, it is extremely difficult for a new leader, however capable, to shift the group's activities. Leaders of small groups tend to direct the group's activities along lines in which they themselves are proficient and away from those areas where they are less competent. The longer the life of the leadership, the less open and free the communication within the group, and probably the less efficient the group in the solution of new problems. The leader of the group will be followed more faithfully if he makes it possible for the members to achieve their private goals along with the group's goals. Democratic leadership appears to be more effective with respect to the durability of the group, the members' satisfaction with it, their independence vis-à-vis the leader, and their productivity on the task.

The amount of interaction among members of a small group varies in relation to the cohesiveness of the group. Interaction decreases as internal dissension rises in a group of high emotional attachment. Interaction increases in small groups of little emotional attachment when the members perceive that there is disagreement within the group on a particular subject. There is an altercation within groups between communications dealing directly with the task and communications dealing with emotional or social relations among members. The former tends to create tensions within the group, and the latter tends to reduce them and achieve harmony. Groups composed of individuals who are compatible in that they all prefer close, intimate relations are more productive than groups in which some individuals are "personal" and some are "counterpersonal." Individuals will also be more effective when playing a role that is similar to their personality type. The most efficient groups are those in which the rules are appropriate for the task, although in general, cooperation results in more individual motivation, division of labor, effective intermember communication, friendliness, and group productivity. When group members expect to cooperate, any behavior that reflects individual, "self-oriented" needs tends to disrupt the group. Proximity in the communication network tends to increase intermember attraction. If there is no opportunity for feedback between members who are close to each other, hostility may appear, and efficiency in problem-solving declines.

Both the effectiveness of the group and the satisfaction of its members are increased when the members see their personal goals being advanced by the group's goals. The more compatible the members are in norms, skills, personality, and status, and the more the procedures of the group are accepted and understood, the more effective and satisfying is the performance of the group in its task. Active discussion by a small group to determine goals, to choose methods of work, to reshape operations, or to solve other problems is more effective in changing group practice than is separate instruction of the individual members, external requests, or the imposition of new practices by superior authority. The discussion by the group regarding goals and procedures is more effective in that it brings about motivation and support for the change and better implementation and productivity of the new practice. The most productive groups are those that can carry out efficiently the major steps in the process of solving tasks and social-emotional problems for the group and for the individual members. To accomplish this, a group must have a combination of members' personalities and skills, group structure, and group problem-solving experiences that are appropriate to the task.

DECISION-MAKING

Decision-making involves more than the simple choice among well-defined alternative solutions to a well-defined problem. It covers several stages, from the discovery and definition of problems and the search for alternatives among which to choose, through commitment, to the implementation of the choice and the evaluation of results. Simon identifies and describes five stages of the decision-making process:

1. The agenda-building phase (intellectual activity) covers the time administrators spend defining goals and tasks and assigning priorities for their completion.

2. The search phase (design activity) encompasses efforts to find or invent alternative courses of action and to find information that can be used to evaluate them.

3. The commitment phase (choice activity) involves testing proposed alternatives to choose one for adoption or to postpone making the choice.

4. The implementation phase includes clarifying the meaning of a commitment for those who are to help carry it out, elaborating the new tasks, and motivating people to help put the commitment into effect.

5. The evaluation phase involves examining the results of previous commitments and actions in order to find new tasks for the agenda and to help the organization learn how to make decisions more effectively [10].

The quality of decision-making in an organization is related to the amount of relevant information available concerning the issues under consideration.

Ordinarily one would wish to maximize the information available to improve the quality of decision-making. Responsibility for organization decisions must be assigned positively and definitely in many cases because the aptness of decisions depends upon knowledge of facts and of organization purpose and is therefore bound up with organization communication. In an attempt to identify alternatives and to arrive at some decision choice, the leader will find it advantageous to use participation whenever such use will lead to increased results at a given or lower cost. Advantages that may stem from the use of participation in decision-making include the following:

1. The improved quality of decisions made. It is seldom if ever possible for leaders to have knowledge of all alternatives and all consequences related to the decisions they must make. Participation tends to break down barriers in communication, making information available to leaders and others that may alter the decisions they make.

2. The improved working relationships of staff. Subordinates who have participated in the process leading toward a determination of matters directly affecting them may have a greater sense of responsibility with respect to the performance of their assigned tasks and may be more willing to accept the authority of their superior.

3. The greater readiness to accept change. When changes are arbitrarily introduced from above without explanation, subordinates tend to feel insecure and to take countermeasures aimed at a sabotage of innovations. When they have participated in the process leading to the decision, they have had an opportunity to be heard. They know what to expect and why, and they may desire the change.

4. The improved staff-leader relationships. There appears to be a reduction in the number of grievances expressed by staff when they are involved in the decision-making process.

5. A higher rate of output and increased quality of work produced. This comes as a result of greater personal effort and attention on the part of subordinates when they are involved in the decision-making process.

6. A reduction in turnover, absenteeism, and tardiness of staff members. Staff members are more interested and involved when they are allowed to participate in the decision-making plans of the group.

Decision-making in organizations involves an understanding of interpersonal as well as intrapersonal aspects of behavior. As subunits interact in considering a decision, there are processes of communication, influence, and negotiation and bargaining that affect the outcome. To understand these, one can draw from a variety of organizational research. For communication processes, the most interesting studies contrast the differences between what one group intends to transmit and what a second receives, explore the effects of different amounts and kinds of information on problem-solving behavior, and investigate the limits on communication imposed by various organizational constraints. There is some indication that individuals approach most decisions with the goal of "satisfying" rather than "optimizing." We make decisions for the present, with the idea that we can remake them in the future. We tend to accept alternates that at most can be described as satisfactory for the time being: we are better judges of what is "better" than of what is "best."

There has been a great deal of discussion about the different distributions of decision-making responsibilities in schools and colleges. Studies have shown that both teachers and students want a more active role in decisions, and there have been a few attempts to measure the effects of participation methods on the educational process [11]. The applicability of ideas about participative decision-making no longer seems as obvious as it once did. Inviting wider involvement does not always bring positive results. Educators have learned that participation generally does not work if other aspects of the environment conflict with the effects it is supposed to produce. They are also discovering that the opportunity to participate in decision-making is not as highly prized by many people as the earlier experiments led them to believe. Administrators are usually not just showing authoritarian attitudes when they complain that the people who work for them are not interested in responsibility. Studies show that employees frequently are quite willing to let superiors make decisions for them. The author saw evidence of this in a university that had developed a faculty organization plan that provided for wide involvement of faculty in decision-making activities regarding university administrative and academic affairs. The faculty found that much time was required for deliberation, negotiation, and problem-solving in areas that were not of primary interest to them. The faculty also found that the responsibility for the consequences of their decisions was painful. Members of the faculty grew reluctant to become involved in university committee activities.

Very little of the basic research on decision-making that has been done has been based in schools and colleges. In building theories, educational administrators have borrowed heavily from ideas that developed from the study of industrial or governmental organizations. Decision-making groups in schools are not the same as customers, suppliers, and directors of business firms. In the case of schools, objections by outsiders are often about the decisions themselves because the basic issue is a contest over whose values, preferences, and subjective experiences will prevail. In a school or college, there are some unusual relations among the major groups involved in its operation. There is often a larger gap between directors or trustees and full-time administrative officers and teachers than there is between directors and management in industry. There are also gaps in many schools between administrators and the teaching and research faculty.

The behavior of group members in relation to each other, to other teachers, and to the administrator changes as needed to influence the decision involved. The teacher who gains the support of his primary group in seeking to influence a decision is engaged in mobilizing power. This involves using his network of interpersonal relations to add group power to his own. The power that a primary group of teachers applies to influence a decision may not be enough. If the decision they seek to influence is important enough for them to invest more energy and time, they can add to their power by obtaining the support of other teachers. This requires communication, persuasion, and mutual adjustments both within and among groups.

Students pose special problems. They are sometimes treated as subordinates, but they are not subordinates in ability and ambition as are some worker groups in industry. Their subordination rests mainly on age and experience, a combination that generates protests and reactions among young persons in business as well as in the educational institution. Students are also transients. The most stable aspect of their experience from year to year lies in their relations with classmates with whom they move from grade to grade rather than with teachers, who change from year to year and from hour to hour. When transient loyalties and strong peer-group ties combine with resentment about subordination, students will keep aggressively raising issues that their predecessors have also raised and pushed.

Educators still have need for considerable amounts of research to find, for different kinds of organizations and different sorts of decisions, patterns of participation that will meet the following goals:

1. Control goal: to insure that decisions do get made and that, for control purposes, there is someone to talk with when it comes time to evaluate decisions or seek explanation for their results.

2. Motivation goal: to bridge the gap that often exists between making and implementing decisions so that people who will have to help carry them out feel identified with their successful implementation.

3. Quality goal: to improve the quality of decisions by involving those who

have most to contribute to the decisions, namely, the experts who have the greatest knowledge of the question under consideration.

4. Training goal: to develop skill for handling problems in those who will eventually move into leadership positions, and to test for the presence of these skills.

5. Efficiency goal: to get decisions made as quickly and with as little waste of manpower as possible.

Goals 1 and 5 suggest fairly limited participation in decision-making. Goals 2, 3, and 4 argue for more extensive participation. Goal 2 requires the participation of people who may be affected by the decision. Goal 3 calls for the participation of people who are expert in solving the problems, and Goal 4 designates the participation of persons who may be neither personally involved nor expert, but who are being prepared for advancement.

If a curriculum decision must be made, it must be explored from the framework of the various goals of decision-making. If, for instance, a decision must be made concerning the development and use of multimedia instruction in the curriculum, the goals and participants may be identified. A pattern of decision-making is suggested in Table 16.

TABLE 16. Goals of and Participants in the Decision-making Process

Goals of Decision-making	Primary Participants in Decision-making		
	Administrators	Teachers	Students
1. Control goal	X	X	
2. Motivation goal	X	X	X
3. Quality goal		X	
4. Training goal		X	X
5. Efficiency goal	X		

This approach to decision-making suggests that for the various decisions to be made, a different pattern of participants will be involved in relation to the several goals of decision-making.

ROLES AND RELATIONSHIPS IN CURRICULUM CHANGE

Curriculum development efforts should be continuous, since they represent study and growth processes. Those involved in the processes become richer through the input from their colleagues, through interaction with peers, students, administrators, and curriculum experts, and through collaborative efforts to design and implement certain innovations in curriculum patterns and activities. The very nature of the processes result in continual modification and change. If there ever is an end product, it is tentative and subject to change.

All professional staff members and students who are to be affected by curriculum decisions should be involved in some way in the decision-making process. The quality of curriculum development efforts is directly related to the input of human and material resources brought to bear on curricular issues. The best curriculum products result from the deliberations of persons representing a variety of roles with various backgrounds of experience. A professional approach to curriculum development allows for a free, open exchange of ideas. It should draw upon the representation of staff members from a variety of roles. A good mix of backgrounds, expertise, and viewpoints can result in improved products. Professionals must be guided by common goals and must constantly remind themselves who is to be the beneficiary of their efforts. In the education business, students are the beneficiaries of curriculum efforts, not the teacher or the administrator. Educators must have a community of purpose. A high degree of mutual trust and respect between and among faculty and students is basic to good working relationships.

ENVIRONMENT FOR CURRICULUM CHANGE

The phenomenon of revolutionary student movements has been a feature of transitional societies, that is, societies in which agrarian-based cultures were breaking down and modern values congenial to industrialization were becoming influential. These societies tend to promote the formation of autonomous student movements. Students are acutely aware of the irrelevance of traditional values transmitted in the relatively cosmopolitan atmosphere of the university and in their training for occupations that represent the emerging social order. Although students are ostensibly being trained for the future, it is usually true that the established elite continue to represent traditional culture, resist modernizing reform, and refuse to redistribute power. Paradoxically, established elites typically sponsor the formation of the university system to promote technical progress while simultaneously resisting the political, social, and cultural transformations that such progress requires. In this situation students almost inevitably come into conflict with established institutions. It appears that student movements tend to arise in periods of transition, when the values inculcated in youth are sharply incompatible with the values they later need for effective participation in the larger society or when values that are prevalent in universities are not supported by established political elites in that society.

During the 1960's the purpose of organized student groups was to develop a radical movement to significantly affect American politics. Although the founders and members of the movement were students, their ultimate concern was not with student issues as such, but rather with the organization of students for social change in the larger society. The thrust of the student movement was toward the reform of society rather than the university. There were protests concerned with removing university restraints on political expression and activity, such as bans on controversial speakers. Students believed that protests against radical and ethnic discrimination 'n fraterni+y systems and against Reserve Officers' Training Corps had a wider political significance than university reorganization. For many students the university represented a kind of social institution in which radical social criticism could be generated and constructive social change promoted. Efforts to utilize the university for this purpose resulted in student reaction in the form of protests and demonstrations. Restrictions were imposed on students who used the campus to support or advocate off-campus political or social action. The struggle on the campus developed into a larger issue: not simply protests against particular violations of student rights, but rather an expression of an underlying conflict between students as a class and the administration, a struggle between two fundamentally opposed orientations toward higher education. Although many disruptions occurred in university life, little effect on university policies was noted. A newer thrust of student activism was an effort to increase the class-consciousness of students and to break down the bureaucratic quality of university life, the paternalistic treatment of students, and the authoritarian pattern of education that was a source of student discontent.

During the past several years resistance and confrontation came to occupy an increasingly prominent position in the strategy of student movement. The conception of the university as a community, sharing common values and culture, and standing apart from both internal political conflict and external political influence, is embedded in academic tradition. The university has long since ceased to be purely a community of shared values. It has become deeply involved in the larger political community without conscious direction and occasionally without careful consideration of the problematic character of its enlarged commitments. The university environment is described from different points of view.

Most universities have developed an ethos of service to the community and the nation. The provision of technical services and trained personnel by institutions of higher learning is indispensible in an advanced society at a high level of technological development. The model of the university as a neutral institution probably describes its pretensions more closely than its uses. It is clear that the university is not and cannot be neutral if this means not to be at the service of any social interests. Nor is the university neutral in the sense of being equally at the service of all legitimate social interests. The university is an important cultural and economic resource; it is also much more fully in the service of some social interests than others. It is understandable that the university has become the scene of conflict and protest focused on control over the nature and direction of the services it provides or fails to provide to the public.

The extension of higher education to lower income and minority groups usually means the attempt to extend norms and values of privileged classes and cultures. Lower income and minority groups may find it difficult to assimilate the cultural traditions of the privileged, at least on a competitive basis. In extending their spheres of interest, influence, and involvement, universities have gained neither clarity of purpose nor direction. The university barely resembles a community if by community is meant a group sharing common interests and values. With such fragmentation of interests, the university is unable to deal effectively with conflict, either internal or external. The university has found it difficult to develop new modes of governance in line with its increased and disparate commitments. It probably will be unable to do so without substantial alteration of its power structure. The attitudes of trustees concerning the locuses of university decision-making tend to be strongly at variance with those of many students and faculty.

Student culture, whether congruent with faculty or administrative goals, has influenced curriculum, university regulations, and policy through informal pressures. This influence has rarely amounted to genuine and formal participation in university governance. Lacking effective representation for the expression and alleviation of grievances, students have resorted to more militant measures. The character of contemporary student protests is seen as a consequence of the lack of genuine political mechanisms within the university. The conditions that appear to mitigate against constructive change are seen as a distant governing board uncommitted to academic values, an administration under pressure and fearful of conservative community reaction, and a faculty concerned with professionalism and retreating from serious involvement in the issues [12]. If order is to be restored to the university community, the university must take major steps toward developing forms of governance appropriate to its implications in the wider social and political order. A prerequisite is the increased participation of students in university decision-making and policy-making. It is neither realistic nor justifiable to expect contemporary students to remain content as second-class citizens within the university.

The description of the university environment in transition conveys the concern of some faculty and students in the field of higher education. The idea that an institution of higher education in a democratic society should be governed democratically raises issues that must also be given thoughtful attention. How sound is the basic premise that a college or university represents a community that, like other political societies, can or should be governed democratically? The position is taken that a university is not simply a microcosm of society; it exists to fulfill several special missions, the most important of which is the advancement and dissemination of knowledge for the benefit of its students as well as the community at large. Given this distinctive purpose, one may argue that the academic government of such an institution cannot simply imitate the political norms that govern society at large.

Another point of view suggests that a university is established to discharge very special functions, and its functioning as a university, like that of other specialized agencies, depends upon an expertise that is inherent in its purpose. The university's special mission requires the authority of the teacher, and the communication of knowledge is impossible without hierarchy and discipline. The different roles of professors and students in the university are built into the essence of the institution. The determination of educational policy, the kind of curriculum to be followed, and the standards to be set for mastery of subject matter are the primary responsibilities of those who have qualified for their standing as scholar-teacher by years of advanced study and experience. The scholar-teacher's professional and personal fitness for her position is to be judged by her peers, the sole criteria of judgment being those of professional competence and personal integrity. Though universities are no more likely than other human institutions to achieve perfection, there is no reason why the principles of academic freedom should be compromised by students whose competence to decide questions of educational policy or academic personnel is no greater than administrators and members of legislatures who earlier challenged academic freedom.

Proponents of this philosophy of educational management believe that the blurring of the distinction between teachers and learners will degrade the learning process. Students should not be taught only what they think they want or what they consider relevant. If students could be relied upon to know what it takes to be an educated person, they would not have to be students. In relation to promotion and tenure of faculty, the students' advisory input can be valuable. But since promotion and tenure depend upon more than classroom performance, and since it is obviously impossible for students to evaluate faculty research and publication, students should not be made members of committees making personnel decisions. Such membership might introduce a serious conflict of roles. Faculty members, entrusted with evaluating the academic performance of students, might become dependent upon the good will of the students in matters of promotion, tenure, and salary increment.

When the consequences of politicizing the life of a university are examined, other compelling reasons for not regarding a university as a democracy are suggested. Since members of the society have to live with the consequences of policies adopted, they can feel the impact and convey their reactions to elected representatives who can alter the course of action. These conditions do not prevail in a college or university. Most students will not have to live for any length of time with the policies their representatives adopt. Given the short period of time they spend at the university, they are in no position to evaluate the legislation enacted by their predecessors.

The larger community in the United States has essentially given real power over curriculum, staff, and teaching methods to the faculty and administration. American society has been convinced that faculties should set educational policies. It has come to accept the notion that while professors may be critical of the values of the larger community, professional rather than ideological standards should determine the content of courses as well as who is hired to teach them. It is unlikely that politicians and the citizenry at large will continue to believe this if universities become politicized, and if substantial power is placed in the hands of students. If such does occur, the larger community may argue that the university belongs to all the people and that the representatives of the people are as well qualified to manage it as are groups of adolescents and young adults.

INDIVIDUAL ROLES

One is thus left with divergent philosophies of educational management. Although it is unlikely that one group will win out completely over the other, some experimentation and changes in academic decision-making is foreseen. It seems obvious to the author that students, faculty, and administration must become the primary participants in making decisions about university affairs. If this is to be realized, students, as well as others in the institution, must be integrated into the system. The channels of communication should be such that all persons receive the necessary information for intelligent responses to the issues and problems confronting the institution. Previous attention to the decision-making process suggested that within any educational institution there are different types of decisions. Who becomes involved in decision-making should be related to the type of decision to be made. More specifically, the determination of roles of the various participants in decision-making should be dependent upon (1) the knowledge and expertise of the participant in relation to the question under consideration, and (2) the impact of the consequences of the decision on the various participants. Although these criteria may be theoretically acceptable, one is aware that colleges and universities are social groups within a larger culture and will probably prescribe roles to its members in keeping with institution custom and tradition. Some general assessment of the roles of administrators, teachers, students, and curriculum coordinators in relation to curriculum development is provided.

ADMINISTRATORS

Administration of student affairs in American colleges and universities until recently has been based on the doctrine of *in loco parentis*. Consequently, the administration was distinctively paternalistic. Some measures of this paternalism were also evident in administrator-teacher relationships, although in some instances teachers possessed the right to initiate programs and instructional and research plans. Both teacher and student demands on administration have increased in recent years and have altered to some degree the role of the administrator in school affairs. While certain roles have remained stable, others have become manifest and have been directed toward establishing and maintaining an environment that is conducive for productive individual and group endeavors. This environment should support and nourish effective administrator-teacher-student relationships that facilitate the decision-making process. The quality of the relationships that the administrator displays will probably have considerable influence upon the kinds of relationships effected by teachers and students.

Attention to certain behavior traits give some indication of the quality of administrator relationships with others in the school environment. The establishment of *trust* is essential to group effort. It is the product of mutual understanding, openly and honestly derived, having some common base, but not necessitating complete agreement. Trust cannot be given, it must be earned. *Reciprocity* in decision-making means that all ideas from all participants are given a fair hearing. Neither trust nor reciprocity is possible unless the blocks to communication are removed. *Respect* and *affection* are terms frequently used in describing personnel relationships for effective group operation. Respect for the office and respect for the individual must be viewed separately. Respect for the individual comes when the individual is perceived to effectively carry out the function of the office. Respect and affection work together as sources of personal influence or power. *Coercion, subversion,* and *persuasion* are behavior traits that characterize the use of power in goal achievement. Coercion and subversion avoid the use of reason, since their use is confined to the implementation of predetermined goals. Coercion is usually easy to observe by the bold and open attempts to induce cooperation through fear. Subversion is at its best when the administrator can gain unity and dependence through the conviction that he is the one best able to protect the group from external dangers and can simultaneously gain the good will of group members so that they are willing to act on his proposals without consideration of the proposals' merits. Persuasion places primary dependence on the power of reason. It is the only control style that could sustain a university climate characterized by intellectual freedom. Restraint is an important aspect of persuasion, but its end is rehabilitation and intelligent change in conduct rather than punishment, which seeks changes in behavior through fear.

Creating an atmosphere where *facts* and *opinions* can be shared and explored is a prime consideration in administration relationships with teachers and students. Facts are considered to be statements of unimpeachable truths, whereas opinions are statements of perceived truth based on the view of a particular person or group. Facts must always be subject to interpretation in terms of the values and purposes of the people interpreting them. The use of factual material of a comprehensive nature can provide a partial basis for mutual agreement among individuals with divergent values seeking to solve a problem. Opinions are interpretations or judgments derived from the application of values to facts which emerge and provide a challenging situation for the development of new ideas. Members of the group should openly and willingly join in the critical examination of all opinions.

Fear, courage, and *commitment* are natural and spontaneous responses in all types of human relationships. Fear should be viewed as a normal response to a situation that an individual comprehends but doubts he can control or that is new to him. In either case he cannot predict what he can do with the situation or what the situation will do to him. Courage is demonstrated in either physical or moral behavior. Physical courage is most easily understood, since it is obvious, dramatic, and widely exploited. The motivation for physical courage may be entirely self-protection or it may include the protection of others, that is, a commitment to do something beyond one's self. Moral courage is a constant in the daily behavior of a professional person, particularly in a university where a high level of commitment to a free marketplace of ideas is required. There is a daily demand on administrators for positive attention to and constructive criticism of conditions that need improvement. There are many sophisticated ways of avoiding responsible expressions of opinion on basic issues and problems: discussing practical affairs without reference to purpose and objectives, disclaiming competence, and declaring the issue to be the prerogative of some other person or group. Sublimated in these attitudes is no small element of fear. It requires courage for an administrator in intellectual controversy to openly confess he was in error.

Educators are becoming increasingly aware of the thrust toward more personal power, power of the individual to direct his own education, shape his own environment, and derive his own value system. On the other hand, administrators are being called to account for time, money, and energy being poured into the educational complex intended to develop "responsible citizens." Some administrators are in a quandry as they anticipate the implications of the quest for more *autonomy* by students and teachers while at the same time they try to satisfy the demands for increased accountability, assessment, and justification. Although autonomy connotes self-governance, auto-regulation, and self-modification, it may be that some students and teachers are demonstrating their interpretation of autonomy to mean immunity. The autonomous person would consciously search for the implications of his behavior on others in order to modify himself; an immune person would feel no obligation to determine the consequences of his actions. The autonomous person would assess the situation to determine appropriate behavior; he would evaluate the power of his decisions in relation to the effect they produced; he would behave in similar situations based on his evaluation of previous performances. An autonomous administrator is one who would be conscious of the educational goals and objectives, and he would be conscious of his own behaviors that facilitate the acquisition of those objectives. Autonomy, like any other behavior, is acquired through practice. Developmental curriculums with corresponding administrative and instructional strategies are being developed, which increasingly trust teachers and students with more decision-making, goal-setting, self-analysis, and sensitization to others. As teachers and students develop increasing autonomy, the administrator needs to alter his own behavior accordingly. As students and teachers become more and more self-directive, the administrator should correspondingly become less and less of the decision-maker for them.

The faculty as a whole is responsible for the total nursing program. The administrator, as a faculty member, shares some responsibilities with the faculty in curriculum development. She has certain responsibilities that are hers as an administrator. The administrator provides leadership for organized curriculum study on an all-school basis. This implies that she has also to give direction to designing and implementing a plan of faculty organization that provides the faculty with the opportunity and responsibility for participating in the development and execution of policies within the school. In order to facilitate the study of curriculum, the administrator provides channels of communication for the faculty to other departments and colleges of the university and to community agencies. The administrator shares her responsibilities with others in the school by delegating certain functions and activities to program chairmen, department heads, and area coordinators and provides guidance and direction to these faculty members in the conduct of their activities. Although individual teachers have the responsibility for recommending to the administrator the use of certain clinical facilities for teaching, the administrator makes the necessary contractual arrangements with community health and/or social agencies for implementing school programs. Periodic review of these contracts is initiated by the school administrator. As the curriculum evolves, the needs for instructional personnel become evident. The administrator must determine priorities in the selection and appointment of new faculty in relation to available budget and the short- and long-term goals of the school. Initial contacts with new instructors are made by the administrator who makes recommendations for their appointment to the faculty. The dean or director is responsible for overall assessment and evaluation of the performance of all faculty members. The administrator, upon the authorization of the faculty, recommends faculty promotion and tenure to the appropriate person(s) in the university hierarchy.

The administrator has the responsibility for providing the faculty and students with appropriate instructional materials and equipment. This task involves the selection of the devices in relation to the extent of usage, the initial purchase of the equipment, and provisions for adequate maintenance. In some instances the acquisition and use of instructional equipment may be a cooperative arrangement of several departments in the college or university. The employment of faculty and the purchase of school equipment is dependent upon budget allocations to the school. The administrator is responsible for preparing, presenting, and justifying budget requests to the college or university officials. Financial support to schools is made available from a number of outside sources (foundations, government). The dean or director in consultation with faculty determines the need for assistance from these sources and makes the necessary contractual arrangements for funding.

The administrator of the school is responsible for providing college or university officials with information about the status of the school, giving attention to the major strengths of the program(s) and the areas of the curriculum(s) that need modification and change. This requires filing a comprehensive report that focuses on the activities and attitudes of students and faculty as well as the physical and social climate of the school. In addition, the dean or director is charged with the responsibility for implementing the overall goals of the university through her leadership activities in university senate and committee endeavors. The administrator is called up to continuously interpret nursing and nursing education to those who have some influence upon the school as well as to the consumers of the school's product. In the transaction of all administrator responsibilities, the essence of quality of performance is determined by the quality of relationships that she establishes with faculty and others in the school environment.

TEACHERS

Teachers devote their talent and training to motivating students, anticipating their learning problems, and clarifying their learning programs. Teachers have the responsibility to make creative and original contributions to the learning dialogue, to guide students to individual solutions of learning problems, and to lead the school and the administration into productive innovations. What is required is a design for teacher participation in curriculum activities, allowing change to be accomplished by involving those most affected by the change (teachers) in planning change. This strategy suggests that involved teachers are probably more committed teachers and also implies enough trust in teachers to allow them to make the best decisions. A teacher in the technological age needs new experiences, encouragement to practice new ways, and freedom to perform, achieve success, make errors, evaluate her learning, and arrive at the best possible decisions for the moment. She needs to be involved directly with the changes in the new age of education and to explore ways that educational media and communications technology can serve herself and the learner.

Broad social forces, technological devices, the behavioral sciences, and other sources of change are modifying the nature of education on almost all fronts. Physical plants, administrators, students, and teachers are in the midst of the change. In particular, the teacher is greatly affected by the many forces impinging upon the school. Each time a change is made in curriculum or organization, the role behaviors of the teacher also change. Little attention is usually given to how an innovation or other change affects the teacher and the teacher's role. The teacher's role is diversified, and it is in a state of transition as a result of the dynamic state of society and the schools. As a result of preliminary studies of the impact of technology on teaching, some teacher role changes are anticipated:

1. Teachers will perform much less of the informational presentation functions. The teacher will become much more involved in the managerial and strategy functions found in the sequencing and evaluation of the instructional process.

2. Teachers will play less of the corrective role in terms of their questioning and evaluative behaviors. This will offer a significant step forward in teacher-student relationships in that much of the negative verbal behavior observed in classrooms will now be shifted to a more individualized and private interaction with instructional media.

3. Teachers will become much more concerned with the host of individual characteristics of students important in designing an instructional strategy. Thus the array of instructional resources and the decision-making found in employing these resources will become more complex and also more frequent in terms of teacher behaviors.

4. The teacher will have a greater involvement in guiding individual students rather than classroom management. She will be able to devote the time usually expended in group communication to individual counseling and advising.

5. Teachers will have to perform a wider range of discussion techniques involving a richer opportunity to affect social and emotional behavior of students. Teachers will have to have greater skill and understanding of human behavior.

6. Teachers will have a greater array of differentiated professionals joining them in the team effort to provide optimal instruction. Some teachers may

become experts in the guidance process, whereas others may become more competent in the application of technological procedures.

7. Teachers may take on many more of the diagnostic assessment and prescriptive functions. Teachers may utilize more group interactive procedures in an attempt to develop latent social and creative talents within their students.

The anticipated role changes of teachers suggest that major attention will be given to individualizing instruction. One of the major reasons for this attention to individualization is the growing recognition that some type of individualized instruction is becoming a necessity in light of the diverse backgrounds, abilities, and motivations of students. The goal of a system of individualized instruction must be to develop persons who seek opportunities to learn and who have the capabilities for setting their own goals, planning an instructional program, and evaluating and monitoring their activities as learning progresses. The teacher's role and all other aspects of instruction must be designed to enhance the achievement of this kind of instructional situation. The desired type of individualized instruction requires a curriculum in which students can take part in meaningful learning activities adopted to their own requirements and to a considerable degree directed and managed by each individual student.

Individualized instruction is not achieved by telling teachers to "pay attention to the individual differences of students." The teacher needs to be assisted by a system that makes individualization feasible. She needs materials that permit a great amount of independent study, diagnostic techniques that provide information as to what a student is ready to study, procedures for monitoring student progress, and guidelines that the teacher and student can follow to make the system operate. The goal of the system is to have each student operating as a self-directed learner within an individualized instructional program. The teacher's role in individualized instruction is to make the system function. The first step in this direction is to evaluate and diagnose the needs and progress of each student to identify where the student is in relation to objectives. Information is obtained that facilitates the development of individual study plans, which include a unique prescription of learning activities developed through cooperative efforts of students and teachers. Helping students to set realistic goals for themselves and to select learning opportunities to achieve these goals are fundamental activities of teachers in individualized instruction. In planning and organizing the classroom and class period to create an effective learning environment, the teacher must allocate time for activities of a general nature, for small-group instruction, for individual instruction, and for counseling. The teacher must be concerned with accessibility of supplies and equipment and the availability of supplementary learning materials. The development of plans for any necessary large-group instruction requires cooperation with other members of the professional staff. The successful operation of individualized instruction demands full cooperation of teachers within the same and in other subject area and on different levels of the instructional program. This calls for regularly scheduled planning sessions involving all teachers who constitute an instructional team. Extensive use of various instructional media requires supervision of the work of certain paraprofessionals, such as the educational media technician. Continuous study and evaluation of the instructional system is necessary in order to improve its functioning and to take steps to correct any instances of malfunctioning.

In addition to the evolving roles of teachers, there are those activities that the teacher performs in the effort to develop and implement the curriculum. The instructor must establish effective relationships with members of nursing-service agencies for the purpose of arranging the clinical opportunities for students. She must also make contacts with community organizations for field trips and for guest lectures. The instructor assumes responsibility of leadership in curriculum development in her specific area of teaching by utilizing the resources of students, physicians, and nursing-service personnel. She also participates as a member of organized curriculum development activities in areas of her competence and expertise. The instructor is responsible for reporting student achievement and learning difficulties to the appropriate sources. The teacher who also has certain administrative responsibilities has some additional functions. This teacher assumes leadership for organized curriculum study within and between various programs (undergraduate, master's, doctoral) including the organization of faculty for study activities. She makes the necessary administrative arrangements with community health and/or social agencies for clinical opportunities for students. As curriculum development proceeds, this teacher identifies the needs for teaching personnel within her area of responsibility and makes recommendations to the dean or director. She provides guidance and direction to teachers in her area of responsibility and makes periodic evaluations of teaching personnel. The master teacher gives direction to the development and implementation of faculty research activities in her area of competence. An important function of this teacher is the career-planning activities of students in her area in relation to professional placement of graduates and the recruitment of faculty. The faculty member who has leadership responsibilities for an area of the curriculum prepares reports and evaluations of her instructional program to keep the dean apprised of the major strengths and needs of the program. The role functions of instructional personnel in a school of nursing vary in relation to the degree of complexity of the decisions to be made. This is determined by the number and categories of persons involved, the temporal characteristics of the decision-making processes, and the nature of the impact of the consequences of certain instructional decisions.

CURRICULUM COORDINATOR (DIRECTOR)

Some schools of nursing employ curriculum coordinators, who give full attention to curriculum development activities. The curriculum coordinator should be more concerned with the macroview of the curriculum. The prime task of the curriculum coordinator is charting and overseeing the master plan. She will need to assume some of the identity of the systems expert in being able to plot the myriad events and activities needed for quality education and the staff needed for new tasks.

The curriculum coordinator also acquires the identity of a communications expert. Effective curriculum processes require an open communication system. Often innovations fail because people, to be affected by the innovation, lack sufficient information. The curriculum coordinator needs to organize a communication network involving teachers and administrators within the school as well as people outside the school who will be involved in curriculum activities. The curriculum coordinator needs to assume responsibility for transmitting and implementing appropriate research findings pertaining to curriculum and instruction. She needs to coordinate research designed to study the process of curriculum development and the effectiveness of specific curriculum changes. How effective is process A in making decisions as compared to process B? How effective is the involvement of certain persons in curriculum decision-making?

In response to the demands for increased accountability and as an integral part of planned change, the curriculum coordinator is responsible for long-range instructional planning and the monitoring of planned changes in the program.

STUDENTS

Students are making unprecedented efforts to influence educational policy. Protests have erupted from student allegations that curriculum is inadequate and/or that teachers or administrators are not attentive to student needs. The current unrest indicates that a new era in student-teacher-administration relations may be forthcoming. One underlying theme in most protests seems to be the insistence that school personnel be more responsive to curriculum needs felt by students.

Instead of being misfits, the student activists are among the most intelligent, the most successful academically, and the most humanitarian, and they exhibit the highest level of moral development within the student body. The sense of boredom, the desire for relevance, the impatience with poor teaching, the duplication of courses and materials, the lack of major attempts to relate subjects and areas and methods, and the continued experience of competition at its worst are legitimate symptoms of need for reform. If these symptoms are to be alleviated, greater participation of students in consultation and decision-making are indicated. Student involvement in school decision-making means that students must exercise a significant degree of control over major portions of the formal activities and events of the school. One of the areas of school life in which students can exercise power could be in curriculum determination. The content of curriculum, the organization of classes, the choice of classroom method, the paths of curriculum sequencing, and the criteria of success should be subject to review, guidance, and management by students. There is little curriculum theory to guide teachers in making decisions about these matters. Although many teachers may have considerable experiential background to assist them in curriculum planning, it must be kept in mind that the students that were taught yesterday are different from those being taught today. And tomorrow's students will be different from those that proceeded them. The changing characteristics of students, their needs, goals, and abilities, require differential approaches to curriculum and instruction. Since there are many ways to accomplish a goal, students should be involved in deciding the routes best suited for them. Student participation in school decision-making also means evaluation of teachers and teaching. Students' exercise of this responsibility is not merely self-serving; many teachers could benefit from knowing how their students experience the classroom and clinical activities and what suggestions or preferences the students have. Student involvement does not have to cause acrimony and distance between students and teachers. Technology has made possible new teaching strategies that enable students to achieve greater independence and more self-direction in their learning. If independence and self-direction are desirable traits for students to acquire, opportunities should be provided for decision-making in other curriculum activities.

Students are the instruments through which the society is changed. The ideas that work within students' lives on the campus are carried into the society, and the society moves from generation to generation with the help of its students. The students are a substantial part of the foundation of the university and must be considered as such because they are the instruments and vehicles of knowledge. The university should be a place where students help their teachers to teach them, where teachers help their students to learn, where administrators help both to accomplish what they have come together to do. This is why the role of the students must now be redefined in order to make clear to them and to others that students are essential constituents of the university. The participation of students in curriculum and instruction involves two processes: consultation and decision-making. Consultation is highly desirable because it enables the faculty to adjust the curriculum to student needs and capacities and to discover the interests that can provide effective motivation. One would not argue that the teacher is more knowledgeable than students about the subject matter of her course and the various teaching stratᴖgies that can be employed to transmit the subject matter. It is also obvious that teachers must set certain goals for instruction that are in keeping with professional and legal standards.

If educators believe that *teachers teach students subject matter,* then they have the responsibility of involving students in the selection of content and learning activities that come within the context of the specific subject matter. Many students today have had wide community contacts and experiences. Very often they can alert teachers to some meaningful opportunities for learning as a means of attaining the course objectives. Students can provide the teacher with the necessary information about the community activity (a new program for juvenile drug users, a clinic for pregnant teenagers, a senior citizen's club) as a potential learning opportunity. Consultation is the appropriate process in this and other similar instances. The utilization of community agencies and voluntary groups requires decision-making on the part of the teacher as it relates to time, costs, and safety factors as well as instructional guidance to make the experience meaningful.

Students should be involved in consultation in determining the general organization of the subject matter of the course. The few studies that are available seem to indicate that students tend to organize the content of the course to be learned in ways different from that of the instructor. Since there appear to be commonalities among students in their patterns of organization, choice by students in the order of presentation of the content seems plausible. The selection of strategies of teaching should also be made in consultation with students. Although consideration must be given to the skill of the teacher, there is ample room for students to suggest the teaching modes that are more compatible with their interests and needs. Although education is a social process, learning is highly individual. Students should indeed have the opportunities to participate in teaching-learning procedures that they consider to be more effective. A graduate student was heard to express her dismay and discouragement concerning the teaching modes in a graduate program in nursing. Among the five courses in which she was enrolled, each course required group projects to be completed outside the class period. Since each group consisted of different students, endless amount of time was spent in arranging times and places for each group to meet. The efforts involved in participating in five groups produced considerable stress. The student observed that the real intent of the various courses was lost in a maze of strained interpersonal relations and began to feel that individual identity was lost to the group.

Evaluation is frequently an emotional process for students. Most students accept the idea and importance of evaluation; however, many express deep concern about the process and techniques. Among the several types of learnings there are many different types of evaluation devices that are available to the teacher. Consultation should be made with students regarding the type of device that would be more acceptable and challenging to them. Where alternates are available, students should be given the opportunity to make certain recommendations. Unless set by university policy, the times for examinations and submission of projects and other assignments should be made in consultation with students. Students are busy people, and every consideration should be given to setting time schedules that will enable them to perform at their best.

The vast array of individual characteristics of students suggests that students participate in decision-making in relation to specific curriculum activities. Decision-making, in this instance, means that students make those decisions that have bearing upon the individual's own learning and progress. Although the teacher must formulate course objectives that are appropriate for the class, modification must be made in the instructional objectives based upon the individual needs, interests, and goals of students. Frequently students are very much aware of certain gaps in their information, and they must be given the opportunity to establish their own objectives for remedial activities. On the other hand, some students may give evidence that they have already attained some of the objectives of the course. Opportunity should then be provided for them to formulate objectives for learning that would enable them to attain greater depth and breadth of content. It is a fact that in a practice field all students must attain an acceptable level of competence. The routes and the amount of time desired within reasonable limits must be decided by the student.

There are many learning opportunities available that are useful to students for the attainment of their objectives. Where there are alternatives, the student should select those that are compatible with their needs and interests. Engaging students in activities that have little interest for them makes for dull and boring learning. The variety of experiences had by students not only enriches the individual student's background but also provides for stimulating experiences for group discussions. Some schools of nursing are giving students the opportunity to decide when they will engage in clinical activities. Students make these decisions in relation to the needs of patients for nursing care and their own learning needs. Decision-making in this case no doubt helps students to mature in relation to their responsibility to patients as well as to themselves.

Students also engage in the organized activities of curriculum study. On all levels of education students have become active and contributing members of curriculum committees. The fresh and creative insights that students offer provide fertile soil for generating new ideas about curriculum and instruction. Their thoughtful and penetrating questions can cause faculty to review and take stock of practices that may no longer serve a useful purpose. The participation of students in organized curriculum activities indicates that they should be full-fledged members of these groups. They should be expected to assume responsibilities similar to other members, prepare for discussion of topics and issues, and express their views openly and intellectually. If voting is inherent in the decision-making process, students should have the right to vote. The experience of the author with students in curriculum study activities has been favorable. In every instance, the students carried their responsibilities equally as well as faculty members. Apart from the useful contributions that students can make, the curriculum study process offers a valuable learning opportunity for students to deal with human relationships in the decision-making process.

ORGANIZATION FOR CURRICULUM CHANGE

The organization for curriculum study and change will assume some different patterns depending upon the internal and external resources of the participants. In selecting certain influence structures and strategies, it is important for the leader to consider among other characteristics the personality system of the members. Some individuals have fairly strong dependence needs and function best when they are closely directed and controlled, whereas others prefer to assume more responsibility, to be given greater freedom, and to rely less heavily on the leader for direction. The knowledge and experience of the members are important considerations in the leader's choice of an influence pattern.

Optimally the leader's degree of directiveness should be conditioned by the resources of the members and by certain other forces existing in the particular situation where her influence is exerted. The time available for making a decision is one variable that must be considered when a leader is deciding to what extent she should engage the participants in making certain decisions. The nature and complexity of specific problems suggest the participation of the members in decision-making. Those decisions that have considerable impact upon a large number of persons should be made by those having the greatest degree of competence and knowledge of the problem(s) under study. The needs and values of the leader may have a considrable influence on the type of leadership pattern that she will choose. The leader's choice of an influence strategy may often be constrained by the nature of her own personality system. The individual who has learned to function in an authoritarian manner may be unable to tolerate psychologically the thought of giving the members latitude in making decisions on their own. Also, confidence in her own abilities to function in uncertain situations is likely to condition the leader's choice of strategies.

These forces are inherent in any group endeavor, including the curriculum and other committees of the school. The organization and membership of the curriculum committee is usually determined by the faculty organization plan that is adopted by the faculty. Whether the chairman and members are appointed or elected will influence the relationships of the members to each other and to the leader. The leader (formal) who is appointed because she holds a particular position in the organization derives power to influence members from the hierarchy. The leader (informal) who is elected by her group derives her power to influence others from the membership of the group itself. The manner in which leadership and membership is obtained will have bearing upon the curriculum study processes.

It is an acceptable notion that all persons who will be involved in curriculum change should participate in the change process. This may be possible where the number of faculty and students is relatively small. The total faculty with representation from the student group may function as a curriculum committee, making individual assignments and reporting back to the total group and the faculty as a whole when making some final decisions.

When the number of faculty is over twenty-five to thirty, more efficient work can take place within smaller groups. The curriculum structure that provides for a steering committee and subcommittee may provide opportunities for more active involvement of faculty members. The steering committee may be charged with the responsibility of designing and directing the general plan for curriculum study, which is reviewed and approved by the total faculty. Subcommittees are formed as the study evolves and as the need for in-depth study of certain problems and issues becomes apparent. The subcommittees report to the curriculum committee, where action is taken on the recommendations. Effort should be exerted to engage all faculty members in committee activities where they can make a significant contribution.

Curriculum committees usually make recommendations for changes to the total faculty group. In the case of some recommendations, faculty approval provides authorization for change. For some changes to be effected, approval by higher authorities may be necessary. Changes involving new courses, employment of additional teaching personnel, and the purchase of new equipment must be reviewed and approved by college or university curriculum committees. Decision-making by the various groups at the different levels is not meant to hinder the creative efforts of faculty but to insure the most efficient and effective use of university resources, giving consideration to the availability of human and material resources.

RESISTANCE TO CHANGE

Curriculum change is complex and perhaps different from changes in some other social endeavors. Most of the significant changes in educational practice require some changes in the attitudes and skills and values of the persons involved for the change to be a successful adoption and adaptation. Most new teaching practice requires significant psychological change and skill acquisition by the adopter and adapter. In the field of education a great proportion of the significant new inventions remain quite invisible, undocumented, and inaccessible for consideration by potential adopters. Educators find a high level of inhibition to communicating ideas about and experiences with new approaches to teaching. They also find in teachers a resistance or an inhibition to adopting another teacher's inventions. The idea of adopting somebody else's practice somehow conveys a notion of imitation and that as such, it is bad. There is in education a significant lack of a professional network of communicators and agents of change. Frequently colleague relations in a school are felt as inhibitions to trying out and adopting new innovations. On occasion, innovative practices utilized by a teacher are viewed as making things difficult for other members of the faculty. For a variety of reasons, there appears to be a lack of creative working relations among the behavioral scientists and the educational specialists and teachers. There is a lack of clear feedback to reinforce the change efforts, to tell the educator and the teacher whether their tryouts are being successful in directions that they had hoped for. Educators find teachers, curriculum coordinators, and administrators quite in the dark about whether there is any evidence that tells them that there has been any payoff at the level of learning efficiency or learning experiences. The process of innovation and diffusion requires different levels of involvement in the process of change in the case of most curriculum practices in order to stimulate and support good quality of change.

NATURE OF RESISTANCE

All of the forces that contribute to stability in personality or in social systems can be perceived as resisting change. In some instances these energies may be seen as obstructions; however, from a broader and more inclusive perspective the tendencies to maintain or to return to a state of equilibrium may be considered to be commendable. Watson describes resistance to change during the life of a typical innovation [13]. In the early stage, when a few pioneer thinkers take the reform seriously, resistance appears massive and undifferentiated. Proponents may be labeled crackpots or dreamers. In the second stage, when the movement for change has begun to grow, the forces for and against become identifiable. Direct conflict and a showdown marks the third stage, as resistance becomes mobilized to crush the proposal. Those who see a favored change as good and needed find it hard to believe the lengths to which opposition will go to curb the innovation. This third stage is likely to mean life or death to the proposed reform. The fourth stage, after the decisive battles, finds supporters of the change in power. The danger of a counterswing of the pendulum remains real and any conspicuous failure of the reform may mobilize latent opposition that could prove sufficient to shift the balance of power. Strategy in the fourth stage requires wisdom in dealing with the overt opponents and with some dissonant elements within the majority who on the whole have accepted the innovation. In the fifth stage, the old adversaries are as few and as alienated as were the advocates in the first stage.

RESISTANCE IN THE INDIVIDUAL

Learning theory suggests that organisms tend to continue to respond in their accustomed way unless the environment changes significantly. Once a habit is established, the behavior pattern becomes satisfying to the organism. The manner in which an organism first successfully copes with a situation sets a pattern that is unusually persistent. It has been observed that many teachers, despite in-service courses and guidance efforts, continue to teach as they themselves were taught.

Once an attitude has been established, a person tends to respond to other suggestions within the framework of his outlook. Experiments with materials and procedures designed to bring about changes in attitude reveal that subjects do not hear clearly or remember well the communications with which they disagree. By reading or listening to what accords with their present views, by misunderstanding communications that, if correctly received, would not be consonant with preestablished attitudes, and by conveniently forgetting any learning that would lead to uncongenial conclusions, subjects successfully resist the possible impact of new evidence upon their earlier views.

The factors that influence resistance to change in the individual may be viewed from the psychological and sociological as well as economic origins. Changes may precipitate organizational redesign, meaning that individuals who have been in association with each other will be assigned to other tasks and relocated to other departments, thereby effecting a disruption of certain interpersonal relationships that have developed over a period of time. The individual may find himself placed in association with new and unknown colleagues whom he may not like or who may like or not like him. Such uncertainties as to how one will be accepted by and fit in with a new group pose a threat to the belongingness needs of the individual.

Organization change or change in the nature of teaching responsibilities may also effect or be perceived to be a threat to the individual's status position and hence to the satisfaction of her esteem needs. Centralization of some activities in a school under one office brings about a realignment of activities of those who previously performed these activities. The utilization of team teaching procedures changes the identity of the teacher vis-à-vis the students when she must share her status position with other teachers.

Changes in curriculum and instruction may be resisted because individuals fear their own inability to handle increased work responsibilities that such modifications may effect. Individuals may refuse to accept promotions to higher organizational levels because of their fears of their inability to deal with increased pressure and job responsibilities. Individuals resisting increases in responsibilities tend to be those whose dependence needs are fairly strong.

Organizational and curriculum restructuring may be viewed as a threat to eeconomic security. Such fears are not without foundation, for technological changes have on many occasions resulted in (1) jobs calling for relatively high-level skills being replaced by lower-skilled work on more highly mechanized equipment, and (2) the total elimination of some jobs. The use of multimedia instruction in nursing curriculums requires the knowledge and expertise of teachers with the utilization of the inherent teaching techniques. Teachers who have neglected to attain the necessary skills may find their teaching outmoded.

A further obstacle to effective participation in social change is the tendency to seek security in the past. When old ways no longer produce desired outcomes, the sensible recourse would be to experiment with new approaches. But individuals are apt at such a time to cling even more desperately to the old and unproductive behavior patterns. The prospect of change arouses anxiety, and they seek to find a way back to the old and more peaceful ways of life.

Schmahl, in describing faculty involvement in her report *Experiment in Change*, identified four stages through which the faculty progressed in a research project in which psychiatric nursing in the curriculum was changed [14]. These stages were as follows:

1. *Stage of impact.* The initial attitudes of the faculty ranged from indifference, surface acceptance, covert hostility to whole-hearted acceptance.
2. *Stage of recoil.* There was an exacerbation of previous problems concerning status differences, attitudes toward authority, the democratic process, and decision-making. Individual defensive patterns emerged, heightening existing tensions.
3. *Early stages of synthesis.* At this stage individuals, as well as groups, shifted from looking for ready-made answers to interest in learning more about the dynamics underlying problematic behavior and a desire to fo-

cus on issues rather than avoid them. The faculty schism between older and younger members of the faculty began to heal.

4. *Later stages of synthesis.* It was in this stage that many of the faculty members discerned something new in concepts they had known before.

It is interesting to note that through all the anxieties and joy of ordering new chaos, new depths of strength, fecundity, and imagination were stirred among faculty members.

RESISTANCE IN THE ORGANIZATION

Any formal organization is constantly subject to competing sets of forces: those that represent inertia or the maintenance of the status quo on the one hand, and those that represent change or innovation on the other. The forces for change represent some sort of dissatisfaction with the status quo. As long as the forces for maintaining the status quo are equal to or greater than the forces to change, the organization is said to be in a state of equilibrium. Disequilibrium occurs when the forces to change become greater than the forces to maintain the status quo. Such disequilibrium represents an occasion for innovation. Persistence or resistance to change may be explained in terms of a lack of dissatisfaction with the present state of affairs and thus with a lack of search for new alternatives.

Assuming that innovations are necessary if the school is to meet the challenge of the social and technological revolution that is taking place in the world today, the problem that confronts us is to identify those elements in the school organization that inhibit such innovations. Attention should be addressed to the following questions: (1) What are the forces operating in the school organization that make it difficult to determine the point at which previously satisfactory programs are no longer satisfactory? (2) Do present organizational arrangements and relationships inhibit the implementation of new programs of action when old ones have been demonstrated to be unsatisfactory?

College and university organization has been previously described as bureaucratic in nature. This organizational pattern has provided the means through which reasonable control might be exercised over the behavior of members of the organization and by which the activities of individuals and groups of individuals with diverse interests and responsibilities might be coordinated. There is belief, however, that rational bureaucratic structure has in many ways increased, rather than diminished the teacher's sense of personal power in the organization. Some observations have been made that seem to indicate that these organizational arrangements and practices produce some seriously dysfunctional consequences in respect to the need for innovative activities in the institution.

In the school organization specialization refers to people, not to tasks. Teachers have developed the competence to perform socially valued functions that other people cannot perform. The bureaucratic pattern provides that authority can be delegated to subordinates in the organization but that the responsibility remains with those in superordinate roles. The administrator must retain the ultimate power to make decisions or to veto the decisions of subordinates. Since the right to make innovations represents a potent source of power in the organization, and since the bureaucratic structure demands that power be concentrated in superordinate roles, innovation from below is difficult to achieve.

Another deterrent to innovation in bureaucratically structured schools grows out of the definition of roles. Although roles in general are defined in terms of both rights and obligations, there is a tendency in bureaucracies, including education, to emphasize rights when referring to superordinate roles and to emphasize obligations when referring to subordinate roles. The rights of those in superordinate roles include the following:

1. The right to veto or affirm proposals of subordinates. This right applies not only to decisions that govern the organization in general but also to decisions that relate to the personal goals of individuals. In one large university, a proposal to introduce an innovative curriculum must run the gauntlet of bureaucratic machinery that contains six decision points (see Diagram 17). At any one of these points, the proposal may be vetoed. Final approval can be given only at the top of the hierarchy. Such a system favors the status quo and inhibits innovations from below. Yet in an organization that consists largely of professionals, meaningful and workable innovations almost necessarily originate at the lower levels of the hierarchy.

2. The right to communicate. The superordinate in the hierarchy has the right to control communication, both to those internal to the organization and to those external to the organization. There is a strong emphasis on following channels in an attempt to communicate, particularly when the communication is upward. Subordinates may be prevented from obtaining sufficient information to enable them to determine accurately the relevance of their immediate activities for achieving the terminal goals of the organization.

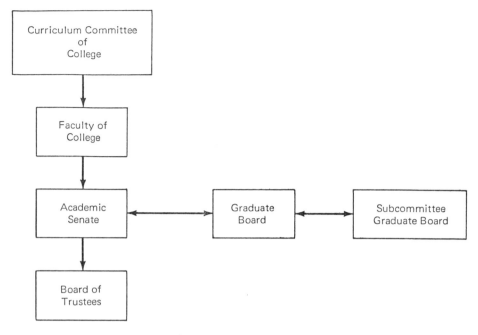

DIAGRAM 17.   Decision-making points in a university.

On the other hand, superordinates may be prevented from obtaining sufficiently accurate feedback from their activities to enable them to assess realistically the effects of their decisions.

3. Organization rights. Superordinates have the right to decide the form of the organization, to determine the types of personnel to be employed, to initiate and assign activities, and to determine agenda for meetings.

Subordinate roles are generally defined in terms of obligations, such as the obligation to follow channels of communication and the obligation to await official approval before engaging in innovative activity.

A final consequence of adhering to rigid bureaucratic structures in the school organization relates to the extent to which such structures impede the professional development of the teaching role. Professions are characterized by a distinctive control structure that is fundamentally different from the hierarchical control of a bureaucracy. The source of discipline in the bureaucratically organized school system is not the colleague group but the authority vested in the hierarchy. It is highly unlikely that innovation will become common among members of a teaching force as long as teachers are subject to rigid hierarchical controls and as long as promotions consist of moving into the hierarchy and are determined by an individual's demonstrated capacity to conform. On recent consultation visits to schools of nursing that were designing innovative approaches to curriculum patterns, the author was told that directives had been sent from top administration indicating that the plans for the innovation must be completed by a specific time, else funding would be curtailed. Innovative ideas are not likely to be nourished under pressures of fixed time schedules.

Shephard has observed that radical innovations are most readily adopted and implemented in times of organizational crisis [15]. During a crisis there is an external threat to the survival of that system; for a moment it is open and searching for new solutions to the basic problems of survival. The state of crisis does not itself generate good innovative ideas. But the uncertainty and anxiety generated by the crisis make organization members eager to adapt new structures that promise to relieve the anxiety.

RESISTANCE IN THE SYSTEM

Norms in social systems correspond to habits in individuals. Members of the organization demand of themselves and of other members conformity to the institutional norms. Teachers have been expected to exemplify certain "proper" behaviors. Norms make it possible for members of a system to work together because each knows what he may expect in the other. Because norms are shared by many participants, they cannot easily change. When one person deviates noticeably from the group norm, a sequence of events may be expected. The group may direct an increasing amount of communication toward him, trying to alter his attitude. If this fails, one after another will abandon him. Communication to him will decrease. He may be ignored or excluded. He no longer belongs. The evidence indicates that if norms are to be altered, this will have to occur throughout the entire operating system. Miles reports the outcomes of experimental programs, which indicate the power of the parent system to impose its norms on units that have been set apart to operate by different standards and expectations [16].

Within the school system it is difficult to change one part without affecting others. Innovations that are helpful in one area may have side effects that are destructive in related areas. Changes in teacher goals and ways of working are dependent upon administrative procedures, policies, and budgets, which in turn require changes in committees and boards. Innovations in any area begin when one or more people perceive that a problem exists, that change is desirable, and that it is possible. These people must decide how best to go about enlisting others to get the information needed to assess the problem further and to develop the strategy leading to implementation of a plan of action. Just as individuals have their defenses to ward off threat, maintain integrity, and protect themselves against the unwarranted intrusions of other's demands, so do social systems seek ways in which to defend themselves against ill-considered and overly precipitous innovations. Individuals and groups constitute the spokesmen for the inner core of tradition and values. They uphold established procedures and are quick to doubt the value of new ideas. They are the ones most apt to perceive and point out the real threats, if such exist, to the well-being of the system that may be the unanticipated consequences of projected changes. They are especially apt to react against any change that might reduce the integrity of the system. They are also sensitive to any indication that those seeking to produce change fail to understand or identify with the core values of tle system they seek to influence.

The existence of interdependence among the subparts of a system and between the system and its environment has many implications for change. It has been noted that interdependence can generate an emergent force toward change if change in one part of a system sets up forces on other parts to match

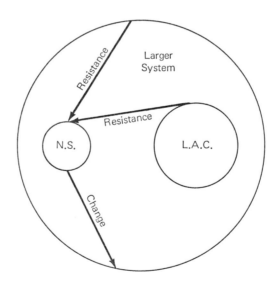

DIAGRAM 18.   Resistance to change exerted by a subunit within the system. N.S. = nursing school; L.A.C. = liberal arts college.

the change or utilize the new resources. Interdependence can serve as a source of resistance. Readiness for change in one part of a system may be negated by the unwillingness or inability of other interdependent parts to change. A change sequence that would be strong enough to modify a subpart if it existed in isolation may have no effect on the system as a whole, and it may consequently fail to have any effect on any part of the system. This situation may be described by Diagram 18, in which a school of nursing in a university attempts to change certain liberal arts requirements of the undergraduate curriculum. Also located in the university is a large, potent college of liberal arts. The college of liberal arts exerts considerable influence on the university as a whole and on its subunits. Efforts to change the liberal arts requirements by the school of nursing are met with resistance from the university (larger system) and the liberal arts college (potent subunit). The change suggested by the school of nursing will have little or no effect on the system or on its subunits.

If the subunit is too small to cope with a given problem, it will be unable to change because of the resistance originating outside the subunit and coming from the larger system in which it is embedded or from parallel systems to which it is related. If the unit is too large and includes semiautonomous

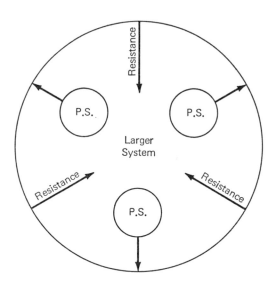

DIAGRAM 19.   Resistance to change exerted by the larger system. P.S. = professional school.

subsystems that are not directly involved in the change process, it may be unable to change because of resistance originating within the system.

In a church-affiliated university, the professional schools believe that the number of courses in religion is too large and may deny the student of opportunities for breadth in their educational program. Efforts are exerted by the professional schools to change this curriculum requirement. The other colleges (subunits) of the university are not interested or involved in this change. The changes suggested by the professional schools may be resisted by the system as a whole because this change may be perceived as attempts to alter the value structure inherent in the system as a whole. A model of this is shown in Diagram 19.

FORCES OPERATING TO PRODUCE CHANGE INFLUENCES
OR RESISTANCE INFLUENCES

In systems consisting of more than one individual, the expectations held by one person or a group about the behavior of other persons or groups serve as important determinants of behavior. People tend to do what others expect them to do. This is true even when people know how to behave differently and in ways that would be more satisfactory but that would run contrary to expectations. Many behavior patterns in a given system will have multiple meanings for that system. A single act may serve several different purposes at the same time. It may be that each purpose or need is anchored in a different subunit of the system. Each subunit has its own impulse to act. The unitary nature of the system makes separate and independent action by the subunits impossible. Some compromise is developed so that the system can act in a way that is generally satisfactory to all of its parts but not exclusively or fully satisfactory to any of them. If change is proposed that would meet some of the needs satisfied by the existing arrangements and ignore others, the subunits whose needs are ignored would oppose the change and insist on preservation of the status quo. If a university endeavored to change its requirements for faculty appointment to insist that all potential teachers possess the doctoral degree, the school of nursing would likely resist the change. In this instance the needs of the school of nursing are being overlooked in view of the supply of nurses holding doctoral degrees. On the other hand, forces toward change would probably be generated if the proposed change seemed likely to give satisfaction to subunits not previously satisfied.

To the extent that one system or subsystem is dependent on another, the one wants to see that the other maintains viability. The vulnerability to threat depends on the extent to which the partners are committed to one another or the degree to which the observing partner has the freedom and ability to terminate the relationship. Resistance occurs when a proposed change seems to promise benefits to one part of the system at the expense of another part. Interdependence among the parts of a system is often associated with a fear that the improvement or change of one part can be gained only at the expense of another, and there is a tendency on the part of a system to feel threatened by any proposal for change except perhaps its own. The recommendations included in the report of the Secretary's Committee to Study Extended Roles for Nurses may be viewed by physicians as a threat to the integrity of the system of medicine. Relinquishing certain roles and activities to the system of nursing may be seen by physicians as an invasion of their territorial rights.

Resistance based on threat is a particular problem because of the psychological concomitants of a state of threat. These include a narrowed field of attention and a need to find some way of controlling whatever it is that threatens. Change is the very thing that is most intolerable to a system or subsystem experiencing a high degree of threat.

PRINCIPLES RELATING TO RESISTANCE TO CHANGE

Few social changes of any magnitude can be accomplished without impairing the life situations of some individuals or groups. There is no doubt that some resistance to change occurs when individuals' livelihoods are affected adversely or when their social or professional standings are threatened. In an effort to reduce or minimize the negative influences of resistance, some principles relating to resistance of change are suggested:

1. Resistance will be less if administrators, teachers, and students feel that the curriculum project is their own, not one devised and controlled by outsiders.
2. Resistance will be less if the project has wholehearted support from top officials of the school.
3. Resistance will be less if participants see the curriculum change as reducing rather than increasing their present burdens.
4. Resistance will be less if the project accords with values and ideals that have been acknowledged by the participants.

5. Resistance will be less if the curriculum offers the kind of new experience that interests the participants.
6. Resistance will be less if participants feel that their autonomy and their security is not threatened.
7. Resistance will be less if participants have joined in diagnostic efforts that lead them to agree on what the basic problem is and to feel its importance.
8. Resistance will be less if the curriculum change is adopted by consensual group decisions.
9. Resistance will be reduced if proponents are able to empathize with opponents, to recognize valid objections, and to take steps to relieve unnecessary fears.
10. Resistance will be reduced if it is recognized that innovations are likely to be misunderstood and misinterpreted and if provision is made for feedback of perceptions of the project and for further clarification as needed.
11. Resistance will be reduced if participants experience acceptance, support, and confidence in their relations with one another.
12. Resistance will be reduced if the curriculum project is kept open to revision and reconsideration if experience indicates that changes would be desirable.

Consideration of these principles in activating curriculum change may make it possible for faculty, students, and administrators to experience professional satisfaction in designing and improving the curriculum of the school.

There is a process of changing the curriculum. This process requires a freeing of faculty to generate new ideas and new approaches and an opportunity to try them out under conditions that will allow them to develop and to be adequately tested and evaluated. An experimental atmosphere is needed with less emphasis upon conforming and standardization and with more attention to meaningful interactions with faculty and students. There must be an appropriate structure within the school for authorizing the curriculum and for giving it validity and sanction. Mechanisms are needed for appropriate committee structures, for interaction among faculty members with different ideas, different persuasions, and backgrounds, and for maintaining an atmosphere for study and consideration and improvement.

The curriculum of a school will be no better than teachers make it. The task of keeping a curriculum up to date and functioning effectively is a day-today, week-by-week, year-by-year responsibility that must be achieved by alert teachers. Curriculum improvement as a process is one that requires skill, knowledge, and wisdom. It is a process that involves reflective thinking, ways of working in professional situations, and the objective identification and systematic study of problems. It is a process of translating educational theory, objectives, and principles into operational learning pathways for students to follow. It is the process of uniting the intellectual contributions of the faculty and others into an effective educational team. It is a process that must be learned and creatively applied by all engaged in defining and developing curriculums for our schools.

SUMMARY

Curriculum change requires that the efforts and activities of teachers, students, administrators, and others be united in planned efforts that have mutually acceptable goals. These efforts must be organized in such a way that the participants have a share in the activities that is commensurate with their knowledge and skills. The organization of individuals in goal-seeking endeavors implies that certain processes are operating in the interest of goal attainment. These organizational processes include authority, leadership, group dynamics, and decision-making.

Authority is institutional power over others and gives that power to one to make decisions that guide the actions of others. Authority functions to enforce the conformity of individuals to the norms laid down by the group. Authority exercised in educational organizations is based upon superior knowledge and technical competence in a particular element in the division of labor. Authority as a process in a social institution may be viewed from the standpoint of administrative authority and legal authority. The university is somewhat unique in its authority process, since it depends upon two structures: the bureaucratic structures and the collegial structures. These two types of authority structures employ different styles of decision-making.

Leadership as an influence process is a function of the characteristics of the leader, those of his followers, and the nature of the specific situation in which the influence efforts take place. There appear to be few generalized personality characteristics that describe a leader. Leadership is primarily a function of the relationship of the individual to the organization and the demand of the individual's organizational role. An individual may be able to influence others because he is in a position to reward them if they accede to his influence efforts. The potential ability of the individual to influence others because he is in a position to reprimand or punish them if they do not follow his wishes is a function of the coercive power of the leader. Expert power refers to the potential ability of one person to influence others because of his superior knowledge of a specific situation. Legitimate power is based on the belief that other individuals holding certain positions have the right to influence behavior. Patterns of leadership behavior may be described as authoritarian, laissez-faire, and democratic.

The study of small groups provides useful information about group dynamics in relation to how groups are formed, how they influence their individual members, and how groups operate internally. These studies reveal the nature of the group and group process as a function of its relationship to its external environment, the characteristics of its leader, the potential for interaction among members, and the goals of the individual members as well as the goals of the total group. The effectiveness of the group and the satisfaction of its members appears to be a function of the enhancement of personal goals by means of group goals. The most productive groups are those that can carry out the major steps in the process of solving tasks and the social-emotional problems for the group.

Decision-making as an organizational process is concerned with the discovery and definition of problems and the search for alternatives among which to choose. It also involves the implementation of the choice and the evaluation of the results of the implementation. Decision-making in organizations involves an understanding of interpersonal as well as intrapersonal aspects of behavior. There has been considerable discussion about the role of different distributions of decision-making responsibilities in schools and colleges. There is little basic research on decision-making to guide educators in the selection of participants who will be effective in making the best decisions. It appears that the participants who are selected should be related to the various goals of the decision-making process, which include control, motivation, quality, training, and efficiency goals.

The major participants in curriculum change include teachers, students, and administrators. The roles that each of these assume should be related to the knowledge and expertise of the participant in relation to the question under consideration and the impact of the consequences of the decision on the various participants. The faculty as a whole is responsible for the nursing curriculum. The administrator, as a faculty member, shares some responsibilities with the faculty. There are, in addition, certain responsibilities that are hers as an administrator. She offers leadership for organized curriculum study by providing the appropriate channels of communication and by delegating certain functions and activities to others. The administrator also provides the faculty and student with appropriate instructional materials and equipment and makes necessary budget requests to the university officials.

Teachers have the responsibility to make contributions to the learning dialogue and to guide students in the solution of their learning problems. Social forces and technological innovations are bringing out changes in the roles and activities of teachers. A teacher in the technological age needs new experiences, encouragement to practice in new ways, and freedom to perform and evaluate her successes and failures. The teacher needs to be directly involved with the changes that are occurring in education and to explore the ways in which technology can serve herself and the learner. Instructors should be actively involved in the process of curriculum change. This implies establishing effective relationships with students, other teachers, community agency personnel, and allied professional colleagues. Teachers assume the major responsibility for curriculum development in their areas of specialization and as a participant member of the organized group for curriculum study.

Students are making unprecedented demands for active participation in curriculum activities. The changing characteristics of students and their needs, goals, and abilities require differential approaches to curriculum and instruction. Since there are many ways to accomplish a goal, students should be involved in deciding the routes best suited for them. The university should be a place where students help their teachers to teach them, where teachers help their students to learn, and where administrators help both to accomplish what they have come together to do. The involvement of students in the curriculum study process offers a valuable learning opportunity for students to deal with human relationships in the decision-making process.

Changes in curriculum frequently require changes in teacher behavior. There is often some inhibition or resistance to change among teachers. Changes are viewed by them as a threat to their security and to their status positions. Changes often require teachers to utilize new skills that are unfamiliar to them. Resistance to change is also seen within the school organization. The bureaucratic structure of most colleges and universities is not always conducive to innovative changes. A recommendation for change that is initiated by a group of teachers must be reviewed and approved by many groups in the university hierarchy. The incentive for innovations is frequently lost before the recommendation gets an initial hearing. Resistance to change in the school system is observed when a change in one part of the system has a profound effect on other parts of the system. School systems seek ways to defend themselves against precipitous changes. Effort is exerted by the system to maintain integrity and to protect itself against unwarranted intrusions of others' demands.

In an effort to minimize the negative influence of resistance, principles relating to resistance to change should be formulated by the faculty of the school. These principles should give consideration to the involvement of teachers and students in the curriculum activities. Participants should be made aware that administrators are giving wholehearted support to their efforts. Mutual trust, cooperation, and support among participants is essential for the security, autonomy, and productivity of teachers and students. Any changes proposed by the participants should be kept open to review and reconsideration if experience indicates that further changes are desirable.

REFERENCES

1. Parsons, T. *Essays in Sociological Theory*. New York: Free Press of Glencoe, 1954. P. 76.
2. Simon, H. A. *Administrative Behavior*. New York: Free Press, 1957. P. 125.
3. Ibid., p. 134.
4. Gross, E. Universities as organizations. *Amer. Sociol. Rev.* 33:518, 1968.
5. Gibbs, C. A. Leadership. In G. Lindzey [Ed.], *Handbook of Social Psychology*. Reading: Addison Wesley, 1954. P. 889.
6. Hemphill, J. K. *Situational Factors in Leadership*. Columbus: Bureau of Educational Research (Ohio State University), 1949. P. 877.
7. Hemphill, J. K. Leadership Behavior Associated with the Administrative Reputation of College Departments. In W. W. Charters, Jr., and N. L. Gage [Eds.], *Readings in the Social Psychology of Education*. Boston: Allyn and Bacon, 1963. P. 319.
8. Berelson, B., and Steiner, G. A. *Human Behavior: An Inventory of Scientific Findings*. New York: Harcourt, Brace & World, 1964. P. 3.
9. Ibid., p. 326.
10. Simon, H. A. *The New Science of Management Decisions*. New York: Harper & Bros., 1960. P. 2.
11. Gregg, R. T. The Administrative Process. In R. F. Campbell and R. T. Gregg [Eds.], *Administrative Behavior in Education*. New York: Harper & Bros., 1957. P. 278.
12. Student protest. *Bull. Amer. Assoc. Univ. Prof.* 55:309, 1969.
13. Watson, G. Resistance to Change. In W. G. Bennis, K. D. Benne, and R. Chen [Eds.], *The Planning of Change*. New York: Holt, Rinehart & Winston, 1969. P. 488.

14. Schmahl, J. A. *Experiment in Change.* New York: Macmillan, 1966. P. 206.
15. Shephard, H. A.   Innovation-Resisting and Innovation-Producing Organizations. In W. G. Bennis, K. D. Benne, and R. Chen [Eds], *The Planning of Change.* New York: Holt, Rinehart & Winston, 1969. P. 521.
16. Miles, M. B. [Ed.].   *Innovation in Education.* New York: Teachers College Bureau of Publications (Columbia University), 1964.

SUPPLEMENTARY READINGS

Berne, E.   *The Structure and Dynamics of Organizations and Groups.* Philadelphia: Lippincott, 1963.
Bush, R.   Redefining the role of the teacher. *Theory Into Practice* 6:246, 1967.
Carver, F. D., and Sergiovanni, T. J. [Eds.].   *Organizations and Human Behavior.* New York: McGraw-Hill, 1969.
Chester, M. A.   Shared power and student decision-making. *Educ. Leadership* 28:9, 1970.
Committee T on College and University Government.   Draft statement on student participation in college and university government. *Bull. Amer. Assoc. Univ. Prof.* 56:33, 1970.
Costa, A. L.   Who's accountable to whom? *Educ. Leadership* 28:15, 1970.
Dubin, R.   *Human Relations in Administration.* New York: Prentice-Hall, 1951.
Fischler, A. S.   The role of the professor and technology in higher education. *Educ. Techn.* 10:21, 1970.
Gardner, E. F., and Thompson, G. C.   *Social Relations and Morals in Small Groups.* New York: Appleton-Century-Crofts, 1956.
Getzel, J. W., Lipham, J. M., and Campbell, R. F.   *Educational Administration as a Social Process.* New York: Harper & Row, 1966.
Golembiewski, R. T.   *The Small Group.* Chicago: University of Chicago Press, 1962.
Graff, O. B.   Value referents in the governance of higher education. *Theory Into Practice* 9:211, 1970.
Griffiths, D. E.   *Behavioral Science and Educational Administration.* Sixty-third Yearbook of the National Society for the Study of Education. Chicago: University of Chicago Press, 1969.
Hare, A. P.   *Handbook of Small Group Research.* New York: Free Press of Glencoe, 1962.
Hare, A. P., Borgatta, E. F., and Bales, R. F.   *Small Groups: Studies in Social Interaction.* New York: Knopf, 1962.
Hook, S.   The architecture of educational chaos. *Phi Delta Kappan* 51:62, 1969.
Hopkins, T. K.   *The Exercise of Influence in Small Groups.* Totowa: Bedminster, 1964.
Lewin, K.   Group Decision and Social Change. In G. E. Swanson, T. M. Newcomb, and E. L. Hartley [Eds.], *Readings in Social Psychology.* New York: Holt, Rinehart & Winston, 1952. P. 463.
Lewey, G., and Rothman, S.   On student power. *Bull. Amer. Assoc. Univ. Prof.* 56:279, 1970.
Likert, R.   *New Patterns of Management.* New York: McGraw-Hill, 1961.

Lindvall, C. M., and Bolvin, J. O.   The role of the teacher in individually prescribed instruction. *Educ. Techn.* 10:37, 1970.

Lippett, R., Watson, J., and Westley, B.   *The Dynamics of Planned Change.* New York: Harcourt, Brace & World, 1958.

Richard, M. D., and Greenlaw, P. S.   *Management Decision-Making.* Homewood: Irwin, 1966.

Smith, B. L.   Educational trends in the seventies. *Bull. Amer. Assoc. Univ. Prof.* 56:130, 1970.

Taylor, H.   The student revolution. *Phi Delta Kappan* 51:62, 1969.

Wilson, G. G., and Weissman, A.   Keeping student participation in its place. *Theory Into Practice* 9:248, 1970.

INDEX

Acceleration, academic, 162–163
Accreditation, of nursing schools, 555–556
Achievement, 400
  academic, influence of, 446
Achievement test, 364, 380
  educational objectives and, 222–223
Activism, 180–181, 619–620
Activities Index, 465, 466
Activity analysis, 545–547
Administrative authority, 602
Administrators
  functions of, 35
  responsibilities of, 627–628
  roles of, in curriculum development, 35–36, 624–628
Admissions policies, 29, 157, 159–160
Adult education, 161–162
Advance organizers, 447–448
Advisor, importance of, to student, 170
Affective behaviors, 250–255
  analyses of, 255
  attempts to identify, 251–253
Aging, nursing of. See Nursing, of aging
Alertness, 441
Alienation, 183
Allied professional personnel in nursing education, 371–373
  criteria for effective use of, 372–373
  purposes of, 372

American College Survey, 172–175
  findings of, 172–173
  implications of, 174–175
  scales used in, 173–174
  Student Orientation Survey of, 174
  Vocational Preference Inventory of, 174
American Council of Education, 44
American Dietetic Association, 43
American Heart Association, 54
American Hospital Association, 42–43
  role of, in curriculum development, 42–43
American Junior College Association, 47
American Medical Association
  opposition of, to social legislation, 41–42
  role of, in nursing education, 40–42
American Nurses Association, 38–39
American Orthopsychiatry Association, 43–44
American Red Cross, 52–53
Amish, 70–71
Analysis
  activity, 545–547
  systems, 580–583
Analytic process, 290, 292
Anecdotal record, 365
Animal psychology, 196
Anxiety, learning and, 440

Applied research, 382
Aptitude test, 364
Army, nursing service in, 568–570
Assessment of student characteristics, 168–175. *See also* Evaluation
comprehensive, 171–175
institutional, 169–171
purposes of, 168–169
Associate degree programs, 565
Association by contiguity, 203
Association of Collegiate Schools of Nursing, 44
Attention, 441, 475–476
Audiotutorial instruction, 512
Authoritarian leadership, 607–608
Authority, 600–604, 651
administrative, 602
and decision-making, 601–602
legal, 602
in universities, 603
Autonomy, 253, 626

Baccalaureate degree programs, 141–143, 566
Bedside nurse, 560
Behavior theories. *See* Learning, theories of
Behavioral analysis, 238–265. *See also* Task description and analysis
of cognitive behaviors, 248–250
of community health nursing, 240–241
of nursing care to tuberculosis patient, 241–243, 244
Behaviorism, 196–197
Behaviors
affective. *See* Affective behaviors
assessment of, 480–481
cognitive. *See* Cognitive behaviors
curriculum and, 13
intermediate, 232–238
modification of, 225
operant. *See* Operant conditioning
personal and interpersonal, 370
psychomotor. *See* Psychomotor behaviors
terminal, 221, 225, 232
Biological system, 577, 578

Branching programs, 498, 503
Broad-fields organization, 552
Bureaucratic authority structure, 603, 643–644
Business and industry, role of, in curriculum development, 55

Career-ladder concepts, 145–147, 571–576
Case method, 365
Case-study analysis, 294–297
of nursing care for hydrocephalus, 296–297
Census, university student. *See* University Student Census
Change
curriculum. *See* Curriculum, change in
directed, 538–539, 558–561
pragmatic approach to, 538–539
resistance to. *See* Resistance to change
social and cultural, 66–72
Childhood development, early, 197
Classroom group
characteristics of, 417–418
dynamics of, 417–421
influence of, on individual learning, 463–465
relationships of, to other groups, 418
as social system, 418–421, 464–465
Coeducation, 159–160
Coercive power, 607
Cognitive behaviors, 245–250
analysis of, 248–250
Cognitive knowledge
classification of, 274–275
as subject matter, 273–274
College. *See* Higher education; University
Collegiate authority structure, 603–604
Commercialization of professions, 83–84
Committee on the Grading of Nursing Schools, 544–545
Common learnings, 278–283
Communication, adequacy of, 590–591
Community, involvement of, in instruction, 373–375
Community curriculum, 6–7

Community junior-college nursing programs, 140–141, 559–561
Community service role of university, 621
Community-teacher-student relationships, 333–336
Comparative evaluation, 356, 383–384
Competence, 117, 441–442
  as learning motive, 441–442
  in professional practice, 117
Competence model, 442
Computer-assisted instruction, 514–516, 518–520
Concepts, 246, 405
  definition of, 284, 286–289
  development and identification of, 283–290
Conditioning, 196
  contiguous, 203–204
  operant, 207–209, 327
Conferences, curriculum, 549–550
Congruence, 347–348, 589–590
Connectionism, 192–194
Consensus, in decision-making, 604
Constructive motivation, 440
Consumer participation in health, 104
Content. See Nursing, content in; Subject matter
Context evaluation, 351
Contiguous conditioning, 203–204
Contingency, 345–347, 349
Continuity of curriculum opportunities, 325–326, 327–328
Contract teaching, 497–498
Control-group evaluation, 384
Cooperative instructional activities, 166–168
Coping, 252–253
  definition of, 252
  worth and, 253
Core, nursing, 278–283
Courage, 626
Credit, course, by examination, 163–164
Cue(s), 473–475
  controlling attention and, 475
  varieties of
    connotative, 473
    denotative prompts, 473, 474

Cultural change
  curriculum and, 330–332
  in technological societies, 67–70
Cultural patterns, 62–63
Cultural pluralism, 71–72
Cultural values, 64–77
  curriculum and, 61–78
  education and, 72–75
  social change and, 66–72
Culture
  definition of, 62–64
  primitive, 72–73
  stability of, within social change, 70–71
Culture lag, 64
Curiosity, 441
Curriculum
  in baccalaureate nursing programs, 141–143
  balance in, 330–333
  career-ladder concepts and, 145–157, 571–576
  change in
    environment for, 619–623
    guidelines for, 584–592
    organization for, 636–638
    organizational processes in, 600–618
      authority, 600–604, 651
      decision-making, 614–618
      group dynamics, 610–614
      leadership, 605–609, 651–652
    process of, 537–539
    resistance to. See Resistance to change
    roles and relationships in, 618–636
      environment, 619–623
      individual, 623–636
    strategies for, 537–594
      activity analysis, 545–547
      definition of content, 563–568
      directed change, 558–561
      establishing new goals, 547–548
      evaluation of innovation, 561–563
      group dynamics, 548–551
      organizational efforts, 542–545
      reform, 540
      standardization, 540–542

Curriculum, change in, strategies for—
   Continued
    studies of nursing, 553–558
    subject reorganization, 551–553
    systems theory, 576–584
  in colleges and universities, 158–159
  components of, 594
  concepts of
    contemporary, 6–8
    past, 3–6
  core, 278–283
  as course of study, 3–4
  cultural values and, 61–78
  defined, 15
  design of, 305–335
    common schemes of, 307
    content vs. process in, 307–308
    functions of, 308–311
    nature of, 305–308
    objectives and. *See* Curriculum,
      objectives of
    questions pertaining to, 306
  development of
    approaches to, 12–14
    basic issues in, 17–31
    influence of psychological and
      learning theories on, 189–216
    participants in, 33–56
      administrators, 35–36, 624–628
      allied professional associations,
        40–47
      business and industry, 55
      external participants, 38–55
      foundations, 47–49
      internal participants, 33–38
      professional nursing associations,
        38–40
      state government, 36–38
      students, 34, 632–636
      teachers, 34–35, 631–632
      voluntary associations, 53–55
  for differentiated student needs, guide
    to, 4
  direction of, 312
  evaluation of, 341–387. *See also* Eval-
    uation
    and research, 381–385
  focus of, 310, 311
    nursing problem as, 321–325

and instructional methodology, 8
as means of achieving "desired learnings," 6
as means to facilitate growth, 5–6
objectives of, 221–267, 311–314
  analysis of, 315–319
  human capabilities as, 315–316,
    317–319
  institutional capabilities and, 316,
    317–319
  material capabilities as, 316, 317–
    319
  and social change, 311
  and student characteristics, 311
  and subject matter, 312
organizing centers of. *See* Organizing
  centers of curriculum
relation of, to society, 330–332
relevance of, 75–77
scope and emphasis of, 312–314
social and scientific forces affecting,
  81–110
state requirements for, 36, 37
structure of, 305–337
student characteristics and, 153–186,
  311
subject matter and, 4, 276–277, 312
Curriculum coordinator, 632
*Curriculum Guide for Schools of Nurs-
  ing, A*, 545
Curriculum opportunities
  continuity of, 325–326, 327–328
  identification and organization of,
    315–333
  integration of, 328–330
  sequence of, 324–325, 326–328
Curriculum for Schools of Nursing,
  544–545
Custom(s)
  definition of, 62
  as role, 63

Dalton Plan, 497
Data-gathering, systematic, 171
Decision-making, 614–618
  and authority, 601–602
  distributions of, in schools and col-
    leges, 616–617

Decision-making—*Continued*
  goals of and participants in, 615, 617–618
  stages of, 614–618
  teaching as, 398–399
Decisions, types of, 292–293
Defensive motivation, 440
Demonstration, 495
Dewey, John, 11, 194–196
Diagnostic test, 365
Directed change, 538–539, 558–561
Discipline, 272–273
Discrimination, 246–247
Discussion
  group, 493–494
  panel, 494
Doctoral programs, 122

Education
  cultural deprivation and, 73–75
  cultural values and, 72–75
  evolution of, in America, 8–12
  general, 118–119
  goals of, 226–227
  graduate, 122
  higher. *See* Higher education
  nursing. *See* Nursing education
  objectives of. *See* Objectives, educational
  in primitive societies, 72–73
  professional. *See* Professional education
  remedial, 164–165
  technical, 123
Educational associations, 44–47
Educational evaluation. *See* Evaluation
Educational management, roles in, 623–624
Educational technology, 526–529
Effective teacher behavior, 429–431, 456–461
  determination of, 458–459
Emotions, 253
Empirical generalizations, 405–406
Empiricism, 190–191
Enlightenment, the, 9
Environment
  influence of, on learning, 212–213
  learning, 461–469

curriculum change and, 588, 619–623
evaluating influence of, 343–348
students in, 584–589
physical, 461–463
  variables in, 462–463
psychological, 465–469
social, 463–465
Environmental dimensions of health, 95–96
Environmental hazards, man-made, 90–92
Equal educational opportunity, 157
Equality
  of opportunity, 73
  in Western tradition, 73
Essay test, 364
Evaluation, 341–387
  administration of, 377
  of allied professional personnel in education, 371–373
  comparative, 356, 383–384
  for congruence, 347–348
  context, 351
  of contingency, 345–347, 349
  control-group, 384
  of curriculum, 351–353
  curriculum change and, 561–563, 589
  defining requirements for, 378
  definition of, 342, 378–379
  of education system, 353–355
  experimental design type of, 381–382
  focusing of, 376
  formative, 356, 382
  generalizability of results of, 383
  goals and roles of, 355–357, 359
  input, 351–352
  institutional, 382
  of instruction
    methodology, 360–75
    purposes, 349–350
  issues and problems in, 377–381
  lack of criteria and instruments in, 379–381
  learning environment and, 343–348
  longitudinal, 363
  methodology of, 355–377
    vs. research methods, 384–385

Evaluation—*Continued*
  norms in, 358–360
  process, 352
  process of, 342–343
  product, 353, 356
  purposes of, 348–355
  roles enacted in, 357–360
  of student progress, 360–366
  summative, 356, 382
  of teacher effectiveness, 366–371
  types of variables in, 344–345
Evaluation decisions, 293
Evaluation design, 375–377
  structure of, 376–377
Examinations for awarding credit, 163–164
Example, 450–451
Execution decisions, 292–293
Experimental design, 381–382
Experimental psychology, 190–191
Expert power, 607
Expression, 253
Expressive role, 129

Faculty, nursing education, 21–22
Faculty psychology, 190
Federal government, role of, in nursing education, 20, 50–52, 568–571
Feelings, 253
Field, description of, 198
  in part-whole phenomena, 198
  physical, 198
Field theory, 200–202
Field trip, 520–521
Flanders' Interaction Analysis Categories (FIAC), 426
Formal instruction, 393
Formative evaluation, 356, 382
Foundations, role of, in curriculum development, 47–49
Frustration, learning and, 440
Functionalism, 194–196

Gagné, R. M., 209–211, 448
Games, 518
  computer-based simulation, 518–520
General education, 118–119
General systems theory, 576–584

Generalization, 246–247, 478–480
Gestalt theory, 198–200
Goals, 195
  congruency of, 589–590
  definition of, 357–358
  of evaluation, 355–357, 359
  teacher-determined, 469–471
Grades, motivation and, 443–444
Graduate education, 122
  nursing, 22, 143, 566–567
Graduation requirements, 162–164
Group discussion, 493–494
Group dynamics, 548–551, 610–614
  in curriculum change, 548–551
Groups
  characteristics of, 417
  formation of, 611
  influence of, 611–612
  internal operations of, 612–614
  standards of, 611–612
  types of, 610
Guthrie, Edwin R., 203–204

Health
  environmental dimensions of, 95–96
  poverty and, 96
Health Amendments Act, 50, 52, 568
Health care
  broadening perspectives of, 87–88
  changes within, 86–88
  consumer participation in, 104
  crisis in, 89–92
  demography and, 84, 93
  facilities, supplies, and equipment in, 98–99
  finances of, 97
  institutionalization of, 86
  interest groups and, 85–86
  manpower needs of, 97–98
  outreach, 98–99
  planning for, 100–109
  population mobility and, 82–83
  prepayment plans and, 88
  problems anticipated in, 93–99
  public accountability for, 101–102
  social changes affecting, 81–86
  sophistication of population and, 83
  specialization of, 87
  strategy for planning, 105–107

Health care—*Continued*
    technical workers in, 123
    trilevel approach to, 107
    urban, 102
Health manpower. *See* Manpower,
    health
Hierarchy of needs (Maslow's), 291
Higher education, 153–168. *See also*
    University
    admission policies of, 157, 159–160
    changing character of, 156–158
    cooperative instructional activities in,
        166–168
    curriculum offerings in, 158–159
    decentralization of, 153–154
    enrollment policies of, 160–162
    graduation policies in, 162–164
    impact of, upon students, 175–179
    impact of student upon, 180–184
    remedial activities in, 164–165
    student-body composition in, 154–
        156
    transfer opportunities in, 165–166
    veterans in, 161
Homeokinesis, 282–283
Homeostasis, 577
Hospital diploma program, 139–140
Hospitals, role of
    future, 99, 102–103
    in nursing education, 18–19, 139–140
Hull, Clark L., 205–207
Human capabilities, as curriculum ob-
    jectives, 315–316, 317–319
Human engineering, 580
Hydrocephalus, case-study analysis of
    nursing care for, 296–297
Hypodermic injection, task description
    and analysis of, 257–259
Hypothesis, model of, 416

Identification decisions, 292
In loco parentis, 624
Individual differences, 445–446
Individualized instruction, 630–631
Inequality
    in health care, 90
    technology and, 73–74
Informal instruction, 393–394
Information, collection of, 376

Initiatory moves
    description of, 422
    and reflexive moves, 422
Innovation, evaluation and, 561–563
Input evaluation, 351–352
Insight, learning through, 199
Institution, 63–64
Institutional capabilities, curriculum ob-
    jectives and, 316, 317–319
Institutional evaluation, 382
Instruction
    analysis of, 392
    audiotutorial, 512
    definition of, 391
    evaluation of
        methodology of, 360–375
        purposes of, 349–350
    formal, 393
    individualization of, 630–631
    informal, 393–394
    laboratory, 495–496
    and learning, 393
    modes of. *See* Instructional modes
        and media; *specific modes*
    nature of, 391–433
    programmed. *See* Programmed in-
        struction
    purpose of, 392
    and teaching, 391–399
    theories of, 214–215, 407–412. *See
        also* Teaching, theories of
        criteria for assessing, 409–410
        current status of, 411–412
        functions of, 408–409
        learning theory and, 402–403
Instructional group. *See* Classroom
    group
Instructional modes and media, 486–
    531. *See also specific modes
    and media*
    curriculum change and, 588
    description of
        media, 498–523
        modes, 490–498
    nature and importance of, 487–490
    rationale for use of, 488–490
    in relation to teaching activities, 524–
        526
    utilization of, 523–526

Instructional process. *See also* Instruction; Teaching
  variables in, 437–484
    learner characteristics, 437–449
    learning environment, 461–469. *See also* Environment, learning
    teacher characteristics, 449–461
    teaching strategies, 469–481
Instructional research, 382
Instructional theory. *See* Instruction, theories of
Integration, of curriculum, 329
Integrative thread, 324, 329–330
Intellectual climate, 466
Interaction analysis, devised by Flanders, 424–428
Interaction analysis matrix, 427, 428
Interest, learning and, 195
Interest groups, 85–86
Intermediate behaviors, 232–238
Inventory, of examinee, 365

Junior colleges, nursing education in, 140–141, 559–561

Kellogg, W. K., Foundation, 45, 48–49
"Knowing how," 274–275
"Knowing that," 274–275
Knowledge, 261–262
  organization of, 272–273
Knowledge requirements, 261–265
  rating scale for, 263–264

Laboratory instruction, 495–496
Laissez-faire leadership, 608
Law
  of closure, 199
  of effect, 193
  of exercise, 193–194
  of good continuation, 199
  of proximity, 199
  of readiness, 193
  of similarity, 199
Leadership, 605–609, 651–652
  authoritarian, 607–608
  characteristics of, 605–606
  effectiveness of, 608–609
  laissez-faire, 608

Learned capabilities, 444–449
  recall of, 476–477
Learner characteristics, 437–449
Learning
  definition of, 211–212
  environment of. *See* Environment, learning
  Gagné's hierarchy of, 209–211
  individual differences and, 445–446
  and instruction, 393
  learned capabilities and, 444–449
  motivation and, 211, 438–444
  nature of, 211–214
  process of, educational objectives and, 224–265
  sequences in, 324–325, 326–328
  teaching and, 399–401
  theories of, 189–216
    applicability of, to classroom, 216
    classification of, 191–192
    current, 202–211
    early, 192–197
    Gestalt and field, 197–202
    historical background, 189–191
    influence of, on education, 191–211
    philosophers, 191
    self-concept, 252
Lecture, as mode of teaching, 491–493
Legal authority, 602
Legitimate power, 607
Lewin, Kurt, 200–202
Liberal studies, 118–119
Life space, 200–201
Linear (single-step) program, 502–503
Locke, John, 10
Longitudinal evaluation, 363

Management Improvement Program (M.I.P.), 502
Manpower, health, 97–98
  education for, 121–125
Manpower Development and Training Act, 50
Material capabilities, as curriculum objectives, 316, 317–319
Matrix of evaluation information, 344–346

Media, instructional. *See* Instructional modes and media
Medical equipment, expansion of, 86
Mennonites, 71
Mobility, population, 82–83
Modeling, 451, 474
Models, 297–298, 302, 522–523
Modes, instructional. *See* Instructional modes and media
Morale, 592
Mother-substitute role, 129
Motion pictures, 507–508
Motivation, 211, 438–444
  to achieve, 439–441
  to attend school, 439
  to continue learning, 443–444
  to engage in learning, 441–443
  extrinsic, 438–439
  intrinsic, 438, 441–442
Murray, H. A., 465

National Association for Mental Health, 54–55
National Committee for the Improvement of Nursing Services, 554–555
National Education Association, 47
National League for Nursing, 39–40
  accreditation and, 555–556
National League of Nursing Education (NLNE), 53, 54
National Nursing Accrediting Service, 555
National Organization for Public Health Nursing (NOPHN), 53, 54
National Tuberculosis Association (NTA), 53
Needs, 465
Negroes, education of, 155–156
Neighborhood health centers, 103–104
New England Council on Higher Education for Nursing, 46–47
Nightingale School, 540
Nonverbal behavior, 429–431
Normative dimension of behavior, 419, 420
Norms, 358–360
  group, 611–613
  in social system, 645

Nurse technician, 132. *See also* Technical nursing
  educational programs for, 139–141
Nurse Training Act, 50
Nursing
  of aging, 233–237
    behavioral analysis of, showing cognitive behaviors, 248–249
    behavioral components and subject matter subtopics in, 235–237
  analysis of, in relation to human, material, and institutional capabilities
    general, 317
    specific, 318–319
  community health, task description and analysis of, 239, 240–241
  conflicts in role expectations of, 419–420
  content in, 270–302, 563–568
    approaches to identifying, 277–302
    analyzing case studies, 294–297
    constructing models, 297–298
    defining and describing concepts, 283–290
    designing nursing core, 278–283
    utilizing nursing process, 290–293
    utilizing science theory, 299–300
  curriculum change and, 585–586
  definitions of, 126–129
  independent functions of, 127
  as learned profession, 22–23, 25
  licensing of, 36
  military, 568–570
  nature of, 125–135
  patient care and, 132
  practical, 144
  preventive aspects of, 25–26
  primary focus of, 131–133
  professional. *See* Professional nurse
  public health, 26
  research in, 25–27, 122
  roles and activities in, 129–131
  self-concept and, 254
  subject matter of, 27–28, 133–135
  technical. *See* Nurse technician; Technical nursing
  theories of, 134

Nursing assistant, programs preparing, 143–145
Nursing associations, professional, 38–40
Nursing curriculum. See Curriculum
Nursing education, 135–147
  accreditation of, 555–556
  administration of, 17–19
  admission policies in, 29
  baccalaureate programs of, 141–143, 566
  career-ladder concept in, 145–147, 571–576
    implementation of, 574–576
  community junior-college programs of, 140–141, 559–561
  computer-assisted, 518–520
  concept of, 22–25
  content of, 27–28
  core concepts in, 278–283
  in early 1900's, 540–542
  faculty in, 21–22
    preparation of, 21
  federal government influence on, 568–571
  financing of, 19–20
    federal role in, 20, 51, 568
  graduate programs of, 22, 143, 567
  hospital diploma programs of, 139–140
  junior colleges in, 140–141, 559–561
  in nineteenth century, 540–541
  programmed instruction in, 499–502
  recent reports on, 556–558
  recommendations concerning, 136–138
  for registered nurse, 572–574
  reports on, in 1948, 553–555
  role of hospitals in, 18–19
  standardization of, 540–542
  tape recordings in, 508–514
  television in, 503–506
  types of programs in, 18, 138–139
  after World War I, 542–545
  during World War II, 547–548
Nursing needs, 294–295
Nursing problems, as focus of curriculum content, 321–325

Objective test, 364
Objectives
  affective, 223–224
  cognitive, 223
  of curriculum. See Curriculum, objectives of
  educational, 221–267
    evaluation of, 350
    informing learner of, 471–472
    initial concern for, 221–224
    levels of, 230–238
    need for reliable observation of, 228
    process of defining, 229–230
    reasons for specifying, 226–229
    types of, 223
  psychomotor, 223
Observations, definition of, 363
Operant conditioning, 207–209, 327
Operations research, 580
Organismic system, 578
Organizing centers of curriculum, 310, 320–325
  characteristics of, 321–322
  promoting mobility as, 322–323, 324–325
Outreach health services, 98–99

Panel discussion, 494
Parsons, Talcott, 577–578
Patient-physician relationships, 105
Pedagogical model of teaching, 395
Peer-group influences, 176–178
Perceptual organization, 199
Performance, 227
  analysis of, 231–238
  self-concept and, 254
Performance test, 365
Personal and interpersonal behavior, 370
Personalistic dimension of behavior, 419–420
Physical environment. See Environment, physical
Physician's assistant, 105–107
Physician-patient relationships, 105
Pictorial presentation, as medium of instruction, 521–522
Planning, 491

Planning decisions, 292
Pluralism, cultural, 71–72
Pollution, 91
Population mobility, 82–83
Poverty, health and, 96
Power, 606–607
Power equalization, 591
Practical nurse, 144
Practice
  description of, 275
  in learning, 214
  and repetition, 204
Pragmatic approach to change, 538–539
Prepayment health plans, 88
Press, 465
Preventive nursing, 26–27
Primitive society, education in, 72–73
Printed language instruction, 522
Problem-solving, 290
Procedural statements, 422–423
Process
  analytic, 290, 292
  nursing, 290–293
Process evaluation, 352
Product evaluation, 353, 356
Professional activity, 114
Professional associations
  allied, 40–47
  educational, 44–47
  nursing, 38–40
Professional education
  aims of, 116–118
  characteristics of, 116
  components of, 118–121
Professional nurse, 132–133, 563–564
  educational programs for, 141–143
Professional studies, 119–121
Professions
  characteristics of, 113–125
  commercialization of, 83–84
  purposes of, 115–116
Programmed instruction, 222, 498–503
  evaluation of, 344, 346
Prompts, and cues, 473–475
Psychiatric concepts, identification of, 283–285
Psychological environment. See Environment, psychological

Psychology
  animal, 196
  experimental, 190–191
  faculty, 190
  Gestalt, 198–200
Psychomotor behaviors, 255–265
  selection of, for teaching, 256
  task description and analysis of, 257–265
Public health nursing, 26

Questionnaire, definition of, 365

Radiation, 91
Radicals, student, 182, 619–620
Ranking, within groups, 612
Rating scale
  knowledge, 263–264
  skill, 264
Rating statements, 422, 423–424
Rationalism, 189–190
Readiness, nature of, 446–447
Recall, 476–477
  concept of spiral curriculum, 477
  techniques and procedures of, 477
  in verbal directions, 476
Reciprocity, in group action, 442
Referent power, 607
Reflexive moves, 422
Reform, strategy of, 540
Reformation, the, 9
Regional accrediting associations, 44
Regional education associations, 44–47, 167
Regional planning, 100–101
Registered-nurse student, 572–574
Reinforcement, 207–208, 228
  intermittent, 208–209
  in programmed instruction, 502
  schedule of, 208
  in teaching, 477–478
Reinforcer, as reinforcing stimulus, 477–478
Relevance, 181–182
  of curriculum, 75–77
Religio-philosophical orientation, 84–85
Remedial education, 164–165

Research
  applied, 382
  curriculum evaluation and, 381–385
  definition of, 414
  need for, 122
  nursing, 25–27
  problems concerning instructional resources, 490
  relationship of, to theory, 416
  on teaching, 413
Resistance to change, 638–639
  individual, 640–642
  interdependence and, 646–648
  nature of, 639–640
  organizational, 642–645
  principles relating to, 649–651
  in social system, 645–649
  stages of, 639–640
  by subunit within system, 646–648
Resources, utilization of, 591–592
Rockefeller Foundation, 48
Role-playing, 517
Roles, 63
  enacted in evaluation, 357–360
  of evaluation, 355–357, 359
  superordinate, 643–644
Romanticism, 67
Rousseau, Jean Jacques, 9

Scholarship, in area of nursing care, 25
Scientific forces affecting curriculum, 81–110
Scientific theory, 406–407
  in curriculum development, 14, 299–300
Scope
  of curriculum, 313
  description of, 313
"Scrambled textbook," 498
Self-appraisal, 365
Self-concept, 252–255
  academic performance and, 254
  nursing and, 254
Seminar, between students and faculty, 494–495
Sequential education, 324–325, 326–328
Simulation, 516–517
  computer-based, 518–520

Skill
  definition of, 256
  in professional occupations, 120
Skill requirements, 261–265
  rating scale for, 264
Skinner, B. F., 207–209, 327, 393
Social action theory (Parson's), 299–300
Social change
  cultural stability within, 70–71
  cultural values and, 66–72
  effects of, on health care, 81–86
Social environment. See Environment, social
Social forces affecting curriculum, 81–110, 311
Social group, as model of classroom, 418–421, 464–465
Social system, 577–578
  norms in, 645
  resistance to change in, 645–649
  school as, 589–592
Sophistication of population, 83
Southern Regional Educational Board, 45–46, 167
Spiral curriculum, 477
Standard Curriculum for Schools of Nursing, 543
Standardization of nursing education, 540–542
Standardized tests, 364
Standards. See Norms
State boards of nurse examiners, 36
State departments of education, 37
State legislatures, role of, in nursing curriculum, 37–38
Status position, 63
Stimulus, 472–473
  and decisions, 472
  definition of, 472
  response to, 472–473
Stimulus-response paradigm, 192–193, 196, 202–203
Stimulus-response techniques, 226
Strategy, for curriculum, 538, 539
Student activism, 180–181
Students
  and admissions policies, 29, 157, 159–160
  alienation of, 183

Students—*Continued*
  characteristics of, 437–449
    assessment of. *See* Assessment of
      student characteristics
  and curriculum, 153–186, 311
  in "high intellectual" environ-
    ments, 466–467
  influence of teachers on, 178–179
  interdependent influences upon,
    176–177
  evaluation of, 360–366
  impact of, upon higher education,
    180–184
  impact of college upon, 175–179
  importance of advisor to, 170
  in learning environment, 584–589
  nursing, characteristics of, 170–171
  peer-group influences on, 176–178
  revolutionary movements of, 619–620
  role of
    in curriculum development, 34,
      632–636
    in decision-making, 617–618
  teacher evaluation by, 368
Student-teacher relationships, 335–
  336
Student-teacher-community relationships, 333–336
Subject matter
  and curriculum, 276–277, 312
  knowledge of, 369–370
  nature of, 271–274
  uses of, 274–276
Subject organization, 551–553
Substantive statements
  classification of, 423
  function of, 422
Subtasks, 257–260
Summative evaluation, 356, 382
Superordinate roles, 643–644
Surgeon General's Consultant Group on
  Nursing, 19–22
System, 578
  characteristics of, 580
Systematic theory of learning, 205–207
Systems approach to curriculum change,
  576–584
  procedures and methods in, 580–583
Systems engineering, 580

Tape recordings, 508–514
  criteria for selection of, 513–514
  for evaluating clinical performance,
    510
  for patient teaching, 509
  television and, 511
Task description and analysis, 222, 238.
  See also Behavioral analysis
  of hot foot-soak, 262–263
  of hypodermic injection, 257–258
    and related psychological require-
      ments, 258–259
  of psychomotor behaviors, 257–265
Tasks
  continuous vs. discontinuous, 260
  related psychological requirements of,
    258–259
Teacher statements, classification of,
  422–424
Teacher-community relationships, 334–
  335
Teacher-made test, 364
Teachers
  activities of, 452–456
    instructional modes and media in
      relation to, 524–526
  behavior of, 457–458. *See also* Effec-
    tive teacher behavior
  characteristics of, 449–461
  as directors of learning, 449–451
  effectiveness of. *See* Effective teacher
    behavior
  effects of, on student characteristics,
    178–179
  evaluation of, 366–371
    by students, 368
  as identifiers of expected outcomes, 453
  as liaison, 451–452
  as models, 451, 474
  procedural methods and management
    techniques of, 226
  as program builders, 452
  roles of, 449–452, 628–632
    in curriculum development, 34–35
  selection of information and materials
    by, 454–455
  superior, characteristics of, 459–461
  tasks of, in behavior modification,
    225–226

Teacher-student conference, 365
Teacher-student interaction, 452–456
Teaching
    analysis of, 414–415, 417–431
        by classification of teacher state-
            ments, 422–424
        by interaction analysis, 424–428
        as social system, 418–421
        by study of effective behavior, 429–
            431
    contract, 497–498
    controlling attention in, 475–476
    cues for learning in, 473–475
    as decision-making, 398–399
    definition of, 391, 413–414
    generalization in, 478–480
    impact of technology on, 629–630
    informing learner of objectives in,
        471–472
    and instruction, 391–399
    learning and, 399–401
    measuring and assessing behavior in,
        480–481
    pedagogical model of, 395
    recall in, 476–477
    reinforcement in, 477–478
    research on, 413
    setting behavioral goals in, 469–471
    stimulus in, 472–473
    strategies of, 469–481
        curriculum change and, 586–587
    study of, 417–431. See also Teaching,
        analysis of
    styles of, 420–421
    as system of actions, 394–398, 414
    team, 497
    theories of, 412–416
        learning theory and, 402–403
    variables in, 396–398
    verbal and nonverbal actions in, 396–
        398, 424–428
Teaching machines, 498
Teaching methods, role of, in curricu-
    lum, 5
Teaching style, 369
Team teaching, 497
Technical education, 123
Technical nursing, 563–564. Se also
    Nurse technician

Technical workers, in health care, 123
Technology
    cultural change and, 67–70
    educational, 526–529
    health effects of, 92
    impact of, on teaching roles, 629–630
    inequality and, 73–74
Television in nursing education, 503–
    506
    effectiveness of, 505–506
    with follow-up sessions, 506
    with tape recordings, 511
Tension, as motivation source, 201
Terminal behaviors, 221, 225, 232
    situations providing for expression of,
        361
Tests, 480
    types of, 364–365
Theories. See specific types
Theory
    characteristics of, 403–404
    nature of, 403–407
    process of development of, 404
    relationship of, to research, 416
Theory-skill spectrum, 124, 256
Therapeutic role, 129
"Thirdness," 401
Thorndike, Edward L., 192–194
Trace theory, 199–200
Transfer student, 165–166
Transparencies, as instructional me-
    dium, 521–522
Trial-and-error learning, 192

United States Office of Education, 51–
    52
Universal education, 156–158
University. See also Higher education
    authority in, 603
    community service of, 621–622
    decision-making points in, 644
    environmental changes in, 619–623
    resistance to change by, 642–645
    student activism and, 619–620
University Student Census, 169–171
Urban health care, 102

Valence, and valence changes, 201

Values, 64–66
    cultural, 64–77
    universal, 65
Verbal behavior, 425–427
    categories of, in classroom, 426–427
    curriculum change and, 587
Verbal interaction, 226
Veterans, in higher education, 161
Videotape, 511
Visual-verbal program, model, 499–500
Vocational training, 123–124

Voluntary associations, 53–55

Watson, John B., 196–197
Western Council for Higher Education for Nursing, 46
Western Interstate Commission for Higher Education (WICHE), 46
Women, education of, 155
Work, changing nature of, 69
Workshop, 548
Worth, description of, 252